Introduction to
Anatomy and Physiology

Susan J. Hall, PhD
Deputy Dean of the
    College of Health Sciences
University of Delaware
Newark, Delaware

Michelle A. Provost-Craig, PhD
Associate Professor of Kinesiology and
    Applied Physiology
University of Delaware
Newark, Delaware

William C. Rose, PhD
Assistant Professor of Kinesiology and
    Applied Physiology
University of Delaware
Newark, Delaware

Publisher
The Goodheart-Willcox Company, Inc.
Tinley Park, Illinois
www.g-w.com

To the Student

Have you ever wondered why you have curly, wavy, or straight hair? Or why you may have to wear corrective lenses for your eyes? Or why diseases strike some people but not others?

Do you ever wonder if certain dietary and health habits might reduce your risk of having diabetes and coronary heart disease in later life? Did you know that it's important to maximize your bone density during early and teenage years to prevent developing osteoporosis? How can your lifestyle choices at 16 affect your body at 60? These are all considerations related to your anatomical and physiological makeup and they are topics discussed in this book.

People have been curious about the human body for centuries. It's quite natural, since it's the body we live in. The more we know and understand about our bodies, the more we can choose to make intelligent choices about our own health and longevity. Knowledge about these topics can also help us to help our family and friends understand their health issues.

This book is your road map to understanding all of the fascinating intricacies of the human body. In addition to providing the basics of how your body works, the text highlights some of the latest research on topics of interest. Since many of you are probably curious about career opportunities in human health and healthcare, this text also features descriptions of job opportunities encompassing the ladder of jobs in healthcare.

This textbook will answer questions you have had and raise questions you have never thought about. As you discover the answers on these pages, we believe you will agree with us that the human body is the most interesting topic in all of science. We wish you happy reading!

Susan J. Hall
Michelle A. Provost-Craig
William C. Rose

Contributors and Reviewers

Contributors

Goodheart-Willcox Publisher would like to thank the following classroom instructors who wrote the Check Your Understanding questions, the Lesson Review and Assessment questions and activities, and the Chapter Review and Assessments.

Karen Cluck, MT (ASCP), RDA
Holland Medical High School
Abilene, Texas

Cory Hubble, MA, ATC/R, CSCS
Instructor: Anatomy & Physiology, Medical Terminology, Sports Medicine Careers
Secondary Technical Education Program (S.T.E.P.), Anoka-Hennepin ISD #11
Anoka-Hennepin, Minnesota

Emma Neil Ogle, RN, RDSC
CTE: Instructional Coordinator
Zebulon B. Vance High School
Charlotte, North Carolina

Tiffany Robertson, RN
Health Careers Instructor
Green Country Technical Center
Okmulgee, Oklahoma

Goodheart-Willcox Publisher also extends a special thanks to Body Scientific International for creating the text's beautiful, expertly drawn illustrations and diagrams.

Reviewers

The author team and Goodheart-Willcox Publisher want to offer a special thank-you to **Professor Robert Neeves**, who carefully read the entire manuscript and reviewed all of the drawings in the text. His comments and suggestions significantly improved the final product.

Goodheart-Willcox Publisher and the authors would also like to thank the following instructors who reviewed selected manuscript chapters and provided valuable input into the development of this textbook program.

Kathy Bonsall, BS, MEd, NBCT, PAEMST
Dual Enrollment Anatomy & Physiology Instructor
McNeese State University, Sulphur High School
Lake Charles, Louisiana

Ernema T. Boettner, BSN
Registered Nurse
Northwest Technical School
Maryville, Missouri

Linda Bradlin, MAT
Science Instructor
Benjamin Carson High School of Science and Medicine
Detroit, Michigan

Matthew Connior, MS Biology
Assistant Professor of Biology
South Arkansas Community College
El Dorado, Arkansas

Erin Dearth, BS Anthropology, MA Biological Anthropology
Science Instructor
Ohio Hi-Point Career Center
Bellefontaine, Ohio

Teri Feierstadt, BSN
Instructor: Health Science Education
JP Taravella High School
Coral Springs, Florida

Cathy German, EdM
Science Teacher
John Glenn High School
Westland, Michigan

Madeline Gervasse, MSN, CCRN, FNP, CNL, PhD(c)
Medical-Legal Forensic Expert, Family/Critical Care, Nurse Practitioner
Georgian Court University
Lakewood Township, New Jersey

Laura Gilpin, RN
Health Science Educator
Cumberland County High School
Crossville, Tennessee

Cheryl Hach, BS Biology/Chemistry, MS Biology
Life Science Instructor
Kalamazoo Area Mathematics and Science Center
Kalamazoo, Michigan

Kyle Harris, MS, LAT, ATC
Instructor/Athletic Trainer
Bucks County Community College
Newtown, Pennsylvania

Dawn Holcomb, MS, MT, ASCP
Instructor
GASC Technology Center
Flint, Michigan

Angela Holland, BSN
Health Science Instructor
Sparkman Medical Academy
Harvest, Alabama

Cory Hubble, MA, ATC/R, CSCS
Instructor: Anatomy & Physiology, Medical
    Terminology, Sports Medicine Careers
Secondary Technical Education Program (S.T.E.P.),
    Anoka-Hennepin ISD #11
Anoka-Hennepin, Minnesota

Detna Kacher
DeBakey High School for Health Professionals,
    Retired
Houston, Texas

**Sue Keppler, RN, DON, DipHSW, CertHlthProm,
CertMgmt, BSc (Hons), MEd**
Health Sciences: Pathway Lead Teacher
Applied Technology College & Career Preparation
    High School
Montebello, California

Jessica Knisley
Biology/Anatomy & Physiology Instructor
Miami Valley Career Technology Center
Clayton, Ohio

Gretchen Kraig-Turner
Science Teacher
Jefferson High School
Portland, Oregon

**Bonnie Lane, BS Health & Physical Education,
MS Exercise Physiology**
Lead Health Instructor, Anatomy & Physiology
    Instructor
2009 Health Professional of the Year (K-12)
Delcastle Technical High School
Wilmington, Delaware

Theresa Mitchell, BS Medical Technology, MAT
New Vision Medical Careers/Science Teacher
Onondaga Cortland Madison BOCES McEvoy
    Campus
Cortland, New York

Emma Neil Ogle, RN, RDSC
CTE: Instructional Coordinator
Zebulon B. Vance High School
Charlotte, North Carolina

**Marilyn Pestano-Harte, EdD(c), MSN, RN, CMAA,
LNC**
Health Science Instructor
Boyd Anderson High School
Lauderdale Lakes, Florida

Sonya Picklesimer, MA Biology
Instructor of AP Biology, Honors Biology, Anatomy
Mingo Central Comprehensive High School
Matewan, West Virginia

Ellie Pribble, RN, BSE, MS
Health Sciences Instructor
Harrison Technology Center
Cynthiana, Kentucky

Cathy Reon, BS, MEd, ADN-RN
Teacher of Nursing Assistant, Biology II, Human
    Anatomy & Physiology
Sulphur High School
Sulphur, Louisiana

Jimmy A. Reyes, DNP, AGNP
Dean of Nursing and Associate Professor
John A. Hartford Foundation BAGNC Scholar
Kirkwood Community College
Cedar Rapids, Iowa

Janet Rittenhouse, MSEd, RN
Health Science Technology Teacher
Central Community High School
Breese, Illinois

Tiffany Robertson, RN
Health Careers Instructor
Green Country Technical Center
Okmulgee, Oklahoma

**Mark Temons, BS Biology/General Science,
MS Biology**
Science Teacher, Retired
Muncy High School
Muncy, Pennsylvania

Mindy Thompson, BS Ecology, MST
Science Instructor
Rockford East High School
Rockford, Illinois

Olga Vega, BS, RRT
Instructor
Carl Wunsche Sr. High School
Spring, Texas

Pam Wilhelm
Health Science Instructor
Daniel Morgan Technical Center
Spartanburg, South Carolina

**Jeanne Zander, MLT, Life Science & Health Science
Certified**
Health Science Instructor and Coordinator
Brenham High School
Brenham, Texas

About the Authors

Susan J. Hall is Deputy Dean of the College of Health Sciences at the University of Delaware. She is a fellow of the American College of Sports Medicine and the AAHPERD Research Consortium, and has served as President of the Biomechanics Academy of AAHPERD, President of the AAHPERD Research Consortium, and Vice President of the American College of Sports Medicine. She is also the author of several successful textbooks and has served on several journal editorial boards. After graduating from Duke University, she began her career as a high school biology teacher. She earned a master's degree from Texas Woman's University and a PhD from Washington State University. She has been teaching at the college level for more than 30 years.

Michelle A. Provost-Craig is an Associate Professor in the Department of Kinesiology and Applied Physiology at the University of Delaware, where she has taught graduate and undergraduate courses in physiology, clinical exercise physiology, and electrocardiogram interpretation for more than 20 years. She is the recipient of the University's most prestigious awards for Excellence in Teaching and Excellence in Advising and Mentoring. She also received a University grant from the Center for Teaching Effectiveness to develop innovative approaches to teaching anatomy and physiology to college students. While at the University of Delaware, she served as the graduate coordinator of the Masters in Exercise Science program and was the founder of their Cardiopulmonary Rehabilitation Program. Dr. Provost-Craig has served in numerous leadership roles for the United States Figure Skating Association (USFSA) and has performed physiological assessments of national and international elite ice figure skaters. She was the Vice President of the Mid-Atlantic Chapter of the Regional American College of Sports Medicine (ACSM) and has participated in several ACSM committees. Dr. Provost-Craig earned a Masters degree from the University of Delaware and a PhD in Exercise Physiology from the University of Maryland.

William C. Rose is an Assistant Professor in the Department of Kinesiology and Applied Physiology at the University of Delaware, where he has taught anatomy and physiology for more than ten years. He is a member of the American Physiological Society and the American College of Sports Medicine. He is the author of textbook chapters and research articles in the fields of cardiovascular physiology and biomechanics. He has served as a grant proposal reviewer for the National Science Foundation and as a manuscript reviewer for scientific journals such as Circulation and the American Journal of Physiology. After graduating from Harvard University with a degree in physics, Rose earned a PhD in biomedical engineering from Johns Hopkins University. He completed a postdoctoral fellowship in cardiology at Johns Hopkins Hospital, and has worked in research and development for the DuPont Company before joining the University of Delaware.

Brief Contents

Table of Contents

WHAT RESEARCH TELLS US

Career Corner
Anatomy and Physiology at Work

How is the human body like a machine?

Andrea Danti/Shutterstock.com

Foundations of Human Anatomy and Physiology

We humans have been interested in our own anatomy and physiology for many centuries. Our bodies have astonishing capabilities, including our abilities to think, speak, move, see, hear, smell, taste, remember, and feel emotions.

Human anatomy and physiology involve the study of the form and function of the human body. These ancient fields of scientific study continue today and are now sufficiently advanced such that we have developed precise terminology to describe what we know. The related, modern-day fields of biology and biomechanics also contribute new knowledge about how our bodies work and interact with the environment.

In this chapter you will learn some of the important, specialized terminology essential for the study of anatomy and physiology. You will also learn the basic, underlying physiological processes essential for life and the different ways in which forces in our environments can cause injury. In addition, we will look back at the historical roots of anatomy and physiology and explore where the exciting fields of science have taken us recently.

Chapter 1 Lessons

Lesson 1.1
The Language of Anatomy and Physiology

Lesson 1.2
Basic Physiological Processes

Lesson 1.3
How Forces Affect the Body

Lesson 1.4
Understanding Science

While studying, look for the online icon to:

- **Practice** with e-flash cards and vocabulary games
- **Review** with interactive art labeling
- **Assess** with online exercises
- **Expand** with interactive activities and animated videos
- **Listen** to pronunciations of key terms in the audio glossary

www.g-wlearning.com/healthsciences

Study on the Go

Use a mobile device to practice vocabulary terms, listen to pronunciations, and review with self-assessment quizzes.

www.m.g-wlearning.com

The Language of Anatomy and Physiology

Try to answer the following questions before you read this lesson.

What body position is considered the "starting point" for describing body positions?

Why is the metric system used in all fields of science?

Lesson Objectives

1. Define *anatomy* and *physiology* and explain the relationship between them.
2. Describe anatomical position and explain why it is useful.
3. Identify the three planes of the body and discuss how they are useful in describing body movements.
4. Identify the major body cavities and the organs that are housed within each cavity.
5. Discuss the choice of the metric system as the international system of measurement for all fields of science.

Key Terms

E-Flash Cards

abdominal cavity	oral cavity
abdominopelvic cavity	orbital cavities
anatomical position	pelvic cavity
anatomy	physiology
anterior (ventral) body cavity	posterior (dorsal) body cavity
cranial cavity	sagittal plane
frontal plane	spinal cavity
metric system	thoracic cavity
middle ear cavities	transverse plane
nasal cavity	

This lesson introduces the study of anatomy and physiology and explains why the two are related. Like all fields of science, anatomy and physiology rely on a specialized set of terminology for accurate descriptions of body structures and functions. This chapter introduces and explains some of the basic terminology that will be used throughout the book.

Introducing Anatomy and Physiology

When a living organism is being described, we often hear the term *anatomy* closely followed by the term *physiology*. Although these concepts are closely related in some respects, they are very different in others.

Anatomy is the study of the form or structure of all living things, including plants and animals. In this book, the living thing we will focus on is the human body, so we will be studying *human anatomy*. The word *anatomy* is taken from Greek words meaning "to cut apart." The study of the body structures we can see with our eyes is called *gross anatomy*. The study of tiny parts seen only with a microscope is termed *microscopic anatomy*.

Physiology (FIZ-ee-AHL-oh-jee) is the study of how living things function or work. This book discusses *human physiology*. Looking through the table of contents, you will see that most of the chapters are about one of the systems of the human body. The muscular system, skeletal system, and cardiovascular system are familiar examples.

Branches of human physiology exist for all of the different systems of the human body, including *muscle physiology*, *skeletal physiology*, and *cardiovascular physiology.* Each system contributes a unique capability to the human body, and some systems also exert influences on other systems.

Why do we combine the study of anatomy and physiology in one book? The answer is that there is a close relationship between how our bodies are structured and how they function.

In a healthy human body all functions are normal and painless. But when a disease or injury causes a breakdown of even a small part of a body structure, abnormal function and pain can result. An obvious example is the case of a broken femur, preventing normal leg movement. Another example is a tumor in the digestive tract that prevents normal passage of materials through the digestive system and rapidly becomes painful and life-threatening. Similarly, inhalation of harmful substances such as tobacco smoke can cause structural changes in the lungs that make breathing difficult. Understanding the normal anatomy and physiology of the human body is the first step in understanding the structures and processes that become dysfunctional with injury and disease.

 Check Your Understanding

1. What is the difference between anatomy and physiology?
2. Why do we study anatomy and physiology together?
3. What is *gross anatomy*?

Describing the Human Body

Throughout this text you will read detailed descriptions of the structures that make up the human body. Learning some specialized terminology will help you picture and understand these structures and their functions.

The body position that serves as a "starting point" for describing positions and directions for the human body is called **anatomical position** (**Figure 1.1**). Anatomical position is a normal standing position, with the feet slightly apart,

the face and shoulders facing forward, and the palms of the hands facing forward.

Planes

To describe the human body and its movements, we imagine that there are three planes, or flat surfaces, passing through the center of the body (**Figure 1.1**). We use these planes to help describe motions of the body and the body segments when they are aligned with the direction of one of these planes.

- The **sagittal plane** divides the body into right and left portions—so forward and backward motions of the body or body parts are said to be *sagittal plane movements.*
- The **frontal plane** divides the body into front and back portions, with sideways movements considered to be *frontal plane movements.*

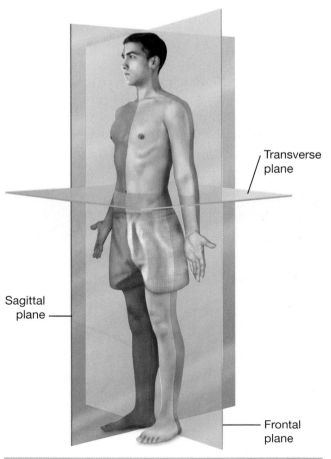

Figure 1.1 Anatomical reference position. Three imaginary planes divide the body into halves in three directions. *Which plane is your body moving along during rotational movements?*

- Finally, the **transverse plane** divides the body into top and bottom portions, and rotational movements are called *transverse plane movements*.

Of course, many movements of our body follow a curved path and are not lined up with any one of these three planes. Movements that do not occur in direction with one of the three planes are described as *nonplanar*.

Directions

Directional terms describe relationships between different body parts. The most commonly used directional terms are paired, describing opposite relationships. For example, the term *superior* means *above* or *over*, whereas *inferior* means *below* or *under*. So it is correct to state that the chin is superior to the knees. Alternatively, we could say that the knees are inferior to the chin (**Figure 1.2**).

Cavities

Inside the human body are a number of open chambers called *cavities* (**Figure 1.3**). These cavities hold the internal organs of the body.

The **posterior (dorsal) body cavity**, located toward the back (or posterior side) of the body,

includes two named cavities—the cranial cavity and the spinal cavity. The **cranial cavity** holds the brain, while the **spinal cavity** surrounds the spinal cord. The delicate brain and spinal cord are protected, respectively, by the bony skull and the bones of the vertebral column.

The **anterior (ventral) body cavity,** located at the front (or anterior side) of the body, also includes subdivisions. A large, dome-shaped muscle called the *diaphragm* separates the **thoracic cavity** and **abdominopelvic** (ab-DAHM-i-noh-PEHL-vik) **cavity**. The thoracic cavity houses the heart and lungs, among other organs. The abdominopelvic cavity includes the **abdominal cavity** and **pelvic cavity**. No structure separates these cavities. The abdominal cavity contains the stomach and other parts of the digestive tract and the liver, as well as other organs. The pelvic cavity holds the reproductive and excretory organs.

The body also includes several small cavities, including the

- **oral cavity**—located within the mouth;
- **nasal cavity**—situated inside the nose;
- **orbital cavities**—hold the eyes; and
- **middle ear cavities**—found in the skull; serve as chambers for transmitting and amplifying sound.

Each of these small cavities is discussed in further detail in chapter 7.

Figure 1.2 Common Directional Terms for Anatomy

Term	Description
superior (cranial)	closer to the head
inferior (caudal)	away from the head
anterior (ventral)	toward the front of the body
posterior (dorsal)	toward the back of the body
medial	toward the midline of the body
lateral	away from the midline of the body
proximal	closer to the trunk
distal	away from the trunk
superficial	toward the surface of the body
deep	away from the surface of the body

The Metric System

Just as there are specific anatomical terms used to describe directions and regions within the human body, there is a system for numerical quantities. This system, known as the **metric system**, is used in all fields of science throughout the world, including the United States. The metric system is also used for everyday measurements by every major country in the world, except the United States.

The metric system originated as the result of a request by King Louis XVI to the French Academy of Sciences during the early 1790s. In 1875, the Treaty of the Meter was signed by 17 countries that agreed to adopt the use of the metric system.

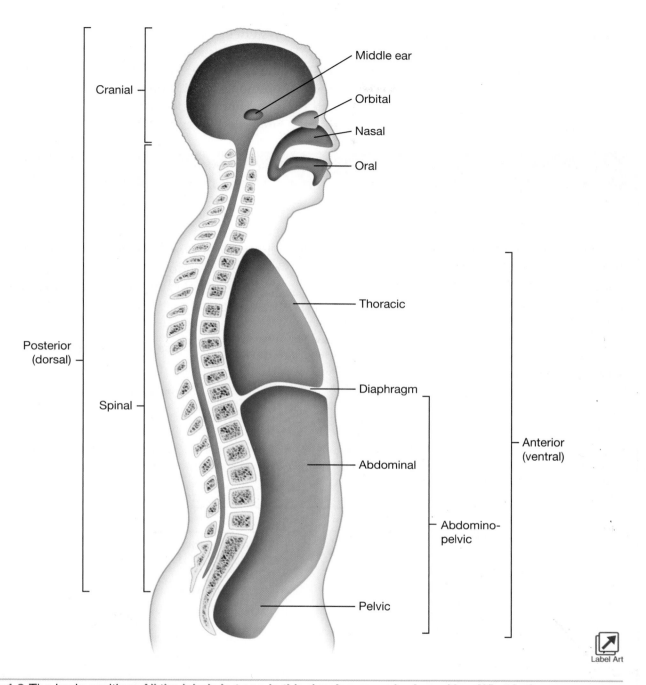

Figure 1.3 The body cavities. *All the labels but one in this drawing name body cavities. What is the one exception?*

Since that time, the metric system has enjoyed worldwide popularity for several reasons:

- It involves only four base units—the meter (of length); the kilogram (of mass); the second (of time); and the degree Kelvin (of temperature).
- The base units are precisely defined, reproducible quantities that are independent of factors such as gravitational force.

- All units (excepting those for time) relate by factors of 10, making conversions between units easy, since you only need to move the decimal point.
- The system is used internationally.

In the United States, the system of measurement used for nonscientific purposes is called the *English system*. The English system of weights and measures arose over the course of several centuries, mainly for purposes of buying and selling goods and dividing parcels of land. Specific units came largely from royal decrees. For example, a yard was originally defined as the distance from the end of the nose of King Henry I to the thumb of his extended arm. The English system of measurement is not regular, or even logical. There are 12 inches to the foot, 3 feet to the yard, 5,280 feet to the mile, 16 ounces to the pound, and 2,000 pounds to the ton.

Metric-English conversion factors are presented in Appendix A.

Lesson 1.1 Review and Assessment

Mini Glossary   Make sure that you know the meaning of each key term.

Build vocabulary with e-flash cards and games

abdominal cavity   space bounded by the abdominal walls, the diaphragm, and the pelvis

abdominopelvic cavity   continuous internal opening that includes the abdominal and pelvic cavities

anatomical position   erect standing position with arms at the sides and palms facing forward

anatomy   the study of the form or structure of living things, including plants, animals, and humans

anterior (ventral) body cavity   continuous internal opening that includes the thoracic and abdominopelvic cavities

cranial cavity   opening inside the skull that holds the brain

frontal plane   an invisible, vertical flat surface that divides the body into front and back halves

metric system   international system of measurement that is used in all fields of science

middle ear cavities   openings in the skull that serve as chambers for transmitting and amplifying sound

nasal cavity   opening within the nose

oral cavity   opening within the mouth

orbital cavities   openings that hold the eyes

pelvic cavity   internal opening that holds the reproductive and excretory organs

physiology   the study of how living things function or work

posterior (dorsal) body cavity   continuous internal opening located near the back of the body that includes the cranial and spinal cavities

sagittal plane   an invisible, vertical flat surface that divides the body into right and left halves

spinal cavity   the internal opening that houses the spinal cord

thoracic cavity   the internal opening that houses the heart and lungs

transverse plane   an invisible, horizontal flat surface that divides the body into top and bottom halves

Know and Understand

Assess

1. Which small cavity is used as a passageway for air and food?

2. Describe three reasons that the English system of measurement is not conducive to use as a universal system of measurement.

3. Name the three anatomical planes and the motions they are correlated with.

4. What are the four base units used in the metric system?

5. What two body cavities are named for directional terms?

Analyze and Apply

6. What is the difference between the terms *superior* and *cranial*?

7. Compare and contrast the metric and English systems of measurement.

8. What is the difference between distal and inferior?

In the Lab

9. With a Twinkie (or similar product) positioned lengthwise (in "anatomical position") on the table in front of you, identify the following locations on the Twinkie: most superior part, anterior, posterior, lateral, most medial aspect. Next, make incisions along the sagittal plane, frontal plane, and transverse plane. How many pieces of Twinkie do you have? Which "structure" would be considered deep to the superficial surface of the Twinkie?

10. Find the most distal aspect of the hand in anatomical position. Is this structure superior or inferior to the elbow? Now, abduct your arm 180 degrees from anatomical position. Is this structure still distal? Is it now superior or inferior?

11. Measure your arm from the tip of your nose to the thumb of your extended arm using the English system. Is your measurement the same as that of King Henry I? Convert your measurement to a metric measurement.

Basic Physiological Processes

Before You Read

Try to answer the following questions before you read this lesson.

What are the major organ systems of the human body?

Why is homeostasis important?

Lesson Objectives

1. Explain how building blocks, beginning with atoms, combine to eventually comprise organ systems.

2. Discuss why the body is organized into systems.

3. Define *homeostasis* and explain how homeostatic mechanisms help maintain health.

4. Explain how the body's metabolism works and what factors can influence metabolic rate.

Key Terms

E-Flash Cards

atoms	metabolism
cells	molecules
control center	negative feedback
effector	organ
homeostasis	organ system
homeostatic imbalance	positive feedback
homeostatic	receptor
mechanisms	tissues
metabolic rate	

The human body is an elegant biological machine. In this lesson you will begin to learn how this machine works.

Structural and Functional Organization of the Body

Our bodies are organized into specialized systems that carry out precise functions. Many of these systems also influence the activities of the other systems. To appreciate these specialized systems, let's start by considering how they are constructed.

At the most basic level, tiny particles called **atoms** combine in different ways to form larger particles known as **molecules**. As you will learn in chapter 2, the human body is dependent on many different kinds of molecules, such as water, proteins, and carbohydrates.

The smallest building blocks of all living beings are **cells**, which are composed of organized groups of specialized molecules. Groups of similar cells with a common function form **tissues**. The four basic types of tissues are *epithelial, connective, muscular,* and *neural*.

The next level of organization is the **organ**. An organ is a body part organized to perform a specific function and is composed of at least two different types of tissue. The heart, lungs, brain, and liver are all critically important organs.

An **organ system** includes two or more organs that work together. The nervous system, for example, includes the brain, spinal cord, and all the nerves located throughout the body. The cardiovascular system includes the heart and all of the blood vessels. Each of the human body's organ systems is discussed in a chapter in this book. **Figure 1.4** and **Figure 1.5** provide an overview of these organ systems.

Figure 1.4 The organ systems of the body. *What are some of the ways in which organ systems work together?*

Figure 1.4 Continued.

Figure 1.5 The Human Organ Systems

System	Major Organs	Primary Functions
Integumentary	layers of skin	protects, eliminates waste, helps regulate body temperature
Skeletal	bones, cartilage, ligaments	supports body, protects organs, produces blood cells
Muscular	cardiac, smooth, and skeletal muscle	pumps the heart, helps move materials through the digestive tract, moves the body
Nervous	brain, spinal cord, nerves, sensory receptors	receives and interprets sensory input, directs body movements, includes memory, emotions, cognition
Special sensory	eyes, ears, organs of smell and taste	enables vision, hearing, smell, and taste
Endocrine	endocrine glands	secretes hormones
Respiratory	lungs, nasal passages, pharynx, larynx, trachea	delivers oxygen and removes carbon dioxide from blood
Cardiovascular	heart, blood vessels	transports oxygen and nutrients to the body's cells and removes waste products
Lymphatic	lymphatic vessels and nodes	returns body fluids to the bloodstream
Digestive	esophagus, stomach, intestines	breaks down foods for absorption of nutrients by the body
Urinary	kidneys, bladder	removes nitrogen-containing wastes from blood
Reproductive	male: testes, scrotum, penis female: ovaries, uterus, vagina	enables production of offspring

Homeostasis

To maintain a healthy environment inside the body, the organ systems work together to control factors such as body temperature, blood pressure, blood sugar, water balance, and sodium levels within normal boundaries. This state of regulated physiological balance is called **homeostasis** (HOH-mee-oh-STAY-sis). The word *homeostasis* comes from Greek words that mean "staying the same."

How does homeostasis work? Organ systems work together to maintain homeostasis through processes called **homeostatic mechanisms**. The body systems that initiate most homeostatic responses are the nervous and endocrine systems. As you will learn in the chapters devoted to these systems, the systems function through a complex combination of chemical and physical processes. To maintain homeostasis, all of the systems must work together and make adjustments when the body's external and internal environments change.

All homeostatic control mechanisms have three elements in common. Changes in the environment stimulate a sensory **receptor** nerve, which relays an informational message to a **control center** along an *afferent pathway*. The control center analyzes the information, and when an action is required to maintain homeostasis, the control center sends a command stimulus to an **effector** along an *efferent pathway*. The effector causes an action that helps maintain homeostasis.

Check Your Understanding

1. List the hierarchy of structure from the smallest living thing to the largest.
2. What are the four basic types of tissue found in the human body?
3. Which body systems typically initiate homeostatic responses?
4. What part of the body is stimulated by changes in the environment, thus beginning the process of maintaining homeostasis?

Negative Feedback

Most homeostatic mechanisms work on the principle of **negative feedback**. In a negative feedback loop, conditions exceeding a set limit in one direction trigger a negative reaction in the opposite direction. This negative reaction restores the system to the set point.

A familiar example of a mechanical system that functions on negative feedback is the thermostat on a home heating or cooling system. If the temperature surrounding the thermostat rises or falls outside the set limits, the thermostat triggers either the furnace or air conditioner to turn on. The furnace or air conditioner stays on until the temperature is restored to the original setting.

In the human body, if the temperature begins to rise above the normal 37°C (98.6°F), the hypothalamus of the brain triggers a series of signals to different organs to cause sweating. The evaporation of sweat on the skin cools the body (**Figure 1.6**). Simultaneously, the blood vessels close to the skin dilate to help release heat.

Alternatively, when the body becomes chilled, the hypothalamus signals the muscles to cause shivering. This increased activity of the muscles produces heat, which helps warm the body. At the same time the blood vessels close to the skin constrict to reduce heat loss through the skin.

Rido/Shutterstock.com

Figure 1.6 Sweating during vigorous exercise helps to cool the body. *Is this homeostatic mechanism an example of negative or positive feedback?*

Positive Feedback

Although most homeostatic mechanisms in the human body operate by negative feedback, positive feedback loops can also occur. In contrast to negative feedback loops that reduce a disruptive influence, **positive feedback** mechanisms *increase* disruptive influences. Positive feedback is involved in accelerating blood clotting, transmitting nerve signals, and stimulating contractions during childbirth.

In the case of body temperature, however, a fever that exceeds 40°C (104°F) can provoke a dangerous positive feedback loop. Body temperature this high increases the body's metabolic rate, which increases body heat still further. This can be fatal if nothing is done to cool the body.

Maintaining Homeostasis

Homeostasis within the human body does not mean that conditions are maintained in a perfectly constant state at all times. Rather, there are routine fluctuations of variables such as blood pressure and body temperature. These normal fluctuations occur in response to a variety of conditions in the external and internal environments. Vigorous exercise, for example, produces a normal elevation in both blood pressure and body temperature. Homeostatic mechanisms, however, work to keep these fluctuations within a normal, healthy range.

Homeostatic Imbalances

A **homeostatic imbalance** occurs when the organ systems have a diminished ability to keep the body's internal environment within normal ranges. For example, the aging process is accompanied by many homeostatic imbalances. These imbalances can lead to changes such as the wrinkling and thinning of skin, reduced muscle mass and strength, and decreased mental acuity.

Homeostatic imbalances can also lead to chronic diseases associated with aging. One such disease is type II diabetes. Type II diabetes develops in adulthood, whereas type I diabetes has its onset in childhood. A brief explanation of diabetes here will help you understand homeostatic imbalances.

When you digest food, the concentration of glucose, a simple sugar in your blood, increases. The pancreas, an organ in the endocrine system, produces a hormone called *insulin* that normally controls blood sugar, keeping it within a healthy range. The insulin does this by moving glucose in the blood into the body's cells, where it can be used for fuel or stored for future use.

People with diabetes, however, are unable to move glucose out of the bloodstream because their pancreas does not make enough insulin or their cells do not respond normally to insulin. The resulting homeostatic imbalance, if not corrected, can lead to serious problems. Among those problems are kidney failure, lower limb amputations, and blindness. You will learn more about diabetes in chapter 8.

Check Your Understanding

1. Explain the difference between positive and negative feedback in maintaining homeostasis. Give an example of each.
2. What is homeostatic imbalance? Include at least one example in your explanation.
3. Is the body always in a homeostatic state? Explain.
4. What are possible consequences of the body's failure to maintain homeostasis?

Metabolism

Metabolism is a term used to describe the multitude of chemical reactions constantly going on within the body's cells. *Metabolism* typically refers to two general types of activity—*anabolism* and *catabolism*. Anabolism is the process through which complex molecules such as proteins are constructed from simpler ones. Catabolism is just the opposite, with complex molecules such as carbohydrates being broken down into simpler molecules.

Through catabolic processes, the complex molecules in the food and drink we consume supply the body with energy in the form of *adenosine triphosphate (ATP)*. ATP, which you will learn more about in chapter 2, powers activities within the cells. Even while sleeping the body needs energy for activities such as breathing, circulating blood, adjusting hormone levels, and growing and repairing cells.

Metabolic Rate

A person's **metabolic rate** is the speed with which the body consumes energy, which is also the rate of ATP production. Approximately 60%–75% of the calories that an average person burns is accounted for by the basal metabolic rate, the energy needed for maintaining basic life functions. About another 10% of the calories burned is used in digesting and processing the food and drink that we consume. (For this reason, diets that are overly restrictive tend to be counterproductive for losing weight—you don't

WHAT RESEARCH TELLS US

...*about* Homeostatic Mechanisms during Distance Running

The number one danger associated with marathons, triathlons, and other long-distance running events is overheating. Overheating is a condition in which the body's homeostatic mechanisms for temperature control are overwhelmed. Overheating begins with heat cramps, which can progress to heat exhaustion, eventually leading to heat stroke and death. How does overheating happen, and what steps can runners take to avoid it?

Researchers have recognized that long-distance running poses a severe challenge to the body's homeostatic processes. One reason for this is that some runners do not drink sufficient fluids during long-distance events. Inadequate water intake impedes the body's ability to sweat—a process that has a cooling effect on the body. An inability to sweat leads to hyperthermia, or dangerously high body temperature. Hyperthermia encompasses both elevated core temperature and elevated skin temperature.

Inadequate water intake can also cause dehydration, which reduces total body blood volume. This limits blood supply to the working muscles, skin, and brain. As a result, the muscles fatigue, the skin is less able to release heat, and the person's judgment may be impaired. Research has shown that dehydration exceeding 3% of the total volume of body water causes increased strain on the cardiovascular system and a marked decline in aerobic performance. This makes it more difficult to sustain exercise at the same pace and increases the perception of effort. Hyperthermia may also directly affect the central

Daniel Korzeniewski/Shutterstock.com

Figure 1.7 It is important to maintain a proper level of hydration during exercise.

nervous system such that it contributes to total body fatigue.

Overheating under any circumstances can lead to heat exhaustion. The symptoms of heat exhaustion can include profuse sweating, weakness, nausea, vomiting, headache, lightheadedness, and muscle cramps. Individuals experiencing any of these symptoms due to overheating should immediately be placed in a cool environment and adequately hydrated. If nausea or vomiting prevents the affected individual from drinking enough water, intravenous fluids may be required.

In cases where the body's homeostatic mechanisms for temperature correction fail, heat exhaustion can progress to heat stroke. Body temperature of 41°C (106°F) and the absence of sweating are signs that the normal

homeostatic processes have been overwhelmed. Individuals under these conditions become confused and lethargic and may have a seizure. These symptoms represent a life-threatening emergency, and immediate medical attention is needed.

Ironically, a related danger during long-distance running can be drinking too much water. Runners in the Boston, Chicago, and Big Sur marathons have died from consuming too much water during the race. The problem is that an excessive amount of water dilutes the blood. This causes the sodium concentration in the blood to fall too low, causing swelling of the brain, which can be fatal.

Under normal conditions, we expel extra water in the form of urine. However, research has shown that during a long-distance endurance event, there is an inflammatory response that can alter hormone levels, reducing the body's ability to produce urine.

Running experts suggest weighing yourself before and after a long training run. If you've gained weight, you've consumed too much water, but if you've lost weight, you need to drink more. The recommended amount of liquid to consume is 3 to 6 ounces for every 20 minutes of vigorous exercise. You must take into account, however, that your sweating rate and the environment may necessitate drinking more or less.

Taking It Further

1. What challenges does long-distance running present to your homeostatic mechanisms?

2. Why is it so important to maintain homeostasis?

burn as many calories because there isn't as much to digest.)

The remainder of the calories burned depends on the amount of physical activity that we engage in. Because muscle requires more energy for maintenance than other tissues, even at rest, muscular individuals burn more calories and are said to have "higher metabolic rates" than others.

✓ Check Your Understanding

1. Which two processes make up metabolism? Define them.
2. What percentage of a person's total calorie consumption is burned performing basic life functions?
3. What powers all activities in a cell?

Lesson 1.2 Review and Assessment

Mini Glossary   Make sure that you know the meaning of each key term.

Build vocabulary with e-flash cards and games

atoms   tiny particles of matter

cells   the smallest living building blocks of all organisms

control center   system that receives and analyzes information from sensory receptors, then sends a command stimulus to an effector to maintain homeostasis

effector   unit that receives a command stimulus from the control center and causes an action to help maintain homeostasis

homeostasis   a state of regulated physiological balance

homeostatic imbalance   a state in which there is a diminished ability

for the organ systems to keep the body's internal environment within normal ranges

homeostatic mechanisms   the processes that maintain homeostasis

metabolic rate   the speed at which the body consumes energy

metabolism   all chemical reactions that occur within an organism to maintain life

molecules   chemical combinations of two or more atoms

negative feedback   mechanism that reverses a condition that has

exceeded the normal homeostatic range to restore homeostasis

organ   body part organized to perform a specific function

organ system   two or more organs working together to perform specific functions

positive feedback   mechanism that further increases a condition that has exceeded the normal homeostatic range

receptor   transmitter that senses environmental changes

tissues   organized groups of similar cells

Know and Understand

Assess

1. Which two factors define whether or not something is an organ?
2. Which two principles form the basics of homeostatic mechanisms?
3. What happens to homeostasis when a person ages?

Analyze and Apply

4. How might the transmission of nerve signals be an example of a positive feedback system?
5. Compare and contrast the signs and symptoms of dehydration with hyponatremia, a condition in which the amount of water in cells exceeds the amount of sodium.
6. Using a hot stove as an example, describe how the afferent and efferent nerves in the body protect us from being burned.

In the Lab

7. Make a collage. Using pictures from magazines, create a collage that helps you remember the function of each organ system. Show and discuss your collage in a group of four to five classmates. Are the other members of your group able to determine the system and functions that you tried to represent?
8. Over the course of one day, keep track of the number of times you notice your body using negative feedback as a response to being out of normal homeostatic range. Record the stimulus and the body's response (for example, you walk into a cold room and get goose bumps).
9. Run up and down some stairs 10 times. What do you notice about how your body responds to this activity? Is this an example of positive or negative feedback? Explain.

Before You Read

Try to answer the following questions before you read this lesson.

Why does the size of the area over which a force is distributed make a difference?

Why does the direction of stress distribution within a tissue make a difference?

Lesson Objectives

1. Explain the kinetic concepts of force, mass, weight, pressure, and torque and explain their effects on the human body.

2. Identify the external forces that can act on the body and explain their effects.

3. Describe the factors that determine whether an external force causes bodily injury.

Key Terms

E-Flash Cards

bending
combined loading
compression
elastic
force
kinetics
mass
net force

pressure
shear
stress
tension
torque
torsion
weight

The human body both generates and resists forces during daily activities. The internal forces produced by our muscles enable body movements, whereas forces such as air resistance and friction may slow us down. Sports may involve applying forces to balls, bats, racquets, or clubs. Sports may also involve absorbing forces from impacts with balls, the ground or floor, and opponents (in contact sports). This lesson introduces key concepts to help you understand the effects that these types of activities have on our bodies.

Basic Kinetic Concepts

Kinetics is the analysis of the actions of forces. The field of human biomechanics is based on analysis of the forces, both internal and external, acting on the human body. A basic knowledge of kinetic concepts will be useful for understanding both the movements of the body and the effects of forces that can potentially cause injury.

Force

Force can be thought of as a push or pull acting on a structure. We describe a force in terms of its size or magnitude, direction, and the point at which it acts on a structure. Body weight, friction, and air or water resistance are all forces that commonly act on the human body.

Because a force rarely acts alone, it is important to recognize that what we see and feel are the effects of what is called **net force**. Net force is the single force resulting from the summation of all forces acting on a structure at a given time (**Figure 1.8**). Thus, net force represents the size and direction of all acting forces.

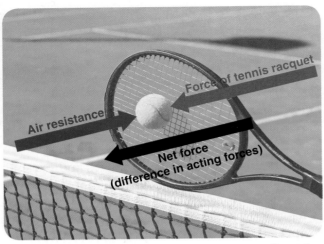

nevenm/Shutterstock.com

Figure 1.8 The net force acting on a tennis ball at the moment of impact with a racquet is the difference between the force exerted by the racquet and the opposing force of air resistance. *How does the net force determine the direction of the resulting motion?*

The size and direction of net force determines the overall effect of the forces acting on a structure. When the forces acting on a structure are balanced, or cancel each other out, there is no net force and no resulting motion. For example, if two people apply equal and opposite forces on the two sides of a swinging door simultaneously, the door won't move. However, if a net force is present, the door will move in the direction of the net force.

Mass and Weight

Mass is the quantity of matter contained in an object. The action of a force causes an object's mass to accelerate, either increasing or decreasing in speed. **Weight** is a force equal to the gravitational acceleration exerted on an object's mass. As the mass of an object increases, its weight increases proportionally. If you were to travel to the moon or another planet with a different gravitational acceleration than on the earth, your weight would be different, but your mass would remain the same.

Pressure

Pressure is defined as the amount of force distributed over a given area. You might wonder how much pressure is exerted on the floor beneath you if you shift your weight to one foot. To find out, divide your body weight by the surface area of the sole of your shoe. Thinking about this, would you prefer to have your foot stepped on by a woman wearing athletic shoes or a woman wearing stilettos (high heel shoes)? The woman's weight would be distributed over a much smaller area in the stilettos, resulting in a much larger pressure against your unfortunate foot.

Torque

When a force causes a structure to rotate, the rotary effect of the force is called **torque**. If you pull or push a suspended bicycle tire, the wheel begins to spin. The harder you pull or push the wheel, the faster it spins. From a mechanical perspective, you are creating torque on the bicycle wheel.

Torque can be quantified as the size of the force multiplied by the perpendicular distance from the line of force application to the center of rotation. In the case of a spinning bicycle wheel, perpendicular distance is the distance from the outside of the tire to the axis of the wheel. The greater the amount of torque acting at the center of rotation, the greater the tendency for rotation to occur.

When a muscle in the human body contracts, it applies a pulling force on a bone. A sufficiently large force causes movement of the bone, with the bone rotating at the nearby joint center. The amount of torque generated at the joint center is the size of the muscle force multiplied by the distance between the muscle attachment and the joint center. You will learn more about how to measure and calculate forces in Chapter 5, *The Muscular System.*

 Check Your Understanding

1. What term defines the process of analyzing actions of forces?
2. Name two forces that commonly act on the body. Define them.
3. What causes an object to rotate?

Forces and Injury to the Human Body

What factors determine whether forces acting on the human body result in injury? The effect of a given force depends not only on its size, direction, and application point but also on the duration of force application.

Directional Force Distribution within the Body

Compressive force, or **compression,** can be thought of as a squeezing force (**Figure 1.9**). An effective way to press wildflowers is to place them inside the pages of a book and to stack other books on top of that book. The weight of the books creates a compressive force on the flowers. Similarly, when you land from a jump, the weight of your body plus the force of landing set up a compressive force on the bones of your skeleton.

Figure 1.9 Compression, tension, and shear represent three directions of stress distribution within a body. *Which directional force would be present during a shoulder dislocation injury?*

The opposite of compressive force is tensile force, or **tension** (**Figure 1.9**). Tensile force is a pulling force that creates tension in the object to which it is applied. When a person hangs from a pull-up bar, tension is created in the arms as they support the weight of the body. A heavier person in this position creates more tension in the arms than a lighter person. Our muscles also produce tensile force that pulls on the attached bones.

A third direction of force is called **shear.** While compressive and tensile forces act along the length of a bone or other object to which they are applied, shear force acts perpendicular to the length of the object (**Figure 1.9**). Shear force tends to cause a portion of the object to slide, or shear, with respect to another portion of the object. Abrasions are caused by shear force acting on the skin. When a baseball player slides into a base, for example, the shear force created by the ground against any exposed skin can cause an abrasion.

The direction of stress distribution within a biological tissue has direct implications for injury potential. Bone, for example, is strongest in resisting compression and the weakest in resisting shear.

Mechanical Stress

Another factor that affects the outcome of forces acting on the human body is the way in which the force is distributed. While pressure represents the distribution of force external to a body, **stress** represents the resulting force distribution inside a body. Stress is quantified in the same way as pressure—the size of the force divided by the area over which the force acts. As **Figure 1.10** on the next page shows, force acting on a small surface produces greater stress than the same force acting over a larger surface.

When a blow is sustained by the human body, the likelihood of injury to body tissue is related to the magnitude and direction of the stress created by the blow. *Compressive stress*, *tensile stress*, and *shear stress* are terms that indicate the direction of the acting stress. The protective pads and helmets worn in many sports are designed to distribute forces over a large area, minimizing the stress sustained by the underlying body parts.

Figure 1.10 When a force of a given size is distributed over an area, the larger the area, the smaller the stress generated. *Which would generate greater amounts of stress—having your hand stepped on by the heel of a stiletto or the heel of a flip-flop sandal?*

Combined Loads

When multiple forces act at once, more complicated force distribution patterns are set up within the body. A combination of off-center forces can create a loading pattern known as **bending** (**Figure 1.11**).

Torsion (TOR-shun) occurs when a structure is caused to twist about its length, typically when one end of the structure is fixed (**Figure 1.11**). Torsional fractures of the tibia can occur in football and skiing accidents in which the foot is held in a fixed position while the rest of the body undergoes a twist.

The simultaneous action of two or more types of forces is known as **combined loading.** Because of the variety of forces that we encounter during daily activities, combined loading patterns are relatively common. Fortunately, they do not usually result in injury.

The Effects of Force Application

When a force acts on an object, there are two potential effects: acceleration and deformation. *Acceleration* is the change in velocity of the object to which the force is applied. The more massive or heavy the object, the smaller the acceleration will be.

The second effect is *deformation*, or change in shape. When a racquetball is struck with a racquet, the ball is both accelerated (put in motion in the direction of the racquet swing) and deformed (flattened on the side that is struck). The amount of deformation that occurs in response to a given force depends on the stiffness of the object acted on.

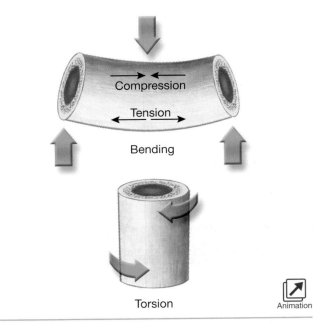

Figure 1.11 Bending and torsion are forms of combined loading.

When an external force is applied to the human body, several factors influence whether an injury occurs. Among these, as discussed, are the size and direction of the force, as well as the area over which the force is distributed. Also important are the material properties of the loaded body tissues.

With relatively small forces, deformation occurs but the response is **elastic**, meaning that when the force is removed, the tissue returns to its original size and shape. Stiffer materials, such as bone, display less deformation in response to a given force. Sometimes the force causes the deformation to exceed the tissue's *elastic limit*. When this occurs the response is *plastic*, meaning that some amount of deformation is permanent. Within the human body, a plastic response translates to injury.

✓ Check Your Understanding

1. What is the difference between compression and tension?
2. Which force is acting between the baseball player and the ground when he slides into home plate?
3. What is the difference between plastic and elastic responses?

Repetitive versus Acute Loads

Yet another factor that influences the likelihood of injury is whether or not the forces sustained by the body are repetitive or acute. When a single force causes an injury, the injury is said to be *acute*. For example, the force produced by a single check in ice hockey or the force resulting from an automobile accident may be sufficient to fracture a bone. These types of forces are acute forces.

Injury can also result from relatively small forces sustained on a repeated basis. For example, each time your foot hits the ground while you are running, a force of approximately two to three times your body weight is sustained. Although a single force of this magnitude is not likely to result in a fracture to healthy bone, many repetitions of such a force may cause a fracture in an otherwise healthy bone of the foot or lower leg. Such injuries are called *chronic injuries* or *stress injuries*.

Lesson 1.3 Review and Assessment

Mini Glossary   Make sure that you know the meaning of each key term.

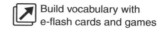 Build vocabulary with e-flash cards and games

bending   a loading pattern created by a combination of off-center forces

combined loading   the simultaneous action of two or more types of forces

compression   a squeezing force that creates compression in the structure to which it is applied

elastic   a response that occurs when force is removed and the structure returns to its original size and shape

force   push or pull acting on a structure

kinetics   the analysis of the actions of forces

mass   the quantity of matter contained in an object

net force   the single force resulting from the summation of all forces acting on a structure at a given time

pressure   force distributed over a given area

shear   a force that acts along a surface and perpendicular to the length of a structure

stress   force distribution inside a structure

tension   a pulling force that creates tension in the structure to which it is applied

torque   the rotary effect of a force

torsion   a loading pattern that can cause a structure to twist about its length

weight   force equal to the gravitational acceleration exerted on the mass of an object

Know and Understand

 Assess

1. List at least three ways that you can describe force. Give examples of how these forces act on the human body.
2. Compare mass and weight.
3. What is net force?
4. Which two forces act along the length of an object such as a bone?
5. What type of force causes rotation?

Analyze and Apply

6. A player gets hit by a lacrosse ball. What is the predominant type of force generated by the ball on the player?
7. Explain how a torn ligament is an example of a plastic response.
8. A linebacker and running back are running toward each other. The linebacker is hit and knocked over by the running back. Using net

force as the basis for your answer, explain why the linebacker was knocked over.

9. Is a stress fracture an acute or chronic injury? Explain your answer.

In the Lab

10. Take a tongue depressor by either end and gently bend it as far as it will go without breaking it; hold that position for 30 seconds. What force is occurring on the top? What force is occurring on the bottom? Now release the tongue depressor. Is the tongue depressor experiencing elasticity or plasticity? Explain.
11. Using a piece of Laffy Taffy®, an Oreo® Cookie, and a soda can, develop a demonstration for the class that depicts tension, compression, and shearing forces. Determine both the causes and effects of the variances in the forces produced. Communicate your findings to the class.

Understanding Science

Lesson Objectives

1. Describe the scientific method and explain why it is important.
2. Discuss the role of data in scientific research.
3. Explain what a scientific theory is and how it is derived.
4. Identify the important early anatomists and physiologists and discuss the impact of their work.

Key Terms

E-Flash Cards

data
research question
science
scientific method
scientific research
  hypothesis

scientific theory
statistical inference
statistical significance

To many, the word *science* creates a mental image of a person wearing safety glasses and a white lab coat, swirling solutions in test tubes and scribbling down equations. But only some scientists wear lab coats and work in laboratories. Others work in a variety of settings as they study plants, animals, birds, insects, volcanos, ocean currents, weather patterns, the earth's solar system, distant galaxies, food safety, human behavior…and human anatomy and physiology.

How can the study of such markedly different topics all constitute science? The word *science* comes from the Latin word *scientia*, which means "knowledge." Thus, **science** is a systematic process that creates new knowledge and organizes that knowledge in the form of testable explanations and predictions about some aspect of our universe. Of course "testable" is a key word in that definition. Some questions are outside the realm of science because they deal with phenomena that are not scientifically testable.

The Scientific Method

The **scientific method** is a systematic process that can be used to answer questions or find solutions to problems in many fields. There are seven steps involved in the scientific method.

Step 1: Identifying a Research Question

All research begins with the identification of a specific **research question** for which someone seeks an answer, or a problem that someone would like to have solved. The research question or problem is the reason for conducting the research.

This means, of course, that the research question or problem must be important. Investigating the research question should be worth an investment of the scientist's time and effort. And keep in mind that almost all scientists today work in teams. Because this type of team research is expensive, investing time and money in an investigation is a substantial commitment.

As mentioned earlier, a sound research question must be sufficiently specific. It should also be possible to investigate the question through the process of using various tools. These tools are used to collect, organize, analyze, and interpret data.

Data are systematically collected and recorded observations of some sort. They may be observations about any topic imaginable. Sometimes the data are quantitative, consisting of numbers. In other cases, they are qualitative, consisting of recorded comments. Sometimes they are a combination of the two (**Figure 1.12**).

Step 2: Formulating One or More Hypotheses

A **scientific research hypothesis** is an *educated guess* as to what the outcome of a research study will be. It is not merely a hunch or a feeling, but an intelligent expectation based on a thorough understanding of the research topic. Researchers usually base their hypotheses

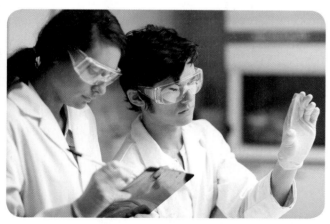
Wavebreakmedia/Shutterstock.com

Figure 1.12 Students collect data during a scientific experiment. *What are some examples of different kinds of data that they might be collecting?*

on related information discovered by scientists in the same field and published in research journals. Scientists are constantly communicating their findings and the information they have extracted from various sources to other scientists. They apply all of this information to refining the question they want to study.

An example of a research hypothesis might be, "We hypothesize that reaction time will be significantly longer following 24 hours of sleep deprivation." Notice that this hypothesis can be confirmed (accepted) or not confirmed (rejected) based on the results of the study. This must be the case for all legitimate scientific research hypotheses. Thus, all hypotheses are tentative, testable statements.

 Check Your Understanding

1. What drives all research?
2. What is an educated guess, as opposed to a hunch or feeling?

Step 3: Planning the Organization of the Study

The organizational aspects of a study involve determining how, where, when, and by whom the data will be collected. In studies involving human participants, organizing the study includes determining

- the criteria to be used for selection of participants;
- the number of participants needed;
- what each participant will be expected to do;
- the equipment or surveys to be used in data collection; and
- the statistical tests that will be used to analyze the data (**Figure 1.13**).

Step 4: Collecting the Data

Empirical research involves the recording of observations, or data. Scientists collect data in many different ways. For example, they can use various tools to take precise, accurate measurements. They can use computer-linked laboratory apparatus to record data

Konstantin Chagin/Shutterstock.com

Figure 1.13 If you enjoy collecting, analyzing, and evaluating data, you might enjoy a career in scientific research. *What are some tools that scientists might use in their work with data?*

values. They can distribute questionnaires or conduct interviews. They use tools as varied as incubators, meter sticks, and calculators.

No matter what the data type or medium for collection, it is essential that all data be collected objectively, using the same procedures. One of the hallmarks of good research is that if other competent researchers were to repeat the study using the same procedures, they would get the same results. For this to be the case, the data collection procedures must be well controlled, and they must be accurately and fully described in the research report.

Step 5: Analyzing and Evaluating the Data with Statistical Tools

The analysis and evaluation of data using statistical tools is a vitally important step in the research process. The statistical tests used in analyzing the data determine whether the findings of a study have **statistical significance**.

When the results of a research study are statistically significant, it suggests that what has been observed from the data collected in the study is also true in general. When data are collected on human participants, statistically significant findings suggest that what is true of the participants sampled is also true of the larger population represented by the participants. This practice of translating the findings of a research study to a large population is known as **statistical inference**.

The ability to accurately predict the characteristics of a very large group based on measurements from a small subset of the large group is a powerful tool. Let's say we would like to know what percentage of US high school students take a course in human anatomy and physiology. We could survey every high school in the country and compile the information, but this would be quite tedious and time consuming. A more efficient method would be to take data from a few representative high schools and then generalize our findings to the entire United States. By looking at such data over a period of years, we could even predict trends in anatomy and physiology enrollment. How would we know that we could legitimately generalize conclusions from our findings? We could do this by making sure that our sample of representative high schools is truly "representative."

Step 6: Interpreting and Discussing the Results

Interpreting and discussing the results of a study are usually the most interesting and challenging components of the scientific research process. Unfortunately, there is no formula for discussing the results of a study. Typically, researchers discuss whether the results do or do not support the original hypotheses and compare the findings of the study to the findings of similar studies. Depending on the nature of the study, it may also be useful to discuss the reasons that the findings are important and to point out practical or clinical applications that may logically follow from the results.

Step 7: Deriving Conclusions from the Results

The conclusions of a study are composed of one or more concise statements that

WHAT RESEARCH TELLS US

...*about* Research

If you were to pursue a career in the health professions, you might become involved in research projects, even if you do not work in a setting in which research is usually done. Scientific investigations happen in laboratories, but research also happens in barns full of cows, community health clinics, pediatricians' offices, and other unconventional places. For example, a pharmaceutical company may work with community healthcare providers to monitor effectiveness and side effects of a new drug. A company that makes dentistry tools may want to get feedback from dental hygienists who have used the tools.

Safety and Resources

Whether the research takes place in the lab or the field, healthcare professionals must be aware of the many safety and resource issues that can arise in research. They must consider how the research could impact their own health, their patients' health, and the environment.

Your Own Health. Ask yourself if the research requires you to change your work routine. If so, are the "usual" steps that you take to ensure workplace safety compromised? Is a new piece of equipment a potential tripping hazard? Are you exposed to potentially hazardous body fluids? Do you have the right personal protective equipment (safety glasses, gloves, lab coat)? If you are working with needles or blades, do you have a safe place (sharps container) to dispose of them? The questions you ask will depend on your situation, but it is important

to anticipate the unexpected when thinking about safety.

Your Patient's Health. The research review process involves extensive consideration of potential risks to patients. Even a research project that has been reviewed and approved could present risks that the reviewers didn't think of. Never hesitate to tell your supervisor if you have a concern about patient safety.

The Environment. Do the potential benefits of the research justify the environmental costs? Most of our activities consume resources and generate waste products. Always try to find ways to minimize the resources needed and the waste created. Also look for ways to recycle resources. Be sure to follow proper procedures for disposing of waste materials.

Types of Research

Just as research occurs in many different settings, it takes many forms. For example, we can classify research projects as descriptive, comparative, or experimental.

Descriptive research means accurately measuring "what's out there." This could mean measuring the height, weight, oral temperature, and age of each child who comes into the clinic. Or it could mean testing saliva samples from adults at the senior center for the presence of a newly discovered virus.

Comparative research involves making comparisons between one group and another. For example, you might want to compare the fitness of the students who take the bus to school to the fitness of those who walk or ride their bicycle to school.

Experimental research is more "active" than descriptive or comparative research. In experimental research, you do something and observe the results. For example, you might ask subjects to complete a math test 15 minutes after drinking coffee, and a week later have them do a similar math test without the coffee. Or you might do an experiment to see whether putting people on a program of regular exercise for two weeks improves their performance on tests of short-term memory.

In all cases, as researchers plan and implement their research, they will ask questions and formulate testable hypotheses. They will select the equipment and technology most appropriate for their particular investigation.

Taking It Further

1. Using the examples above, work in groups to plan and implement descriptive, comparative, and experimental investigations. Brainstorm, asking questions that lead to a testable hypothesis. Then select the appropriate equipment and technology for your investigation. Describe your plan to the class.

2. Demonstrate your safety awareness by creating a poster that highlights what you believe are the most important safety precautions for both lab and field investigations. Include information about the use and conservation of resources and proper disposal and recycling of materials.

communicate the key findings of the study. Legitimate, valid conclusions are directly related to the original hypotheses of the study and explain whether or not the hypotheses were supported by the data collected.

When scientists read the conclusions of a study, they may or may not agree with or accept the conclusions. Scientists are trained to carefully analyze, evaluate, and critique scientific explanations. They do this by considering the empirical evidence (data) presented as the result of the experimental or observational testing. They also consider the logical reasoning behind the interpretation of the study results. A knowledgeable scientist will also examine all sides of the scientific evidence presented in the study by considering whether the results presented are in agreement or conflict with the published results of other similar studies.

 Check Your Understanding

1. How do you determine whether a research project is worthwhile?
2. How are statistical significance and statistical inference related?
3. The conclusion of a research project needs to be related back to which part of the study?

Developing Scientific Theories

We often hear the word *theory* used when the speaker really means a *guess* or a *hunch*. For example, "My theory is that our teacher will give us a pop quiz tomorrow if his football team loses this evening." Sometimes the word *theory* is also used when the speaker really means an *educated guess*, or a *hypothesis*.

A **scientific theory** is an explanation of some aspect of the natural world that is based on rigorously tested, repeatedly confirmed research. When a hypothesis has been thoroughly tested through a variety of conditions and is found to accurately explain a natural or physical phenomenon, it becomes a theory.

The strength of a scientific theory is based on the extent to which it explains a diverse set of circumstances. Theories can be improved and refined as more research is conducted and new areas of science and new technologies are developed. Scientists use theories to advance our scientific knowledge, to create new inventions, and treat diseases.

The Impact of Scientific Research: A Historic Journey

To appreciate the development of science, it is interesting to consider a brief historical perspective. The history of scientific research dates back to the dawn of civilization. One of the earliest topics of interest was the anatomy and physiology of humans.

Early Greek and Roman Anatomists

One of the first to systematically study topics related to anatomy was the well-known early Greek philosopher Aristotle (384–322 BCE). Aristotle studied and wrote about more than 540 species of animals in his anatomy book, *On the Parts of Animals.*

Another early anatomist and physiologist was the Roman physician, surgeon, and philosopher Galen (129–c.200 CE). While serving as the personal physician to several Roman emperors, Galen compiled numerous anatomical reports on his dissections of pigs and monkeys. During Galen's life, dissection of human cadavers was prohibited, so many of his assumptions about human anatomy were based on animal anatomy.

Based on his experiments, Galen was the first to advance the notion that the brain controls the muscles through signals from nerves. Galen also, however, advocated the notion that arteries carry the purest blood to the brain and lungs from the left ventricle of the heart, while veins carry blood to the other organs from the right ventricle. This notion is, of course, incorrect. For his belief to be true, some openings were needed in the walls of the ventricles, which Galen incorrectly claimed to have found.

Anatomists in the Renaissance

Spanning the mid-fourteenth to the mid-seventeenth centuries, the Renaissance was a period of significant cultural and scientific developments. Interest in science increased during this era, leading to new and exciting discoveries. Let's discuss some of the key anatomists of the Renaissance and the contributions they made to the study of anatomy and physiology.

Leonardo da Vinci. During the Renaissance period, the renowned artist Leonardo da Vinci (1452–1519) also distinguished himself as a scientist, engineer, and inventor. Among his many contributions was advancing knowledge of human anatomy and physiology.

To better understand the human body for his paintings, da Vinci was given permission to dissect human corpses at hospitals in Rome, Florence, and Milan. He was known to have dissected at least 30 corpses, including males and females of different ages. From his studies, he prepared a theoretical work on human anatomy with more than 200 drawings, including individual bones, muscles, tendons, ligaments, veins, and arteries.

The Vitruvian Man by da Vinci is one of the best known drawings in the world (**Figure 1.14**). This drawing represents what were considered to be the ideal proportions of man, and illustrates the blending of science and art that was an important trend during the Renaissance.

Andreas Vesalius. A Flemish physician, Andreas Vesalius (1514–1564) is regarded as the founder of modern human anatomy. Vesalius authored a comprehensive and influential work on human anatomy entitled *De Humani Corporis Fabrica (On the Structure of the Human Body)*.

In the course of his work, Vesalius proved that some views of human anatomy proposed by Aristotle and Galen were incorrect. Vesalius correctly observed, for example, that the human heart has four chambers, the liver has two lobes,

Reed/Shutterstock.com

Figure 1.14 Leonardo da Vinci's famous anatomical drawing, *The Vitruvian Man*.

and the blood vessels originate in the heart, not the liver. These findings were all in contrast to the assertions of Aristotle and Galen.

Vesalius did, however, support Galen's views on bloodletting, which was the standard treatment of the day for most illnesses. The classical Greek procedure, advocated by Galen, was to drain blood from a site near the part of the body believed to be associated with an illness.

Using knowledge gained from dissecting human cadavers, Vesalius was able to construct anatomical drawings of the human body that were more detailed than other medical illustrations of the day. One of Vesalius' anatomical drawings is shown in **Figure 1.15**.

William Harvey. One of the first accurate descriptions of human physiology was provided by William Harvey (1578–1657), a physician to two kings of England. Harvey and his colleague Michael Servetus (1511–1553) were the first to understand that blood circulates continuously through the body, with the heart serving as the pump.

Suzan Oschmann/Shutterstock.com

Figure 1.15 An early anatomical drawing from Vesalius' 1543 text, *De Humani Corporis Fabrica.*

Robert Hooke and Antonie van Leeuwenhoek. Science took another large step forward thanks to the work of the Englishman Robert Hooke (1635–1703) and a Dutch textile merchant named Antonie van Leeuwenhoek (1632–1723). Hooke made a number of improvements to the microscopes of the day, which magnified only about 30 times (as opposed to modern microscopes, some of which can magnify up to 10 million times). Using his improved microscope, Hooke was the first to view and name cells. He published a book about microscopy called *Micrographia* in 1665.

Leeuwenhoek further advanced the quality of the microscope, designing an instrument with a magnification of about 200 times for the purpose of close examination of the weave of fabrics. With the new power of his microscope, however, he was soon examining drops of water, blood, sperm, muscle tissue, and bacteria, and confirming that many biological materials are made of cells.

Looking Ahead

We have come a long way in advancing scientific knowledge since the discovery of cells. As is clear from reading about some of these early scientists, the prevailing views of human anatomy and physiology have changed greatly over time. This is true of all fields of science, and change continues today. As new discoveries are made and current assumptions are challenged, we continue to advance our knowledge of many phenomena.

In modern times, researchers investigating topics related to human health often use animal models to test new hypotheses. Depending on the nature of the research, scientists may use rats, chickens, cats, dogs, sheep, or chimpanzees to first test new drugs or other experimental interventions that we ultimately hope could be used with humans. In this type of research the animal serves as a model of a human.

Rats, for example, are mammals, as are humans. There are, of course, obvious differences between rats and humans: rats have four legs, they have a much shorter life span, and they have a much higher metabolic rate. So, although rats are not perfect models, they do provide meaningful opportunities to test and try remedies that we would not want to first test on people. Scientists using animal models in their research must interpret their research findings in light of the differences between the animal model and human anatomy and physiology.

Today the scientific discoveries being made dramatically impact our lives and improve our environment. Recent scientific breakthroughs as a result of research sponsored by the National Aeronautics and Space Administration (NASA) have contributed to the development of many products related to human anatomy and physiology. Examples include memory foam for comfortable seating, scratch-resistant lenses and cochlear implants, software for viewing partial blockages of the carotid artery, and insulin pumps. Research by NASA scientists has also improved our environment. They have made discoveries leading to technology for superior water filters and a compound called *emulsified zero-valent iron* that can be injected into groundwater to neutralize toxic chemicals. Their research has also led to solar-powered appliances, improved insulation materials for residential and commercial buildings, and better fertilizer for plants.

 Check Your Understanding

1. What has to happen for a hypothesis to become a scientific theory?
2. Who was the first to assert that the brain controls muscles?
3. Evaluate the benefits and limitations of using mice as models for studying aspects of human anatomy and physiology.

Lesson 1.4 Review and Assessment

Mini Glossary   Make sure that you know the meaning of each key term.

 Build vocabulary with e-flash cards and games

data systematically collected and recorded observations

research question a question to be answered or a problem to be solved in a research study

science a systematic process that creates new knowledge and organizes it into a form of testable explanations and predictions about an aspect of our universe

scientific method a systematic process that can be used to answer questions or find solutions to problems

scientific research hypothesis an educated guess about what the outcome of a study will be

scientific theory an explanation of some aspect of the natural world that is based on rigorously tested, repeatedly confirmed research

statistical inference the practice of generalizing the findings of a research study to a large population

statistical significance an interpretation of statistical data indicating that the results of a study can legitimately be generalized to the population represented in the study sample

Know and Understand

 Assess

1. Which famous artist was also a preeminent anatomist?
2. The improvement of which scientific tool produced significant advancements in the study of anatomy and physiology?
3. List, in order, the steps of the scientific method.
4. Elaborate on the definition of *hypothesis*. What are the characteristics of a hypothesis?

Analyze and Apply

5. Working with the definition of *science* and the information about science provided in this lesson, explain the limitations, if any, of science.
6. Give an example of a scientific theory that has been refined or improved since it was first established as a theory. Begin with a comprehensive list of the characteristics of a scientific theory. Be sure to show the difference between a hypothesis and a theory.

7. Assume that Aristotle and Galen had been able to dissect cadavers. How do you think that advancement in the study of anatomy might have been different?
8. Explain how da Vinci's study of anatomy influenced the future of anatomical science and art.
9. How would you evaluate the impact of scientific research on a society and the environment in your city, state, or region of the country?

In the Lab

10. Make a time line. Research scientific advancements and the scientists who brought about these changes. Create a 10-point time line from Aristotle through today showing significant milestones that have led to new discoveries and theories. Use the historical information in the text as a starting point. Describe your findings to the class.

Career Corner
Anatomy and Physiology at Work

Studying anatomy and physiology provides a foundation of knowledge that you may use in an exciting and rewarding career in the future. Let's take a look at two such career possibilities.

Biologist

A biologist is a scientist who studies living organisms (**Figure 1.16**). The field of biology comprises numerous subfields. Some examples include

- botany, the study of plants;
- ecology, the study of the interrelationships between living organisms and the environment;
- entomology, the study of insects;
- marine biology, the study of saltwater organisms;
- microbiology, the study of microscopic organisms;
- physiology, the study of the functions of living organisms;
- wildlife biology, the study of wild animals and their habitats; and
- zoology, the study of animals.

Many biological scientists conduct research to advance our knowledge of living organisms, with some working primarily in a laboratory and others primarily in the field. Research biologists are hired by universities, government agencies, and industrial facilities. Topics studied may be basic or applied. The general goal of basic research is to discover the mechanisms underlying various functions of an organism. Examples of applied research outcomes include improved medical treatments, crop yields, and wildlife management.

A bachelor's degree in biology typically requires courses in math, chemistry, and physics as well as coursework in biology. A career as a biological scientist requires a PhD. Most PhD programs in a field of biology require four to six years of training beyond the bachelor's degree. Many individuals with a PhD in biology then go on for another two to three years of specialized training in a postdoctoral fellowship.

Biomechanist

A biomechanist is a scientist who investigates the mechanical aspects of living organisms. Although biomechanics is a relatively young, recognized field of scientific inquiry, biomechanical considerations are of interest in a number of scientific disciplines and professional fields. Biomechanists may have academic backgrounds in zoology, biomedical or biomechanical engineering, physical therapy, or kinesiology, with the commonality being an interest in the biomechanical aspects of the structure and function of living things.

Given the different scientific and professional fields represented, it is no surprise that biomechanists study diverse questions or problems. Biomechanists who study humans may analyze elite performances in different sports to determine which movement characteristics enable some athletes to excel. They also investigate topics such as balance and falling in elderly individuals, bone and muscle loss in astronauts, prevention of low back pain, and design of more efficient and safe sports apparel. Every major athletic shoe company today employs biomechanists to participate in product design (**Figure 1.17**).

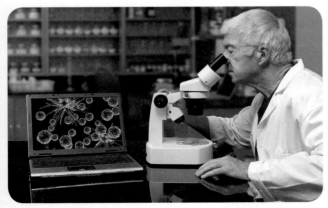

Figure 1.16 A biologist examines spores under a microscope.

Maridav/Shutterstock.com

Figure 1.17 Biomechanists are instrumental in the design of athletic shoes.

Biomechanics is a quantitative field of study, so education for a career in biomechanics requires a bachelor's degree that includes courses in math, physics, engineering, and computer science. To be a research biomechanist, one must earn a PhD or DPT (Doctor of Physical Therapy) degree. PhD programs in biomechanics typically require four to five years of work.

Planning for a Health-Related Career

Do some research on career options for a biologist or biomechanist. Keep in mind the many specialties available within these fields. For example, a marine biologist studies saltwater organisms, and an entomologist studies insects. A biomechanist might, for example, study ways to prevent low back pain or design athletic apparel and equipment optimized for performance.

Alternatively, select a profession from the list of **Related Career Options**. Using the Internet or resources at your local library, find answers to the following questions:

1. What are the main tasks and responsibilities of a biologist or biomechanist?
2. What is the outlook for the career that you have chosen to research? Are workers in demand, or are jobs dwindling? For complete information, consult the current edition of the *Occupational Outlook Handbook*, published by the US Department of Labor. This handbook is available online or at your local library.
3. What special skills or talents are required? For example, do you need to be good at biology, chemistry, or physics? Do you need to enjoy interacting with other people?
4. What personality traits do you think are needed to be successful in this career?
5. Does the job involve a great deal of routine, or are the day-to-day responsibilities varied?
6. Does the work require long hours, or is the career of a biologist or biomechanist a standard, "9-to-5" job?
7. What is the salary range for this job?
8. What do you think you would like about this career? Is there anything about it that you might dislike?

Related Career Options

- Animal Scientist
- Bioengineer
- Biologist
- Biomechanist
- Biomedical Engineer
- Botanist
- Ecologist
- Entomologist
- Forest and Conservation Technician
- Marine Biologist
- Microbiologist
- Natural Science Manager
- Physiologist
- Range Manager
- Soil and Water Conservationist
- Wildlife Biologist
- Zoologist

Chapter Summaries

Lesson 1.1 The Language of Anatomy and Physiology

 Build vocabulary with e-flash cards and games

Key Points

- Anatomy and physiology are studied together because the structure of a cell, tissue, or organ is closely related to its function.
- Scientists use universal terminology for anatomical positions, planes, and directions to accurately describe body positions and movements.
- The body is divided into cavities that contain various bones and organs.
- The metric system is used throughout the world in all fields of science to measure numerical quantities.

Key Terms

abdominal cavity	oral cavity
abdominopelvic cavity	orbital cavities
anatomical position	pelvic cavity
anatomy	physiology
anterior (ventral) body cavity	posterior (dorsal) body cavity
cranial cavity	sagittal plane
frontal plane	spinal cavity
metric system	thoracic cavity
middle ear cavities	transverse plane
nasal cavity	

Lesson 1.2 Basic Physiological Processes

Key Points

- The human body is comprised of a hierarchy of structures, from atoms at the most basic unit to organ systems at the highest level.
- Each body system fulfills a vital function, independent from the other systems, to keep the human body viable.
- Although the human body is in a constant state of flux, it is kept in balance and healthy by maintaining homeostasis.
- Metabolism is the constant breaking down and building up of molecules to provide energy, create cells, and perform bodily functions needed to sustain life.

Key Terms

atoms	metabolism
cells	molecules
control center	negative feedback
effector	organ
homeostasis	organ system
homeostatic imbalance	positive feedback
homeostatic mechanisms	receptor
metabolic rate	tissues

Lesson 1.3 How Forces Affect the Body

Key Points

- Kinetics is the study of forces on the human body. These forces include pressure, compression, torque, shearing, and stress.
- Forces can cause tissues to experience acceleration and deformation. Deformation may be either elastic or plastic.
- Injuries can occur when a structure experiences a significant force all at once or a smaller amount of force repetitively over time.

Key Terms

bending	pressure
combined loading	shear
compression	stress
elastic	tension
force	torque
kinetics	torsion
mass	weight
net force	

Understanding Science

Key Points

- Scientific knowledge is increased via research conducted using the scientific method to ensure uniformity in experimentation.
- A statistically significant finding is one that is true of the participants sampled in a research study and the larger population represented by the participants.
- A scientific theory emerges from a hypothesis that has been rigorously and repeatedly researched and tested such that all evidence points to the accuracy of the theory in explaining a natural occurrence. A scientific theory can be strengthened through continued research.
- Scientific knowledge continues to grow with advancements in research methods and tools.

Key Terms

data
research question
science
scientific method
scientific research
  hypothesis

scientific theory
statistical inference
statistical significance

Chapter Assessments

Assess

Lesson 1.1

The Language of Anatomy and Physiology

Learning Key Terms and Concepts

1. The _____ cavity contains the skull and brain.
2. The universal starting point for describing positions and movements of the human body is _____.
3. _____ is the study of the functions of the human body.
4. Which of these organs is found in the thoracic cavity?
   A. heart
   B. stomach
   C. liver
   D. kidneys
5. The knee is _____ to the ankle.
   A. lateral
   B. posterior
   C. distal
   D. proximal
6. A cut that would divide the body into right and left parts is a(n) _____ cut.
   A. sagittal
   B. transverse
   C. frontal
   D. coronal
7. When we refer to the dorsal surface of a person or object, we are talking about the _____.
   A. superior surface
   B. inferior surface
   C. posterior surface
   D. anterior surface

Thinking Critically

8. What plane(s) can the shoulder move in? Explain your answer.

9. Using the common directional terms for anatomy that you learned in lesson 1, provide a written description for the location of the index finger of the left hand.
10. Describe which planes the legs of a sprinter move in. Explain your answer.

Lesson 1.2

Basic Physiological Processes

Learning Key Terms and Concepts

11. The smallest living structure is the _____.
12. The body maintains a stable internal environment via _____.
13. _____ nerves carry a signal from the external environment to the control center.
14. The lungs are part of the _____.
    A. circulatory system
    B. integumentary system
    C. endocrine system
    D. respiratory system
15. The next and most complex level after the cellular level in organisms is the _____.
    A. organ
    B. tissue
    C. body system
    D. chemical
16. Which of the following is *not* one of the four main types of tissue in the body?
    A. muscle tissue
    B. connective tissue
    C. alveolar tissue
    D. nerve tissue

17. Cells are composed of organized groups of specialized _____.
    A. tissues   C. proteins
    B. organs   D. molecules
18. Which of the following is the best example of homeostasis?
    A. storage of food in the form of excess body fat
    B. sexual reproduction
    C. regulation of body temperature
    D. growth of underarm hair

Thinking Critically

19. You have a very muscular friend who needs to reduce his weight for wrestling. What advice would you give him about eating while trying to lose weight? Explain your answer.
20. It is a hot, dry day, and you are going to be running a race in the middle of the afternoon. What challenges does your body face in trying to maintain homeostasis while you run?

Lesson 1.3

How Forces Affect the Body

Learning Key Terms and Concepts

21. _____ is a force that pulls or stretches the tissue.
22. _____ is a force that, with enough energy, crushes tissue.
23. _____ is a force that moves parallel with tissue.
24. _____ is caused by a combination of off-center forces.
25. A bruise is caused by _____.
    A. compression   C. shearing
    B. tension   D. torque
26. _____ is the single force resulting from the summation of all forces acting on an object at a given time.
    A. Net mass   C. Net torque
    B. Net force   D. Net weight
27. A tissue is said to be _____ when a force is removed and the object returns to its original shape.
    A. plastic   C. efferent
    B. torqued   D. elastic

Thinking Critically

28. A football player's foot is planted, and he is in the process of turning when his knee is hit from the side, resulting in a serious injury to the ligaments of the knee. Which two forces acted on the knee to produce this injury?
29. Assume that your body is struck by a baseball and a basketball of the same weight traveling at the same speed. Which will exert more pressure on your body—the baseball or the basketball? Why?
30. Is skin or bone more elastic? Why?

Lesson 1.4

Understanding Science

Learning Key Terms and Concepts

31. All research begins with the identification of a(n) _____.
32. Early anatomists studied _____ because of religious or political influences prohibiting the dissection of _____.
33. The key to collecting data is that it must _____.
    A. be collected objectively using the same procedures every time
    B. be collected objectively and obtained in the largest quantities possible
    C. be collected subjectively using the same procedure every time
    D. be collected subjectively and obtained in the smallest possible quantities
34. Step 2 of the scientific method is _____.
    A. formulating a hypothesis
    B. planning the organization of the study
    C. identifying a research question
    D. collecting the data
35. When a hypothesis has been thoroughly investigated and found to accurately explain a natural or physical phenomenon, it is _____.
    A. a hunch   C. a hypothesis
    B. a guess   D. a theory

Thinking Critically

36. Create a measurable hypothesis about study time and its relationship to success on exams. Make precise, accurate measurements of both time and grades. What can you infer from your data? What trends can you predict? Communicate your conclusions to your classmates.
37. Suppose that a hypothesis is proven incorrect. Does this mean that the research was a waste of time? Defend your answer.
38. With the students in your anatomy and physiology class as the participants, research the impact of exercise on the homeostatic state of the respiratory system. Collect, organize, analyze, and evaluate both quantitative and qualitative data using appropriate tools. Will this population sample be considered statistically significant? How could you improve this experiment?

Building Skills and Connecting Concepts

Analyzing and Evaluating Data

The graph at the right shows the average number of steps (foot contacts) resulting in chronic injury, as they occur in groups of people in different weight categories. Use the graph to answer the following questions.

39. How many foot contacts is the group with a body weight of 160 pounds able to make before an injury occurs?

40. Which group is generating the most pressure per foot contact?

41. What prediction would you make about the number of foot contacts leading to injury for people in the 170- to 175-pound range?

42. Based on the data provided in the graph, write a hypothesis about body weight and foot contacts resulting in chronic injuries.

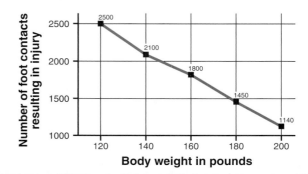

Communicating about Anatomy and Physiology

43. **Speaking and Listening**   Working in small groups, create a poster that illustrates the anatomical planes and directional movements of the human body. Have a volunteer briefly stand before the class as a "visual aid" to help you accurately capture and represent anatomical position and directional relationships.

First, draw a figure in anatomical position with the body erect, the arms at the sides, and the palms facing forward. Then, label the three anatomical planes: *sagittal*, *frontal* (coronal), and *transverse*. Within each of the planes, add labels to show the directional relationships among body parts and the different positions of movement: *superior* (cranial), *inferior* (caudal), *anterior* (ventral), *posterior* (dorsal), *medial*, *lateral*, and *proximal*. Use different-colored markers to outline and label each anatomical plane and directional relationship.

As you work with your group, discuss the meaning of each term. If necessary, a member of your group might stand and demonstrate directional movements to confirm your understanding of the terms. Afterward, display your posters in the classroom as a convenient reference aid for discussions and assignments.

Lab Investigations

44. Working in groups of two or three students, create a three-dimensional anatomical man and label your creation using the terms that you have learned in this chapter. If you created a poster in the "Communicating" activity above, use it as a guide as you label your "anatomy man."

Work with your group members to organize your project. Be creative in deciding what materials you will use to create your figure. Delegate responsibility to team members for bringing each of the needed materials. As much as possible, use materials that are readily available in your home (for example, boxes, string, balloons, plastic bottles, paper, tape, glue, or pipe cleaners). Do *not* use any sharp objects. Also refrain from using manufactured figures such as dolls, action figures, or stuffed animals.

Incorporate into your anatomical man the directional and body cavity terms that you learned in this chapter. Include all the terms in **Figures 1.2** and **1.3**. You must be accurate in your placement of each term. You may use arrows, and you may create several layers on your anatomy man.

Expand your learning with additional online resources
- Supplemental Lab Activities
- Interactive Exercises
- Animations

www.g-wlearning.com/healthsciences

What will be the next breakthrough as scientists study human cells?

Cells and Tissues

*O*ur bodies are made of cells—trillions of them. Although scientists have yet to come up with a satisfactory definition of life, it seems clear that our individual cells are alive. They reproduce, by mitosis. They transmit information from one generation to the next, using DNA. They transform energy from one form to another, and they use energy to maintain their internal environment in the face of outside pressures.

Our cells cannot survive independently; they need one another to stay alive. Each cell is a specialist with its own job to do. Certain tasks, such as maintaining an internal environment different from that of the surrounding fluid, are performed by *all* cells. Other tasks, such as making ATP, are done by *most* cells. And some tasks, such as making circulating antibodies, are done by *only one* type of cell.

We must understand how cells work, and how they work together, to understand anatomy and physiology. An understanding of cells and the tissues made from cells is also necessary for understanding diseases and their treatment. This is even truer now than it was a generation ago because modern medicine relies more than ever on therapies targeted at cellular processes.

In this chapter we will learn about the parts of a cell and how those parts cooperate to keep cells alive, reproduce, and accomplish specialized tasks. We will also learn about the types of tissues that combine to make organs and organ systems.

Chapter 2 Lessons

Lesson 2.1
Molecules of Life

Lesson 2.2
Cells

Lesson 2.3
Tissues

While studying, look for the online icon to:

- **Practice** with e-flash cards and vocabulary games
- **Review** with interactive art labeling
- **Assess** with online exercises
- **Expand** with interactive activities and animated videos
- **Listen** to pronunciations of key terms in the audio glossary

www.g-wlearning.com/healthsciences

Study on the Go

Use a mobile device to practice vocabulary terms, listen to pronunciations, and review with self-assessment quizzes.

www.m.g-wlearning.com

Molecules of Life

Before You Read

Try to answer the following questions before you read this lesson.

What are the major types of large organic molecules in the human body?

What molecule is the universal source of energy for cellular reactions?

What properties of water make it essential for life?

Lesson Objectives

1. Name and explain the functions of several major organic molecules, including carbohydrates, proteins, lipids, nucleic acids, and water.

2. Describe amino acids and give examples of types, structures, and functions.

3. Discuss the advantages and disadvantages of glycogen and glycerides with regard to energy storage.

4. Know the differences between the structures of DNA and RNA.

5. Explain the importance of ATP.

6. Describe polarity and pH balance.

Key Terms

E-Flash Cards

amino acids	nucleic acids
ATP	nucleotides
base pairs	peptide bond
DNA	phospholipids
enzymes	polymer
fatty acid	polypeptide
glucose	RNA
glycogen	steroids
human genome	triglycerides
lipids	

An almost countless number of different types of molecules exists in the human body. *Biochemistry* is the detailed study of the molecules of life, how they are made, how they interact, and how they are broken down. In this lesson you will receive a short summary of the key molecules of life, the ones that will be important in your study of anatomy and physiology.

Many chemicals important for life are organic molecules. Organic molecules always contain carbon and hydrogen. They usually contain oxygen, and they sometimes contain nitrogen, phosphorous, sulfur, and other elements. Major classes of large organic molecules in the body include carbohydrates, proteins, lipids, and nucleic acids. Important small molecules and atoms include ATP, sodium, potassium, chloride, calcium, phosphate, and, of course, water.

Carbohydrates

Carbohydrates, also known as *saccharides* (SAK-a-righdz), are "sugar and starch" molecules. Carbohydrates made of just one or two simple subunits are called *simple carbohydrates*, or sugars. **Glucose** ($C_6H_{12}O_6$) (**Figure 2.1**) is a monosaccharide (simple sugar) and is the main form of sugar that circulates in the blood. Sucrose (table sugar) is a disaccharide made of two monosaccharides: glucose and fructose.

Simple sugars can join together into long chains known as *complex carbohydrates*. A molecule made of many similar subunits is called a **polymer**. **Glycogen** (GLIGH-koh-jehn) is a polymer of glucose and is found in animals; starch is a polymer of simple sugars and is found in plants.

A. **Diagram of a glucose molecule.** The black spheres are carbon atoms, red are oxygen, and blue are hydrogen.

B. **Standard representation of a glucose molecule.**

Figure 2.1 Glucose, shown here in two ways, is an organic molecule. Notice the difference in the number of carbon atoms in A as opposed to B. The reason for this difference is that, in the standard method of representing the molecular structure of glucose (B), a carbon atom is assumed to be present at each unlabeled "corner" where two or more lines (bonds) meet.

Liver and muscle cells make glycogen molecules (**Figure 2.2**) from glucose. The glycogen granules are a form of stored fuel. When a muscle cell needs fuel, it can break glucose molecules off of the glycogen and use the glucose for energy. If blood sugar becomes too low, liver cells break glucose molecules off of the glycogen and release the glucose into the blood. A single glycogen molecule may contain hundreds of thousands of glucose subunits.

The main function of carbohydrates in the body is to serve as a source of chemical energy, or fuel. The body can quickly utilize this fuel to make ATP, which you will learn about later in this chapter.

 Check Your Understanding

1. What subunits form carbohydrates? What does the word *carbohydrate* mean?
2. What is the term for simple sugars that join together in long chains?
3. Where in the body are glycogen molecules made from glucose?

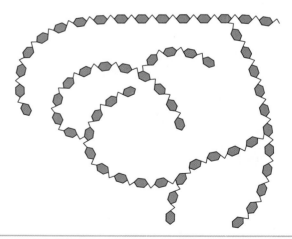

Figure 2.2 Glycogen structure. Glycogen is a polysaccharide made of glucose monomers, which are shown here as hexagons. Glycogen has many branches. *What would you need to remove from this drawing to change the complex carbohydrate to many simple carbohydrates?*

 Memory Tip

The name *carbohydrate* is derived from the elements that go together to make up a carbohydrate. The name also provides a clue to the atomic formula for carbohydrates. All carbohydrates are made of carbon, hydrogen, and oxygen atoms. The hydrogen and oxygen are usually present in a two-to-one ratio, like water (H_2O). *Hydrate* is a chemical term for water. So carbohydrate means "carbon plus water."

WHAT RESEARCH TELLS US

...*about* Glycogen Storage Diseases

Glycogen storage diseases are a class of disorders in which either the formation or the breakdown of glycogen does not work properly (**Figure 2.3**). In healthy individuals, the liver and muscles perform two different processes involving glycogen and glucose. They synthesize glycogen from glucose, and they break down glycogen to release glucose. Glucose from the liver is released into the bloodstream. Glucose

found in the muscle is used to make ATP for energy.

In hepatic types of glycogen storage diseases, the liver does not release glucose into the blood as it should. The liver is often enlarged due to an abnormal accumulation of glycogen granules in its cells. In myopathic types of glycogen storage diseases, the storage or breakdown of glycogen in muscles does not work properly. (The combining form *myo* means

"muscle" and the combing form *path-* means "sickness.")

Glycogen storage diseases are usually inherited. They are caused by genetic mutations that affect enzymes (proteins) that catalyze biochemical reactions involving glycogen. There is no cure, but in many cases, symptoms can be lessened by dietary changes, drugs, or a liver transplant.

A. Normal formation and breakdown of glycogen

B. Hepatic form of glycogen storage disease

C. Myopathic form of glycogen storage disease

Figure 2.3 Glycogen storage disease. *If everything is working properly, does the liver turn glucose to glycogen, glycogen to glucose, or both?*

Proteins

Proteins are large biological molecules made of chains of dozens to hundreds of **amino acids**. Some proteins help form the structure of cells, while other proteins, called **enzymes**, catalyze (speed up) specific biological reactions. Still others (notably hemoglobin) act as carriers (hemoglobin carries oxygen in red blood cells).

Amino Acids

There are 20 common amino acids, which are the building blocks of proteins. All 20 amino acids share a common design: each has an identical "backbone" consisting of an amino group (-NH$_2$), an acid group (-COOH), and a central carbon in between, as shown in **Figure 2.4**. The central carbon has a hydrogen and a variable group of atoms attached to it. The variable group is what varies from one amino acid to another. Biochemists call the variable group the *residual group*, so we use an R to indicate this group in **Figure 2.4**.

Glycine (GLIGH-seen), the simplest amino acid, has a residual group consisting of a single hydrogen atom. Tryptophan (TRIP-toh-fan) has the largest residual group (C$_9$H$_4$N). Some amino acids have residual groups that are acidic, some have residual groups that are basic, and two amino acids have residual groups that contain sulfur. The sulfur residual group is important because disulfide bonds, which connect sulfurs of different amino acids, are essential contributors to the structure of some proteins.

Peptide Bonds

Amino acids join together by forming a **peptide bond**, a bond linking the amino group of one amino acid to the acid group of another.

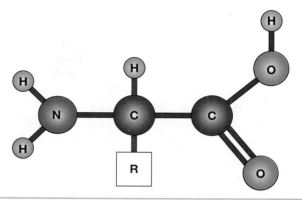

Figure 2.4 An amino acid has a "backbone" made of an amino group, which consists of -NH$_2$ (to the left in the drawing), a carboxylic acid group -COOH (to the right), and a central carbon. A residual group (R) is attached to the central carbon. The residual group varies from one amino acid to another.

Short chains of amino acids (fewer than 50) are often referred to as *peptides*. Examples include the octapeptide (8 amino acids) oxytocin (AHK-see-TOH-sin), a hormone that is important in childbirth, and enkephalin (ehn-KEHF-a-lin), a pentapeptide (5 amino acids) that acts in the brain to inhibit the perception of pain.

A longer chain of amino acids is called a **polypeptide**. Many proteins, such as actin (275 amino acids long) and titin (more than 33,000 amino acids long), are made of a single polypeptide chain. Both actin and titin are found in muscle tissue. Other proteins are made of multiple polypeptide chains. The oxygen-carrying protein hemoglobin (HEE-moh-GLOH-bin) is made of four polypeptide chains, each between 140 and 150 amino acids long.

Structure of Proteins

The structure, or shape, of a protein is determined by the sequence of amino acids it contains (**Figure 2.5**). The amino acid sequence is known as the *primary structure* of a protein. The polypeptide chain folds up into a specific shape that is determined by its primary structure.

This folding process occurs because it allows the protein to reduce its potential energy. Just as a marble "wants" to roll downhill, a polypeptide "wants" to fold. It wants to fold because folding allows energetically favorable interactions of

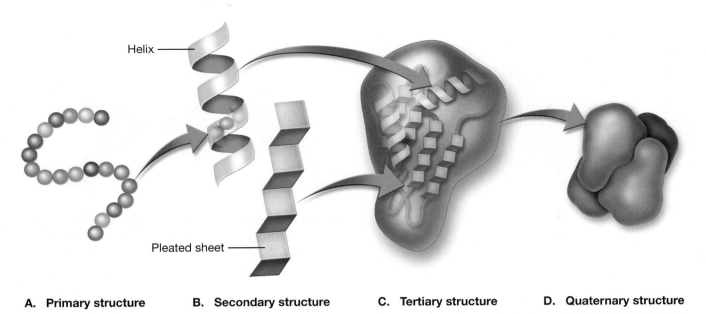

A. **Primary structure**   B. **Secondary structure**   C. **Tertiary structure**   D. **Quaternary structure**

Figure 2.5 Levels of protein structure. *How are these different levels of protein structure related to energy?*

residual groups of amino acids with one another and with surrounding molecules, including water.

The first level of folding is called *secondary structure*. One common form of secondary structure is the alpha helix, in which part of the polypeptide chain assumes a spiral conformation. Another common form of secondary structure is the beta-pleated sheet, in which part of the chain assumes a "flat with slight folds" conformation.

The next level of folding is the *tertiary* (meaning "third level") *structure*. At this level, helical sections, pleated sheet sections, and other sections fold together into a three-dimensional whole. If the protein is made of a single polypeptide, the tertiary structure is the final level of protein structure. For proteins made of multiple subunits, the arrangement of subunits into a whole, or *quaternary* (meaning "fourth level") *structure*, is the final step in determining the protein's shape.

Functions of Proteins

As mentioned earlier, proteins have many functions in the body, including acting as structural elements, enzymes, and carriers. Collagen, which gives strength to ligaments and tendons, is an example of protein with a structural function.

An enzyme is a molecule that participates in a chemical reaction without being consumed or destroyed in the reaction. An enzyme is a molecular facilitator, which allows a specific reaction to occur much faster than it would if the enzyme were not present. For example, the enzyme *salivary amylase*, found in saliva, is a protein that breaks down carbohydrate molecules into smaller sugar molecules.

Myoglobin (MIGH-oh-GLOH-bin) and hemoglobin are proteins that act as carriers. Myoglobin carries oxygen in muscle; hemoglobin carries oxygen in blood.

 Check Your Understanding

1. What three components form the backbone of all 20 amino acids in the body?
2. What are the functions of proteins in the body?
3. What is the difference between a peptide bond and a polypeptide?
4. What is an enzyme?

Lipids

Lipids are "fats and oils" and related molecules. They are rich in carbon and hydrogen, usually with a ratio of about two

Memory Tip

The ability to carry a reserve fuel supply has a survival benefit if food becomes scarce. The body stores chemical energy for future use in the form of carbohydrates (especially glycogen) and fats (especially triglycerides). Which is the better way to store energy?

Each form of stored chemical energy has advantages and disadvantages. For example, glycogen can be turned into usable chemical energy more quickly than triglycerides, because glycogen provides glucose directly to cells. This glucose can then be used rapidly by virtually all body cells to make ATP (discussed later). The breakdown of triglycerides, however, yields fatty acids, which cannot be used by as many cells and, in addition, cannot be used as quickly as glucose.

Glycogen, but not triglycerides, can provide energy fast enough to sustain prolonged rigorous exercise—at least it can until the glycogen stores run out. It should be noted, however, that exercise does help consume unwanted fat because fat is used to some extent during exercise itself. Fat is also used during recovery from exercise to restock the body's storehouse of glycogen.

The big advantage of fat over glycogen is that it stores about twice as much energy per kilogram (or pound) as glycogen or other carbohydrates. A gram of glycogen stores about four to five kilocalories of chemical energy. A gram of fat stores about nine kilocalories of energy. There is obviously a benefit to carrying the same amount of energy reserves with fewer pounds. That is why, if one consumes more calories than are needed to meet the demands of living, the body stores the excess energy as fat.

hydrogen atoms for every carbon atom. They also contain oxygen atoms and sometimes other types of atoms.

Lipids do not dissolve well in water or blood, although there are special proteins that help carry lipids in the blood. Lipid molecules do not get as big as the large proteins and carbohydrates, but they have a wide range of structures and functions.

Fatty Acids

A **fatty acid** is a hydrocarbon chain with a carboxylic acid group (COOH) at one end. Fatty acids may have all single bonds, in which case they are called *saturated*. Fatty acids with one or more double bonds are called *unsaturated*. Stearic acid ($C_{18}H_{36}O_2$) and oleic acid ($C_{18}H_{34}O_2$) are examples of saturated and unsaturated fatty acid, respectively.

The presence of double bonds in a fatty acid often puts a "kink" in the molecule. Fatty acids in their "pure" form are not that common in the body, but they are key building blocks for other lipids, particularly glycerides and phospholipids (FAHS-foh-LIP-idz).

Glycerides

Glycerides are composed of a glycerol molecule (a simple sugar) with one, two, or three fatty acids attached, to make mono-, di-, and **triglycerides** (trigh-GLIS-er-ighdz) (**Figure 2.6**). Glycerides are important energy storage molecules in the body. Most of the fat in fat cells is in the form of triglycerides.

Figure 2.6 A triglyceride has a glycerol head (blue) and three fatty acid chains (red). The triglyceride shown here has two saturated fatty acids (top two chains) and one unsaturated fatty acid (bottom chain), which is a result of the double bond.

Phospholipids

Phospholipids are similar to glycerides. The phosphate-bearing head of the phospholipid is *hydrophilic* (HIGH-droh-FIL-ik), which means that it can form energetically favored hydrogen bonds with water molecules. The fatty acid tails are *hydrophobic* (HIGH-droh-FOH-bik), which means they cannot form favorable hydrogen bonds with water. As a result, phospholipids in a watery environment tend to form bilayers, liposomes (LIGHP-oh-sohmz), or *micelles* (migh-SELZ) ("little spheres") with the heads facing the water and the tails adjacent to one another (**Figure 2.7**).

A. Atomic structure of a phospholipid molecule

Bilayer

Liposome

Micelle

B. Phospholipids in water

Figure 2.7 A—The atomic structure of a phospholipid includes a "head" (blue outline) containing glycerol, a polar group (red) that includes phosphate, and two fatty acid tails (green). The head is hydrophilic and the tails are hydrophobic. B—Phospholipids in water can form a bilayer, a liposome, or a micelle. In each of these arrangements, the hydrophilic phosphate heads face outward, toward water, and the hydrophobic tails "hide" themselves by facing inward.

Memory Tip

Molecules, or parts of molecules, differ in how well they bond with water. Molecules that easily bond with water are called *hydrophilic*, which means "water-loving." Molecules that do not bond well with water are called *hydrophobic*, or "water-fearing." Most lipids, including fatty acids, triglycerides, and steroids (discussed in the next section), are significantly hydrophobic. That's why oil and water don't mix. Phospholipids are different: they have hydrophilic heads and hydrophobic tails. This makes them ideally suited for making cell membranes, as shown in **Figure 2.7**.

Steroids

Steroids are a class of lipids whose structure is very different from that of other lipids. Three well-known steroid molecules—cholesterol, testosterone, and estrogen—are shown in **Figure 2.8**. All steroids have the same four-ring backbone but differ in the attached side groups. Cholesterol is a component of cell membranes. Testosterone and estrogen are hormones that regulate the reproductive system.

✔ Check Your Understanding

1. Identify the four types of lipids.
2. What are the two classes of fatty acids?
3. What does it mean when a molecule is hydrophilic?
4. Name three well-known steroid molecules.

Nucleic Acids

Nucleic acids are key information-carrying molecules in cells. Some nucleic acids also function as enzymes. The two kinds of nucleic acids found in cells are ribonucleic acid (RNA) and deoxyribonucleic acid (DNA). Like proteins and complex carbohydrates, nucleic acids are polymers.

The subunits that make up nucleic acids are called **nucleotides** (NOO-klee-oh-tighdz). Each nucleotide is made of a phosphate group, a sugar group, and a nitrogenous (nitrogen-containing) *base* (**Figure 2.9**). Two nucleotides join together by forming a bond between the phosphate of one nucleotide and the sugar of another, with the

Figure 2.9 A nucleotide is made up of a phosphate group, a sugar group, and a nitrogenous base. Adenine is the base shown here, and the entire molecule—base plus sugar plus phosphate—is called *adenosine monophosphate*.

A. **Cholesterol**

B. **Estrogen**

C. **Testosterone**

Figure 2.8 Steroid molecules: cholesterol, estrogen, and testosterone. *Which of the three steroids shown are hormones?*

bases "hanging off" to the side. A water molecule is produced and released in the process—as it was in the formation of a disaccharide and in the formation of a peptide bond.

Just as different side chains distinguish different amino acids, different bases distinguish different nucleotides. However, there are only 5 kinds of nucleotides, as opposed to 20 different amino acids. The bases are *adenine*, *guanine*, *cytosine*, *thymine*, and *uracil*, each of which is commonly abbreviated by its first letter. DNA is made of nucleotides containing A, G, C, and T. RNA is made of nucleotides containing A, G, C, and U.

DNA

In **DNA**, shown in **Figure 2.10**, two nucleotide chains coil around each other to form a double helix, which is similar in structure to a twisted ladder. The sugar and phosphate groups form the sides of the ladder. The bases from each side meet in the middle to form the rungs.

Each base can join with only one other base to form a rung: A and T form **base pairs**, and C and G form base pairs. Thus, if you know the base sequence of one strand, you can predict the base sequence of the complementary strand.

Base pairs are joined in the middle by hydrogen bonds, but the sugar-phosphate backbone is held together by covalent bonds. Because hydrogen bonds are weaker than covalent bonds, a DNA molecule can "unzip" down the middle with relative ease, while the backbone on each side remains intact. As we shall see, the ability of DNA to unzip is crucial for two processes: making a copy of the DNA before a cell divides and making transcripts of short segments of the DNA.

Chromosomes. One DNA molecule and the proteins around which it coils make up one chromosome. Almost every human cell has 46 chromosomes—23 from each parent. There are 22 pairs of similar chromosomes (numbered 1 through 22), plus one X and one Y chromosome (in males) or two X chromosomes (in females).

Two exceptions to the 46-chromosomes-per-cell rule are sperm cells and egg cells, each of which has just 23 chromosomes. Another exception is red blood cells, which do not have nuclei or chromosomes.

Glycogen is a very large molecule, with a molecular weight in the tens of millions, but DNA is much bigger. Chromosome 1, with about 250 million base pairs, has a molecular weight of about 150 billion atomic units, which does not include proteins that bind to it and help it coil. The 46 DNA molecules in a single cell, if laid out straight, would have a length of about 2 meters. The extreme thinness of DNA allows it to fit in a nucleus of 10 micrometers in diameter or smaller. This is similar to the ability of a fisherman to keep a quarter mile or more of fine fishing line (preferably on a spool) in a small tackle box.

Human Genomes. The DNA sequence of a human is referred to as the **human genome**. All humans (except identical twins, whose genomes are essentially the same) have very similar, but

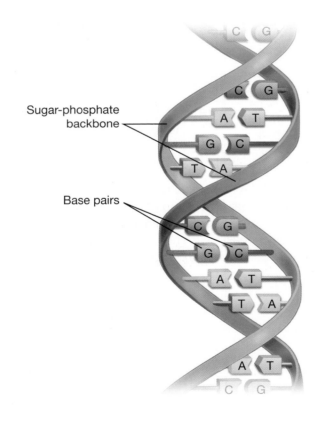

Sugar-phosphate backbone

Base pairs

A.   DNA molecule

Figure 2.10 A DNA molecule. *What joins the base pairs and how does this affect cell replication?*

not quite identical, genomes. On average, about one base in every thousand bases is variable.

Certain base locations are much more likely to differ between individuals than other base locations. The base locations that tend to vary are called *single nucleotide polymorphisms*, or SNPs (pronounced "snips"). SNPs are the subject of much study given that they account for the genetic differences among individuals, including innate differences in athletic ability, disease susceptibility, and other inherited tendencies.

DNA Blueprints. It is interesting to note that cells can be very different even though they all contain the same DNA. For example, the bone cells, muscle cells, skin cells, and nerve cells in one person all contain complete and identical genetic blueprints, yet the cells are very different in structure and function. This brings us to the subject of the information stored on the DNA.

DNA provides the blueprint for making proteins. The sequence of bases along DNA molecules specifies which amino acids to arrange in a particular order to make the proteins needed for life. It takes three bases of DNA to specify one amino acid in a protein. A set of three bases that specifies one amino acid in a protein is called a *codon*. A segment of DNA containing all the codons to make one polypeptide chain is called a *gene*.

RNA

RNA, like DNA, is a polymer of nucleotides. Its bases are adenosine, guanine, cytosine, and—instead of thymine, which is found in DNA—uracil. An RNA molecule is a single chain of nucleotides, as shown in **Figure 2.11**. In some RNA molecules, part of the chain forms a "hairpin" that doubles back on itself. When it does, the bases form pairs analogous to the pairs seen in the DNA double helix: C and G form pairs, and A and U form pairs.

There are several forms of RNA: messenger RNA (mRNA), transfer RNA (tRNA), *ribosomal RNA* (rRNA), and the most recently discovered and least well understood—regulatory RNA. Here is a brief description of the functions of each type of RNA:

- Messenger RNA functions as an information carrier in the manufacture of proteins.

- Transfer RNA assists in the manufacture of proteins.
- Ribosomal RNA forms ribosomes, large enzymes that act as catalysts for protein synthesis.
- Regulatory RNA helps regulate which proteins are produced.

The ability of RNA to function as both an information carrier (mRNA) and as an enzyme (rRNA) has led biologists to speculate that RNA may have been the first self-replicating molecule and, thus, a key molecule in the development of life. We will examine the functions of DNA and RNA in more detail later in this chapter.

ATP

Adenosine triphosphate (a-DEHN-oh-seen trigh-FAHS-fayt), also known as **ATP**, is a nucleotide composed of an adenine base, a sugar, and three phosphate groups. ATP is a common energy source used in many cellular processes. A significant amount of chemical potential energy is stored in the bonds between the phosphates.

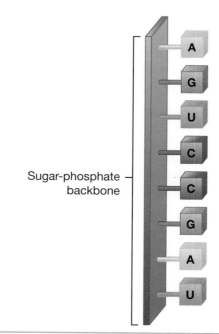

Figure 2.11 An RNA molecule is a chain of nucleotides. The four nucleotides—abbreviated A, C, G, and U—can occur in varying order. The chain can "fold up" in many possible ways, depending on the molecule's function.

The energy in the bond between the last and middle phosphates can be released by splitting off the last phosphate. This process yields adenosine diphosphate (ADP) and inorganic phosphate, abbreviated P_i. (It is called inorganic phosphate because the molecular fragment contains no carbon.) This reaction is shown in **Figure 2.12** by the arrow on the left. ATP can be resynthesized by combining ADP and P_i and adding energy. This process is shown by the arrow on the right-hand side of **Figure 2.12**.

To understand the role that ATP plays in cells, consider the role that money plays in our economy. If there were no money, we would have to trade certain items to get those that we needed. If Alice raises goats, for example, she could trade goat's milk to get bread from Bob the bread maker. In an economy without money, Alice will have a hard time getting bread, if Bob doesn't like goat's milk. But in an economy with money, Alice can convert something valuable into money (by selling it), and she can use that money to get something that she wants. Money carries value and is accepted by everyone.

ATP plays a similar role in the energy economy of cells. Cells take chemical potential energy stored in molecules (for example, in glucose or glycogen or triglycerides), and exchange it for ATP, by breaking down the energy-containing chemical (glucose, for example) and using the energy to make ATP. ATP is a carrier of energy accepted by all kinds of enzymes that need a source of energy. Those enzymes work by breaking down ATP to ADP plus P_i, and using the energy obtained to accomplish some other energy-requiring process.

✓ **Check Your Understanding**

1. Identify the three components of a nucleotide.
2. How many chromosomes does each parent contribute to its offspring?
3. What is the human genome?
4. Name the four forms of RNA.
5. What does *ATP* stand for and what is it composed of?

Figure 2.12 Breakdown and formation of ATP. ATP (top) can be broken down to yield ADP plus phosphate plus energy (bottom). *Why is ADP so important in the human body?*

Water

Another molecule of life is dihydrogen oxide, more commonly known as water. All life as we know it is water-based. Water makes up about two-thirds of the mass of the human body.

Polarity of Water

Water is a polar molecule, which means that it has a negatively charged region (the end of the oxygen atom that is situated away from the hydrogen atoms) and positively charged regions (at the far ends of the hydrogen atoms). The molecular configuration of water is shown in **Figure 2.13A**.

Hydrogen Bonding. The polarity of water molecules allows them to form *hydrogen bonds* with one another or with other charged or polar molecules. Hydrogen bonds are electrical interactions between the positive region around the hydrogen atom of a water molecule and the negatively charged region of another molecule.

Hydrogen bonds are relatively weak chemical bonds, but they are responsible for several biologically important properties of water. These properties of water include its high heat capacity, its relatively high boiling point, and its excellent solvent properties.

Water molecules also form short-lived hydrogen bonds with one another, as shown in **Figure 2.13B**. Hydrogen bonds in water quickly form, then break, and then reform as the molecules move around in a solution.

Hydrogen bonding gives water the ability to absorb or release a great deal of energy without much of a change in temperature. It is this property of water that creates the high *heat capacity* of water. Water's high heat capacity, and the fact that we are made mostly of water, means that our body temperature doesn't change much when we gain or lose heat energy.

Hydrogen bonding also makes it energetically difficult for a water molecule to leave the liquid environment because it cannot form hydrogen bonds in the gaseous state. Thus, water has a high heat of vaporization (it takes a lot of energy to boil water) and a high boiling point. This high heat of

A. Water molecules have polarity

B. Water molecule forming hydrogen bonds

Figure 2.13 A—A water molecule is polar. That is, it has one side that is positively charged and one side that is negatively charged. B—A water molecule can form hydrogen bonds with other water molecules by orienting oppositely charged regions toward each other. In this diagram the central water molecule is forming hydrogen bonds with surrounding water molecules.

vaporization means that we can rid ourselves of much heat when water evaporates from our skin, which occurs when we sweat.

Water as a Solvent. The polar nature of water makes it a good solvent for many compounds. For example, ionic compounds, such as sodium chloride, dissolve well in water. This happens because the positively charged sodium ions are attracted to the negative parts of water molecules, and the negatively charged chloride ions are attracted to the positive parts of water molecules.

Other hydrophilic but uncharged compounds, such as glucose, have positive and negative regions. This means that they can interact favorably with opposite-charged parts of water molecules.

pH

A small fraction of water molecules in solution dissociate to make hydrogen ion (H^+) plus hydroxide ion (OH^-). A substance that, when added to water, increases its hydrogen ion concentration is called an *acid*. A substance that reduces the hydrogen ion concentration of a solution and increases its alkalinity is called a *base*. In short, acids are neutralized with bases, and bases are neutralized with acids. *pH* is a measure of the acidity or alkalinity of a solution.

Carbonic acid (H_2CO_3) is an important acid in the body. It dissociates to form H^+ and bicarbonate (HCO_3^-). It is considered a weak acid because, when added to water, not all of it dissociates. You may have the sodium salt of bicarbonate ($NaHCO_3$) in your kitchen. It is the white powder in the box labeled *baking soda*.

 Check Your Understanding

1. What is a polar molecule?
2. Name three important properties of water that result from water's weak hydrogen bond.
3. Would you characterize water as a good or a poor solvent?
4. What does pH measure?

Lesson 2.1 Review and Assessment

Mini Glossary   Make sure that you know the meaning of each key term.

 Build vocabulary with e-flash cards and games

amino acids   the building blocks of proteins

ATP   adenosine triphosphate; a nucleotide composed of an adenine base, a sugar, and three phosphate groups

base pairs   pairs of complementary nucleic acid bases; that is, A and T or C and G

DNA   a polymer of nucleotides with the bases adenosine, guanine, cytosine, and thymine; deoxyribonucleic acid

enzymes   proteins that speed up specific biological reactions

fatty acid   a hydrocarbon chain with a carboxylic acid group at one end

glucose   the main form of sugar that circulates in the blood

glycogen   a polymer of glucose found in animals; stored form of glucose

human genome   the DNA sequence of a human

lipids   fatty molecules that dissolve poorly in water but dissolve well in a nonpolar solvent; fats and oils

nucleic acids   key information-carrying molecules in cells

nucleotides   subunits that make up nucleic acids

peptide bond   the chemical bond that links two amino acids by connecting the amino group of one amino acid to the acid group of another

phospholipids   a lipid-containing phosphate group

polymer   a molecule made of many similar subunits

polypeptide   a long chain of amino acids

RNA   one of two kinds of information-carrying nucleic acids found in cells; ribonucleic acid

steroids   a class of lipids with a structure that is different from other lipids; cholesterol, testosterone, and estrogen are three well-known steroids

triglycerides   compounds composed of a glycerol molecule with three fatty acids attached

Know and Understand

 Assess

1. Organic chemicals always include _____ and _____.
2. The main purpose of carbohydrates in the body is to provide a source of _____.
3. A long chain of amino acids is called a(n) _____.
4. Amino acids join together by forming a(n) _____.
5. What does an enzyme do and what happens to it in a chemical reaction?
6. Fats and oils in the body are known as _____.
7. Phospholipids are ideally suited for making _____.
8. List the three nucleotides found in both DNA and RNA. Then identify the nucleotide found only in DNA and the one found only in RNA.
9. What property of a water molecule allows it to form hydrogen bonds?
10. Describe the way ATP is used to create energy in the body.

11. What property does pH measure?

Analyze and Apply

12. Is life possible without water? Why or why not?
13. Is DNA essential for multicellular life? Explain and defend your answer.

In the Lab

14. Working with a partner, create a model of ATP. Use the information in this lesson and do any research necessary. Be sure to represent molecules of adenosine, a sugar, and three phosphates. Create the model so that the parts can be removed. Use your model to demonstrate to the class how ATP provides energy when the bond between the second-to-last and the last phosphate molecules are broken.

Lesson 2.2 Cells

Before You Read

Try to answer the following questions before you read this lesson.

How do cells control what goes in and what comes out?

How do cells move and change their shape?

How do cells obtain and use energy to accomplish tasks?

Lesson Objectives

1. Identify the major parts of a typical cell, including the plasma membrane, cytoskeleton, mitochondria, Golgi apparatus, ribosomes, endoplasmic reticulum, and nucleus.

2. Explain the functions of proteins in the cell membranes and the processes of active and passive transport.

3. Describe the importance of mitochondria.

4. Explain the relationship among DNA, RNA, and proteins.

5. Identify the phases and subphases in the life cycle of a cell.

Key Terms

E-Flash Cards

centrioles
channel proteins
cilia
codon
cytoplasm
cytoskeleton
endoplasmic reticulum
extracellular fluid
extracellular matrix
glycoproteins

Golgi apparatus
messenger RNA
microvilli
mitochondria
mitosis
nucleus
plasma membrane
ribosomes
RNA polymerase
transfer RNA

Let's take a tour of a typical cell in the human body. We will begin our tour on the outside and work inward toward the middle. We will also examine the life cycle of a cell.

Anatomy and Physiology of a Cell

The cells of the human body are surrounded by **extracellular fluid**, which is mostly water, and an **extracellular matrix**. The extracellular matrix may be solid or gel-like and differs depending on the type of tissue. The **plasma membrane** defines the outer shell of a cell. Inside the membrane is the **cytoplasm** (SIGH-toh-plazm)—which contains everything except the nucleus—and the **nucleus**. Please refer to **Figure 2.14** as we take our tour of a cell.

Plasma Membrane

The plasma membrane keeps the inside of the cell in and the outside of the cell out, and controls what passes through (**Figure 2.15**). It is a phospholipid bilayer, as shown in **Figure 2.7**. In addition to phospholipids, the membrane contains cholesterol and a variety of proteins. The proteins include structural proteins, ion and water channels, and glycoproteins.

Proteins in the Cell Membrane. Structural proteins such as cadherin, integrin, and spectrin connect the cell to neighboring cells, to the extracellular matrix, and to the cytoskeleton inside the cell. In this way these structural proteins form a link between the inside and the outside of the cell.

Channel proteins have a hollow central pore, or channel, that allows water or small, charged particles such as sodium, potassium,

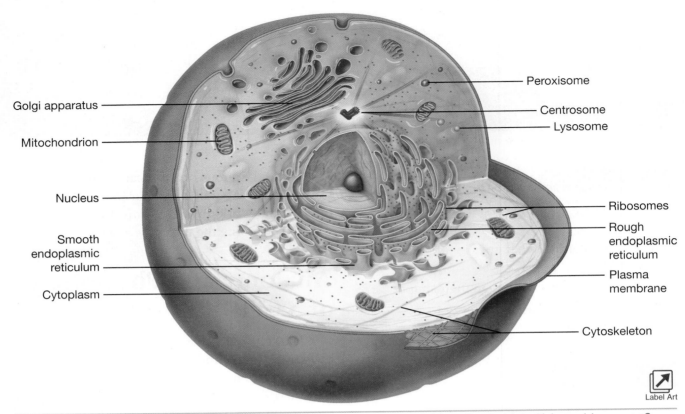

Golgi apparatus

Mitochondrion

Nucleus

Smooth
endoplasmic
reticulum

Cytoplasm

Peroxisome

Centrosome

Lysosome

Ribosomes

Rough
endoplasmic
reticulum

Plasma
membrane

Cytoskeleton

Label Art

Figure 2.14 A typical cell. *If your job were to label the area outside of this cell, what label(s) would you use?*

calcium, and chloride to pass into or out of the cell. These substances cannot enter or leave the cell without channels because their polarity, or charge, makes them unable to penetrate a lipid bilayer.

Channels are extremely selective about which substances they allow to cross the membrane, and when. For example, water channels, known as *aquaporins* (ah-kwah-POR-inz), will let H_2O cross but will not let H^+ or OH^- cross, even though these two substances are smaller. This selective property is important for helping the cell control its pH.

Other channels allow potassium ions to cross, but they do not let smaller sodium ions through. This ability of the channels to be so selective is trickier than it might seem given that potassium and sodium ions are electrically similar (both have a single positive charge), but sodium ions are smaller. It is not obvious how one would design a channel that would let a large, similarly charged ion to pass through yet prevent a smaller ion from passing through.

Glycoproteins (GLIGH-koh-PROH-teenz) are proteins with carbohydrate groups attached. These proteins are usually found in the plasma membrane, with the carbohydrate group projecting into the extracellular fluid.

The layer of carbohydrate groups surrounding a cell is called the *glycocalyx* (GLIGH-koh-KAY-liks). The glycocalyx helps cells bind to extracellular substances, which is important for cell recognition. Immune system cells of the body, for example, are always on the lookout for foreign cells and will try to destroy those cells when they are found. The glycocalyx helps to identify our own cells as friend, not foe, to the immune system.

Membrane Transport. As you have just read, living cells take in substances (such as oxygen and glucose) and move out substances (such as carbon dioxide and other metabolic wastes). *Membrane transport* is the movement of these substances across the plasma membrane. Membrane transport can occur in one of two basic ways: by passive transport or active transport.

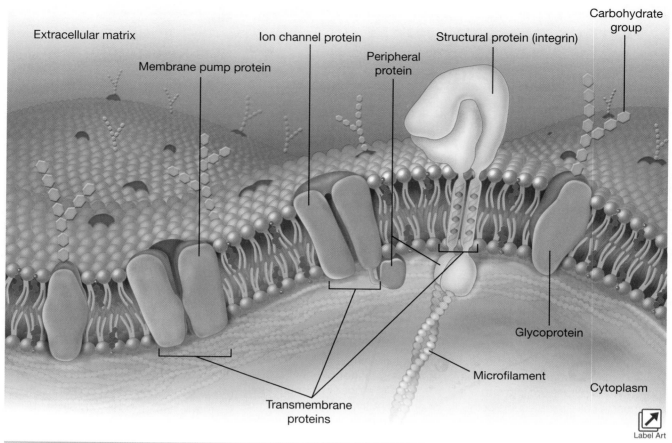

Figure 2.15 The plasma membrane. *What is the major purpose of the structural proteins?*

Passive transport does not require the expenditure of any extra energy. Passive transport usually involves *diffusion*—the movement of material from a place where it is concentrated to a place where it is less concentrated. For example, if you drop food coloring into a pot of water, the coloring is initially concentrated at the point where it hits the water. Gradually, however, the food coloring spreads and evens out—the result of diffusion.

Channel proteins provide pathways across a cell membrane that allow specific substances to diffuse into or out of the cell. Aquaporin channels, for example, allow water to enter and leave cells by passive transport. Dissolved gases such as oxygen and CO_2 also enter and leave cells by passive transport, but they do not need a channel pathway. In some cells, glucose enters by passive transport.

Active transport requires energy because it involves making a substance go where it "doesn't want to go." The most important and widespread examples of active transport are the movement of sodium *out* of a cell and potassium *into* the cell. Because a resting cell has much less sodium inside than it does outside, energy is required to move the sodium out. Similarly, a cell with more potassium inside than outside needs energy if it wants to move potassium in. For this purpose, the cell membrane has a sodium-potassium pump protein. The pump breaks down the high-energy molecule ATP, and it uses the energy from the ATP to pump sodium out of the cell and potassium into the cell.

✓ Check Your Understanding

1. Where are glycoproteins usually found?
2. How does glycocalyx help the immune system?
3. What is the difference between active and passive transport?

WHAT RESEARCH TELLS US

...*about* Integrating Physical and Chemical Processes

As you know, different processes and control systems interact with one another to maintain homeostasis—ongoing balance within the body's internal environment. This happens even when the body faces extreme challenges. Let's look at some examples.

Active and Passive Transport

Active and passive transport are inherently stable processes. "Inherently stable" means that small disturbances to the body's internal environment naturally tend to be corrected because of the way in which a process works. The movement of potassium into and out of a muscle cell illustrates this point.

Research has shown that during exercise a small amount of potassium leaves a muscle cell with each muscle twitch. During intense exercise the amount of potassium inside the cell may start to drop slightly, and the amount outside the cell may start to rise. This change in potassium balance across the cell membrane causes more potassium to enter the cell by passive transport because there is more potassium outside the cell and less inside the cell than usual. The passive transport process tends to bring the cell back to its normal, steady state.

The lower levels of potassium also cause the sodium-potassium pump, which actively transports sodium out of the cell and potassium into the cell, to run a bit faster. This active transport process, like the passive process described before, also helps to correct the potassium imbalance.

You might think that pushing the sodium out of the cell would disrupt its sodium balance. This is not the case, however, because exercise also causes excess sodium accumulation inside the cell. Thus, speeding up the pump helps to fix the sodium imbalance as well as the potassium imbalance. In short, both the active and passive transport processes, working together, naturally tend to correct temporary imbalances.

Equilibrium

A cell maintaining homeostasis is in a steady state, but it is *not* at equilibrium. The difference between a steady state and equilibrium is important. In fact, it is a matter of life and death.

Life is a nonequilibrium state of affairs. A living organism is not in equilibrium with its surroundings. However, an organism that is no longer living is, or soon will be, in a state of equilibrium.

Body temperature is a good example of this concept. Humans and other mammals are warm-blooded. The scientific term for this is *homeothermic* (from the Greek word for "same temperature"). Our nervous system and endocrine system are control systems that help us to maintain a constant internal body temperature, which is in a steady state but not at equilibrium with our surroundings. If core body temperature starts to deviate from the norm, the nervous system and the endocrine system initiate responses that bring the temperature back to normal.

pH Balance

pH is, like temperature, a closely regulated internal property of the body. For example, the pH of arterial blood is about 7.35 to 7.45. Chemicals in the blood, especially bicarbonate ions (HCO_3)

and circulating proteins, act as buffers that tend to prevent pH from changing. In addition, the respiratory system and the urinary system help to regulate blood pH via mechanisms that will be discussed in later chapters.

Biofeedback

The regulation of sodium concentration, body temperature, pH, and other physiological states occurs subconsciously, for most people, most of the time. In other words, one does not have to consciously think about the levels of these substances to control them. It is possible, however, to learn how to consciously control some of these variables. With training, some people have learned how to control their heart rate, blood pressure, and even body temperature. *Biofeedback* and *neurofeedback* both refer to the ability to control such variables. Biofeedback has been shown to be useful in treating certain medical conditions, including some types of headaches.

Taking It Further

1. In lessons 2.1 and 2.2 you have read several examples of the integration of chemical and physical processes to achieve homeostasis. Select one of these examples or choose one of your own, do further research on the integrated processes, and then prepare a detailed description for your class.

Cytoskeleton

The **cytoskeleton** is a network of proteins that defines the shape of a cell and gives it mechanical strength (**Figure 2.16**). The cytoskeleton rearranges itself when necessary to change the shape of the cell or to allow the cell to move to a new location.

The cytoskeleton contains three types of long fibers, or struts:

- *Microfilaments*, the thinnest of these fibers, are made of actin subunits. They are found

in most cells and are especially prominent in muscle cells.

- *Intermediate filaments* are made of keratin. They extend across a cell and give the cell strength to resist external pulling forces.
- *Microtubules* (MIGH-kroh-TOO-byoolz) are the largest-diameter cytoskeletal fibers. They are composed of tubulin subunits. They help to separate and organize chromosomes during cell division. Motor proteins, such as kinesin and dynein,

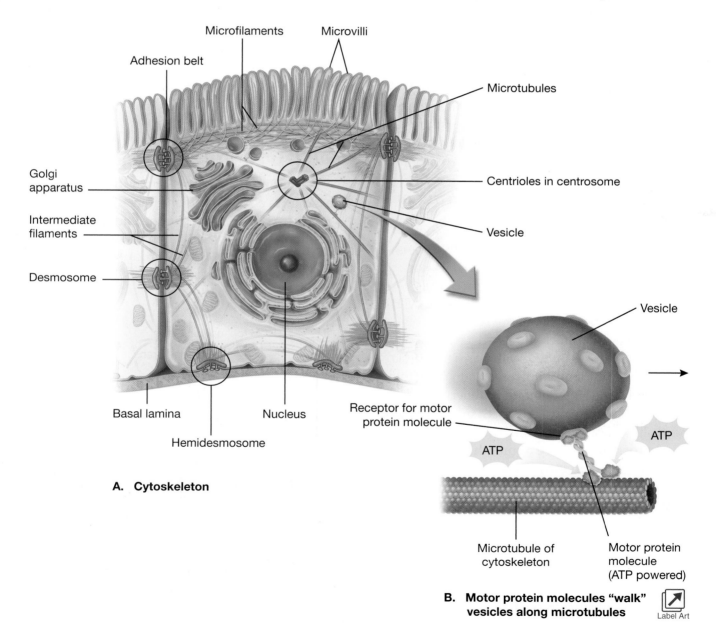

A. Cytoskeleton

B. Motor protein molecules "walk" vesicles along microtubules

Figure 2.16 The cytoskeleton and the role of microtubules in cell division. *If you were to compare motor proteins and microtubules to automobiles and highways, which structure is the automobile and which is the highway?*

move along microtubules as they transport vesicles and other structures inside the cell (**Figure 2.16B**).

Some cells have **microvilli** (MIGH-kroh-VIL-ee), finger-like extensions that increase the surface area of a cell. Microfilaments, stringy proteins inside the microvilli, provide structural support.

Other cells have hair-like projections called **cilia** (SIL-ee-a), which are longer than microvilli. Cilia actively flex back and forth to move fluid or mucus across the outside of the cell. The active beating of cilia is caused by microtubules that run inside them.

Most cells have a pair of **centrioles** (SEHN-tree-ohlz) in the *centrosome* (SEHN-troh-sohm), an area of the cell near the nucleus. Each centriole is a short cylinder made of nine triplets of parallel microtubules. The centrioles help guide the movement and separation of chromosomes during cell division.

Mitochondria and the Making of ATP

Mitochondria (MIGH-toh-KAHN-dree-a) are organelles ("little organs"), tubular-shaped structures in the cytoplasm of cells. Mitochondria are responsible for making ATP, the universal carrier of energy within cells. For this reason, mitochondria are often called the "powerhouses" of the cell. Cardiac muscle cells have abundant mitochondria to meet their large and unending demand for energy to drive muscular contraction. Cells with minimal energy needs have few mitochondria.

Mitochondria have a smooth outer membrane and an inner membrane with many cristae (folds) that increase its surface area, as shown in **Figure 2.17**. The synthesis of ATP begins with *glycolysis* (gligh-KAHL-i-sis), the breakdown of a glucose molecule into two pyruvate (PIGH-roo-vayt) molecules. Glycolysis occurs in the cytoplasm, outside the mitochondrion.

The pyruvates pass from the cytoplasm into the mitochondrial matrix, the space inside the inner membrane. Enzymes in this space catalyze

the reactions of the *citric acid cycle* (also known as the *Krebs cycle* or the *tricarboxylic acid cycle*). As a result, each pyruvate is broken down into individual carbon atoms, which combine with oxygen molecules to make CO_2.

The energy from pyruvate breakdown is used to pump hydrogen ions into the intermembrane space, which is, not surprisingly, the space between the inner and outer membrane of the mitochondrion. *ATP synthase*, an enzyme present in large numbers in the inner membrane, captures the energy from the hydrogen ions escaping from the intermembrane space. It then uses that energy to add inorganic phosphate to ADP, thus completing the synthesis of ATP (**Figure 2.12**). The newly formed ATP leaves the mitochondrion and enters the cytoplasm, where it can be used as an energy source for many different processes.

Golgi Apparatus

The **Golgi** (GOHL-jee) **apparatus**, also called the Golgi, is a set of membranous discs in the cytoplasm, usually between the endoplasmic reticulum and the plasma membrane of the cell (**Figure 2.14**). The Golgi produces small membranous spheres called *vesicles*.

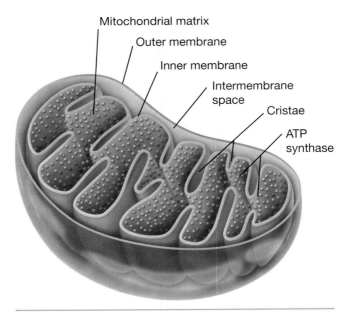

Mitochondrial matrix
Outer membrane
Inner membrane
Intermembrane space
Cristae
ATP synthase

Figure 2.17 A mitochondrion. *Why is this structure called a "powerhouse"?*

Some of the vesicles deliver new membrane, perhaps with newly embedded proteins, to the cell's plasma membrane. Some vesicles are packed with proteins or glycoproteins that are destined for secretion from the cell. Other vesicles are *lysosomes* (LIGH-soh-sohmz), compartments in which reactions involving potentially dangerous enzymes and reactants can be conducted in isolation from the rest of the cytoplasm.

All the vesicles may need proteins, which are received at the inner side of the Golgi (the forming face) as transport vesicles from the endoplasmic reticulum. The proteins may be modified or sorted in the Golgi before they are released in vesicles from the outer side of the Golgi (the maturing face).

Ribosomes and Endoplasmic Reticulum

Ribosomes (RIGH-boh-sohmz) are very large enzymes that make polypeptides. A ribosome is made up of a small and a large subunit. Each subunit includes ribosomal RNA and protein subunits. Even the small subunit is large by molecular standards, with thousands of bases of RNA and dozens of protein subunits.

The small and large subunits are assembled separately in the nucleolus (part of the nucleus). They then move out to the cytoplasm, where they join to form a functional ribosome. Some ribosomes are found free in the cytoplasm; others are attached to the rough endoplasmic reticulum.

Endoplasmic reticulum (ER), shown in **Figure 2.18**, is a network of membranes in the cytoplasm. The ER is near, and connected to, the *nuclear envelope* (the membrane that defines the boundary of the cell nucleus). Rough ER, when viewed through an electron microscope, is (as the name implies) rough looking because it has ribosomes attached to it. It often has flattened or sheet-like chambers, or *cisternae* (sis-TER-nee). Smooth ER does not have ribosomes attached to it, and it often has tubular cisternae.

The rough endoplasmic reticulum is a site for protein production and modification. Ribosomes on rough ER make polypeptides and secrete them into the cistern of the rough ER. Here the polypeptides may join with other polypeptides to form a multi-subunit protein, or they may be modified by chemical reactions

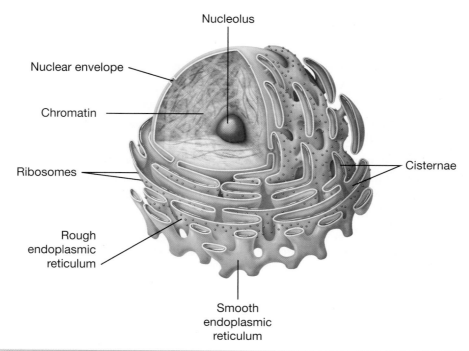

Nucleolus

Nuclear envelope

Chromatin

Ribosomes

Rough endoplasmic reticulum

Cisternae

Smooth endoplasmic reticulum

Label Art

Figure 2.18 The nucleus and associated endoplasmic reticulum. *What creates the difference in appearance between smooth and rough endoplasmic reticulum?*

that alter their size or shape. Not all proteins are made on the rough ER, however. Free ribosomes in the cytoplasm also make many proteins.

Smooth ER is a site where "replacement" membrane is made for membranous structures in the cell, including the plasma membrane, the nuclear envelope, mitochondria, ER, and Golgi. It is also a site of steroid hormone production in cells of the reproductive organs and of triglyceride formation in *adipocytes* (AD-i-poh-sights), which are fat cells, and *hepatocytes* (HEHP-a-toh-sights), which are liver cells. A *cistern* is a chamber or tank for holding water. The corresponding Latin words are *cisterna* (singular) and *cisternae* (plural). Besides referring to the interior of the endoplasmic reticulum, these words refer to the interior of the Golgi apparatus membrane compartments and to the interior of the sarcoplasmic reticulum in muscle.

Check Your Understanding

1. What are two functions that a cytoskeleton performs for a cell?
2. What is the function of the mitochondria?
3. What are lysosomes?
4. Where are ribosomes located?

The Nucleus: Home of DNA

The cell nucleus, shown in **Figure 2.14**, contains the cell's genetic information—its DNA. It also contains RNA (but not all RNA) and many proteins that are involved with the coiling, uncoiling, copying, and maintaining of DNA.

The nuclear envelope is a lipid bilayer folded over to form a double membrane. It contains protein-lined pores that allow small molecules to pass in and out of the nucleus. The nucleolus is an area in the nucleus where ribosomal RNA is made and packaged with protein subunits to make the small and large ribosomal subunits. Nucleoli are not present in all cells all the time.

All of a cell's DNA resides in the nucleus. When a cell is neither dividing nor about to divide, the DNA is spread throughout the nucleus. It wraps around small proteins called *histones* (HIS-tohns). The mixture of DNA and

associated protein is called chromatin (KROH-ma-tin).

When cell division is about to begin, the DNA becomes much more organized. It wraps into tight bundles called *chromosomes*. Each chromosome contains one DNA molecule plus the many proteins that enable it to coil.

DNA, RNA, and Proteins

Three biological polymers—DNA, RNA, and proteins—are made up of similar but not identical subunits, which must be present in a specific order to work correctly. DNA and RNA are made of nucleotides, which come in four varieties. Proteins are made of amino acids, which come in 20 varieties. The order of subunits is a form of information; the use and continuation of this information is essential for life.

Let's look at how these molecules are made—or to put it another way—how information is transferred among the molecules. The quick explanation is that DNA makes RNA, and RNA makes protein. This fundamentally important concept is regarded as the core principle of molecular biology.

Making RNA from DNA

The sequence of bases in DNA contains the information essential for making the proteins and RNA needed for life. The production of RNA from DNA is shown in **Figure 2.19**. This process is called *transcription*.

RNA polymerase (pahl-IM-er-ays) is the enzyme that makes an RNA molecule complementary to a gene on DNA. RNA polymerase binds to a region of DNA at the starting point of a gene. The DNA "unzips" in the region where the RNA polymerase binds. The RNA polymerase then starts moving along the DNA, one base at a time. As it moves, it generates an RNA strand whose nucleotides are complementary to the DNA nucleotides. RNA uses uracil (U) as the base complementary to adenine (A). In DNA, thymine (T) is the base complementary to A.

A. RNA polymerase binds to DNA

B. RNA polymerase "unzips" the DNA and begins forming mRNA

C. RNA polymerase continues to form mRNA as it moves along the DNA

Animation

Figure 2.19 Transcription, which occurs in the nucleus, is the creation of a new RNA molecule. A—The enzyme RNA polymerase binds to DNA. B—RNA polymerase partially unwinds the DNA double helix and begins to form a molecule of messenger RNA (mRNA). The arrow shows the direction of RNA polymerase movement. C—RNA polymerase continues along the DNA, adding new bases to the growing mRNA molecule.

As the RNA polymerase moves along, the DNA strands reclose behind it. When the RNA polymerase encounters the end of the gene, it detaches from the DNA and releases the RNA strand. The RNA strand is called **messenger RNA** (mRNA) because it carries a message: the base sequence information that will be used to make a protein. This mRNA leaves the nucleus through a *nuclear pore*.

Memory Tip

Transcription and translation—which comes first and what does each accomplish? It helps to remember that "DNA makes RNA makes protein" and to think of the everyday meaning of *transcribing* and *translating*.

Transcribing is copying words (or numbers) from one place to another, without changing them. Someone taking precise notes in class is transcribing the teacher's words. If you copy a line from a book into an e-mail, you are transcribing. And when a cell makes RNA from DNA, it is simply copying, or transcribing, the information from one nucleic acid molecule to another.

Translating involves converting information from one language to another. When we translate, the meaning is the same, but the words are not exactly the same. When a cell makes protein from RNA, it is converting from the language of nucleotides to the language of amino acids.

So, transcription is making RNA from DNA, and translation is making protein from RNA.

Making a Polypeptide from mRNA

The mRNA molecule made by transcription leaves the nucleus via a pore. Every three bases along the mRNA specifies, or codes for, one amino acid in the polypeptide. A **codon** (KOH-dahn) is a set of three bases in the mRNA that codes for one amino acid. It takes a 300-base (100-codon) mRNA to code for a protein 100 amino acids long. An mRNA molecule is like a blueprint for making a polypeptide.

In the cytoplasm, a small ribosomal subunit attaches to the beginning of the mRNA. A **transfer RNA** (tRNA) molecule also binds to the mRNA-ribosome complex. Each tRNA can bind to one and only one amino acid, and each tRNA has a specific *anticodon*, a set of three bases that are complementary to a three-base codon on mRNA. The tRNA that binds to the ribosome and mRNA has its specific amino acid attached.

With the help of the ribosome, the tRNA aligns its three-base anticodon with the complementary three-base codon of the mRNA. Then the large ribosomal subunit binds, and a second tRNA arrives with a codon complementary to the next codon on the mRNA. We now have a complex incorporating mRNA, tRNA, and rRNA (in the ribosome).

The ribosome now catalyzes the formation of a peptide bond between the two amino acids of the two tRNAs. It also catalyzes the breaking of the bond connecting the first amino acid to its tRNA. Then the first tRNA detaches from the mRNA-ribosome complex, and the ribosome moves over by one codon on the mRNA.

Now another tRNA, complementary to the third codon of the mRNA and loaded with its amino acid, arrives at the complex and aligns its anticodon with the third codon of the mRNA. The ribosome joins the three amino acids to the 2:1 chain, and this process continues until the ribosome reaches the end of the mRNA. Then the large and small ribosomal subunits detach from one another and from the mRNA, and the complete polypeptide is released.

The Life Cycle of a Cell

Do you have any idea how long a cell lives? You might be surprised to learn that most cells in the human body have a life span that is considerably shorter than that of humans.

For example, the cells lining your intestines have a life span of just 2 to 7 days. Your red blood cells live for about 120 days (4 months). Many of the nerve cells in your brain, on the other hand, are as old as you are.

Because most cells have shorter lives than we do, they must divide to make new cells for our bodies. This division takes place during one of the two major phases—the *interphase* or the *mitotic phase*—of a cell's life cycle. During interphase, the cell performs its usual functions and prepares for cell division. It is during the mitotic phase that the cell actually divides. The diagram in **Figure 2.20** illustrates the phases and subphases in the life cycle of a cell.

Interphase

Interphase is divided into three subphases. It includes two "gap" phases, G_1 and G_2. Between the gap phases is a synthetic (S) phase.

Of these three phases, the duration of G_1 varies the most between different cell types. G_1 is long— sometimes years long—in cells that have a long life span, and short in cells that have a brief life span. The other two phases of the cycle—G_2 and S—are usually short (just minutes or hours).

Each of the 46 chromosomes in a typical human cell is duplicated in the S phase. The *synthesis* of new DNA is what gives this phase its name. You might want to review the process of DNA replication (**Figure 2.19**).

After the S phase, the cell enters the second gap phase (G_2). During G_2 the cell completes its preparations for cell division.

Multiple "checkpoints" occur during interphase. At a checkpoint a cell verifies that it has successfully completed the appropriate steps for that phase of the cycle and is, therefore, ready to progress to the next phase. This verification process often involves checking for DNA damage and repairing any damage, if found, before clearing the checkpoint.

It should be noted that some cells will never divide. Examples include red blood cells and most nerve cells in the brain. Cells such as these are said to be in *phase G_0*.

Mitotic Phase

The mitotic phase can be divided into two types of division: mitosis and cytokinesis. **Mitosis** is the division of a cell nucleus and chromosomes into two nuclei, each with its own set of identical chromosomes. *Cytokinesis* is the division of the cytoplasm. Mitosis followed by cytokinesis results in the formation of two identical daughter cells.

Mitotic cell division is the process by which a single fertilized egg cell develops into an adult made of trillions of cells. Meiosis, a different kind of nuclear division, will be discussed in chapter 15. Here we will take a closer look at mitosis—divided into prophase, metaphase, anaphase, and telophase—and cytokinesis (**Figure 2.21**). Keep in mind that when mitosis begins, the DNA has already been duplicated.

Prophase. In *prophase*, the chromatin (DNA plus associated proteins) "condenses" to form

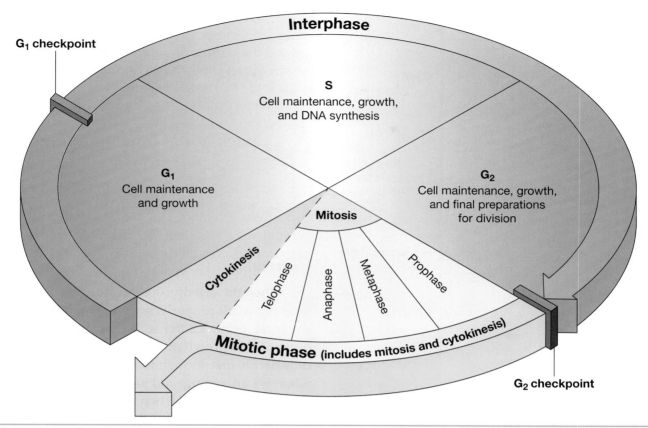

Figure 2.20 The two phases in the life cycle of a cell are interphase, when it is not dividing, and the mitotic phase, when it is dividing. Each of these phases is divided into subphases. *What is the last phase of mitosis?*

chromosomes, which are visible in the light microscope. Each chromosome is made of two identical DNA molecules, which are joined to each other at the *centromere*. As a result, each chromosome resembles a narrow X, and the centromere is the center of the X.

The two DNA molecules in a chromosome are called *sister chromatids*, and they form the two sides of each X-shaped chromosome. At the same time the chromosomes are forming, the nuclear membrane is breaking down, and the centrioles are migrating to opposite sides of the cell. Microtubules start to grow away from the centrioles, forming spindle fibers. The spindle fibers form *asters* (from the Latin for "star").

Metaphase. In *metaphase*, some spindle fibers "lock on" to the centromeres of the chromosomes. At least one spindle fiber from each of the two centrioles attaches to each centromere. Then the spindle fibers pull in a balanced way on each chromosome, causing all the chromosomes to be positioned along the midline of the cell.

Anaphase. In *anaphase*, the enzyme *separase* (sehp-a-RAYS), which functions like a molecular scissors, cuts each centromere in half. Now the sister chromatids are free to move apart. Each chromatid pulls itself along the spindle toward the centriole. As a result, 46 chromatids go to one side, and the other 46 chromatids go to the other side.

Telophase. In *telophase*, the chromosomes gather around each centriole, where they "decondense," which means that they spread out and are no longer visible in the light microscope. The spindles disappear, and a new nuclear membrane forms around the DNA. Mitosis is now complete. One nucleus has become two, and the DNA has been equally divided.

Cytokinesis. During telophase, *cytokinesis* begins. Cytokinesis is the division of the cytoplasm into two parts—the final step in cell division. A ring of actin microfilaments forms a circle around the cell. Myosin proteins pull on the actin filaments, making them shorten, much like what happens when you pull on a purse

A. Prophase

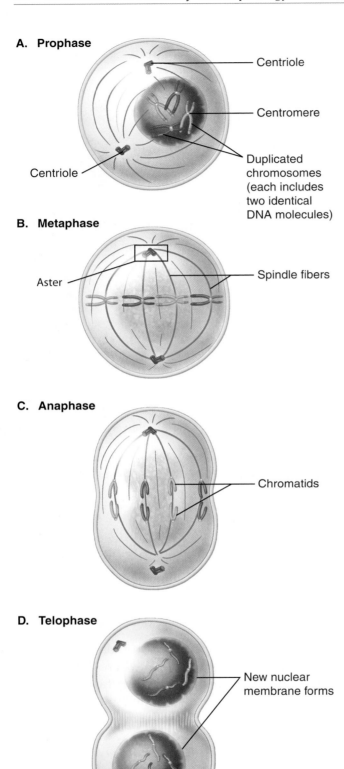

- Centriole
- Centromere
- Duplicated chromosomes (each includes two identical DNA molecules)
- Centriole

B. Metaphase

- Aster
- Spindle fibers

C. Anaphase

- Chromatids

D. Telophase

- New nuclear membrane forms

Animation

Figure 2.21 Mitosis. During telophase another process—cytokinesis—is starting. *How many chromosomes would be shown if this were a human cell?*

string. As a result of this pulling process, a *cleavage furrow*, or deepening groove, forms around the middle of the cell. The cleavage furrow gets tighter and tighter, until the cell splits into two daughter cells. Now cell division is complete.

> ✓ **Check Your Understanding**
>
> 1. Describe the transcription process.
> 2. Explain the life cycle of a cell, including all the phases and subphases.

Cancer

When the cell division process just described does not work properly, serious problems, such as cancer, occur. *Cancer* is the uncontrolled division and growth of abnormal cells. Normal cells divide just enough to allow us to grow when we are young, and just enough to replace dead or injured cells when we are mature.

Normal cells grow only where they are supposed to grow. This means that muscle cells do not grow in our brain, nor do brain cells grow in our muscles. A normal cell will notice if its DNA is damaged and will try to repair the damage. If the cell can't repair the DNA, it will, in a sense, "commit suicide," a process called *apoptosis*. In general, cancer cells grow more than they should, they grow in places where they don't belong, and they don't commit suicide when they should.

Cancer is caused by damage to a cell's DNA molecules. A mutation is damage to DNA that changes the genetic code—the pattern of As, Ts, Cs, and Gs. A mutation will not always, or even usually, cause cancer.

But certain mutations can put a cell on the pathway to cancer. Mutations to genes that govern DNA repair, cell-cycle checkpoints, and apoptosis have all been implicated in cancer. For example, if a cell's DNA repair mechanism is damaged, more and more mutations will tend to accumulate.

Cancer is caused by damage to DNA, but what causes damage to DNA? Some mutations seem to occur by random chance, or for reasons whose cause is thus far unknown. But we do know that various chemicals, cigarette smoke, alcohol, sunlight, X rays, and viruses can cause mutations. This means, of course, that we can reduce our risk of cancer by not smoking, limiting alcohol intake, wearing sunscreen, and being vaccinated for human papillomavirus, for example.

Some chemicals that disrupt the cytoskeleton are useful in cancer treatment because they interfere with mitosis. For example, paclitaxel interferes with microtubules and, therefore, prevents cells from segregating their chromosomes during mitosis. Paclitaxel is used as a chemotherapy drug for cancers of the lung, breast, and other organs.

You will learn more about various types of cancer in chapters throughout this text.

Lesson 2.2 Review and Assessment

Mini Glossary   Make sure that you know the meaning of each key term.

 Build vocabulary with e-flash cards and games

centrioles   short cylinders made of nine triplets of parallel microtubules

channel proteins   molecules with a hollow central pore that allows water or small, charged particles of certain substances to pass into or out of the cells

cilia   a hair-like projection that actively flexes back and forth to move fluid or mucus across the outside of a cell

codon   a set of three bases in DNA or RNA that codes for one amino acid

cytoplasm   the part of the cell that contains everything inside the cell membrane except the nucleus

cytoskeleton   a network of proteins that defines the shape of a cell and gives it mechanical strength

endoplasmic reticulum   a network of membranes in the cytoplasm

extracellular fluid   the liquid—consisting of mostly water—that surrounds a typical cell

extracellular matrix   the solid or gel-like substance that surrounds a typical cell

glycoproteins   proteins with carbohydrate groups attached

Golgi apparatus   a set of membranous discs in the cytoplasm

messenger RNA (mRNA)   single-strand RNA molecule whose base sequence carries the information needed by a ribosome to make a protein

microvilli   finger-like extensions that increase the surface area of a cell

mitochondria   organelles in the cytoplasm that make ATP

mitosis   the division of a cell nucleus and chromosomes into two nuclei, each with its own set of identical chromosomes

nucleus   a rounded or oval mass of protoplasm within the cytoplasm of a cell that contains the cell's DNA and is bounded by a membrane

plasma membrane   the membrane that defines the outer shell of a cell

ribosomes   very large enzymes that make polypeptides

RNA polymerase   the enzyme that makes an RNA molecule complementary to a gene on DNA

transfer RNA (tRNA)   a molecule that binds to the mRNA-ribosome complex and helps assemble amino acids into polypeptides

Know and Understand

 Assess

1. The material outside of and between cells is called _____.
2. What is the glycocalyx?
3. In what part of the cell can you find mitochondria?
4. Vesicles are produced in the _____.
5. DNA is contained in the _____ of a cell.
6. How does mRNA leave the nucleus?

Analyze and Apply

7. How might the human body be different if our cells had walls instead of membranes?
8. Explain the relationship between sodium and potassium in active transport.

In the Lab

9. Working with a partner, create a model of a typical cell. Include the following structures, making sure to place them properly if this lesson provides information about placement: *centriole, channel protein* (just one as an example), *cilia, cytoplasm, endoplasmic reticulum, Golgi apparatus, microvilli* (just a small section as an example), *mitochondria, mRNA, nucleus, DNA, plasma membrane,* and *ribosomes.* Be creative in selecting materials for the various structures. Options include Jello with toothpicks for labels of structures, a shoebox with structures attached and labeled inside the box, or an opened beach ball with structures labeled inside.

Lesson 2.3

Tissues

Before You Read

Try to answer the following questions before you read this lesson.

What are the major tissue types in the body?

What are the functions of connective tissue?

What does muscle tissue do that other tissue does not do?

Lesson Objectives

1. Identify and describe the functions of the four main types of body tissue.
2. Describe the various types and functions of epithelia.
3. Explain the properties and functions of different types of connective tissue.
4. Identify the major types of muscle tissue.
5. Describe the basic types and functions of nerve tissue.

Key Terms

E-Flash Cards

cardiac muscle
cartilage
chondroblasts
compressive strength
connective tissue
elasticity
endocrine gland
epithelial tissue
exocrine gland
glands
histology

lumen
muscle tissue
nerve tissue
neurons
osseous tissue
reticular connective
  tissue
skeletal muscle
smooth muscle
tensile strength

Tissues are concentrations of cells with a similar structure that join together to accomplish a common function. The many different tissues in the body have been classified into four main types: epithelial, connective, muscle, and nervous. Each of these has its own subtypes. The study of tissues is called **histology**.

Epithelial Tissue

Epithelial (EHP-i-THEE-lee-al) **tissue** includes epithelia and glands. *Epithelia* (singular: *epithelium*) are tissues that cover the body and line cavities within the body. Glands secrete chemicals, either to the outside world (exocrine glands) or within the body (endocrine glands). Epithelial tissues form the interface between the body and its surroundings. The design of epithelial tissues allows them to accomplish several functions. They

- protect the body from physical damage;
- control what substances enter and leave the body;
- provide sensory information; and
- secrete various substances.

Epithelia: Inside and Outside

All epithelia have an inside and an outside, usually referred to as the *apical* (think *apex*, or *top*) and *basal* surface (think *base*). The apical surface faces the outside world, or the **lumen** (hollow inside portion) of a body cavity or tube, and the basal surface faces deeper body cells.

The surface of the skin is an epithelium that faces the outside world. It obviously forms a barrier separating the inside of the body from the external environment.

But it is not obvious whether epithelial tissues inside the body separate the inside from

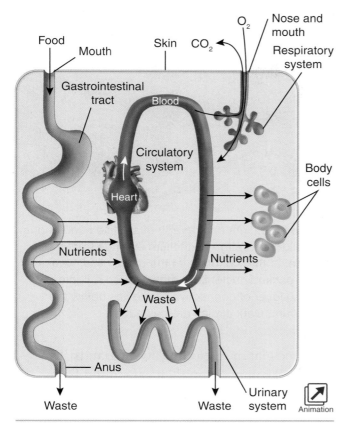

Figure 2.22 This diagram represents the human body's relationship to the outside world. *Explain how epithelial cells inside the body separate the internal environment from the external world.*

the outside. In fact, most epithelia *do* separate inside from outside, if you define "outside" as a place that is connected to the external world, without any intervening tissues.

Figure 2.22 above illustrates this concept of inside and outside. The figure shows the body as a rectangle penetrated by tubes that connect to the outside. The gastrointestinal tract (GI tract) runs through the body, from mouth to anus, so the lumen of the GI tract is all "outside." The respiratory system, the urinary system, and the reproductive system (not shown) also connect to the outside. The only epithelia that do not separate outside from inside are the linings of the cardiovascular system and endocrine glands (which are not shown in the figure).

Epithelia: Cell Layers and Shapes

Epithelia are classified according to how many cell layers they have and the shape of

those cells, as shown in **Figure 2.23**. *Simple epithelia* have a single layer of cells, and *stratified epithelia* have multiple layers of cells. The cell shapes that are observed include *squamous* (almost flat), *cuboidal* (height about equal to width), and *columnar* (tall and skinny). If an epithelium has multiple layers of cells that are not all the same shape, it is classified according to the shape of the most apical cells (that is, those on the top, facing outside).

Simple Epithelia. A ***simple squamous*** (SKWAH-mus) ***epithelium*** has a single layer of flattened cells. Examples of simple squamous epithelia in the body include

- the gas-exchanging cavities (alveoli) of the lungs;
- the lining of the abdominal cavity; and
- the endothelium, a single layer of cells that lines the blood vessels and the inside of the heart.

Simple squamous epithelia allow rapid diffusion of substances because of their thinness.

Simple cuboidal epithelia have a single layer of cuboidal cells. They surround tubules in the kidneys and are present in various secretory

	Simple	Stratified
Squamous		
Cuboidal		
Columnar		

Figure 2.23 Types of epithelia. Some intermediate types, not shown, also exist.

glands. They are typically involved with secretion or absorption.

Simple columnar epithelia have a single layer of columnar cells. They are found in the lining of some ducts in the kidneys and in the stomach and intestines, among other places. They sometimes have microvilli on their apical surfaces to increase surface area. **Figure 2.24** shows the simple columnar epithelium in the stomach. Like simple cuboidal epithelia, these epithelia have secretory and absorptive functions.

Stratified Epithelia. *Stratified squamous epithelia* are found where chemical and mechanical protection are most needed. The most familiar stratified squamous epithelium is the surface of the skin. Stratified squamous epithelia are also found in areas that are closely connected to the outside of the body, including the mouth and throat and anus and rectum.

The most apical cells in the epithelium of the skin are actually dead and dying skin cells filled with the protein keratin (which also is a key constituent of hair and fingernails). The layer of keratinized cells helps prevent loss of water through the skin and provides additional protection. **Figure 2.25** shows the stratified epithelium of the esophagus.

Stratified cuboidal and stratified columnar epithelia are relatively rare. The stratified cuboidal epithelia are found in the ducts of some

Figure 2.25 Light micrograph of stratified squamous epithelium. Here the epithelium extends from the surface, at the top, down to the basal cells, whose tightly packed nuclei form a dark layer. A lighter-staining layer of connective tissue lies below the epithelium. Dark circles are cell nuclei.

exocrine glands, including sweat glands. The stratified columnar epithelia are found lining ducts of the pancreas and salivary glands.

Other Epithelia. Some epithelia do not fit into the tidy classification scheme described so far. *Transitional epithelia*, for example, are stratified epithelia found in the lining of hollow organs that can stretch. For example, when the bladder is empty, or nearly so, it is relaxed, and the cells near the surface are rounded or cuboidal. When the bladder is full, however, the apical cells are stretched and have a more squamous appearance.

Glands

Epithelial cells that are organized to produce and secrete substances are called **glands**. A gland may have just a handful of cells, or it may be large and complex, with blood vessels and connective tissue, in which case it is considered a *glandular organ*.

An **exocrine gland** secretes its product to the outside world, as noted earlier. An **endocrine gland** secretes its product into the interstitial space. The secretion then diffuses from the interstitial space into the blood and is carried to the rest of the body. You will learn about the endocrine glands in chapter 8.

Figure 2.24 Light micrograph of a simple columnar epithelium. The purple ovals are cell nuclei.

Exocrine glands are classified by their structure. *Unicellular* (single-cell) *exocrine glands* are isolated secretory cells in an epithelium. In humans, unicellular exocrine glands are found in portions of the linings of the respiratory and digestive tracts. These cells secrete mucus, which forms a protective covering over the epithelial surface.

Multicellular exocrine glands (*multicellular* means "multiple cells") have two basic parts. One part is a secretory unit composed of cells that make and secrete a glandular product. The other basic part is a duct that connects the secretory unit to the surface of the epithelium.

An exocrine gland is *simple* if it has a single, unbranched duct and *compound* if the duct branches as it travels from the surface to the secretory units. The secretory units of a gland may be tubular (tube-shaped) or alveolar, which is a more spherical shape. Some secretory units have both shapes and are therefore called tubuloalveolar (TOO-byool-oh-al-VEE-oh-lar). **Figure 2.26** shows examples of different types of exocrine glands.

Check Your Understanding

1. Where in the body are epithelial tissues found?
2. What are the two surfaces of an epithelium?
3. What four functions do epithelial tissues perform?
4. What is the difference between an exocrine gland and an endocrine gland?

Surface of epithelium

Duct

Secretory unit

Tubular shaped

Alveolar (spherical) shaped

A. Simple duct structure. A single duct to the secretory unit.

Compound tubular

Compound alveolar

Compound tubuloalveolar (both tubular and aveolar shaped)

B. Compound duct structure. The duct branches before reaching the secretory units.

Figure 2.26 The different basic structures of multicellular exocrine glands.

Connective Tissue

Connective tissue is found throughout the body. Its functions include

- giving the body and organs the strength to resist external forces, including gravity;
- protecting internal organs;
- maintaining the proper shape of organs (to keep the trachea, or windpipe, from collapsing, for example);
- providing a rigid framework on which muscle can pull, allowing movement.

Connective tissue comprises several major classes: connective tissue proper, cartilage, bone, and blood. Blood connects distant body areas by circulating to all regions and carrying substances from place to place. You will learn about blood in more detail in chapter 10.

All forms of connective tissue include both cells and extracellular material, or extracellular matrix. The types of cells, and the nature of the extracellular matrix, differ among the major classes of connective tissue (**Figure 2.27**).

Extracellular fibers are an important part of connective tissue, helping to determine its mechanical properties (strength and elasticity, for example). Three types of fibers are found in connective tissue, although not all connective tissue has all types of fibers.

Collagen fibers are formed from tropocollagen (TROH-poh-KAHL-a-jehn) proteins that link together. Collagen fibers are strong and resistant to stretch. They give **tensile strength** to tissue.

Reticular fibers are thinner and less strong than collagen fibers. They help to provide a structural framework that keeps cells in place.

Elastic fibers can lengthen considerably when stretched, and then spring back to their original length when the stretching force is removed. Elastic fibers give springiness, or elasticity, to tissues.

Tension, Compression, and Elasticity

Before *tension* was used to describe an emotional state, it had, and still has, another meaning: a force that pulls something apart (which gives some insight into why it is now also a name for an emotional state). Tensile strength is the ability to withstand a pulling force without stretching much or breaking. The opposite of tension is *compression*: a force that pushes in. **Compressive strength** is the ability to withstand compression.

As an example of the difference between these two types of forces, consider a rope. When a rope is used in a tug-of-war, its tensile strength is evident. However, the rope does not have any significant compressive strength. If you try to compress a rope by pushing the ends together, it does not resist; it simply folds and buckles.

Elasticity is the ability to stretch when tension is applied, and then spring back to the original length when the tension is withdrawn. Elastic fibers give elasticity to skin. Unfortunately, elastic fibers in skin, like the elastic fibers in the waistband of a favorite pair of athletic shorts, tend to lose their elasticity as they get older. As a result, the skin (and the shorts) tend to get more baggy and wrinkly, and less elastic.

Connective Tissue Proper

Connective tissue proper includes loose and dense subtypes. *Loose connective tissue* has cells and an extracellular matrix with fibers running through it. Dense connective tissue has relatively few cells and an extracellular matrix composed mainly of fibers and little else.

Types of Loose Connective Tissue. Loose connective tissue includes areolar, reticular, and adipose connective tissue.

Areolar connective tissue is found throughout the body, typically as a layer beneath epithelial tissues (**Figure 2.28** on page 70). It holds water in its gel-like extracellular matrix. Areolar connective tissue provides support, strength, and elasticity to overlying epithelia, thanks to collagen, reticular, and elastic fibers. It plays a role in inflammation and immune system defenses because it contains most of the cells—mast cells, macrophages, and the occasional white blood cells (lymphocytes)—involved in the inflammation process and immune system function.

Figure 2.27 Major Classes of Connective Tissue

Class	Subclasses	Cells	Extracellular Matrix	Extracellular Fibers	General Features
Connective tissue proper	loose • areolar • reticular • adipose dense • regular • irregular • elastic	fibroblasts adipocytes mast cells macrophages lymphocytes	loose includes fibers; areolar is gel-like; adipose has very little dense is mainly fibers; little else	all three • collagen • reticular • elastic	wide variety of locations and functions; loose tissue provides support, strength, and elasticity; plays a role in immune defenses dense fibers provide tensile strength and elasticity; resist stretching
Cartilage	hyaline elastic fibrocartilage	chondroblasts chondrocytes	secreted by chondroblasts; contains proteoglycan molecules, which blend to immobilize water molecules	collagen in all; elastic in some	provides support and flexibility; minimizes friction
Bone (osseous) tissue	cortical (compact) trabecular (spongy)	osteoblasts osteocytes (see chapter 4 for more information)	secreted by osteoblasts	collagen	provides framework; protects organs; supports body
Blood	no major classes; see cell types at right and chapter 10 for more detailed information about blood	red blood cells (erythrocytes); white blood cells (leukocytes); platelets	plasma	none	provides transportation, regulation and protection; carries oxygen and nutrients to cells; carries away wastes and carbon dioxide

Reticular connective tissue, which contains reticular fibers, is found in lymph nodes, bone marrow, and the spleen. In all these locations it provides a loose framework for blood–forming cells (in bone marrow) or immune system defenses (in the spleen and lymph nodes).

Adipose tissue consists almost entirely of cells—adipocytes, or fat cells—and very little extracellular matrix (**Figure 2.29**). It provides a reservoir of metabolic fuel as well as thermal insulation and cushioning for organs.

Types of Dense Connective Tissue. As mentioned on the previous page, dense connective tissue has few cells, and its extracellular matrix is made up primarily of fibers. Dense tissue can be of three types: regular, irregular, or elastic.

Regular dense connective tissue consists of collagen fibers that are mostly parallel to one another (**Figure 2.30**). It contains occasional fibroblasts, which secrete collagen. Regular dense connective tissue is found in tendons and

Figure 2.28 Areolar connective tissue is found below the epithelium of the skin and below the epithelial tissues of the respiratory and digestive tracts. In this image cell nuclei appear as round or oval dark spots, and fibers appear as dark lines.

Figure 2.29 Light micrograph of adipose connective tissue.

Figure 2.30 Dense regular connective tissue is found in ligaments and tendons. In this light micrograph, the parallel collagen fibers in the extracellular matrix stain pink. The nuclei of spindle-shaped fibroblast cells stain dark purple. The cell bodies of the fibroblasts are not visible because they do not contain material that stands out with this stain.

ligaments. Its abundant collagen fibers give it great tensile strength, particularly when pulled parallel to the fiber direction.

Irregular dense connective tissue, like regular dense connective tissue, is composed primarily of collagen fibers. Unlike with regular dense connective tissue, the fibers are not all parallel; they run in all directions. As a result, irregular dense connective tissue is good at resisting stretching forces from a variety of directions. It is found in the dermis, in the deep layer of the skin, and in the fibrous capsule around joints, among other places.

Dense elastic connective tissue has an extracellular matrix full of elastic fibers (**Figure 2.31**). Not surprisingly, it is highly elastic. It is found in the walls of airways and large arteries.

Cartilage

Cartilage is part of the skeleton. It is found on the ends of bones and between bones. It provides support and flexibility, and it minimizes friction.

Chondroblasts (KAHN-droh-blasts) secrete the extracellular matrix of cartilage. The extracellular matrix contains collagen fibers and proteoglycan (PROH-tee-oh-GLIGH-kan) molecules (proteins with carbohydrates added), including hyaluronic acid and chondroitin (kahn-DROH-i-tin). These large molecules bind to and immobilize many water molecules. The high water content of cartilage helps to account for its high resistance to compression (given that water is incompressible) and for its low friction.

Figure 2.31 Light micrograph of dense elastic connective tissue.

Check Your Understanding

1. What four functions do connective tissues perform in the body?
2. Identify the four classes of connective tissue.
3. What is the difference between loose connective tissue and dense connective tissue?
4. What is the function of chondroblasts?

The most common form of cartilage is *hyaline* (HIGH-a-lin) *cartilage*, shown in **Figure 2.32**. The smooth, shiny substance at the end of a chicken or turkey leg bone is hyaline cartilage. Hyaline cartilage forms a smooth covering on the ends of long bones, and it forms the ends of the ribs where they connect to the sternum, or breastbone. It is also found in the nose, trachea (windpipe), and larynx (voicebox).

Elastic cartilage is similar to hyaline cartilage but contains more elastic fibers. Its elastic fibers allow it to bend and spring back into its original shape. Elastic cartilage is found in the external ear and the epiglottis, a flap of tissue in the throat that prevents food and water from entering the lungs.

Fibrocartilage (FIGH-broh-KAR-ti-lij) has more collagen fibers than hyaline or elastic cartilage. Therefore, it has more tensile strength than other types of cartilage. It is found in the discs between vertebrae and in the discs in the knee joint.

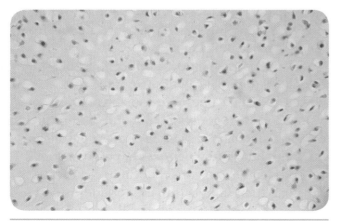

Figure 2.32 Light micrograph of hyaline cartilage.

Bone

Bone, also known as **osseous** (AHS-ee-us) **tissue**, protects organs and supports the body, providing a rigid framework on which muscles can pull (**Figure 2.33**). Osteoblasts secrete the extracellular matrix of bone. The extracellular matrix contains collagen fibers, which give bone its tensile strength, and calcium salts, which

Memory Tip

The combining forms *-blast* and *-cyte* are used in cell names. The combining form *–blast* is derived from the Greek word for "bud," and has been traditionally used to denote a *precursor* cell that can give rise to (precede) a variety of daughter cells. The words *blastula* and *blastocyst*, which refer to early stages in the development of an embryo, are based on this combining form.

Blast cells are sometimes called *stem cells*, which seems reasonable given the close relationship between buds and stems. Their descendant cells can *branch* out and develop into various subtypes of specialized mature cells.

The combining form *-blast* has also come to be used, especially with regard to connective tissues, when referring to a cell that actively secretes components of the extracellular matrix. Fibroblasts secrete collagen (which is used to make fibers—hence the combining form *fibro-*). Chondroblasts secrete proteoglycans in cartilage, and osteoblasts secrete osteoid, which hardens into bone.

The combining form *-cyte* comes from the Greek word for "container" and is used to refer to cells in general. *Cytology* is the study of cells. When compared to the traditional use of *-blast* to denote a stem cell, *-cyte* usually denotes a mature cell that, unlike a blast cell, can only produce descendants that are just like the parent, or that cannot divide at all. For example, lymphoblasts give rise to lymphocytes, and erythroblasts give rise to erythrocytes. In connective tissue, we also find *-cyte* used to denote a cell that is quiescent— that is, it does not actively secrete extracellular matrix content. Thus we have osteocytes, fibrocytes (rare), and chondrocytes.

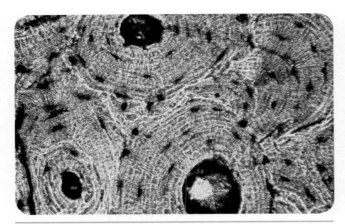

Figure 2.33 Cross section of a bone.

Figure 2.34 Skeletal muscle.

make it hard and give it compressive strength. You will learn more about the structure and function of bone in chapter 4.

Muscle Tissue

Muscle tissue allows our bodies to move. The distinguishing property of muscle is its ability to generate force on command. All muscle cells use intracellular filaments made of *actin* and *myosin* proteins to generate force, and they all require ATP as fuel for contraction.

The three kinds of muscle tissue are skeletal, cardiac, and smooth muscle. Skeletal and cardiac muscle are both called *striated muscle* because they have striations, or stripes, when viewed through a light microscope. Following is a brief introduction to the types of muscle tissue. You will learn more about these tissues in various chapters throughout this text.

Skeletal muscle is by far the most common type of muscle (**Figure 2.34**). Skeletal muscle pulls on bones to make us move. Skeletal muscle cells are long and thin. They have multiple nuclei because they are formed from the merging of multiple embryonic cells. The striations in skeletal muscle are at right angles to the long axis of the cells.

Cardiac muscle is the major tissue of the heart. It is similar to skeletal muscle, but its cells are much shorter. Because the heart never stops working, cardiac muscle must generate ATP continuously. As a result, cardiac muscle cells have many mitochondria.

Smooth muscle is found in the walls of hollow organs, including the blood vessels, airways, gastrointestinal tract, bladder, and uterus. As its name implies, the cytoplasm of smooth muscle cells appears uniform, or smooth, under the light microscope.

Nerve Tissue

Nerve tissue is a class of tissue that has the unique ability to convey information by electrical signaling. Nerve tissue is concentrated in the brain and spinal cord, which comprise the central nervous system. However, nerves extend throughout the body.

The nerves outside the central nervous system comprise the *peripheral nervous system*. The peripheral nervous system has separate nerve fibers for sending out signals (motor commands to the muscles and glands) and for receiving incoming signals (sensory signals from the eyes, ears, skin, etc.).

Nerve tissue includes supporting cells, called *glial* (GLIGH-al) *cells* (from the root word for "glue"), and **neurons**, the nervous system cells that generate, transmit, and receive electrical signals. **Figure 2.35** shows neurons in the brain. Individual neurons have a compact cell body and extensions that carry electrical signals to their targets (muscles, glands, or other neurons, for example), and receive input from other neurons.

Figure 2.35 Light micrograph of a neuron. The dark-staining soma, or cell body, has dendrites and an axon extending from it.

 Check Your Understanding

1. The distinguishing property of muscle is its ability to generate _____ on command.
2. Identify the three types of muscle tissue.
3. What kind of signals does nerve tissue use to convey information?
4. Identify the two types of nerve tissue.

Lesson 2.3 Review and Assessment

Mini Glossary   Make sure that you know the meaning of each key term.

📲 Build vocabulary with e-flash cards and games

cardiac muscle   the major tissue of the heart

cartilage   a connective tissue that provides support and flexibility to parts of the skeleton

chondroblasts   cells that secrete the extracellular matrix of cartilage

compressive strength   the ability of a material to withstand compression (inward-pressing force) without buckling

connective tissue   supporting tissue, which consists mainly of an extracellular matrix

elasticity   the ability of a material to spring back to its original shape after being stretched

endocrine gland   a gland that secretes its product into the interstitial space

epithelial tissue   a class of tissue that includes epithelia and glands

exocrine gland   a gland that secretes its product to the outside world

glands   epithelial cells that are organized to produce and secrete substances

histology   the study of tissues

lumen   the hollow inside portion of a body cavity or tube

muscle tissue   a type of tissue that generates force and allows the body to move

nerve tissue   a type of tissue that conveys information by electrical signaling

neurons   the cells that make up nerve tissue

osseous tissue   bone tissue

reticular connective tissue   a type of tissue that contains reticular fibers and is found in lymph nodes, bone marrow, and the spleen

skeletal muscle   voluntary muscle that is usually attached to bone and helps us to move

smooth muscle   involuntary muscle found in the walls of hollow organs

tensile strength   the ability to withstand tension (outward pulling force) without tearing or breaking

Know and Understand

Assess

1. What are the two types of glands and how do they differ?
2. What shape does an alveolar gland have?
3. What service do collagen fibers provide to tissues?
4. The most common type of cartilage is _____.
5. Bone is also known as _____ tissue.
6. Identify the two types of protein that make up the intracellular filaments in muscle.

Analyze and Apply

7. Compare and contrast skeletal and cardiac muscles. What do they have in common? How are they different?

8. What would be the consequences if the human body lacked internal epithelial tissues?
9. Assume that you are looking at cell cultures from the lining of the stomach, the wall of the heart, and a leg muscle, but the slides are not labeled. How can you identify each cell structure?

In the Lab

10. Do some research to learn more about the effects of the aging process on the bodily tissues. Select a type of tissue and create models to represent that tissue as it exists in a young person and a senior citizen. Explain to the class how and why you have represented the tissue in the two different ways.

Career Corner
Anatomy and Physiology at Work

A variety of career options are available to those interested in studying and working with human cells and tissues. Because modern medicine continues to develop new and improved diagnostic tests and technologies, career opportunities in this dynamic field are flourishing.

Cytotechnologist

A cytotechnologist (SIGH-toh-tehk-NAHL-oh-jist) is a laboratory specialist who studies human tissues under a microscope for signs of abnormality or disease (**Figure 2.36**). In short, a cytotechnologist is a "cell detective" who works both independently and as part of a team to identify viral and bacterial infections, cancerous growths, and precancerous changes in cells.

Perhaps you have heard of the Pap test. The field of cytotechnology is responsible for developing this test, which is used to check cervical cells for changes that potentially indicate infection, cancer, or precancerous cell growth.

A career as a cytotechnologist requires a high school diploma and completion of a four-year training program endorsed by the Commission on Accreditation of Allied Health Education Programs (CAAHEP), in conjunction with the Cytotechnology Programs Review Committee of the American Society of Cytopathology. Typically, students are admitted to a cytotechnology program in their junior or senior year of college. Although specific course requirements vary, it is recommended that students complete 20 semester hours of biological science, 8 semester hours of chemistry, and 3 semester hours of higher mathematics or statistics.

After completion of a CAAHEP-accredited program in cytotechnology, students must pass a national examination administered by the American Society for Clinical Pathology Board of Certification (ASCP BOC). With successful completion of this exam, a student has achieved entry-level proficiency and is recognized as a CT (ASCP), or certified cytotechnologist.

Cytotechnologists are typically employed in private medical laboratories, hospitals,

michaeljung/Shutterstock.com

Figure 2.36 Cytotechnologists are "cell detectives," searching for harmful bacteria and viruses.

university medical centers, government agencies, and industrial settings. Within these environments, cytotechnologists may have opportunities in education, supervision, and administration, some of which may require additional experience or education.

Pathologists' Assistant

A pathologists' assistant (PathA) is a health professional who prepares and examines human tissues under the direction and supervision of a pathologist (a medical doctor). Pathologists' assistants are responsible for tissue banking, examination of surgical pathology specimens, and assisting with complex surgeries and post-mortem examinations (**Figure 2.37**).

A career as a pathologists' assistant requires a bachelor's degree from a college or university program recognized by the National Accrediting

Agency for Clinical Laboratory Sciences (NAACLS). The educational curriculum, which is rigorous, includes coursework in clinical anatomy, systemic pathology, autopsy pathology, and neuroscience. In addition, students must complete anatomic pathology clerkships in any of a number of medical specialties, such as neurosurgery, oncology, cardiothoracic surgery, and more.

Those with a bachelor's degree in the field and three years' continuous work experience can become an Affiliate member of the American Association of Pathologists' Assistants. As an Affiliate, a pathologists' assistant is eligible to take the certification examination given by the ASCP BOC. Upon successful completion of the exam, a pathologists' assistant achieves the status of a Fellow.

Pathologists' assistants work in community, government, and university hospitals; medical laboratories; medical schools; and within the Medical Examiner (ME) system. In the United States, the ME system partners with law enforcement to investigate unusual, suspicious, violent, and sudden and unexplained deaths that may pose a threat to public health.

Pathologists' assistants are qualified to teach courses in subjects such as anatomy and physiology, histology, gross pathology, and gross dissection skills for surgical and autopsy pathology.

luchschen/Shutterstock.com

Figure 2.37 If you enjoy studying anatomy and physiology, you might want to consider a career as a pathologist's assistant.

Planning for a Health-Related Career

Do some research on the career of a cytotechnologist or pathologists' assistant. Alternatively, select a profession from the list of **Related Career Options**. Using the Internet or resources at your local library, find answers to the following questions:

1. What are the main tasks and responsibilities of the career that you have chosen to research?
2. What is the outlook for this career? Are workers in demand, or are jobs dwindling? For complete information, consult the current edition of the *Occupational Outlook Handbook*, published by the US Department of Labor. This handbook is available online or at your local library.
3. What special skills or talents are required? For example, do you need to be good at biology, chemistry, and anatomy and physiology? Do you need to thrive under the pressure of intense working conditions?
4. What personality traits do you think are needed to be successful in this job?
5. Does this career involve a great deal of routine, or are the day-to-day responsibilities varied?
6. Does the work require long hours, or is it a standard, "9-to-5" job?
7. What is the salary range for this job?
8. What do you think you would like about this career? Is there anything about it that you might dislike?

Related Career Options

- Clinical Lab Technologist
- Histotechnician
- Histotechnologist
- Medical Laboratory Technician
- Phlebotomy Technician
- Specialist in Cytotechnology
- Technologist in Molecular Biology

Chapter Summaries

Lesson 2.1 Molecules of Life

⬈ Build vocabulary with e-flash cards and games

Key Points

- Carbohydrates, which always contain carbon and hydrogen, are the sugar and starch molecules that provide fuel for the body's work.
- Proteins, which help form the structure of cells or speed up biological processes, are made up of long chains of amino acids.
- Lipids are fats and oils in the body; they store energy or regulate the reproductive system.
- DNA and RNA are nucleic acids that contain the body's genetic information or carry it from cell to cell.
- Water is essential to life, comprising about two-thirds of body mass.

Key Terms

amino acids	nucleic acids
ATP	nucleotides
base pairs	peptide bond
DNA	phospholipids
enzymes	polymer
fatty acid	polypeptide
glucose	RNA
glycogen	steroids
human genome	triglycerides
lipids	

Lesson 2.2 Cells

Key Points

- The plasma membrane controls what is contained inside a cell and what moves in and out of the cell.
- Active and passive transport are different methods for moving substances inside and outside of a cell.
- The cytoskeleton is a network of proteins that defines the shape of a cell, gives it strength, and helps it to move to a new location.
- The life cycle of a cell consists of two major phases—interphase and the mitotic phase—both of which are divided into several subphases. Cell division occurs in the mitotic phase.
- The nucleus of a cell contains the DNA that makes it possible for the cell to transmit information to new cells.
- Mitochondria are small structures (organelles) within a cell that produce ATP, the source of the cell's energy.

Key Terms

centrioles	Golgi apparatus
channel proteins	messenger RNA
cilia	microvilli
codon	mitochondria
cytoplasm	mitosis
cytoskeleton	nucleus
endoplasmic reticulum	plasma membrane
extracellular fluid	ribosomes
extracellular matrix	RNA polymerase
glycoproteins	transfer RNA

Lesson 2.3 Tissues

Key Points

- Epithelial tissues include epithelia, the skin and linings of internal body cavities, and glands, which secrete chemicals.
- Connective tissues protect the body and give it strength, help the body maintain its shape, and provide the structure against which muscles pull.
- Muscle tissues generate force to move the body.
- Nerve tissue conveys information through the body via electrical signals.

Key Terms

cardiac muscle
cartilage
chondroblasts
compressive strength
connective tissue
elasticity
endocrine gland
epithelial tissue
exocrine gland
glands

histology
lumen
muscle tissue
nerve tissue
neurons
osseous tissue
reticular connective tissue
skeletal muscle
smooth muscle
tensile strength

Chapter Assessments

Assess

Lesson 2.1

Molecules of Life

Learning Key Terms and Concepts

1. Glucose is the main form of _____ that circulates in the blood.

2. As the word carbohydrate indicates, the elements that make up these molecules include _____ and _____.

3. A molecule made up of many similar subunits is called a(n) _____.

4. Adenosine triphosphate (ATP) provides _____ for many cellular processes.

5. Fatty acids are key building blocks for other lipids, especially _____ and _____.

6. The bond that links the amino group of one amino acid to the acid group of another is called _____.
   - A. an acid bond.
   - B. an amino bond.
   - C. a peptide bond.
   - D. a residual bond.

7. Identify the three types of glycerides. Explain the relationship between fatty acids and the different types of glycerides.

8. DNA is formed in the shape of a(n) _____.
   - A. double pleat
   - B. double helix
   - C. triple helix
   - D. pleated helix

9. Glycine and tryptophan are both amino acids. Based on your reading of the lesson, name characteristics that they have in common and a key difference between them.

10. Identify and describe the four levels of protein structure.

Thinking Critically

11. Consider the enzymes discussed in this lesson. Which bodily functions might *not* be possible in their absence?

12. Using the information and figures in this lesson, analyze at least two different types of chemical reactions that provide the body with energy.

13. What might be the consequences of DNA damage in a person's cells?

Lesson 2.2

Cells

Learning Key Terms and Concepts

14. Charged particles can only enter or leave a cell via _____.

15. Glycoproteins are proteins with _____ groups attached.

16. Located near the nucleus, the _____ help to guide the movement and separation of chromosomes during cell division.

17. Because of their great need for energy to power muscle contractions, cardiac muscle cells have a high number of _____.

18. The breakdown of a glucose molecule into two pyruvate molecules is called _____.

19. Because it carries the basic information that will be used to make a protein, an RNA strand is often called _____.
   - A. +RNA
   - B. rRNA
   - C. mRNA
   - D. none of the above

20. The cytoskeleton does *not* include _____.
    A. cytofilaments
    B. intermediate filaments
    C. microfilaments
    D. microtubules

21. Which of the following is a set of membranous discs in the cytoplasm?
    A. ATP
    B. endoplasmic reticulum
    C. Golgi apparatus
    D. vesicles

22. Which of the following does *not* describe a ribosome?
    A. It is a very large enzyme.
    B. It is found in the nucleus.
    C. It makes polypeptides.
    D. It includes a large and a small subunit.

23. The enzyme that unzips DNA to produce an RNA molecule is called _____.
    A. adenine
    B. transfer RNA
    C. adipocyte
    D. RNA polymerase

24. Describe the differing functions of the rough and smooth endoplasmic reticulum.

Instructions: Write the **letter** of the name of the cell structure on your answer sheet next to the corresponding number.

_____ 25. Mitochondrion
_____ 26. Ribosomes
_____ 27. Golgi apparatus
_____ 28. Cytoskeleton
_____ 29. Centrosome
_____ 30. Nucleus
_____ 31. Plasma membrane
_____ 32. Cytoplasm

Thinking Critically

33. Compare and contrast microvilli and cilia.

34. Investigate the physical and chemical processes that contribute to homeostasis, including equilibrium, temperature, pH balance, chemical reactions, active and passive transport, and biofeedback. In an oral presentation, describe how these processes are integrated.

Lesson 2.3

Tissues

Learning Key Terms and Concepts

35. The study of tissues is called _____.

36. Epithelial tissues accomplish which of the following functions?
    A. protect the body from physical damage
    B. provide sensory information
    C. determine which substances enter and leave the body
    D. all of the above

37. The apical and basal surfaces are the two sides of all _____.

38. The hollow inside portion of a body cavity or tube is called the _____.

39. Which of the following is a *true* statement?
    A. All epithelia separate inside from the outside.
    B. The linings of the cardiovascular system separate inside from outside.
    C. Most epithelia separate inside from outside.
    D. none of the above

40. An exocrine gland is called _____ if its duct branches out as it travels from the surface to the secretory units.

41. *True or False?* Blood is a type of connective tissue.

42. The fibers that help to keep cells in place are called _____.

43. *True of False?* Collagen fibers are very elastic.

44. Which of the following is *not* a connective tissue?
    A. cartilage
    B. epithelia
    C. blood
    D. bone

45. What kind of epithelia make up alveoli?

46. Which of the following is *not* a form of loose connective tissue?
    A. adipose
    B. areolar
    C. columnar
    D. reticular

47. Identify three types of cartilage.

48. The target of a neuron's electrical signals can be _____.
    A. muscles
    B. glands
    C. other neurons
    D. all of the above

49. What is the difference between simple and stratified epithelia?

Thinking Critically

50. Review the general properties of epithelial tissue and connective tissue. Then explain why connective tissue is better suited than epithelial tissue for constructing cartilage.

51. Evaluate the cause and effect of cancer on the structure and function of cells, tissues, organs, and systems.

Building Skills and Connecting Concepts

Analyzing and Evaluating Data

The chart at the right lists 12 elements in order of their percentage of total body weight. Use the chart to answer the following questions.

52. Elements not shown in this chart that play a role in human physiology and contribute to total body weight are called *trace elements*. What percentage of body weight is made up of these trace elements? Round your answer to the nearest hundredth of a percent.

53. What percentage of your body weight is made up of the two elements contained in every organic molecule?

54. How much more nitrogen than potassium does your body contain?

Element	Percentage of total body weight
Oxygen	65%
Carbon	18%
Hydrogen	10%
Nitrogen	3%
Calcium	1.5%
Phosphorous	1%
Sulfur	0.25%
Potassium	0.20%
Sodium	0.15%
Chlorine	0.15%
Magnesium	0.05%
Iron	0.006%

Communicating about Anatomy and Physiology

55. **Speaking and Reading** In lesson 2.1, you learned that molecules, or parts of molecules, differ in how well they bond with water. Molecules that bond easily with water are called *hydrophilic*, from the combining forms *hydr-* ("water") and *phil-* ("loving"). By contrast, molecules that do not bond well with water are called *hydrophobic* (the combining form *-phobia* means "fearing").

With a group of classmates, make a list of other words you know that contain the combining forms *hydr-*, *phil-*. and *phob-*. The words may be used in everyday language or in the fields of science or medicine. You may use a dictionary or online etymology resource to locate words that contain these combining forms.

Here are some examples to help you get started: *dehydration* (loss of bodily fluids); *hydrogen* (one of the elements; a colorless, odorless gas); *philosophy* (love of wisdom); *arachnophobia* (fear of spiders); *claustrophobia* (fear of closed or narrow spaces).

With your group, review the list for words that can be used in the subject area of anatomy and physiology. Break each word into its combining form, practice pronouncing the word, and discuss its meaning. As a fun challenge, work together to compose a creative narrative using as many words as you can from your new list.

Lab Investigations

56. Working in groups of three or four students, build a clay model of one of the different types of epithelial tissue listed below. Use modeling clay of various colors, index cards or paper and scissors, and transparent adhesive tape. Use the appropriate illustration(s) in this chapter as a guide while preparing your model.

- Simple squamous
- Simple cuboidal
- Simple columnar
- Stratified squamous
- Stratified cuboidal
- Stratified columnar

When you have finished your model, create a label for the type of epithelial tissue that

the model represents, and specify where the epithelial tissue is located in the body. Display your model in the classroom as a reference for discussion and study.

Expand your learning with additional online resources
- Supplemental Lab Activities
- Interactive Exercises
- Animations

 Companion Website

 Expand

www.g-wlearning.com/healthsciences

What determines whether we have straight, wavy, or curly hair?

Membranes and the Integumentary System

We tend to think about our skin mainly when we are interested in getting a tan or avoiding sunburn. Consider, however, that the skin is actually a body organ like the heart or lungs. In fact, this organ called *skin* makes up approximately 15 percent of your total body weight!

The skin is quite a remarkable organ. It is far more than just an outer layer of covering. The skin contains glands and sensory receptors that perform specialized functions; it also grows hair and nails. For these reasons, we refer to the skin and its contents as a body system—the *integumentary system*.

In this chapter we will examine the anatomy and functions of the integumentary system, including associated structures and membranes. We will also discuss some of the common injuries and disorders of the skin and membranes, along with their symptoms and current treatments.

Chapter 3 Lessons

Lesson 3.1
Body Membranes

Lesson 3.2
The Integumentary System

Lesson 3.3
Injuries and Disorders of the Skin

While studying, look for the online icon **to:**

- **Practice** with e-flash cards and vocabulary games
- **Review** with interactive art labeling
- **Assess** with online exercises
- **Expand** with interactive activities and animated videos
- **Listen** to pronunciations of key terms in the audio glossary

www.g-wlearning.com/healthsciences

Companion Website

Study on the Go

Use a mobile device to practice vocabulary terms, listen to pronunciations, and review with self-assessment quizzes.

www.m.g-wlearning.com

G-W Mobile

Lesson 3.1

Body Membranes

Before You Read

Try to answer the following questions before you read this lesson.

Do all membranes secrete some type of fluid?

What is the common name for the integumentary system?

Lesson Objectives

1. Identify the different types of body membranes and explain their functions.

2. Explain the purposes of serous fluid and synovial fluid.

Key Terms

E-Flash Cards

cutaneous membrane
epithelial membranes
membranes
mucous membranes
pericardium
peritoneum

pleura
serous fluid
serous membranes
synovial fluid
synovial membrane

The body **membranes** surround and help protect the body's surfaces. These surfaces include cavities that open to the outside world, internal cavities that house body organs, capsules that surround ball-and-socket synovial joints, and the skin. This lesson explores the similarities and differences among the membranes that cover these different body surfaces.

Epithelial Membranes

The **epithelial** (EHP-i-THEE-lee-al) **membranes** provide a lining, or covering, for the internal and external surfaces of the body. These membranes include both a sheet of epithelial cells and an underlying layer of connective tissue. There are several categories of epithelial membranes.

Mucous Membranes

The **mucous membranes** line the body cavities that open to the outside world (**Figure 3.1**). These cavities include all the hollow organs of the respiratory, digestive, urinary, and reproductive tracts. The mouth, nose, lungs, digestive tract, and bladder are examples of hollow organs lined with mucous membranes.

The structure of the mucous membranes comprises a layer of epithelium on top of loose connective tissue called *lamina propria*. The mucous membranes are all moist: the membranes of the digestive and respiratory tracts secrete mucus, and glands in the urinary tract add mucus there. Mucus is a slippery solution that protects the mucous membranes and aids in transporting substances.

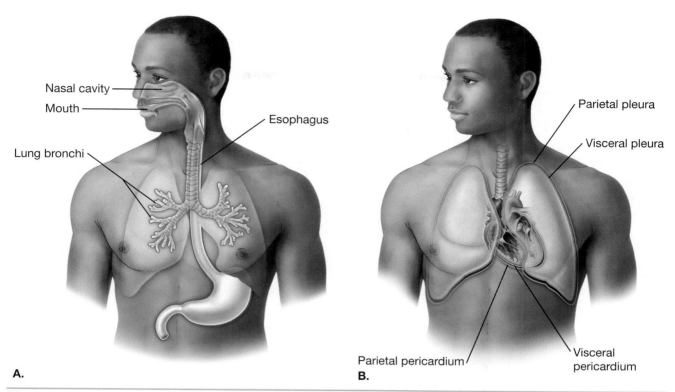

Figure 3.1 Two classes of epithelial membranes. A—Mucous membranes line body cavities that open to the outside world. B—Serous membranes line body cavities that are closed to the outside world.

Serous Membranes

Serous (ser-us) **membranes** line body cavities that are closed to the outside world (**Figure 3.1**). Examples are the **pleura** (PLOO-ra), which encloses the lungs; the **pericardium** (PER-i-KAR-dee-um), which surrounds the heart; and the **peritoneum** (PER-i-toh-NEE-um), which lines the abdominal cavity (see **Figure 13.10** on page 463).

The structure of serous membranes is an outer layer of simple squamous (flattened) epithelium on a thin layer of loose connective tissue. Each serous membrane forms a double lining with an outer lining and an inner lining. The outer lining of each body cavity is called the *parietal layer*. The inner lining that covers each organ within a body cavity is called the *visceral layer*.

Serous membranes secrete a thin, clear fluid called **serous fluid**. This fluid serves as a lubricant between the parietal and visceral membranes to minimize friction and "wear and tear" on organs that move within the linings, such as the beating heart.

Cutaneous Membrane

The **cutaneous** (kyoo-TAY-nee-us) **membrane** is the name for what we know as skin. The basic structure of skin is a keratinizing, stratified (layered) squamous epithelium over dense, fibrous connective tissue. Although the skin contains sweat glands, it is a dry membrane when sweat is not present. The integumentary system, which encompasses the skin and its related structures, is discussed in detail in the next lesson.

Connective Tissue Membranes

Only one type of membrane in the body is composed solely of connective tissue and includes no epithelial cells: **synovial** (si-NOH-vee-al) **membrane**. Synovial membranes line the capsules that surround synovial joints, such as the shoulder and knee (**Figure 3.2**). They also line tendon sheaths (the connective tissue that

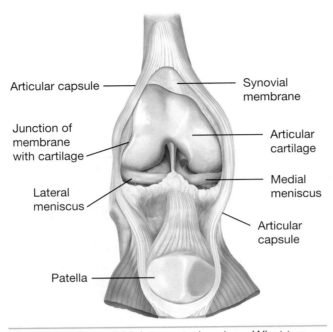

Articular capsule

Junction of membrane with cartilage

Lateral meniscus

Patella

Synovial membrane

Articular cartilage

Medial meniscus

Articular capsule

Figure 3.2 Synovial joint—anterior view. *What two important purposes does synovial fluid serve?*

surrounds tendons) as well as *bursae*, the small, connective tissue sacs that serve as cushions for tendons and ligaments surrounding the joints. Synovial membranes in all these locations secrete a clear **synovial fluid**, which provides cushioning and reduces friction and wear on moving structures.

✓ Check Your Understanding

1. Where are epithelial membranes located? Name at least three locations for mucous membranes and three for serous.
2. What percentage of your body weight is made up of the skin?
3. What is the difference between mucous membranes and serous membranes?
4. Which two components make up epithelial membranes?

Lesson 3.1 Review and Assessment

Mini Glossary   Make sure that you know the meaning of each key term.

 Build vocabulary with e-flash cards and games

cutaneous membrane   another name for skin

epithelial membranes   thin sheets of tissue lining the internal and external surfaces of the body

membranes   thin sheets or layers of pliable tissue

mucous membranes   thin sheets of tissue lining the body cavities that open to the outside world

pericardium   the membrane that surrounds the heart

peritoneum   the membrane that lines the abdominal cavity

pleura   the membrane that encases the lungs

serous fluid   a thin, clear liquid that serves as a lubricant between parietal and visceral membranes

serous membranes   thin sheets of tissues that line body cavities closed to the outside world

synovial fluid   a clear liquid secreted by synovial membranes that provides cushioning for and reduces friction in synovial joints

synovial membrane   the lining of the synovial joint cavity that produces synovial fluid

Know and Understand

 Assess

1. List the two main categories of body membranes.
2. List the subcategories of the epithelial membranes.
3. Describe the basic structure of skin.
4. Are synovial membranes composed of epithelial tissue or connective tissue?
5. Name three examples of serous membranes.
6. List the areas of the body in which mucous membranes are found.

Analyze and Apply

7. What is the primary purpose of fluid that is produced by serous membranes?

8. If synovial fluid were not present, what would happen to the joints in the body?

In the Lab

9. Using the information that you have learned about membranes, examine your mouth and nose. What do you see? Is the skin that lines your mouth pink or red? moist or dry? How would you describe the skin around your nose? Be as detailed as possible in your description. Do the characteristics that you noted match the information presented in this lesson?

Lesson Objectives

1. Explain how the skin continually regenerates.
2. Describe the processes by which the skin helps to regulate body temperature.
3. Explain the different protective functions of the skin.
4. Identify the different glands and sensory receptors present in skin and describe their functions.

Key Terms

E-Flash Cards

dermis
epidermal dendritic cells
epidermis
hypodermis
integumentary system
keratin
keratinocytes
melanin
melanocytes
Merkel cells

papillary layer
reticular layer
sebaceous glands
sebum
stratum basale
stratum corneum
stratum granulosum
stratum lucidum
stratum spinosum
sudoriferous glands

Why do we refer to the skin as the **integumentary** (in-TEHG-yoo-MEHN-ta-ree) **system**? The term *integumentary* comes from the Latin word *integumentum*, which means "covering." However, the skin is not simply a membranous covering like those discussed in the previous lesson. It is an entire system that includes a cutaneous membrane, sweat and oil glands, and nails and hair. Working together, these structures perform critically important functions that are not only convenient but also essential for life.

Functions of the Integumentary System

The skin forms a protective cover that serves a variety of purposes. When you sustain a cut or an abrasion, your skin acts as the first line of defense in protecting the underlying tissues. The skin's outermost layer contains **keratin** (KER-a-tin), a tough protein also found in hair and nails that adds structural strength. In addition, keratin helps to protect the skin against damage from harmful chemicals.

Keratin and naturally occurring oils in the skin assist in serving as a water barrier. The skin substantially lessens the evaporation of water and essential molecules that the water carries from inside the body. Furthermore, keratin prevents water from entering the body during bathing or swimming.

The skin is also critically important in regulating body temperature, due to the extensive array of tiny capillaries and sweat glands that lie near the surface of the skin. When the body is overheated, the capillaries dilate (expand), enabling body heat to dissipate. Likewise, during heat conditions, the sweat glands become active, producing sweat that evaporates and has a cooling effect on the skin. When the environment is cold, the capillaries constrict (tighten), and blood flow moves to deeper vessels away from the skin to minimize heat loss.

Skin is also involved in certain chemical processes in the body. Specialized cells in the skin called **melanocytes** (MEHL-a-noh-sights) produce **melanin**, a pigment that protects the body against the harmful effects of ultraviolet ray damage from sunlight. Exposure to the ultraviolet-B (or UVB) rays from sunlight causes the conversion of modified cholesterol molecules called *provitamin D3* in the skin to vitamin D. Vitamin D is essential for bone health. In addition, during the process of sweating the body eliminates chemical waste products, including urea, uric acid, and salts. And, because the fluid secreted by the sweat glands is acidic, it helps to protect the body against bacterial infections.

Finally, the skin contains specialized *cutaneous sensory receptors* that are part of the nervous system. These receptors transmit nerve signals that contain information about the environment, including touch, pressure, vibration, pain, and temperature.

The table in **Figure 3.3** summarizes the functions of the integumentary system.

✓ Check Your Understanding

1. Why is the skin called the *integumentary system*?
2. How do sweat glands protect against bacterial infections?

Anatomy of the Skin

The skin has two layers—an outer **epidermis** (EHP-i-DERM-is) and an underlying **dermis** (**Figure 3.4**). A blister is produced when a burn or friction causes these two layers to separate, forming a fluid-filled pocket. The epidermis and dermis are thick over areas such as the soles of the feet and thin in delicate areas such as the eyelids.

Memory Tip

The word dermis means "true skin." The prefix epi- means "upon" or "over." The prefix hypo- means "below," or "under." Thus, the epidermis lies above the dermis, and the hypodermis lies below the dermis.

Beneath the dermis is the **hypodermis**, or *subcutaneous fascia*, which serves as a storage

Figure 3.3 Functions of the Integumentary System

Function	Mechanisms
Protection	Tough keratin protects against mechanical injury and chemical damage. Melanocytes produce melanin to protect against UV ray damage. Acidic sweat protects against bacterial infections.
Water barrier	Keratin and oils in the skin reduce water loss through evaporation and form a barrier against water infusion.
Temperature regulation	Capillaries dilate to dissipate heat and constrict to conserve heat. Sweat evaporation provides a cooling effect.
Vitamin D production	Sunlight converts modified cholesterol molecules to vitamin D, which is essential for bone health.
Waste elimination	Urea and uric acid are eliminated in sweat.
Sensory perception	Receptor cells transmit information about touch, pressure, vibration, pain, and temperature to the central nervous system.

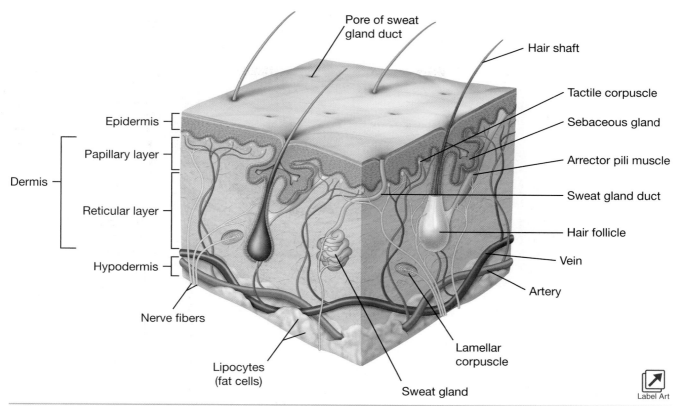

Figure 3.4 The integumentary system, as represented by a section of skin.

repository for fat. The hypodermis is not part of the skin, but it connects the skin to the underlying tissues. It also provides cushioning and insulation against extreme external temperatures.

Epidermis

The outer layer of skin, the epidermis, is the skin that we see. The epidermis contains five layers of tissue (**Figure 3.5** on the next page). From superficial to deep (the outside going in), these are named the **stratum corneum**, **stratum lucidum**, **stratum granulosum**, **stratum spinosum**, and **stratum basale**.

All epidermal layers consist of cells, but they do not include a blood supply that provides nutrients to the skin. The innermost layer, the stratum basale, absorbs nutrients from the adjacent, underlying dermis. The cells in the stratum basale are constantly producing new skin cells. As new cells germinate, they are pushed toward the surface and away from nutrients. Eventually, they die.

Most of the cells within the epidermis are **keratinocytes** (keh-RAT-i-noh-sights), which produce keratin. Moving up through the stratum spinosum and stratum granulosum, cells become progressively flatter and more filled with keratin, which makes them tough and water resistant. The stratum lucidum is a clear layer of thick skin found only on the palms of the hands, fingers, soles of the feet, and toes.

The outer layer of the epidermis, the stratum corneum, consists of dead cells that are completely filled with keratin and are continually shedding. You might be surprised to learn that the epidermis completely replaces itself every 25 to 45 days.

The stratum basale contains melanocytes. As you learned in the section entitled "Functions of the Integumentary System," these specialized cells produce the pigment melanin. Melanin, which ranges in color from reddish yellow to brown and black, is primarily responsible for human skin color. Exposure to sunlight causes melanocytes to produce more melanin. As *melanin granules* are pushed out into the neighboring skin cells, the result is *tanning*.

Figure 3.5 The layers of the epidermis. *Which layer continually replaces itself?*

Labels on the figure:
Stratum corneum
Stratum lucidum
Stratum granulosum
Stratum spinosum
Stratum basale
Dermis
Dermal blood vessels
Sweat pore
Shedding keratinocytes
Dead keratinocytes
Living keratinocytes
Dendritic cell
Stem cell
Merkel cell
Sweat duct
Melanocyte
Dermal papilla
Tactile nerve fiber
Label Art

The presence of extra melanin in the skin functions as a sunscreen, which is why sunburn is more likely to affect individuals with light skin. Sunburn is also less likely once a light-skinned person has a tan.

An inherited condition called *albinism* (AL-bi-nizm) prevents the normal production of melanin. Albinism produces very little pigment in the skin, hair, and eyes. Individuals with albinism have extremely pale skin and white hair.

The epidermis contains specialized cells associated with the immune and nervous systems. **Epidermal dendritic cells** respond to the presence of foreign bacteria or viruses by initiating an immune system response, which brings in other specialized cells to attack the foreign invaders. There are as many as 800 dendritic cells per square millimeter of skin to help ward off infections.

Merkel cells (also called *Merkel-Ranvier cells*), located in the stratum basale, function as touch receptors. These cells form junctions with sensory nerve endings that relay information about touch to the brain.

Dermis

The dermis, or "true skin," is a dense, fibrous connective tissue composed of *collagen* and elastic fibers. The collagen fibers provide toughness and also bind with water molecules to help keep the inner skin moist. The elastic fibers are what keep the skin looking young, without wrinkles or sagging.

During the normal course of aging, the numbers of collagen and elastic fibers decrease. The dermis has a rich supply of blood vessels, which, as previously discussed, dilate or constrict to help dissipate or retain body heat, respectively. Also present throughout the dermis is a variety of specialized sensory receptors for touch, vibration, pain, and temperature. These receptors communicate with nerve endings to transmit information to the brain about what the body is sensing. Specialized white blood cells called *phagocytes* (FAG-oh-sights), which are distributed throughout the dermis, are responsible for ingesting foreign material, including bacteria as well as dead cells.

The outer layer of the dermis is the **papillary** (PAP-i-LAR-ee) **layer**, after the *dermal papillae* (pa-PIL-ee) that protrude from its surface up into the epidermis (**Figure 3.6**). Some of the dermal papillae contain capillaries that supply nutrients to the epidermis. Other dermal papillae contain nerve endings involved in sensing touch and pain. These papillae form genetically determined, ridged patterns on the palms of the hands, fingers, toes, and soles of the feet. It is from the papillae patterns on the fingers that each person's unique fingerprints are derived.

Underneath the papillary layer lies the **reticular layer** of the dermis. As **Figure 3.6** shows, the collagen and elastic fibers in this region have an irregular arrangement. The reticular layer includes blood and lymphatic vessels, sweat and oil glands, involuntary muscles, hair follicles, and nerve endings.

Hypodermis

The hypodermis, or subcutaneous fascia, includes fibrous connective tissue and adipose (fatty) tissue. It is within the hypodermis that *lipocytes* (LIP-oh-sights), or fat cells, reside. Some amount of body fat is important for padding and insulating the interior of the body. Fat also serves as a source of energy.

Jubal Harshaw/Shutterstock.com

Figure 3.6 Light micrograph showing the two regions of the dermis below the epidermis. *Why do you think the dermis is called the "true skin"?*

 Check Your Understanding

1. What are the two layers of skin?
2. Where does the body store fat?
3. How does the epidermis receive nutrients?
4. What specialized cells are responsible for human skin color?

Appendages of the Skin

Structures considered to be appendages of the skin include the sudoriferous (sweat) glands, sebaceous (oil) glands, hair, and nails.

Sudoriferous (Sweat) Glands

Sweat glands, or **sudoriferous** (SOO-doh-RIF-er-us) **glands**, are distributed in the dermis over the entire body, with larger concentrations in the axilla (under the arms), on the palms of the hands and soles of the feet, and on the forehead. Each person has approximately 2 to 3 million sweat glands. There are two types of sweat glands: eccrine glands and apocrine glands (**Figure 3.7** on the next page).

The *eccrine* (EK-rin) *glands* are the major sweat glands of the body. They cover most of the body and open directly onto the skin. The sweat secreted by eccrine glands is a clear, acidic fluid that consists of approximately 99% water, but it also contains waste products such as urea, uric acid, salts, and vitamin C.

Sweat is odorless, but if it is left on the skin, bacteria can chemically change it to produce an unpleasant odor. Sweat glands contain nerve endings that cause sweat to form when body temperature or external temperature is elevated. Evaporation of sweat from the skin's surface is very effective in dissipating body heat. However, during periods of physical activity in a hot environment, we can lose as much as a liter of liquid per hour in the process of sweating. In such circumstances, it is important to drink appropriate amounts of fluids to avoid serious, potentially life-threatening conditions.

The *apocrine* (AP-oh-krin) *glands*, which begin to function during puberty, are located in the genital and axilla (armpit) areas. The apocrine

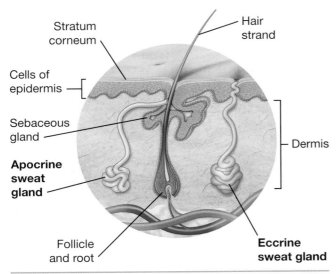

Figure 3.7 The eccrine and apocrine sweat glands. *What is the difference between the eccrine and the apocrine glands?*

glands are larger than the eccrine glands. They secrete a milky fluid consisting of sweat, fatty acids, and proteins. Unlike the eccrine gland ducts, which open directly onto the skin, the apocrine gland ducts empty into hair follicles.

Sebaceous Glands

Sebaceous (seh-BAY-shus) **glands**, located all over the body except for the palms of the hands and soles of the feet, produce an oily substance called **sebum** (SEE-bum). Most sebaceous glands empty into a hair follicle, though some secrete directly to the skin. Sebum helps to keep the skin and hair soft and also contains chemicals that kill bacteria. Because the sebaceous glands are particularly active during adolescence, teenagers' skin tends to be oily.

Hair

Hair *follicles* (FAHL-i-kuhlz) are bulb-shaped structures within the dermis that produce hair (**Figure 3.8**). The base of the follicle is "invaded" by a papilla of connective tissue containing a rich capillary supply, which provides nourishment for hair cell formation. In the *matrix*, or growth zone, within the base of the follicle are specialized cells that divide and generate living hair cells. But, like the epithelial cells generated in the stratum basale, as these cells are pushed up

toward the scalp, they become filled with keratin and die. Most of a shaft of hair is, therefore, nonliving material composed mainly of protein.

What gives a person's hair a particular color and texture (straight, wavy, or curly)? Melanocytes within the follicle produce the pigment that gives hair its color. As a person ages, the melanocytes produce less pigment, resulting in gray or white hair.

The shape of the hair follicle is genetically determined. A round hair follicle produces straight hair; an oval follicle causes hair to be wavy; and a flat-shaped follicle produces curly hair.

What causes the familiar "goose bumps" that are part of an involuntary reaction when we are cold or frightened? Tiny muscles called *arrector pili* (ah-REHK-tor PIGH-ligh) connect either side of the hair follicle to the epidermis. When stimulated, these muscles contract, pulling the hair upright and causing the appearance of goose bumps on the skin. The erect hair traps a layer of air close to the skin, which adds insulation and helps to warm the body.

Nails

Underlying each nail is a specialized region of the stratum basale known as the *nail bed*.

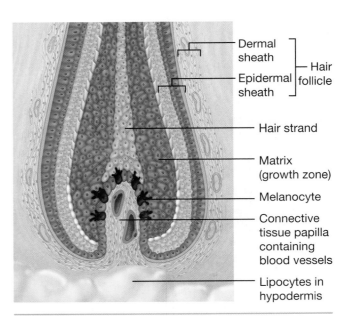

Figure 3.8 The base of a hair follicle—longitudinal section view. *If you were to ask a stylist or barber to trim all the "dead ends" from your hair, you would be practically bald. Why?*

The proximal end of the nail bed is a thickened region called the *nail matrix*, or growth zone. As with hair, it is within the matrix that nail growth occurs, with new cells rapidly becoming keratinized and dying.

Nails are transparent, but they appear pinkish in color because of the capillary supply beneath the stratum basale. The white, crescent moon-shaped region at the base of the nail, which is positioned over the thickened nail matrix, is called the *lunule* (LOO-nyool). The word *lunule* gets its name from the Latin word *luna*, which means "moon." The lunule has a curved shape like that of a crescent moon.

Lesson 3.2 Review and Assessment

Mini Glossary   Make sure that you know the meaning of each key term.

 Build vocabulary with e-flash cards and games

dermis   layer of skin between the epidermis and hypodermis; includes nerve endings, glands, and hair follicles

epidermal dendritic cells   skin cells that initiate an immune system response to the presence of foreign bacteria or viruses

epidermis   the outer layer of skin

hypodermis   the layer of skin beneath the dermis, which serves as a storage repository for fat

integumentary system   enveloping organ of the body that includes the epidermis, dermis, sudoriferous and sebaceous glands, and nails and hair

keratin   a tough protein found in the skin, hair, and nails

keratinocytes   cells within the epidermis that produce keratin

melanin   a pigment that protects the body against the harmful effects of ultraviolet ray damage from the sun

melanocytes   specialized cells in the skin that produce melanin

Merkel cells   touch receptors in the skin

papillary layer   the outer layer of the dermis

reticular layer   the layer of skin superficial to the papillary layer

sebaceous glands   glands located all over the body that produce sebum

sebum   an oily substance that helps to keep the skin and hair soft

stratum basale   the deepest layer of the epidermis

stratum corneum   the outer layer of the epidermis

stratum granulosum   a layer of somewhat flattened cells lying just superficial to the stratum spinosum and inferior to the stratum lucidum

stratum lucidum   the clear layer of thick skin found only on the palms of the hands, fingers, soles of the feet, and toes

stratum spinosum   the layer of cells in the epidermis superior to the stratum basale and inferior to the stratum granulosum

sudoriferous glands   sweat glands that are distributed in the dermis over the entire body

Know and Understand

 Assess

1. List the important features of the epidermal dendritic cells and Merkel cells of the epidermis.
2. Describe collagen fibers.
3. Describe elastic fibers and list the different areas of the body in which they are located.
4. Describe two ways that skin helps to protect the body.
5. What is the other name for sweat glands?
6. What are the two types of sweat glands? Describe them both.
7. Where does hair and nail growth occur?

Analyze and Apply

8. As you learned in lesson 3.2, the epidermis completely replaces itself every 25 to 45 days. Describe the process of skin shedding and how the body constantly supplies nutrients to the outer layers of the skin.

9. In the summer months, exposure to extreme temperatures can be life threatening, but specialized glands close to the surface of the skin help to keep the body cool. What are these specialized glands and how do they help to regulate body temperature?

10. The skin is involved in chemical processes. Which vitamin is essential to bone health and what role does the skin play in producing that vitamin?

In the Lab

11. Using the information that you have learned about the layers of skin, examine your hands, arms, and feet. Describe what the skin looks like on these areas. Does the skin of your hands and feet have a different color, thickness, or design than that of your arms? Describe in detail why this is or is not the case.

Lesson 3.3 Injuries and Disorders of the Skin

Before You Read

Try to answer the following questions before you read this lesson.

Why are the worst skin burns not painful?

Which common viral infection never completely goes away?

Lesson Objectives

1. Describe how a bedsore forms and what can be done to prevent its development.
2. Explain the differences between first-, second-, and third-degree burns.
3. Explain the difference between herpes simplex virus type 1 and herpes simplex virus type 2.
4. Explain how fungal infections can be prevented.
5. Explain the difference between benign and malignant cancer.

Key Terms

E-Flash Cards

basal cell carcinoma
cellulitis
common warts
first-degree burns
herpes simplex virus
  type 1 (HSV-1)
herpes simplex virus
  type 2 (HSV-2)
herpes varicella
  (chickenpox)
herpes zoster (shingles)
impetigo

malignant melanoma
peritonitis
plantar warts
pleurisy
psoriasis
rule of nines
second-degree burns
squamous cell
  carcinoma
third-degree burns
tinea

As the first "line of defense" in protecting the body from the external environment, the skin is routinely subject to minor injuries and is exposed to a variety of common infections. Fortunately, the skin is a multilayered system with a remarkable capacity for self-healing.

Injuries of the Skin

The skin commonly sustains minor cuts, abrasions, and blisters that tend to heal quickly. This healing is aided immensely by the skin's normal self-renewal process. Every 25 to 45 days, new epithelial cells reach the surface of the skin.

With all minor skin injuries, infection is a major concern. Injuries to the skin that penetrate the underlying tissues are more complicated, and infection is still the most significant concern.

Decubitus Ulcers

Decubitus (deh-KYOO-bi-tus) *ulcers* or *pressure ulcers*, commonly known as *bedsores*, are skin injuries caused by an area of localized pressure that restricts blood flow to one or more areas of the body. Without the normal blood supply to provide nutrients and oxygen, the skin cells die. These skin injuries typically occur in people who undergo prolonged bed rest. When a bedridden patient is not turned often enough, sustained pressure over an area can result in a bedsore. Bedsores can occur anywhere on the body, but most form over bony areas such as the lower back, coccyx (tailbone), hips, elbows, and ankles.

A bedsore begins as an area of reddened skin, but as cells start to die, small cracks or openings in the skin appear. As the condition progresses, the tissue continues to degenerate and an open ulcer forms. If not treated, tissue degeneration can progress all the way to the bone and eventually can be fatal.

Although the term *bedsore* suggests that these injuries affect only bedridden individuals, bedsores can develop in any situation in which the blood supply to the tissues is restricted. People who use wheelchairs, for example, can develop bedsores over pressure points. Individuals with numbness in parts of the body from a spinal injury or diabetes mellitus must be particularly careful to avoid remaining in the same position for prolonged periods.

Bedsore treatment includes prescription of oral antibiotics to address or prevent infection. Removal of damaged tissues is another component of treatment. Because dead tissue prevents healing, it must be removed for proper healing to occur.

There are two approaches to removing bedsore-damaged tissues—*debridement* and *vacuum-assisted closure*. Debridement is the removal of dead tissue using a surgical or chemical procedure. In vacuum-assisted closure, a vacuum tube is attached to the wound. The vacuum draws moisture from the ulcer, thereby shortening the healing process and reducing the risk of infection.

Proper nutrition is an important factor in both the prevention and healing of bedsores. Vitamins A, B, C, and E and the minerals magnesium, manganese, selenium, and zinc all contribute to skin health. Sufficient amounts of dietary protein are also important.

✔ Check Your Understanding

1. What causes decubitus ulcers, or bedsores?
2. Where on the body do bedsores commonly occur?
3. Describe two types of treatment for removal of bedsore-damaged skin tissue.

Burns

Burns are injuries that can arise from exposure to excessive heat, corrosive chemicals, electricity, or ultraviolet radiation (from sunburn, for example). Burns, which vary considerably in severity, cause tissue damage and cell death.

First-degree burns affect only the epidermal layer of skin (**Figure 3.9A**). These burns involve reddening of the skin and mild pain, and they tend to heal in less than a week. Most types of sunburn are first-degree burns.

Second-degree burns involve damage to both the epidermis and the upper portion of the underlying dermis (**Figure 3.9B**). Second-degree burns are characterized by blisters, fluid-filled pockets that form between the epidermal and dermal layers. These types of burns are painful and take longer to heal than first-degree burns. An even longer period of healing is required for larger blisters.

Third-degree burns are the most serious type of skin burn (**Figure 3.9C**). Because these

A **B** **C**

Suzanne Tucker/Shutterstock.com, JTeffects/Shutterstock.com, Naiyyer/Shutterstock.com

Figure 3.9 Different types of burns. A—First-degree burn. B—Second-degree burn. C—Third-degree burn.

burns destroy the entire thickness of the skin, they are also called *full-thickness burns*. (First- and second-degree burns are called *partial-thickness burns*.)

The area affected by a third-degree burn appears grayish-white or blackened. Although a third-degree burn is a serious injury, it is initially not painful because the nerve endings in the skin have been destroyed. Later, scarring and pain will occur. A third-degree burn cannot heal on its own because the stratum basale, which generates new skin cells, has been destroyed. Treatment involves grafting skin over the damaged area.

When a large region of skin has been burned, clinicians use the **rule of nines** to estimate the extent of burned tissue. **Figure 3.10** illustrates the rule of nines.

According to the rule of nines, the percentage of total body surface area covered by burns is approximated as follows:
- 9% for both the anterior (front) and posterior (back) of the head and neck;
- 18% for the anterior and 18% for the posterior of the torso;
- 9% for both the anterior and posterior of each arm;
- 18% for both the anterior and posterior of each leg; and
- 1% for the genital region.

Using this approach for both the anterior and posterior surface areas of the body, the total is 100%. For example, if the anterior of the torso and the anterior of one arm were burned, the affected surface area would be approximately 23% (4.5% for the anterior of the arm and 18 percent for the anterior of the torso).

Infections of the Skin and Membranes

Skin infections can be caused by contact with an infectious agent that is present on another person or a surface. They can also be caused by airborne particles such as viruses or bacteria or by contamination introduced by a foreign object into a penetrating wound.

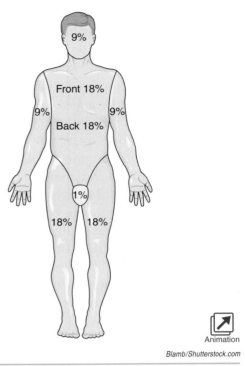

Animation

Blamb/Shutterstock.com

Figure 3.10 The rule of nines. *How is the rule of nines useful in helping a physician determine how to treat a patient with burns on her body?*

Viral Infections

Herpes. *Herpes* is a viral infection that produces small, painful, blister-like sores. Once a herpes infection is present, it lasts for the rest of a person's life. Fortunately, herpes infections tend to stay dormant most of the time, with no noticeable sign of infection. Occasional flare-ups do occur, however; the resurgence of symptoms usually accompanies periods of stress or sickness. Several different varieties of the herpes virus are known to exist.

Herpes varicella (VAIR-i-SEHL-a), better known as *chickenpox*, is a common childhood disease. Because chickenpox is highly contagious, it tends to spread quickly and widely. The fluid-filled blisters caused by chickenpox are extremely itchy. They can spread over most of the body, or they can be limited in scope. A vaccine is available for chickenpox that decreases the chances of infection or reduces the seriousness of the virus if infection does occur.

Once a person infected with chickenpox has recovered, the virus lies dormant. In an adult, the virus can recur as **herpes zoster** (ZAHS-ter), commonly known as *shingles* (**Figure 3.11A**). Shingles involves an extremely painful, blistering rash accompanied by headache, fever, and a general feeling of unwellness. The shingles virus may trigger more serious symptoms, such as chronic nerve pain. In the United States, approximately 50% of people older than 80 years of age have had shingles at least once. A vaccine for shingles is recommended for adults older than 60 years of age.

Herpes simplex virus type 1 (HSV-1), sometimes associated with the common cold, generates "cold sores" or "fever blisters" around the mouth (**Figure 3.11B**). **Herpes simplex virus type 2 (HSV-2)** is the genital form of herpes. Both types of the herpes simplex virus are highly contagious and can be transmitted to the mouth or genital area. In the US, about one in six people has genital herpes.

Transmission of the herpes simplex virus from an infected male to a female partner occurs with greater ease than from an infected female to a male partner. Thus, more women than men are infected with the virus.

During the first outbreak of genital herpes, a person may experience flu-like symptoms such as fever, body aches, and swollen glands. Repeat outbreaks are common, particularly during the first year of infection. Symptoms during repeat outbreaks are usually shorter in duration and

less severe than those in the first outbreak. As with all herpes infections, once a person has been infected by a herpes simplex virus, it remains dormant, with the potential to reactivate, throughout the remainder of the person's life. However, the number of outbreaks tends to decrease over time.

 Check Your Understanding

1. Describe a first-degree burn.
2. Which layers of skin does a second-degree burn involve?
3. Explain why third-degree burns are usually not painful.
4. What is herpes?
5. Are fever blisters generated by herpes simplex type 1 or herpes simplex type 2?

Human Papillomavirus (HPV). Warts are raised, typically painless growths on the skin that vary in shape and size. Warts can spread from one part of the body to another. Less commonly, warts can spread from one person to another. All types of warts are caused by the *human papillomavirus (HPV)*.

HPVs are a group of more than 150 related viruses. **Common warts** typically appear on the hands or fingers and tend to disappear without treatment (**Figure 3.12**). It is important, however, to make sure that a wart-like growth on an adult

A   **B**

Figure 3.11 Two different types of herpes infections. A—Herpes zoster (shingles) infection. B—Herpes simplex (cold sore) infection.

Maksym Bondarchuk/Shutterstock.com

Figure 3.12 Common warts.

is not a form of skin cancer. **Plantar warts**, which develop on the soles of the foot, grow inward and can become painful. When warranted, warts can be removed by surgery, cryotherapy (freezing), and topical medications such as salicylic acids.

Genital warts caused by HPV infections are the most common sexually transmitted infections in the US. More than 40 of the HPVs can be easily spread through direct, skin-to-skin contact during vaginal, anal, and oral sex. More than 50% of all sexually active people are infected with an HPV at some point during their life.

There are two major categories of HPVs: *low risk* and *high risk*. HPVs are identified by number, and your physician can discuss with you whether a possible HPV infection is categorized as low risk or high risk.

Low-risk HPVs can cause warts on the skin around the genital area and anus but are not known to cause cancer. High-risk HPV infections, however, do cause nearly all cervical cancers, which is why some healthcare

professionals advocate the papillomavirus vaccine for teenage girls and boys. High-risk HPV infections also cause most anal cancers and about 50% of all vaginal, vulvar, and penile cancers. In addition, HPV infections cause cancer of the soft palate, the base of the tongue, and the tonsils. High-risk HPVs account for about 5% of all cancers.

Fungal Infections

Fungal infections, or **tinea** (TIN-ee-a), tend to occur in areas of the body that are moist. They, therefore, tend to be more prevalent during warm weather, and they are more common in individuals whose work or sporting activities involve frequent periods of sweating.

Athlete's Foot. *Tinea pedis* (athlete's foot) is the most common fungal infection. It is characterized by cracked, flaky skin between the toes or on the side of the foot. The skin may also be red and itchy. Because tinea pedis is highly contagious, it spreads rapidly on locker room and shower floors. Treatment and prevention includes keeping the feet clean and dry, especially between the toes, and using over-the-counter, antifungal powder or cream that contains clotrimazole, miconazole, or tolnaftate.

Jock Itch. *Tinea cruris*, or *jock itch*, primarily affects males around the groin and scrotum. It is caused by the combination of prolonged sweating and friction from clothes. It can be spread through direct contact with infected skin or unwashed clothing. Tinea cruris typically is treated by keeping the skin clean and dry, wearing loose clothing, and applying a topical antifungal or drying powder that contains clotrimazole, miconazole, or tolnaftate.

Ringworm. *Tinea corporis*, more commonly known as *ringworm*, does not actually involve any type of worm. However, the characteristically red, ring-shaped rash with a pale center somewhat resembles the shape of a worm.

Tinea corporis, which is usually caused by prolonged sweating and poor hygiene, is especially common in children. It is highly contagious and can be spread through direct contact with the infection on someone's body or through contaminated areas such as pool

WHAT RESEARCH TELLS US

...*about* High-Risk HPVs and Cancer

The human papillomavirus (HPV) infects epithelial cells on the skin and in the membranes that line areas such as the genital tract and anus. When an HPV enters an epithelial cell, the virus begins making specialized proteins. Two of these proteins initiate cancer by interfering with the cell's normal functions, enabling the cell to grow in an uncontrolled manner and resist cell death (**Figure 3.13**).

When the immune system recognizes HPV-infected cells, it attacks and attempts to destroy them. When the immune system fails, however, these infected cells continue to grow, and infection takes root. As the cells multiply, they can develop mutations that further promote cell growth, sometimes leading to tumor development.

Researchers believe that some 10 to 20 years can pass

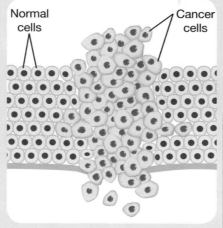

Normal cells / Cancer cells

Alila Sao Mai/Shutterstock.com

Figure 3.13 Development of cancer cells. *Explain how HPV-infected cells can develop into a tumor.*

between the initial HPV infection and tumor formation. They estimate, however, that less than

50% of high-grade HPV infections lead to cancer. Fortunately, because HPVs do not enter the blood stream, an HPV infection in one part of the body should not spread to other parts of the body.

Taking It Further

1. Working with a group of classmates, design a brochure to raise HPV awareness. Your brochure should address these questions: What is HPV? How do people become infected with this virus? How is HPV diagnosed? What treatments are available? What is the link between HPV and certain cancers? How can HPV be prevented? You might include separate discussions for HPV in women and HPV in men. Share your brochure with the rest of the class.

surfaces. Treatment involves keeping the skin clean and dry and applying an over-the-counter, antifungal cream that contains clotrimazole, miconazole, ketoconazole, or oxiconazole.

Toenail Fungus. *Tinea unguium* is a fungal infection under the nails of the fingers or toes (**Figure 3.14** on the next page). It causes discoloration and thickening of the infected nail. In general, over-the-counter antifungal creams do not help this condition. A prescription antifungal medication must be taken orally for several weeks.

Bacterial Infections

Impetigo (IM-peh-TEE-goh) is a highly contagious staphylococcus infection common in elementary school children. Its symptoms are pink, blister-like bumps, usually on the face

around the mouth and nose, that develop a yellowish crust before they rupture.

Cellulitis (SEHL-yoo-LIGH-tis), another staphylococcus infection, is characterized by an inflamed area of skin that is red, swollen, and painful. The origin of cellulitis often is an open wound or ulceration. Cellulitis is a serious condition that can become life threatening if not treated with antibiotics.

 Check Your Understanding

1. What causes warts?
2. Where do common warts typically appear?
3. What are the most common sexually transmitted infections in the US?
4. Is athlete's foot contagious?
5. What is impetigo?

Figure 3.14 Tinea unguium, or toenail fungus.

Inflammatory Conditions of the Skin and Membranes

Inflammation is a general response of bodily tissue to any injury or disease that damages cells. It is a protective response that involves increased blood flow to the distressed area, along with marshalling of specialized cells that attack infectious agents and destroy dead tissue. The increased blood flow causes redness; major inflammation also causes pain and swelling.

Although most infections and disorders of the skin and membranes provoke an inflammatory response, those discussed in this section are specific inflammatory conditions that may have different causes.

Pleurisy

Pleurisy (PLOOR-i-see) is an inflammation of the *pleura*, the membrane that lines the thoracic (chest) cavity and lungs. It can be caused by an infection, such as pneumonia or tuberculosis. It can also be caused by cancer, rheumatoid arthritis, lupus, injury to the chest, a blockage in the blood supply to the lungs, or the harmful presence of inhaled asbestos.

Pleurisy causes the normally smooth surfaces of the pleura to become rough. With each breath, the pleura lining the chest cavity

and the pleura lining the lungs rub against each other, producing a grating sound called a "friction rub" that can readily be heard with a stethoscope (**Figure 3.15**).

The primary symptom of pleurisy is chest pain that sharpens with inhalation or coughing. The pain may radiate to one or both shoulders. Pleurisy can cause an accumulation of fluid in the thoracic cavity. This fluid accumulation can make breathing difficult and may cause a bluish skin color (due to reduced oxygen circulation in the blood), shortness of breath, rapid breathing, and coughing.

The course of treatment for pleurisy depends on the cause. Bacterial infections are treated with antibiotics. When fluid has accumulated in the chest cavity, it can be drained through a surgical procedure. Anti-inflammatory drugs can help control the pain caused by pleurisy.

Peritonitis

Peritonitis (PER-i-toh-NIGH-tis) is an inflammation of the peritoneum, the membrane that lines the inner wall of the abdomen and covers the abdominal organs. Peritonitis is caused by the accumulation of blood, bodily fluids, or pus in the abdomen. Symptoms include abdominal pain and tenderness that may worsen with movement or touch. The abdomen may also be swollen. Other symptoms may include fever and chills, nausea and vomiting,

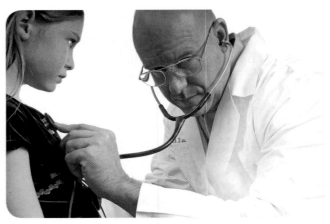

Figure 3.15 Doctor examining patient. *Why will the doctor be able to determine whether or not the young girl has pleurisy?*

fatigue, shortness of breath, rapid heartbeat, and decreased urine and stool output.

Peritonitis is a serious, potentially life-threatening condition. Medical treatment typically involves surgery to repair the internal damage that caused the condition, along with a course of strong antibiotics.

Psoriasis

Psoriasis (soh-RIGH-a-sis) is a common skin disorder that involves redness and irritation. The condition is characterized by regions of thick, red skin with flaky, silver-white patches called *scales* that itch, burn, crack, and sometimes bleed (**Figure 3.16**).

According to the prevailing hypothesis, psoriasis has its roots in an autoimmune disorder, an inappropriate immune response to a substance or tissue that is present in the body. In the case of psoriasis, the body's immune system causes skin cells to be produced too quickly. This overproduction of skin cells yields raised patches of skin, or scales.

Psoriasis is not contagious and may be hereditary. It typically develops between 15 and 35 years of age and can progress quickly or slowly. It may disappear and return, or it may persist indefinitely. Outbreaks of psoriasis most commonly affect the elbows, knees, and trunk region, although they can occur anywhere on the body.

A variety of conditions can trigger or exacerbate psoriasis. These conditions include bacterial or viral infections, minor injuries to the skin, dry skin, stress, too little or too much sunlight, excessive alcohol consumption, and certain medications. Psoriasis is also worsened by a weakened immune system due to AIDS, chemotherapy, or autoimmune disorders such as rheumatoid arthritis.

The goal of psoriasis treatment is to control symptoms and prevent infection. Three treatment approaches are available: topical treatments, systemic treatments, and light therapy. Topical treatments include special skin lotions, ointments, creams, and shampoos that are applied to the affected area. Systemic treatments, which treat the whole body, include medications that can be injected or taken orally.

Light therapy, also called *phototherapy*, is a medical treatment in which the skin is carefully exposed to ultraviolet light. The UVB in natural sunlight is an effective treatment for psoriasis. It penetrates the skin and hinders the growth of skin cells affected by the condition. In light therapy, the skin is exposed at regular intervals to a source that delivers artificial UVB.

 Check Your Understanding

1. What causes the redness associated with inflammation?
2. What is pleurisy?
3. What skin disorder is characterized by regions of thick, red skin with flaky, silver-white patches?

Cancers of the Skin

As described earlier in this lesson, many skin conditions involve bumps or small, noncancerous lesions. Common warts are an example. Thus far, we have discussed conditions that are *benign*—that is, they involve tumors that do not *metastasize*, or spread, to remote regions of the body.

When a tumor is *malignant*, or cancerous, it tends to metastasize to other body parts. Skin cancer is the most common type of

Kenxro/Shutterstock.com

Figure 3.16 Psoriasis.

cancer in the US; at some point, about one-fifth of the population experiences skin cancer. Overexposure to the sun is a major risk factor. The three most common forms of skin cancer follow.

Basal cell carcinoma (KAR-si-NOH-ma) is the most common form of skin cancer and, fortunately, is also the least malignant (**Figure 3.17**). It is caused by overproduction of cells in the stratum basale that push upward, forming dome-shaped bumps. These bumps most often appear on areas of the face that have been exposed to the sun. Slow-growing basal cell carcinomas are usually noticed and surgically removed before they can spread and become dangerous.

Squamous cell carcinoma is caused by overproduction of cells in the stratum spinosum layer of the epidermis. These cancers appear as a scaly, reddened patch that progresses to an ulcer-like mass with a raised border. The most commonly affected locations are the scalp, ears, lower lip, and backs of the hands among fair-skinned people. Dark-skinned people, however, typically develop this condition in areas not exposed to the sun, such as the legs or feet. Squamous cell carcinomas grow rapidly and can easily spread to nearby lymph nodes. With early removal by surgery or radiation treatment, these cancers can be completely cured.

The most serious form of skin cancer is **malignant melanoma** (MEHL-a-NOH-ma),

cancer of the melanocytes (**Figure 3.18**). Although typically dark colored and irregular in shape, a malignant melanoma can appear pink, red, or "fleshy." Change in the size, shape, color, or elevation of a mole are typical warning signs of a malignant melanoma.

The American Cancer Society advocates the *ABCD rule* for determining the presence of melanoma:

A. **Asymmetry**: The shape of the mole is irregular.
B. **Border irregularity**: The outside borders are not smooth.
C. **Color**: More than one color is present. Melanomas may contain different shades of black and brown, blues, reds, or pinks.
D. **Diameter**: The mole size is larger than about one-quarter of an inch in diameter, or larger than the diameter of a pencil.

It is important to see a healthcare provider immediately if malignant melanoma is suspected. Although these cancers comprise only about 5% of all skin cancers, they can be deadly.

✓ **Check Your Understanding**

1. Squamous cell carcinoma is an overproduction of cells in which layer of the epidermis?
2. What is the ABCD rule for detecting melanoma?

Figure 3.17 Basal cell carcinoma. Although this common form of skin cancer is less likely than other forms to be malignant, it should not be ignored. *How are slow-growing basal cell carcinomas often treated?*

Librakv/Shutterstock.com

Figure 3.18 Malignant melanoma. *What is the ABCD rule for determining the presence of a malignant melanoma?*

Lesson 3.3 Review and Assessment

Mini Glossary   Make sure that you know the meaning of each key term.

Build vocabulary with
e-flash cards and games

basal cell carcinoma   the most common form of skin cancer and the least malignant type

cellulitis   a bacterial infection characterized by an inflamed area of skin that is red, swollen, and painful

common warts   warts that typically appear on the hands or fingers and disappear without treatment

first-degree burns   burns that affect only the epidermal layer of skin

herpes simplex virus type 1   the form of herpes that generates cold sores or fever blisters around the mouth

herpes simplex virus type 2   the genital form of herpes

herpes varicella (chickenpox)   a highly contagious, common childhood disease that is characterized by extremely itchy, fluid-filled blisters

herpes zoster (shingles)   a disease that involves a painful, blistering rash accompanied by headache, fever, and a general feeling of unwellness

impetigo   a bacterial infection common in elementary school children that is characterized by pink, blister-like bumps, usually on the face

malignant melanoma   cancer of the melanocytes; the most serious form of skin cancer

peritonitis   inflammation of the peritoneum, the membrane lining the inner wall of the abdomen and covering the abdominal organs

plantar warts   warts that develop on the soles of the foot, grow inward, and can become painful

pleurisy   inflammation of the pleura, the membrane that encases the lungs

psoriasis   a common skin disorder that involves redness, irritation, and scales (flaky, silver-white patches) that itch, burn, crack, and sometimes bleed

rule of nines   a method used in calculating body surface area affected by burns

second-degree burns   burns that involve damage to both the epidermis and the upper portion of the underlying dermis; characterized by blisters

squamous cell carcinoma   a type of rapidly growing cancer that appears as a scaly, reddened patch of skin

third-degree burns   burns that destroy the entire thickness of the skin

tinea   a fungal infection that tends to occur in areas of the body that are moist

Know and Understand

Assess

1. Describe how the skin regenerates.

2. Name two interventions that can help to reduce a bedridden patient's risk for developing bed sores.

3. Describe each of the three types of skin burns.

4. List and describe two types of skin infections common in school-age children.

5. List the medical treatments for warts.

6. List and briefly describe four common fungal infections.

Analyze and Apply

7. Why are third-degree burns not painful? Why are they not able to heal on their own?

8. What is the connection between herpes varicella (chickenpox) and herpes zoster (shingles)?

9. Assume that you are a doctor, and one of your elderly patients has bedsores in the coccyx area of her body. When you inform the patient of your diagnosis, she seems confused, saying that she sleeps fewer hours per night than most people

she knows. What explanation would you give your patient so that she could better understand her condition?

In the Lab

10. Go to the Centers for Disease Control (CDC) website and search *herpes varicella*, *herpes zoster*, *herpes simplex type 1*, and *herpes simplex type 2*. What characteristics are similar among all of these herpes viruses? What characteristics, if any, are different? Prepare a short written report of the differences and present your report to the class.

11. Using the rule of nines, calculate the percentage of total body surface area covered by burns for each of the following burn victims:
    A. burns on one leg: all of the front, half of the back
    B. burns in the genital area and all of the lower limbs
    C. burns to just the front of the body: the head, right arm, and torso
    D. burns over the entire body except for the head

Dermatology is the field of medicine that deals with the anatomy, functions, and diseases of the skin. A career in dermatology can be challenging, profitable, and rewarding.

Dermatologist

A dermatologist is a medical doctor (MD) who specializes in treating diseases and disorders of the skin through medicine and surgery (**Figure 3.19**). Many dermatologists also perform cosmetic procedures.

To become a dermatologist, one must earn a college degree and complete four years of medical school followed by a residency in dermatology. In the US, residency training typically takes four years to complete. The first year of residency usually consists of a supervised internship in medicine or surgery. During the following three years, residents receive specialized training in dermatology. Further specialization can be acquired through an additional two-year fellowship.

The following specialized procedures are generally performed by dermatologists:

- Photodynamic therapy for treatment of skin cancer and precancerous growths
- Cryosurgery for treatment of warts and skin cancers
- Laser therapy for management of unwanted birth marks or tattoos and for cosmetic resurfacing
- Hair removal
- Hair transplantation
- Injections of cosmetic filler substances
- Liposuction
- Allergy testing for allergies caused by skin contact
- Topical therapies for various skin conditions

Dermatology Technician

A dermatology technician, also called a *dermatology assistant*, usually provides patient support and performs specialized medical technical tasks for a licensed dermatology practice. Some dermatology technicians, however, choose to work independently in salons or spas, providing services such as hair removal, facials, and skin-care treatments. Because dermatology technicians work directly with patients or clients and handle a variety of duties, they must have strong communication skills and the ability to multitask (**Figure 3.20**).

At minimum, dermatology technicians must have a high school diploma or GED, although most businesses prefer candidates who have earned a certificate or associate's degree in medical assisting. Community colleges offer certificate and associate's degree programs in medical assisting accredited by the Commission on Accreditation of Allied Health Education Programs (CAAHEP) or the Accrediting Bureau of Health Education Schools (ABHES). In addition, most college programs offer internships beyond traditional coursework.

Medical Assistant Certificate. A one-year medical assistant certificate program prepares students for clinical and administrative duties in a variety of healthcare settings. Coursework typically includes medical terminology, anatomy, dermatology, and pharmacology. Administrative subjects

Dean Bertoncelj/Shutterstock.com

Figure 3.19 A dermatologist evaluates a patient's skin for melanoma. *Based on what you have read on this page, do you think you would enjoy a career as a dermatologist? Why or why not?*

Figure 3.20 This dermatology technician works in a nail salon. Here she is removing calluses from a customer's feet.

wavebreakmedia/Shutterstock.com

include clerical functions, basic accounting, and insurance billing.

Associate of Applied Science for Medical Assistants. An associate's degree program in medical assisting takes 18 to 24 months to complete. Most programs include externships in a clinical setting in which students are trained in drawing blood, giving injections, preparing and maintaining patients' medical records, and using appropriate telephone techniques. Coursework covers computer software applications, medical office procedures, biology, microbiology, and hematology.

Planning for a Health-Related Career

Do some research on the career of a dermatologist or dermatology technician.

Alternatively, select a profession from the list of **Related Career Options**. Using the Internet or resources at your local library, find answers to the following questions:

1. What are the main responsibilities of the career that you have chosen to research?
2. What is the outlook for this career? Are workers in demand, or are jobs dwindling? For complete information, consult the current edition of the *Occupational Outlook Handbook*, published by the US Department of Labor. This handbook is available online or at your local library.
3. What special skills or talents are required? For example, do you need to be good at biology and anatomy? Do you need to enjoy interacting with other people?
4. What personality traits do you think are needed to be successful in this job? For example, a dermatology career involving laboratory research requires collaboration with other people. Do you enjoy teamwork?
5. Does this career involve a great deal of routine, or do the day-to-day responsibilities vary?
6. Does the work require long hours, or is it a standard, "9-to-5" job?
7. What is the salary range for this job?
8. What do you think you would like about this career? Is there anything about it that you might dislike?

Related Career Options

- Dermatologist
- Dermatology Technician
- Immunodermatologist
- Medical Aesthetician
- Medical Assistant
- Pediatric Dermatologist
- Teledermatologist
- Veterinary Dermatologist

Chapter Summaries

Lesson 3.1 Body Membranes

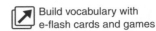
Build vocabulary with
e-flash cards and games

Key Points

- The body membranes surround and help protect the body's surfaces.
- Epithelial membranes line or cover the internal and external surfaces of the body.
- Mucous membranes line the body cavities that open to the exterior; examples include the linings of the mouth, nose, lungs, digestive tract, and bladder.
- Serous membranes line the body cavities that are closed to the exterior; examples include the pleura, the pericardium, and the peritoneum.

Key Terms

cutaneous membrane
epithelial membranes
membranes
mucous membranes
pericardium
peritoneum

pleura
serous fluid
serous membranes
synovial fluid
synovial membrane

Lesson 3.2 The Integumentary System

Key Points

- The integumentary system includes a cutaneous membrane, sweat and oil glands, and nails and hair.
- Keratin is a tough protein found in hair and nails; it also adds to the structural strength of the skin.
- The skin protects the body against damage from harmful chemicals and ultraviolet rays from sunlight, serves as a water barrier, and helps to regulate body temperature.
- The two layers of the skin are the epidermis (outer layer) and the dermis (underlying layer).
- The appendages of the skin include the sweat glands, the sebaceous glands, hair, and nails.

Key Terms

dermis
epidermal dendritic cells
epidermis
hypodermis
integumentary system
keratin
keratinocytes
melanin
melanocytes
Merkel cells

papillary layer
reticular layer
sebaceous glands
sebum
stratum basale
stratum corneum
stratum granulosum
stratum lucidum
stratum spinosum
sudoriferous glands

Injuries and Disorders of the Skin

Key Points

- In the skin's normal self-renewal process, new epithelial cells reach the surface of the skin every 25 to 45 days.
- Decubitus ulcers, or bedsores, are skin injuries caused by an area of localized pressure that restricts blood flow to one or more areas of the body.
- The three categories of skin burns are first-degree burns, second-degree burns, and third-degree burns.
- Viral infections of the skin include herpes and warts.
- Fungal infections of the skin tend to occur in areas of the body that are moist.
- Cancers of the skin are the most common type of cancer in the US; about one-fifth of the population experiences skin cancer at some point in their lives.
- The three types of skin cancer are basal cell carcinoma, squamous cell carcinoma, and malignant melanoma.

Key Terms

basal cell carcinoma
cellulitis
common warts
first-degree burns
herpes simplex virus type 1
herpes simplex virus type 2
herpes varicella (chickenpox)
herpes zoster (shingles)

impetigo
malignant melanoma
peritonitis
plantar warts
pleurisy
psoriasis
rule of nines
second-degree burns
squamous cell carcinoma
third-degree burns
tinea

Chapter Assessments

Assess

Lesson 3.1

Body Membranes

Learning Key Terms and Concepts

1. Membranes surround and protect which of the following surfaces?
   A. ball-and-socket synovial joints
   B. internal cavities housing organs
   C. cavities open to the outside world
   D. all of the above
   E. none of the above

2. _____ line or cover the internal and external surfaces of the body.

3. The _____ line the body cavities that open to the exterior surfaces.

4. The mucous membranes line which of the following hollow organ tracts?
   A. digestive tract
   B. urinary tract
   C. respiratory tract
   D. all of the above
   E. none of the above

5. *True or False?* Mucous membranes tend to be dry.

6. Which type of membrane is composed only of connective tissue and includes no epithelial cells?

7. The pleura, pericardium, and peritoneum are all examples of which type of membranes?

8. *True or False?* Cutaneous membrane is the name for what we know as skin.

9. *True or False?* The visceral layer is the outer lining of each serous membrane.

10. *True or False?* The epithelial membranes line or cover the internal surfaces of the body only.

11. *True or False?* The body membranes surround and help to protect the body's surfaces.

Thinking Critically

12. Explain the main difference between a mucous membrane and a serous membrane. Discuss examples of both membrane types in your explanation.

13. Assume that someone challenges you when you tell them that skin is a membrane. Explain why they might think that but why they would be wrong.

Lesson 3.2

The Integumentary System

Learning Key Terms and Concepts

14. Which type of protein, found in the outermost layer of the skin, adds structural strength to the skin?

15. What is the name of the receptors that transmit nerve signals containing information about the environment, including touch, pressure, vibration, pain, and temperature?

16. The skin is made up of which two layers?
    A. epidermis and hypodermis
    B. epidermis and dermis
    C. hypodermis and dermis
    D. dermis and underlying tissues

17. Which of the following are considered to be appendages of the skin?
    A. sweat glands
    B. hypoglands
    C. hair
    D. both A and C
    E. all of the above

18. Collagen and elastic fibers make up the dense, fibrous connective tissue called _____.

19. *True or False?* Keratin is primarily responsible for human skin color.

20. *True or False?* The epidermis completely replaces itself every 25 to 45 days.

21. *True or False?* The skin has two layers, the outer epidermis and the underlying dermis.

Instructions: Write the **letter** of the integumentary system structure on your answer sheet next to the corresponding number.

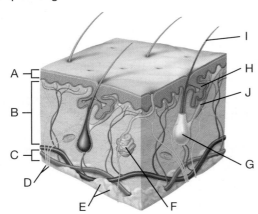

_____ 22. lipocytes	_____ 26. dermis
_____ 23. hypodermis	_____ 27. hair follicle
_____ 24. sebaceous gland	_____ 28. epidemis
	_____ 29. sweat gland
_____ 25. arrector pili muscle	_____ 30. hair shaft
	_____ 31. nerve fibers

Thinking Critically

32. Explain the skin's function in regulating body temperature. Compare and contrast the ways in which the skin helps the body cool to the way it helps the body warm.

33. Explain to an imaginary person why his or her hair color and texture (straight, wavy, or curly) have developed as they have.

34. The skin is described as keratinizing stratified squamous epithelial tissue. Describe what each of these terms means in relationship to the structure and function of the skin. (You may need to refer to the discussion in chapter 2 on types of epithelial tissue.)

Lesson 3.3

Injuries and Disorders of the Skin

Learning Key Terms and Concepts

35. Which type of burn, referred to as a full-thickness burn, destroys the entire skin?

36. Which of the following is not a type of viral infection?
    A. herpes   C. plantar warts
    B. psoriasis   D. genital warts

37. *True or False?* Psoriasis is a highly contagious disease characterized by scaly skin patches that itch, burn, crack, and sometimes bleed.

38. _____ is a highly contagious staphylococcus infection that is common in elementary school children.

39. _____ is a common skin disorder characterized by regions of thick, red skin with flaky, silver-white patches.

40. The most serious form of skin cancer is _____.
    A. basal cell carcinoma
    B. squamous cell carcinoma
    C. malignant melanoma
    D. none of the above

41. *True or False?* Burns can be caused by exposure to electricity.

42. *True or False?* First-degree burns damage the epidermis and parts of the underlying dermis.

Thinking Critically

43. Name the two major categories of HPVs and explain how they differ.

44. Which form of skin cancer is the most serious? What are some of its typical characteristics?

45. Describe the effects of decubitus ulcers, or pressure ulcers (bedsores), on the body.

Building Skills and Connecting Concepts

Analyzing and Evaluating Data

Using the information that you learned in this chapter about skin burns and the rule of nines, look at the figure below to answer the following questions.

46. What percentage of burned tissue would you assign to a patient who suffered burns to the anterior and posterior portions of the head and the anterior portion of both arms?

47. What percentage would you assign to a patient who suffered burns to the anterior portion of the left leg and the anterior portion of the torso?

48. What percentage would you assign to a patient who suffered burns to the anterior and posterior right leg, the anterior portion of the torso, and the posterior portion of the right arm?

Communicating about Anatomy and Physiology

49. **Writing** Go to the Centers for Disease Control (CDC) website and research skin injuries and disorders that commonly occur in the work environment. After reading the information, list steps that you can take at your workplace to prevent possible dermal exposure to yourself. Develop a plan that could be used to help yourself and others in the event of dermal exposure at work. Be sure to use key terms from this chapter in explaining how the exposure could occur. Write your plan and present it to the class. If you do not have an actual workplace to use for this activity, specify a place you would like to work.

50. **Writing** Research the effects of chemicals on the skin. Then write a three-paragraph summary about how a worker in a chemical plant might be exposed to chemicals through the different layers of the skin. Incorporate information that you learned in this chapter into your summary.

Lab Investigations

51. Working in a small group, use the following general procedure to design a laboratory experiment and test a hypothesis developed by your group. **Materials**: White UV beads, petri dishes, sunscreen. **Note**: Specific procedures will vary depending on the hypothesis that you test.

Place 5 to 7 UV beads in a petri dish. Apply a thin, even layer of sunscreen (as appropriate based on your group's hypothesis) to the exterior of the petri dish. Then place the petri dish outside in a sunlit or shaded location (based on your group's hypothesis) for 15 to 20 minutes.

Reminders:
- List and number the steps in your experiment;
- The experiment must be repeatable;
- Your directions must be very clear so that someone else could repeat the experiment exactly as your group did; and
- The data collected must be measurable.

On a sheet of paper, summarize the procedure that your group used. Next, record your observations (a description of what you notice during the experiment) as accurately and in as much detail as possible. Then summarize the results of your experiment.
- Was your hypothesis correct?
- What problems did you encounter?
- What did you learn from this experiment?

Expand your learning with additional online resources
- Supplemental Lab Activities
- Interactive Exercises
- Animations

Companion Website

www.g-wlearning.com/healthsciences

Why is it important for astronauts to exercise in space?

The Skeletal System

We tend to think of bone as a hard, dried-up chunk of mineral that a dog would enjoy chewing. While this is true of dead bone, the living bones inside our bodies are made up of amazing, complex living tissues. Our bones are not only hydrated (containing water), but also very dynamic, continually changing in size, shape, and strength over time.

How and why do these processes of change occur? In this chapter we will explore the characteristics of living bone and describe the well-tailored functionality of the major bones and joints in the human skeleton. We will also discuss some of the common injuries and disorders of the bones and joints, how these problems tend to occur, and in some cases, how their likelihood can be reduced.

Chapter 4 Lessons

Lesson 4.1
Bone as a
Living Tissue

Lesson 4.2
The Axial Skeleton

Lesson 4.3
The Appendicular
Skeleton

Lesson 4.4
Joints

Lesson 4.5
Common Injuries
and Disorders of
the Skeletal System

While studying, look for the online icon to:

- **Practice** with e-flash cards and vocabulary games
- **Review** with interactive art labeling
- **Assess** with online exercises
- **Expand** with interactive activities and animated videos
- **Listen** to pronunciations of key terms in the audio glossary

www.g-wlearning.com/healthsciences

Companion Website

Study on the Go

Use a mobile device to practice vocabulary terms, listen to pronunciations, and review with self-assessment quizzes.

www.m.g-wlearning.com

G-W Mobile

Bone as a Living Tissue

Before You Read

Try to answer the following questions before you read this lesson.

Do all bones have the same internal structure?

When and why do bones stop growing?

What practices can make bones stronger or weaker?

Lesson Objectives

1. Describe the functions of the skeletal system.
2. Identify the two types of bone tissue and explain the differences between them.
3. Describe the anatomical structure of a typical long bone.
4. Explain the processes through which bones grow in length and diameter during normal human development.
5. Discuss bone remodeling, including the cells responsible and the practices and environments that can dramatically influence remodeling.

Key Terms

E-Flash Cards

articular cartilage
bone marrow
cortical bone
diaphysis
epiphyseal plate
epiphysis
Haversian canals
Haversian system
hematopoiesis
lacunae
medullary cavity

ossification
osteoblasts
osteoclasts
osteocytes
osteon
perforating
  (Volkmann's) canals
periosteum
remodeling
trabecular bone

Functions of the Skeletal System

The approximately 206 individual bones comprising the human skeleton come in many different sizes and shapes, each uniquely well designed to serve a particular function. The skeletal system, in general, performs the following important functions.

Support

It's hard to imagine humans without bones because, like the wooden framework of a house, our bones form the internal support system that provides shape and support to our trunk and limbs. The bones in your legs enable you to stand upright, and your ribs support your chest cavity.

Protection

Our bones surround and support the body's delicate internal organs. For example, the ribs serve as bony protectors of critical organs such as the heart and lungs nestled in the thoracic cavity. Equally important, the skull provides protection for the brain, and the vertebral column surrounds and protects the delicate spinal cord.

Movement

What produces human movement? It is our muscles, which attach to bones. When muscles contract or shorten, they pull on the attached bones, thereby causing movement.

The design of the skeletal system, with bones able to rotate or glide in certain ways around joints, is extraordinarily functional. This amazing design enables walking, running, jumping, pushing, pulling, and throwing, as well as all of the routine activities that we take for granted every day.

A joint such as the shoulder allows movement in multiple directions, while movement at the knee is largely constrained to one direction. These movement capabilities are favorably designed for the ways in which we humans move. You will learn more about the muscles and how they work in the next chapter.

Storage

Bones also serve as a storage repository for minerals, notably phosphorous and calcium. Phosphorus plays a vital role in the development and maintenance of healthy bones and teeth, and it also plays a role in the chemical reactions that release energy from stored fat in the body. Calcium is essential for normal functioning of the neuromuscular system, as well as for blood clotting. Through a chemical balancing procedure known as homeostasis (HOH-mee-oh-STAY-sis), discussed in chapter 1, the body is able to draw upon the stored phosphorous or calcium in bone if the levels of these minerals in the bloodstream should fall below normal.

Another storage site in our skeletal system is the **medullary** (MEHD-oo-LAIR-ee) **cavity,** a central hollow space inside most of the long bones, such as those of the arms and legs. The medullary cavity is also known as the *marrow cavity* because it stores **bone marrow**, a specialized flexible tissue found inside bones.

There are two types of bone marrow—yellow and red. Both types contain a rich blood supply. Yellow marrow, found within the medullary cavity, is a major storehouse for fat within the body. Red marrow is found in the cavities of many bones, including flat and short bones, bodies of the vertebrae, sternum, ribs, and articulating ends of long bones.

Blood Cell Formation

It is in the red marrow that the critically important function of **hematopoiesis** (HEE-ma-toh-poy-EE-sis), or blood cell formation, occurs. As you will learn in chapter 8, our blood cells deliver oxygen to tissues throughout the body

and also transport waste in the form of carbon dioxide to the lungs, where it can be breathed out.

Check Your Understanding

1. List the five functions of the skeletal system.
2. What are two functions of bone marrow?

Structures and Classifications of Bones

The composition and structure of bone make it remarkably strong and resilient given its relatively light weight. Beyond this, bones assume very specialized shapes in accordance with their specific functions.

Composition of Bones

Cells are the structural building blocks of bone, as they are in other kinds of tissues in the body. **Osteocytes** are mature bone cells.

One factor that distinguishes bone from other tissues, however, is that 60–70% of bone weight comes from its mineral content—primarily calcium carbonate and calcium phosphate. The remaining 30–40% of bone weight comes from collagen, a protein that provides bone's flexibility, and water. Both the mineral and water content contribute to bone strength. The bones of children tend to be more flexible than the bones of adults due to higher collagen and water content.

Organization of Bones

Bone is structurally organized into two different types of tissue—cortical and trabecular bone. Whereas **cortical** (KOR-ti-kal) **bone** tissue is relatively dense, **trabecular** (tra-BEHK-yoo-lar) **bone** tissue, also known as *spongy* bone, is relatively porous, with a honeycomb structure (**Figure 4.1**). Cortical bone is stiffer due to its higher mineral content, so it is generally stronger than trabecular bone. Trabecular bone, with its spongy structure, is more flexible than cortical bone.

Figure 4.1 A micrograph of trabecular bone tissue. *How would you describe the difference between trabecular and cortical bone to someone who knew nothing about these two types of bone tissue?*

Memory Tip

The word *cortical* (coming from *cortex*) pertains to the outer layer of something. For example, the outer layer of the brain is known as the *cerebral cortex*. The outer layer of many structures and objects, including a plant stem or even a rock, is also known as its *cortex*. The type of bone tissue forming the outer layer of bone is therefore called *cortical* bone.

Shape Categories of Bones

Most bones include both cortical and trabecular tissue. The function of a given bone determines whether it is composed mostly of cortical or trabecular bone. The outer layer of a bone is always composed of hard, protective cortical bone, with spongy trabecular bone present to varying degrees in the interior of bones.

The long bones in the arms and legs are primarily composed of strong cortical bone tissue, although there is trabecular bone inside the ends. The bones in the spinal column contain a large amount of trabecular bone inside their cortical encasings, giving them a certain amount of shock-absorbing capability. **Figure 4.2** compares the properties of these two types of bone tissue.

Because of the large variety of sizes and shapes of the bones in the human skeleton, for purposes of discussion bones are traditionally divided into four categories (**Figure 4.3**):

1. *Long bones* have a long, somewhat round shaft made of cortical bone, with bulbous knobs of trabecular bone encased in cortical bone at both ends. The shafts enclose the central hollow medullary cavity or canal. The major bones of the arms and legs are long bones.
2. *Short bones* are shaped like a cube and are composed mainly of trabecular bone. The bones of the wrists and ankles are short bones.
3. *Flat bones* are thin, relatively large in surface area, and generally curved to some extent. Structurally, they consist of two thin layers of cortical bone with a layer of trabecular bone in between. These bones function to protect underlying organs and also provide

Figure 4.2 Properties of the Two Types of Bone Tissue		
	Cortical Bone	**Trabecular Bone**
Structure	dense	porous (honeycomb structure)
Mineral content	relatively high	relatively low
Strength	relatively high	low
Flexibility	low	relatively more
Shock-absorbing ability	low	relatively more
Primary locations	outer surface of all bones, long bones of limbs	interior of vertebrae, femoral neck, wrist, and ankle bones

Figure 4.3 The four shape categories of bones.

large areas for muscle attachments. The scapula (page 131) and the bones of the skull are considered flat bones.

4. *Irregular bones* are all those bones that do not fit into one of the preceding categories. They have individualized shapes to fulfill specific functions. The bones of the spinal column and hip girdle are in this category.

✔ Check Your Understanding

1. What percentage of bone weight comes from its mineral content?
2. What is collagen?
3. Where is cortical bone typically found?
4. Where is trabecular bone typically found?
5. List the four shape categories of bone.

Anatomical Structure of Long Bones

The **diaphysis** (digh-AF-i-sis) of a long bone is the hollow shaft of the bone composed of cortical bone (**Figure 4.4** on the next page). A fibrous connective tissue membrane called the **periosteum** (PER-ee-AHS-tee-um) surrounds and protects the diaphysis. The periosteum contains blood and lymph vessels, as well as nerves. It is involved in bone growth, repair, and nutrition.

The hollow center of the diaphysis, as discussed, is the medullary canal, or cavity. Beginning when a person is about five years old, this cavity is filled with yellow bone marrow, which has a rich supply of blood vessels and is a storehouse for fat. The medullary cavity is lined by a membrane known as the *endosteum* (ehn-DAHS-tee-um).

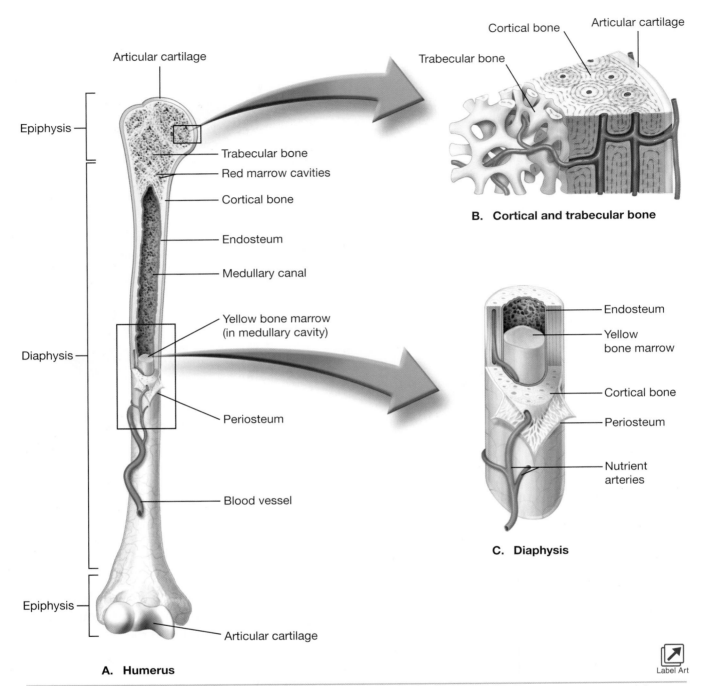

Figure 4.4 The anatomical structure of a long bone. A—Anterior view of the humerus with the interior of the top half exposed. B—Cortical and trabecular bone of the epiphysis. C—Enlargement of the diaphysis.

The bulbous endings of the long bones are known as **epiphyses** (eh-PIF-i-seez). These regions are composed of trabecular bone that contains red marrow, which participates in the formation of red blood cells, or erythrocytes (e-RITH-roh-sights), and some white blood cells, or leukocytes (LOO-koh-sights). Each epiphysis is surrounded by a protective covering of **articular** (ar-TIK-yoo-lar) **cartilage**. You may have noticed the shining white covering of articular cartilage over the ends of the bone in chicken drumsticks.

How does living bone receive nourishment and get rid of waste products? Bone has what you might think of as its own subway system. An intricate array of passageways exists at a microscopic level inside the mineralized part of bone. Blood vessels and nerves course through these tiny tunnels (**Figure 4.5**). Major passageways running in a lengthwise direction through the bone are called **Haversian** (ha-VER-zhen) **canals.** Tiny cavities called **lacunae** (la-KOO-nee) are laid out in concentric circles called *lamellae* (la-MEHL-ee) around the Haversian canals, and it is the lacunae that provide homes for the osteocytes.

Each Haversian canal, with its surrounding layers of lacunae, forms a structural unit called an **osteon**, or **Haversian system**. Within the system there are tiny sideways canals called *canaliculi* (kan-a-LIK-yoo-ligh). The canaliculi connect with the lacunae, forming a comprehensive transportation matrix for supply of nutrients and removal of waste products throughout the Haversian system. The multiple Haversian systems are joined by **perforating (Volkmann's) canals**, also running sideways, that interconnect the Haversian canals.

Growth and Development of Bones

Over the course of the lifespan from birth through old age, some parts of our bodies grow, while others tend to shrink. Knowledge of the processes by which bones grow and develop is the key to understanding why these phenomena occur.

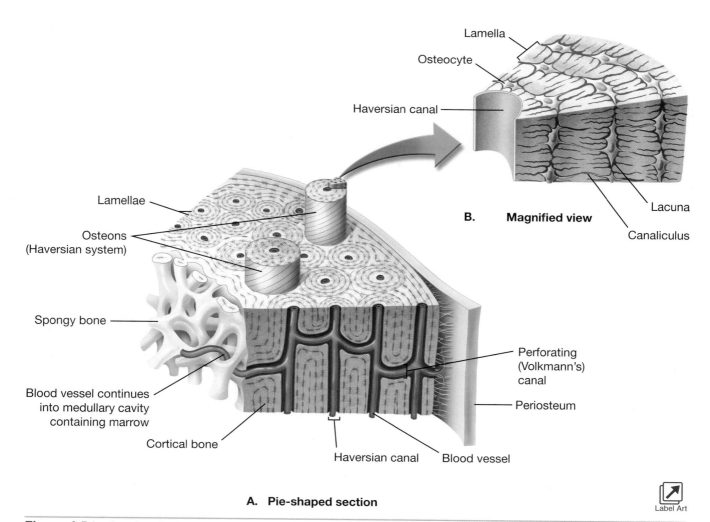

Figure 4.5 In drawing A above, you see a microscopic view of the inside of bone tissue; in B, you see an even more magnified view. *Why might someone compare the inside of living bone to a subway system?*

Osteoblasts and Osteoclasts

Specialized bone cells called **osteoblasts** (AHS-tee-oh-BLASTS) carry out the work of building new bone tissue. When there is a need to resorb or eliminate weakened or damaged bone tissue, that work is accomplished by other specialized cells called **osteoclasts** (AHS-tee-oh-KLASTS).

Bone growth clearly involves more osteoblast activity than osteoclast activity. However, both osteoblasts and osteoclasts remain extremely busy over the course of a normal person's life. In healthy adult bone, the activity of osteoblasts and osteoclasts is balanced. As a result of this balance, our bones stay strong and optimally designed for their various functions.

Memory Tip

Osteoblast and *osteoclast* are very similar-sounding names for these specialized bone cells. An easy way to avoid confusing them is to remember the "b" in *osteoblast* is the same as the "b" in *build*. Similarly, the "cl" in *osteoclast* is the same as the "cl" in *clear*. Osteoblasts *b*uild bone and osteoclasts *cl*ear away old or damaged bone.

Bone Formation

Bone *modeling* is the process in which new bone is created through osteoblast activity during the formation and growth of immature bones. The skeleton of early-developing embryos is composed mainly of a flexible tissue called *hyaline cartilage*. Although cartilage forms parts of the adult nose, ribs, and some joints, there is a rapid replacement of cartilage with bone even within the developing fetus.

The process of bone formation is called **ossification** (AHS-i-fi-KAY-shun). Before birth this occurs in two phases. During the first phase, a bone matrix shell covers the hyaline cartilage through the activity of osteoblasts. Next, osteoclasts resorb the enclosed hyaline cartilage, creating a medullary cavity within the bony superstructure.

Longitudinal Growth

Bones grow in length at the **epiphyseal** (EHP-i-FIZ-ee-al) **plates**, located close to the ends of long bones (**Figure 4.6**). During childhood growth, osteoblasts on the central side of the epiphyseal plate produce new bone cells, resulting in an increase in bone length. At the end of the growth period, occurring during or shortly after adolescence, the plate dissolves and the bone on either side of the plate fuses, effectively ending the longitudinal growth of the bone.

Circumferential Growth

Although most bone growth occurs during childhood, bones actually grow in diameter, or width, throughout most of life (**Figure 4.7**). Osteoblasts in the internal layer of the periosteum build concentric layers of new bone on top of existing ones. To understand the process, it helps to visualize the way in which the rings on a cross-cut tree stump reveal the tree's growth.

At the same time that the osteoblasts are doing their work, the osteoclasts resorb layers of bone inside the medullary cavity, causing the diameter of the cavity to be progressively enlarged. This beautifully engineered process occurs in such a way that a healthy bone remains optimally functional, lightweight, and strong enough to resist daily stresses.

Figure 4.6 Bones grow in length at the epiphyseal plates (the dark blue area). *When will this plate dissolve?*

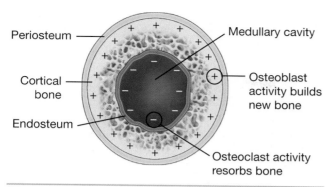

Figure 4.7 Cross section of a long bone showing normal bone throughout life. *Is it the circumference or the length of bones that continues to grow throughout life?*

Adult Bone Development

While osteoblast and osteoclast activity tends to maintain bones at functional sizes and shapes throughout life, age-related changes in the proportion of mineralized to nonmineralized bone do occur. As we age, there is a progressive loss of collagen (which provides elasticity) and an increase in bone brittleness. This means that children are often able to successfully sustain falls and other accidents without harm, while older adults tend to be increasingly vulnerable to bone fractures.

Bone mineral normally peaks in women at about 25 to 28 years of age and in men at about 30 to 35 years of age. Thereafter, bone mass is progressively lost. Because women tend to have smaller bones than men, the loss of bone mass and bone mineral density is generally more problematic for women.

 Check Your Understanding

1. What is the periosteum? Name at least three functions of the periosteum.
2. Where is the endosteum found? Is it inside or outside the periosteum?
3. What covers the ends of long bones?
4. Describe the functions of osteoblasts and osteoclasts.
5. Describe and analyze the effects of less elasticity on the body as people age.

Remodeling of Bones

As we have seen, bones grow and change dramatically during childhood and adolescence. Living adult bone is also a very active tissue, always changing at a microscopic level in bone mineral content (and thereby strength) and sometimes in size or shape. This occurs through osteoblast and osteoclast activity during a process called **remodeling**.

Forces, such as gravitational force, muscle forces, forces received when we push or pull on something, and impact forces when we bump into something, all influence our bones. The remodeling process converts the size and direction of the forces acting on bone to changes in bone mineral density. In some circumstances, the remodeling process also causes changes in the size or shape of bone.

Hypertrophy of Bones

Generally, when bone is subjected to larger (stronger) forces it tends to *hypertrophy* (high-PER-troh-fee), with increases in density and growth at the sites of force applications (often muscle attachments). As a result, the bones of people who are physically active are usually denser and stronger than the bones of people who are sedentary.

Because gravity is also a force that continuously acts on bones, people who are heavier tend to have greater bone mass and density than people who are lightweight for their heights. Dynamic activities such as running and jumping involve landing impacts, which cause motion of fluid within the bone matrix. This motion is particularly effective at triggering the actions of osteoblasts to build bone.

Altogether our bones account for only about 15% of body weight. This tends to be true whether a person is underweight, of average weight, or overweight. No one is overweight because of heavy bones, however. Being overweight is almost always the result of carrying excess body fat.

WHAT RESEARCH TELLS US

...*about* Physical Activity and Bones

There are many documented examples of bone remodeling, and hypertrophy, in response to regular physical activity. Sports that require repeated, forceful use of a certain limb promote not only muscle hypertrophy, but also bone hypertrophy, in the stressed area. For example, clinical case studies have shown increased bone mass, circumference, and mineralization in the dominant forearm of professional tennis players and in the dominant upper arm of baseball players.

It also appears that the larger the forces habitually encountered, the more dramatic the effect. In one interesting study, researchers measured the density of the femur among 64 nationally ranked athletes from different sports. The densest femurs were those of the weight lifters, followed by hammer and discus throwers, runners, soccer players, and swimmers. As you might expect from this research, the size of the regularly acting forces on the body is one factor that appears to be related directly to bone mass.

The other important factor contributing to increased bone mineral density is absorption of repeated impacts, such as those routinely encountered during

Pete Saloutos/Shutterstock.com

Figure 4.8 *Where would you expect this pitcher's bone mass to be greater than the average person's?*

running and landings from jumps. In an investigation involving collegiate female athletes, those participating in high-impact sports (basketball and volleyball) were found to have much higher bone mineral densities than the swimmers, with the soccer and track athletes having intermediate values. Another study compared the bone mineral densities of trained runners and cyclists to those of sedentary individuals of the same age. Not surprisingly, the runners were found to have increased bone density, but the cyclists did not.

On the whole, the evidence suggests that physical activity involving impact forces is necessary for maintaining or increasing bone mass. One need not be an athlete, however, to exercise for bone health—even vigorous walking generates bone-building impact forces.

Competitive swimmers, who spend a lot of time in the water where the buoyant force counteracts gravity, may have even less bone mineral density than that of sedentary individuals. It is important for competitive swimmers to also participate in activities such as weight training and running to maintain normal bone density.

Taking It Further

1. Explain in your own words the relationship between physical activity, bone remodeling, and hypertrophy.

2. Create a continuum, placing activities that negatively impact bone mass, such as swimming, on one end and those that increase bone mass (for example, basketball and volleyball) on the other end. Plot your daily activities on the continuum. Could you change your routine in a way that would increase your ability to build bone mass?

Atrophy of Bones

The opposite of what you just read about hypertrophy is also true. People who are subject to reduced forces are prone to bone *atrophy*, or loss of bone mineral density and strength. This has been observed, for example, in individuals who are bedridden for long periods of time.

Somewhat surprisingly, it has also been observed in elite swimmers who spend hours a day training in a swimming pool. Swimming involves a large amount of muscle activity, but the buoyancy of the water counteracts much of the force of gravity. So, while swimmers are in the water, their bones are subjected to greatly reduced stresses.

Loss of bone mass and strength is an even more significant problem for astronauts, who spend time completely out of the earth's gravitational field. The loss of bone in astronauts in space is so rapid that it is currently one of the major factors preventing a manned space mission to Mars.

 Check Your Understanding

1. What factors can cause bone to hypertrophy, increasing mass, density, and sometimes circumference?
2. What factors can cause bone to atrophy, losing mass and mineralization?

Lesson 4.1 Review and Assessment

Mini Glossary   Make sure that you know the meaning of each key term.

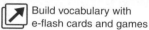 Build vocabulary with e-flash cards and games

articular cartilage   dense, white, connective tissue that covers the articulating surfaces of bones at joints

bone marrow   material with a rich blood supply found within the marrow cavity of long bones; yellow marrow stores fat, and red marrow is active in producing blood cells

cortical bone   dense, solid bone that covers the outer surface of all bones and is the main form of bone tissue in the long bones

diaphysis   the shaft of a long bone

epiphyseal plate   growth plate near the ends of long bones where osteoblast activity increases bone length

epiphysis   the bulbous end of a long bone

Haversian canals   major passageways running in the direction of the length

of long bones, providing paths for blood vessels

Haversian system   (also called an *osteon*) includes a single Haversian canal along with its multiple canaliculi, which branch out to join with lacunae, forming a comprehensive transportation matrix for supply of nutrients and removal of waste products

hematopoiesis   process of blood cell formation

lacunae   tiny cavities laid out in concentric circles around the Haversian canals

medullary cavity   central hollow in the long bones

ossification   process of bone formation

osteoblasts   specialized bone cells that build new bone tissue

osteoclasts   specialized bone cells that resorb bone tissue

osteocytes   mature bone cells

osteon   a Haversian system

perforating (Volkmann's) canals   large canals that connect the Haversian canals; also known as *perforating canals*; oriented across bones and perpendicular to Haversian canals

periosteum   fibrous connective tissue membrane that surrounds and protects the shaft (diaphysis) of long bones

remodeling   process through which adult bone can change in density, strength, and sometimes shape

trabecular bone   interior, spongy bone with a porous, honeycomb structure

Know and Understand

 Assess

1. List each of the five functions of the skeletal system and describe how they benefit the body.
2. Explain the differences between cortical bone and trabecular bone.
3. Describe where the diaphysis of a long bone is in relation to the epiphysis; the periosteum in relation to the endosteum.

Analyze and Apply

4. Compare and contrast osteoblasts and osteoclasts and explain how they work together to reshape and remodel bones.

5. Explain why a doctor would be worried about a child who broke a long bone close to the epiphyseal plate.

In the Lab

6. Before reading further in this chapter, make labels for all the bones that you can name. Quickly research the bones identified on your labels. Taking turns with your classmates, place your labels on the correct bones of the classroom skeleton and tell what category (long, short, flat, irregular) each bone belongs to.

The Axial Skeleton

Before You Read

Try to answer the following questions before you read this lesson.

Why is the skull composed of multiple bones?

Why is the spine curved instead of straight?

Lesson Objectives

1. Explain the ways in which the skull of an infant is similar to and different from an adult skull.

2. Identify the bones of the cranium and face and describe their locations.

3. Describe the structure of a typical vertebra and explain how the atlas, axis, and other cervical, thoracic, and lumbar vertebrae are specialized for their specific functions.

4. Identify and describe the normal spinal curves and the abnormal spinal curvatures that can develop.

5. Discuss the functional importance of the intervertebral discs, including which practices can help keep them healthy.

Key Terms

E-Flash Cards

atlas	mandible
axial skeleton	maxillary bones
axis	sacrum
cervical region	skull
coccyx	sternum
cranium	sutures
facial bones	thoracic cage
fontanel	thoracic region
intervertebral discs	vertebra
lumbar region	

Anatomists divide the body into the axis, consisting of the head and trunk, and the appendages—the arms and legs (**Figure 4.9**). Consequently, the major bones of the axis are known as the **axial skeleton**, which includes three major parts—the skull, vertebral (spinal) column, and thoracic cage. The axial skeleton is designed to provide stability to the core of the body. We will discuss the axial skeleton in this section. In lesson 4.3 we will learn about the appendicular skeleton.

The Skull

The 22 bones of the **skull** are divided into two groups: the cranial and the facial bones (**Figure 4.10**). The thin, curved bones of the **cranium** surround and protect the delicate brain. The round shape of the cranium is structurally strong in resisting impact forces and tends to absorb less force than if it were composed of flat surfaces. The **facial bones** protect the front of the head, give our faces their individual shapes, protect and orient the eyes, and allow chewing of food.

Most of the bones of the skull and face are joined together by irregularly shaped, interlocking, and immovable joints called **sutures**. A suture is a joint in which bones of the skull are bound together by strong, tiny fibers. The sutures permit a very small amount of movement, which contributes to the compliance (ability to change size and shape in response to force) and elasticity of the skull. The one exception is the mandible, or jaw bone, which is attached to the skull by a movable joint (for obvious reasons!)

The skull of a newborn infant is quite different from the adult skull. Compared to adults, babies have big heads relative to the size

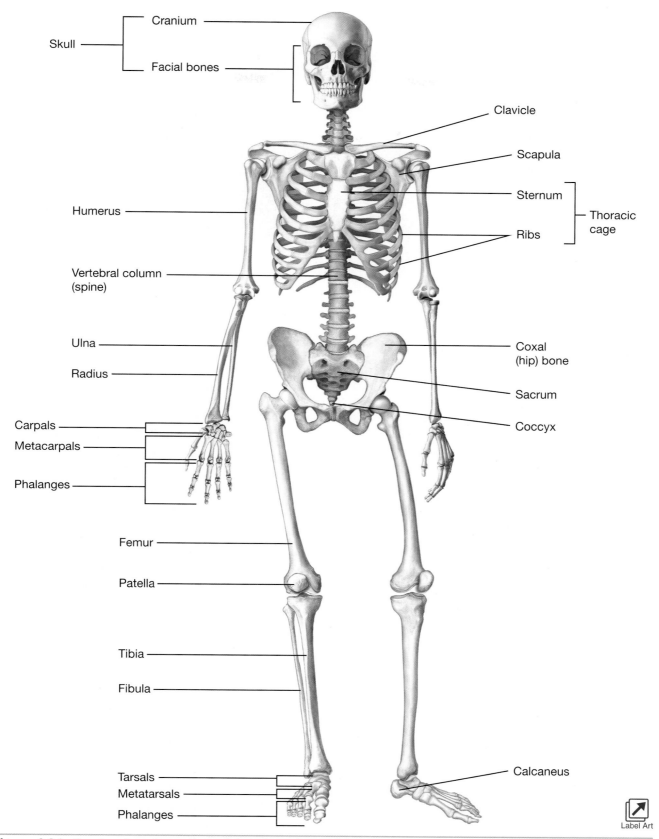

Figure 4.9 In the drawing above, the axial skeleton is a reddish color to distinguish it from the appendicular skeleton.

A. Side view

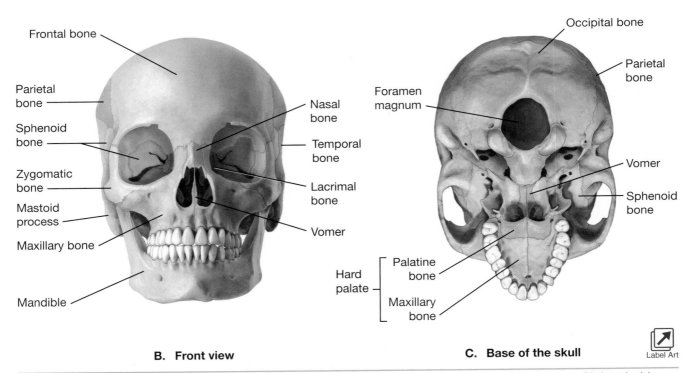

B. Front view

C. Base of the skull

Label Art

Figure 4.10 Bones of the skull. *How many bones go together to make up the skull? What type of joints hold these bones together?*

of their bodies. Whereas the skull of an adult accounts for about one-eighth of total body height, the skull of a newborn represents about one-fourth of body height.

As previously discussed, the skeletal system

of children includes regions of hyaline cartilage. The sutures of the skull in infants are composed of this soft, connective tissue, which will ossify (turn to bone) in early childhood. In regions of the infant skull where several bones join together, there are openings connected only by pockets of fibrous membranes. Because the baby's pulse can be felt through these "soft spots," they have been given the name **fontanel** (FAHN-ta-NEHL), which is French for "little fountain."

The soft sutures and fontanels serve two important functions. They enable some compression of the skull (the largest part of the body) during birth. Equally important, they enable brain growth during late pregnancy and early infancy. The fontanels ossify to bone by 22 to 24 months following birth.

The Cranium

The cranium includes eight bones. There are two sets of paired (left and right side) bones; the rest are single bones. Following is a list of the bones making up the cranium.

- the *frontal bone*, which forms the forehead;
- the two paired *parietal* (pah-RIGH-eh-tal) *bones*, which form the majority of the top and sides of the skull;
- the two paired *temporal* (TEHM-poh-ral) *bones*, which surround the ears;
- the *occipital* (ahk-SIP-i-tal) *bone*, which forms the base and lower back portions of the skull;
- the *ethmoid* (EHTH-moyd) *bone*, which forms part of the nasal septum; and
- the *sphenoid* (SFEE-noyd) *bone*, which is butterfly shaped and centrally located within the skull. The sphenoid bone supports part of the base of the brain, forms part of the orbits of the eyes, and is connected to all of the other bones of the skull.

The Facial Bones

A total of fourteen bones form the face, including the mandible (MAN-di-buhl), *vomer* (VOH-mer), and six pairs (left and right) of bones. The facial bones include

- the two fused **maxillary** (MAK-si-lair-ee) **bones**, which form the upper jaw, house the upper teeth, and connect to all other bones of the face, with the exception of the mandible;
- the two *palatine* (PAL-a-tighn) *bones*, which form the posterior part of the hard palate, or roof of the mouth;
- the two *zygomatic* (ZIGH-goh-MAT-ik) *bones*, or cheekbones, which also form much of the sides of the orbits, or eye sockets;
- the two *lacrimal* (LAK-ri-mal) *bones*, tiny bones connecting to the orbits and surrounding the tear ducts;
- the two *nasal bones*, forming the bridge of the nose;
- the vomer (plow-shaped) bone, comprising most of the bony nasal septum;
- the two *inferior concha* (KAHN-ka) *bones*, forming the sides of the nasal cavity; and
- the **mandible**, or lower jaw bone, which is the largest facial bone, as well as the only movable facial bone.

✔ Check Your Understanding

1. Scientists often divide the human skeleton into two parts. What are these parts called?
2. Which bones make up the axial skeleton?
3. What holds the bones of the skull together? Is movement possible at these joints? Why is this important?
4. List the two functions of the fontanels in a baby's skull.
5. List the eight cranial bones and tell where each is found.
6. List the fourteen facial bones and tell where each is found.

The Vertebral Column (Spine)

Although the word *spine* suggests a straight, rigid bar, the human spine, or vertebral column, is anything but straight and rigid. The human spinal column is well designed to perform its functions of protecting the extremely delicate spinal cord, while supporting the weight of the trunk and allowing flexibility in multiple directions.

Thirty-three stacked, individual bones called **vertebrae** (VER-teh-bray) comprise the spine. The vertebrae differ in size and shape in the different regions of the spine to best fulfill their respective functions (**Figure 4.11**).

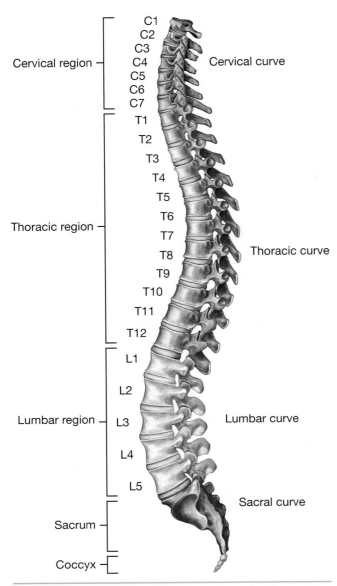

Figure 4.11 The vertebral column (spine). *How many bones make up the sacrum? the coccyx? How do these bones differ from the bones of the other three regions of the vertebral column?*

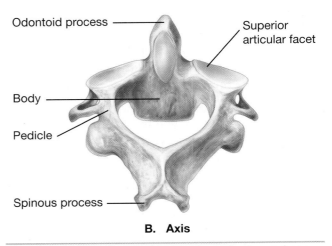

Figure 4.12 The first and second cervical vertebrae, the atlas and the axis.

Regions of the Spine

There are five named sections of the spine:

1. The **cervical** (SER-vi-kal) **region** (or neck) includes the upper seven vertebrae that enable nodding the head up and down, as well as rotation to the right and left. The first cervical vertebra, the **atlas**, is specialized to provide the connection between the occipital bone of the skull and the spinal column (**Figure 4.12**). The second cervical vertebra, the **axis**, is also specialized, with an upward projection called the *odontoid process*, on which the atlas rotates.

2. The **thoracic** (thoh-RAS-ik) **region** encompasses the next 12 vertebrae, which extend through the chest region and articulate (connect) with the ribs.

3. The **lumbar** (LUM-bar) **region** includes the 5 vertebrae found in the lower back.

4. The **sacrum** (SAY-krum) consists of 5 fused vertebrae that form the posterior portion of the pelvic girdle.

5. The **coccyx** (KAHK-siks), or tailbone, located at the bottom of the spine, includes 4 fused vertebrae.

Structures of the Vertebrae

Although no two vertebrae are exactly alike, most of the vertebrae have several structural features in common (**Figure 4.13**):

- The *vertebral body* is the thick, disc-shaped portion that bears weight and forms the anterior portion of the vertebra.
- The *vertebral* (VER-teh-bral) *arch* is the round projection of bone on the posterior aspect of the vertebra. It surrounds a hole known as the *vertebral foramen* (foh-RAY-mehn), through which the spinal cord passes.
- The *transverse processes* are bony projections on the lateral sides of the vertebral arch.
- The *spinous process* is a bony projection that extends posteriorly.
- The *superior* and *inferior articular processes* are indentations or facets where a vertebra articulates, or joins, with the vertebrae immediately above and below. These articulations are called *facet* (FAS-eht) *joints.*

There is a progressive increase in vertebral size from the cervical region down through the lumbar region (**Figure 4.14** on the next page). This gradual size increase serves a functional purpose.

When the body is in an upright position, each vertebra must support the weight of all of the body parts positioned above it. Think about what this means. While a cervical vertebra supports only the weight of the head and neck, a lumbar vertebra supports the weight of the head, neck, arms, and all of the trunk positioned above that vertebra.

The size and angulation of the vertebral processes also vary throughout the spinal column. This changes the orientation of the facet joints, which interconnect the vertebrae and serve to limit range of motion in the different spinal regions.

The Spinal Curves

The characteristic shapes of the vertebrae in the different spinal regions also form the normal spinal curves. As **Figure 4.11** shows, the cervical and lumbar curves are posteriorly concave, while the thoracic, sacral, and coccyx curvatures are anteriorly concave. These alternating curves make the spine stronger and better able to resist potentially injurious forces than if it were straight.

The thoracic and sacral curves are known as *primary spinal curves* because they are present at

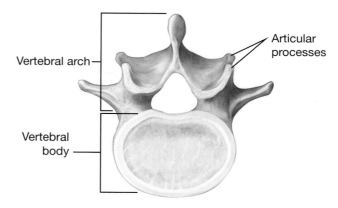

A. The major components of a typical vertebra (superior view)

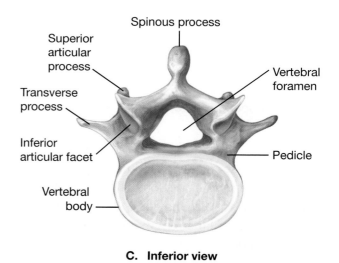

B. Lateral and slightly inferior view

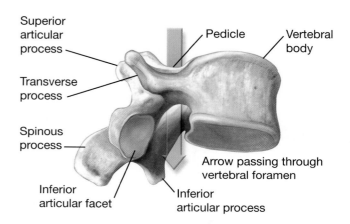

C. Inferior view

Figure 4.13 Three views of a typical vertebra. *What are the names of the indentations on the articular processes?*

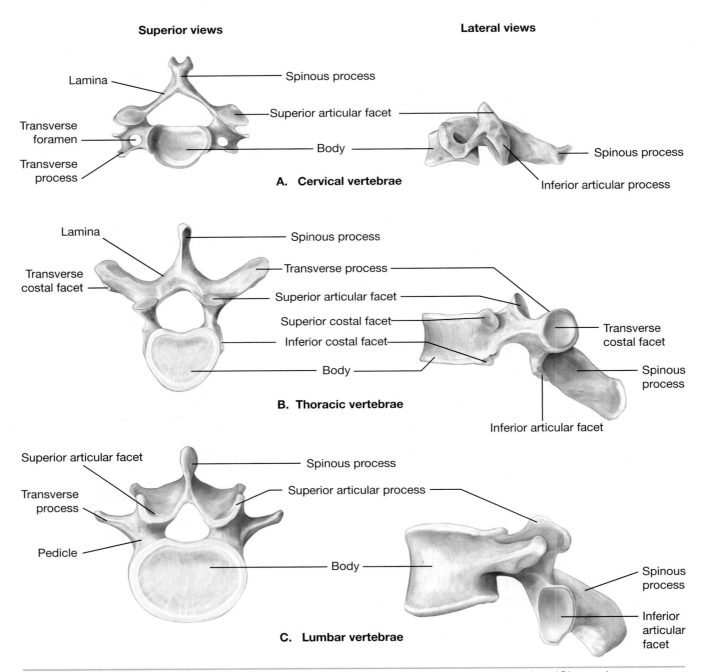

Superior views

Lateral views

Lamina

Spinous process

Superior articular facet

Transverse foramen

Body

Spinous process

Transverse process

A. Cervical vertebrae

Inferior articular process

Lamina

Spinous process

Transverse process

Transverse costal facet

Superior articular facet

Superior costal facet

Transverse costal facet

Inferior costal facet

Body

Spinous process

B. Thoracic vertebrae

Inferior articular facet

Superior articular facet

Spinous process

Transverse process

Superior articular process

Pedicle

Body

Spinous process

Inferior articular facet

C. Lumbar vertebrae

Figure 4.14 Superior and left lateral views of typical cervical (A), thoracic (B), and lumbar (C) vertebrae.

birth. The lumbar and cervical curves are referred to as *secondary spinal curves*. They develop after the baby begins to raise the head, sit, and stand, as increased muscular strength enables the young child to shift body weight to the spine.

Abnormal spinal curvatures can develop due to genetic or congenital abnormalities or when the spine is habitually subjected to asymmetrical forces (**Figure 4.15**). Exaggeration of the lumbar curve is termed *lordosis* (lor-DOH-sis), accentuation of the thoracic curve is called *kyphosis* (kigh-FOH-sis), and any lateral deviation of the spine is known as *scoliosis* (SKOH-lee-OH-sis).

The Intervertebral Discs

Intervertebral (IN-ter-VER-teh-bral) **discs** composed of fibrocartilage provide cushioning between all of the articulating vertebral

Exaggerated lumbar curve —

Accentuated thoracic curve —

Lateral deviation of spine

A. Lordosis

B. Kyphosis

C. Scoliosis

Figure 4.15 Three types of abnormal spinal curvature. *What are some causes of abnormal curvature?*

bodies that are not fused. These discs serve as shock absorbers and allow the spine to bend. The differences in the anterior and posterior thicknesses of these discs produce the normal cervical, thoracic, and lumbar curves.

In a normal adult, the discs account for approximately one-quarter of the height of the spine. When a person is lying in bed during overnight sleep, the discs absorb water and expand slightly. During periods of upright standing and sitting, when the discs are bearing weight, they lose a small amount of fluid and are compressed. For this reason, people are as much as three-fourths of an inch taller when they first arise in the morning. Injury and progressive aging reduce the water retention capability of the discs, accounting for diminished standing height in elderly individuals.

Because the discs receive no blood supply, they must rely upon changes in posture and body position to produce a pumping action that brings in nutrients and flushes out metabolic waste products with an influx and outflux of fluid. Because maintaining a fixed body position curtails this pumping action, sitting in one

position for a long period of time can negatively affect disc health.

 Check Your Understanding

1. List the five regions of the vertebral column, from upper to lower.
2. What is the functional purpose of the vertebrae increasing in size from the cervical region down to the lumbar region?
3. What is the function of the intervertebral discs?

The Thoracic Cage (Bony Thorax)

The ribs, sternum, and thoracic vertebrae are collectively known as the **thoracic cage**. Why are these bones given this name? It is because together they form a protective, bony "cage" that surrounds the heart and lungs in the thoracic cavity, as shown in **Figure 4.16**. You can also see this in **Figure 11.1.** The breastbone, or **sternum** (STER-num), includes three regions:

- The *manubrium* (ma-NOO-bree-um) is the upper portion of the sternum. It has articulations to the left and right bones of the clavicle, or collarbone, as well as to the first and second ribs.
- The remainder of the bony portion of the sternum is often referred to as the *body* of the sternum.
- At the lower end of the sternum is a projection called the *xiphoid* (ZIGH-foyd) *process*.

There are 12 pairs of ribs in the thoracic cage, as shown in **Figure 4.16**.

- The first 7 pairs (1–7) attach directly to the sternum and are, therefore, called *true ribs*.
- The next 3 pairs of ribs (8–10) are called *false ribs* because they have cartilaginous (KAR-ti-LAJ-i-nuhs) attachments to the cartilage of the seventh rib, rather than attaching directly to the sternum.
- The lowest 2 pairs of ribs (11–12) are known as *floating ribs*, because they do not attach to bone or cartilage in front of the body.

 Check Your Understanding

1. Which bones make up the thoracic cage?
2. List the three regions of the sternum.
3. How many pairs of ribs are in the thoracic cage?
4. How many ribs do *not* attach directly to the sternum?

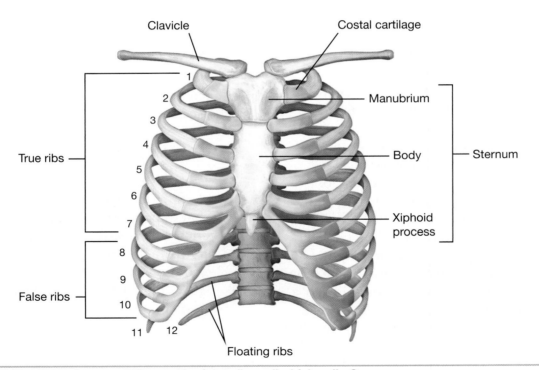

Figure 4.16 The thoracic cage. *Why are the false ribs called false ribs?*

Lesson 4.2 Review and Assessment

Mini Glossary   Make sure that you know the meaning of each key term.

 Build vocabulary with e-flash cards and games

atlas   the first cervical vertebra; specialized to provide the connection between the occipital bone of the skull and the spinal column

axial skeleton   central, stable portion of the skeletal system, consisting of the skull, spinal column, and thoracic cage

axis   the second cervical vertebra; specialized with an upward projection called the *odontoid process*, on which the atlas rotates

cervical region   the first 7 vertebrae, comprising the neck

coccyx   4 fused vertebrae at the base of the spine forming the tailbone

cranium   fused, flat bones surrounding the back of the head

facial bones   bones of the face

fontanel   openings in the infant skull through which the baby's pulse can be felt; these openings enable compression of the skull during birth and brain growth during late pregnancy and early infancy

intervertebral discs   fibrocartilaginous cushions between vertebral bodies that allow bending of the spine and help to create the normal spinal curves

lumbar region   low back region of the spine composed of 5 vertebrae

mandible   jaw bone

maxillary bones   two fused bones that form the upper jaw, house the upper teeth, and connect to all other bones of the face, with the exception of the mandible

sacrum   five fused vertebrae that form the posterior of the pelvic girdle

skull   the part of the skeleton composed of all of the bones of the head

sternum   breastbone

sutures   joints in which irregularly grooved, articulating bone sheets join closely and are tightly connected by fibrous tissues

thoracic cage   bony structure surrounding the heart and lungs in the thoracic cavity; composed of the ribs, sternum, and thoracic vertebrae

thoracic region   the 12 vertebrae in the middle of the back

vertebra   one of the bones making up the spinal column

Know and Understand

 Assess

1. Explain the function of the axial skeleton and which bones are included in it.

2. The bones of the skull are often divided into two groups. Name those two groups.

3. Describe how sutures and fontanels relate to each other.

4. List the five named sections of the spine and tell how many vertebrae are included in each of these sections.

5. Name at least five structural features common to most vertabrae.

6. Which bone of the skull is freely movable?

Analyze and Apply

7. Why is it important to protect and cradle a baby's head when you are holding the baby?

8. Compare and contrast the conditions of lordosis, kyphosis, and scoliosis.

9. How does the structure of an intervertebral disc (made of fibrocartilage) relate to its function (acting as a shock absorber and allowing the spine to bend)?

10. Explain the different ways in which ribs are attached to the sternum.

11. What are the primary and secondary spinal curves? Explain why and distinguish between them.

In the Lab

12. Using different colors of clay, construct a model of the axial skeleton. Be sure to label all of the bones included. You will add to this skeleton in a later section in this chapter.

The Appendicular Skeleton

Lesson Objectives

1. Discuss the joints of the shoulder girdle, including the names of the articulating bones, their locations, and their functions.
2. Identify the bones and joints of the arm and describe their motions.
3. Identify the bones of the pelvis and explain their functions.
4. Identify the bones and joints of the leg and describe their motions.
5. Discuss the structure of the ankle and foot, including the names of the joints, their locations, and their functions.

Key Terms

E-Flash Cards

appendicular skeleton	pelvis
carpal bones	phalanges
clavicle	radius
femur	scapula
fibula	shoulder complex
humerus	shoulder girdle
lower extremity	tarsals
metacarpals	tibia
metatarsals	ulna
patella	upper extremity

The **appendicular skeleton**, as the name suggests, includes the body's appendages. These include both the bones of the **upper extremity** (the shoulder complex, arms, wrists, and hands) and those of the **lower extremity** (the pelvic girdle, legs, ankles, and feet). Altogether, there are approximately 126 bones in the appendicular skeleton. The appendicular skeleton is built for motion.

The Upper Extremity

The upper extremity is well designed for all of the tasks that we routinely ask it to perform. The muscles, bones, and joints of the upper extremity enable movements as diverse as carrying a load, throwing a ball, and threading a needle. The different movements of hammering a nail, texting on a cell phone, and performing a handspring are also made possible by this unique design.

The Shoulder Complex

The bones surrounding the shoulder are referred to as the **shoulder girdle**, or *pectoral* (PEHK-toh-ral) *girdle*, and include the left and right **clavicles**, or collarbones, and a left and right **scapula** (SKAP-yoo-la), or shoulder blade (**Figure 4.17**). These bones serve as sites for attachment of the numerous muscles that enable motion of the arms at the shoulders in so many different directions.

As **Figure 4.18** shows, there are two bony projections on the scapula, known as the *acromion* (a-KROH-mee-ahn) and the *coracoid* (KOR-a-koyd) *process.* The lateral end of the clavicle attaches to the acromion process to form the *acromioclavicular* (a-KROH-mee-oh-kla-VIK-yoo-lar) *joint* (**Figure 4.17**). The medial end of the clavicle

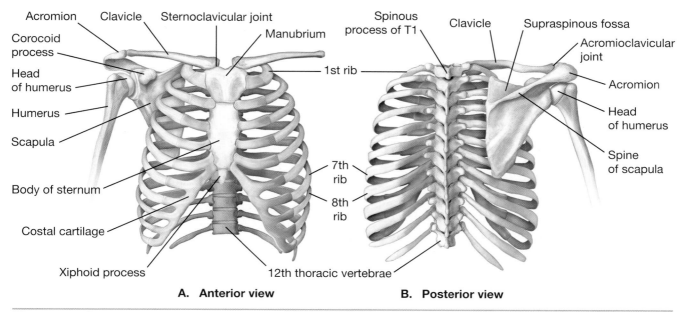

Figure 4.17 Anterior and posterior views of the shoulder girdle, ribs, and humerus.

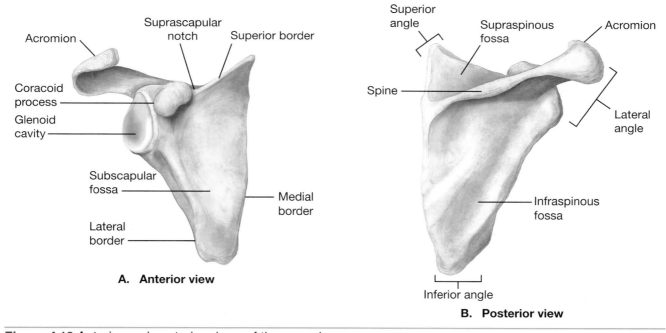

Figure 4.18 Anterior and posterior views of the scapula.

attaches to the sternum to form the *sternoclavicular* (STER-noh-kla-VIK-yoo-lar) *joint*.

The acromioclavicular joint primarily allows you to raise your arm so that you can perform movements overhead. The sternoclavicular joint enables you to move your clavicle and scapula for motions such as shrugging the shoulders, raising your arms, and swimming.

As **Figures 4.17** and **4.18** show, the clavicle serves as a brace for positioning the shoulder laterally away from the trunk. Although there are no bony articulations between the scapulae and the posterior aspect of the trunk, the region between each scapula and the underlying tissues is sometimes referred to as the *scapulothoracic* (skap-yoo-loh-thoh-RAS-ik) *joint*.

The *glenoid* (GLEE-noyd) *fossa* of the scapula is a relatively shallow indentation that articulates, or joins, with the head of the **humerus** (HYOO-mer-us), the bone in the upper arm, to form the *glenohumeral joint*, or shoulder joint. Because the glenoid fossa (socket) is less curved than the humeral head, the humerus is able to glide against the glenoid fossa, in addition to rotating. As a result, the glenohumeral joint allows motion in more directions than any other joint in the body.

The glenohumeral joint, along with the bones and joints of the shoulder girdle, are referred to as the **shoulder complex**. Together these joints provide the significant range of motion present in a healthy shoulder. This large degree of mobility, however, comes at the cost of instability: the shoulder is one of the most frequently dislocated joints in the human body. **Figure 4.19** summarizes the joints of the shoulder complex.

The Arm

The single bone of the upper arm is the humerus (**Figure 4.20**). The humerus is a large, strong bone, second in size only to the major bone of the upper leg. The upper end of the humerus forms a rounded head, which, as mentioned, articulates with the glenoid fossa of the scapula to form the glenohumeral joint.

As **Figure 4.21** shows, the framework for the forearm consists of two bones—the **radius** (RAY-dee-us) and **ulna** (UHL-nuh). The radius is the bone that articulates with the wrist on the thumb side. The name *radius* comes from the ability of this bone to "radially" rotate around the ulna. This radial rotation is the familiar motion that enables the forearm and hand to freely rotate.

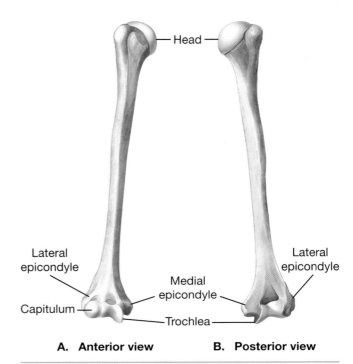

Figure 4.20 Anterior and posterior views of the humerus.

The ulna is larger and stronger than the radius, and it articulates with the humerus at the humeroulnar joint (elbow). The ulna attaches to the wrist on the "little finger" side. The bony projection at the upper end of the ulna, called the *olecranon* (oh-LEHK-ra-nahn) *process*, is what we refer to as the *elbow*.

The radius and ulna are connected along their entire lengths by an *interosseus* (IN-ter-AHS-ee-us) *membrane*. The two bones articulate at both ends, and these joints are known as the *proximal* and *distal radioulnar* (RAY-dee-oh-UHL-nar) *joints*.

At the distal (lower) ends of both the radius and ulna are *styloid* (STIGH-loyd) *processes* that

Figure 4.19 Articulating Bones of the Shoulder Complex		
Joint	*Notched Bone*	*Joining Bone or Region*
acromioclavicular joint	acromion of the scapula	clavicle
sternoclavicular joint	sternum	clavicle
scapulothoracic joint	scapula	thorax
glenohumeral (shoulder) joint	glenoid fossa of the scapula	humerus

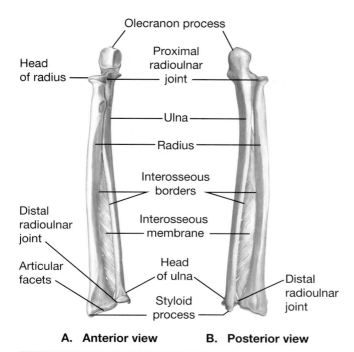

A. **Anterior view**   B. **Posterior view**

Figure 4.21 Anterior and posterior views of the radius and ulna. *Which of these two bones allows your forearm and hand to rotate freely?*

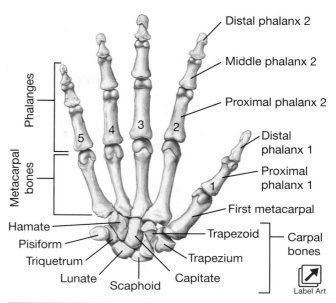

Figure 4.23 Anterior view of the bones of the right hand. *Look ahead to Figure 4.28, which shows the bones of the right foot. Describe at least two similarities and two differences between the bones of the hand and the foot.*

are easy to see and feel with your fingers. The distal end of the radius unites with several of the carpal bones of the wrist to form the *radiocarpal* (RAY-dee-oh-KAR-pal) *joint* (**Figure 4.22**).

The Wrist and Hand

Collectively, there are 54 bones in the wrists and hands—27 on the left and 27 on the right. This large number of bones enables a wide range of precise movements along with the important ability to grasp objects.

As **Figure 4.23** shows, the wrist includes eight **carpal** (KAR-pal) **bones** that are roughly arranged in two rows. The carpal bones are

bound together by ligaments that allow a small amount of gliding motion at the intercarpal joints. However, the main function of the carpals is to provide a base for the bones of the hand.

Five **metacarpal** (meht-a-KAR-pal) **bones** in each hand articulate with the carpal bones within each wrist. The **phalanges** (fa-LAN-jeez)—or fingers—consist of 14 bones. Each of the four fingers has proximal, medial, and distal phalanges, but the thumb has only two.

Whereas the joints of the fingers permit motion in only one plane, the thumb has the ability to freely rotate and to stretch across the palm of the hand. This capability, known as an *opposable thumb*, is shared only by humans and other primates.

Figure 4.22 Articulating Bones of the Arm and Wrist		
Joint	*Notched Bone*	*Joining Bone*
humeroulnar (elbow) joint	humerus	ulna
radioulnar joints (proximal and distal)	radius	ulna
radiocarpal (wrist) joint	radius	three carpal bones

Check Your Understanding

1. Which bones make up the appendicular skeleton?
2. Which bones are included in the shoulder complex?
3. Which forearm bone enables rotation of the hand around the longitudinal axis of the arm?
4. How many bones are in each wrist and hand?

The Lower Extremity

The lower extremity is well designed for its functions of weight bearing and gait, including walking and running. During sporting activities the muscles, bones, and joints of the lower extremity also enable movements involved in jumping, skating, surfing, skiing, and dancing, for example.

The Pelvic Girdle

As the name suggests, the *pelvic* (PEHL-vik) *girdle* is a bony encasement of the pelvic region that shelters the reproductive organs, bladder, and part of the large intestine. It is formed by two large, strong *coxal* (KAHK-sal) *bones* (hip bones) and the sacrum (**Figure 4.24**). These three bones, with the addition of the coccyx, comprise the **pelvis**. The female pelvis is wider than the male pelvis to enable pregnancy and childbirth. The pelvis is one of the hallmark differences that allows classification of a skeleton as male or female.

Each coxal bone is formed by the fusion of the ilium, ischium, and pubis. During childhood these are three separate bones.

The *ilium* (IL-ee-um) comprises most of each coxal bone, connecting posteriorly to the sacrum at the *sacroiliac* (SA-kroh-IL-ee-ak) *joint*. The prominent upper edge of the ilium, which can usually be palpated (examined or felt by touch), is called the *iliac crest*.

The *ischium* (IS-kee-um), forming the inferior (lowest) portion of each coxal bone, is the bone that supports the weight of the upper body during sitting. Within each coxal bone lies an *acetabulum* (as-eh-TAB-yoo-lum), a deep, bony socket that receives the head of the thigh bone.

The *pubis* (PYOO-bis) is the anterior (front) portion of each coxal bone. The two pubic bones fuse in the center front of the body at the *pubis symphysis* (SIM-fi-sis), where the bones are joined by a disc of hyaline cartilage.

A. Pelvis

B. Coxal bone, right lateral view

Figure 4.24 Bones of the pelvis. *Why are these bones important when classifying skeletons?*

The Leg

The single bone of the upper leg, or thigh, is the **femur** (FEE-mer), which is the longest and strongest bone in the body. **Figure 4.25** shows the anatomical features of the femur. The head of the femur fits snugly into the acetabulum of the hip, making the joint extremely stable. The most vulnerable part of the femur is the neck, the site where hip fractures occur.

The lower leg has two bones: the tibia and fibula **(Figure 4.26)**. The thick, strong **tibia** (TIB-ee-a)—or shinbone—is the bone that bears most of the weight of the body above it.

Unlike the radius in the forearm, the **fibula** (FIB-yoo-la) has no special motion capability and serves primarily as a site for muscle attachments. The fibula is not part of the articulation with the femur at the knee joint, but the distal (lower) end of the fibula has a bony prominence called the *lateral malleolus* (mal-LEE-oh-lus), which you can readily touch and feel on the lateral (outer) side of the ankle.

Like the radius and ulna in the forearm, the tibia and fibula are connected along their lengths by an interosseous membrane, and they articulate at both ends of the fibula. The **patella** (pa-TEHL-a), or kneecap, is a small, flat, triangular-shaped bone that protects the front of the knee **(Figure 4.27)**.

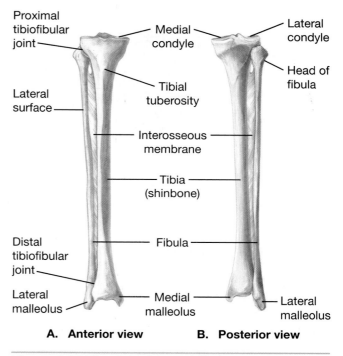

A. Anterior view **B. Posterior view**

Figure 4.26 The right tibia and fibula, anterior and posterior views.

Figure 4.25 The right femur and the patella. *Although the femur is the strongest bone in the body, one part is vulnerable to fracture. What is the most vulnerable part of the femur?*

Figure 4.27 Articulating Bones of the Leg and Ankle		
Joint	*Notched Bone or Socket*	*Joining Bone or Region*
iliofemoral (hip) joint	acetabulum	femur
tibiofemoral (knee) joint	tibia	femur
patellofemoral joint	patella	anterior knee
tibiofibular joints (proximal and distal)	tibia	fibula

Distal phalanx 1

Proximal phalanx 1

Distal phalanx 5

Middle phalanx 5

Proximal phalanx 5

Metatarsal

Medial cuneiform

Intermediate cuneiform

Lateral cuneiform

Navicular

Cuboid

Talus

Trochlear surface
of talus

Calcaneus

Tuberosity of calcaneus

Phalanges

Head

Body

Base

Metatarsal
bones

Tarsal bones

A. Superior view   **B. Inferior view**

Figure 4.28 Superior and inferior views of the bones of the right foot.

The Ankle and Foot

The ankle and foot serve the critically important functions of supporting body weight and enabling locomotion. The foot is so well designed that it assists with walking and running by acting like a spring that stores and releases energy.

As **Figure 4.28** shows, the hindfoot is constructed of **tarsal** (TAR-sal) **bones**, with the two largest, the *talus* (TAY-lus) and *calcaneus* (kal-KAY-nee-us)—or heel bone—bearing most of the weight of the body. The five **metatarsals** (meht-a-TAR-salz) that support the midfoot region are similar to the metacarpals of the hand. Like the fingers, each toe is comprised of three phalanges, and like the thumb, the big toe has only two phalanges. The toes function by increasing the area of the foot during weight-bearing activities such as walking and running—thereby increasing body stability.

The configuration of the metatarsal bones forms two important arches (**Figure 4.29**).

Medial
longitudinal arch

Transverse arch

Lateral
longitudinal arch

Figure 4.29 Arches of the foot, inferior view. *How do these arches contribute to our ability to walk with a smooth, easy gait?*

The *longitudinal arch* runs lengthwise from the calcaneus to the heads of the metatarsals. The *transverse arch* runs sideways (perpendicular to the longitudinal arch), and in most people causes the medial (inside) center of the bottom of the foot to be slightly elevated. It is these arches that compress somewhat during the weight-bearing phase of your gait, but then act as springs when they rebound to their original shape during the propulsive (push-off) phase of the gait.

 Check Your Understanding

1. Which bones make up the pelvic girdle?
2. Which three bones fuse to form each coxal bone?
3. What is the longest and strongest bone in the body?
4. Although relatively small bones, the bones of the toes serve what important function?

Lesson 4.3 Review and Assessment

Mini Glossary   Make sure that you know the meaning of each key term.

 Build vocabulary with e-flash cards and games

appendicular skeleton   the bones of the body's appendages; the arms and legs

carpal bones   bones of the wrist

clavicle   doubly curved long bone that forms part of the shoulder girdle; the collarbone

femur   thigh bone

fibula   bone of the lower leg; does not bear weight

humerus   major bone of the upper arm

lower extremity   bones of the hips, legs, and feet

metacarpals   the five interior bones of the hand, connecting the carpals in the wrist to the phalanges in the fingers

metatarsals   small bones of the ankle

patella   kneecap

pelvis   bones of the pelvic girdle and the coccyx at the base of the spine

phalanges   bones of the fingers

radius   smaller of the two bones in the forearm; rotates around the ulna

scapula   shoulder blade

shoulder complex   all joints surrounding the shoulder,

including the acromioclavicular, sternoclavicular, and glenohumeral joints

shoulder girdle   bones surrounding the shoulder, including the clavicle and scapula

tarsals   bones of the ankle

tibia   major weight-bearing bone of the lower leg

ulna   larger bone of the lower arm

upper extremity   bones of the shoulders, arms, and hands

Know and Understand

 Assess

1. Explain how the bones of the pectoral girdle, along with various muscles and joints, allow movement in many different directions.
2. Which bone of the forearm, the radius or the ulna, is larger and stronger than the other?
3. Why is the pelvis of a female wider than the pelvis of a male?
4. Which bone of the lower leg, the tibia or the fibula, is the stronger bone that bears most of the weight of the body above it?

Analyze and Apply

5. Functionally, why does the pectoral girdle have much more range of motion than the pelvic girdle?

6. Why are there two bones in the forearm rather than just one?
7. Why would you not be able to walk properly if you had a fracture in one of the metatarsals or phalanges?

In the Lab

8. Using different colors of clay, construct a model of the appendicular skeleton, labeling all of the bones included. Attach your appendicular skeleton to the axial skeleton you constructed in lesson 4.2.

Lesson 4.4 Joints

Before You Read

Try to answer the following questions before you read this lesson.

Why do some joints permit little to no movement?

How do joints avoid damage from frictional wear over time?

Lesson Objectives

1. Describe the general structures and functions of the three major categories of joints.
2. Identify several examples of each of the three major categories of joints.
3. Identify and explain the functions of the six types of diarthrodial joints.
4. Discuss the ways in which joint structure governs movement capability.
5. Describe and explain the functions of joint-related structures, including tendons, ligaments, bursae, and articular cartilage.

Key Terms

E-Flash Cards

amphiarthrosis
articular fibrocartilage
ball-and-socket joint
bursae
condyloid joint
diarthrosis
gliding joint
hinge joint
ligament

pivot joint
saddle joint
symphysis
synarthrosis
synchondrosis
syndesmosis
synovial joint
tendon
tendon sheath

The joints of the human body govern the extent and directions of movement of the bones that articulate (come together) at the joint. Although the range of motion at a given joint is affected by the tightness of the soft tissues crossing that joint, it is the structure of the bony articulation that determines the directions of motion permitted.

Anatomists classify joints in different ways based on joint complexity, the number of axes present, joint structure, and joint function. Joint function determines movement capability and is the most easily remembered; therefore, this classification is used in this section.

There are three main categories of joints with regard to function: the immovable joints, the slightly movable joints, and the freely movable joints. Most of the joints of the body appendages are freely movable, because moving is the function of the arms, hands, legs, and feet. The joints of the axial skeleton are primarily immovable or slightly movable, because stability and protection of vital organs are its functions.

Immovable Joints (Synarthroses)

The immovable joints are called **synarthroses** (SIN-ar-THROH-seez). The prefix *syn-* means "together" and the root word *arthron* means "joint." Synarthroses are fibrous joints that can absorb shock but permit little or no movement of the articulating bones. There are two types of immovable joints: sutures and syndesmoses.

Sutures, which you read about earlier in this chapter, are joints in which irregularly grooved, articulating bone sheets join closely and are tightly connected by fibrous tissues. The fibers

138

begin to ossify (turn to bone) in early adulthood and are eventually replaced completely by bone. The only sutures in the human body are the sutures of the skull.

Syndesmoses (SIN-dehz-MOH-seez), meaning "held by bands," are joints where dense, fibrous tissue binds the bones together, permitting extremely limited movement. Examples include the coracoacromial (KOR-a-koh-a-KROH-mee-al) joint and the distal (lower) tibiofibular (TIB-ee-oh-FIB-yoo-lar) joints.

Slightly Movable Joints (Amphiarthroses)

The **amphiarthroses** (AM-fee-ar-THROH-seez)—the prefix *amphi-* means "on both sides"—are joints that permit only slight motion. These cartilaginous joints allow more motion of the adjacent bones than do the synarthrodial joints and are, therefore, somewhat better able to absorb shock. The two types of amphiarthroses are synchondroses and symphyses.

Synchondroses (SIN-kahn-DROH-seez), meaning "held by cartilage," are joints in which the articulating bones are held together by a thin layer of hyaline cartilage. Examples include the sternocostal joints (between the sternum and the ribs) and the epiphyseal plates (or growth plates).

Symphyses (SIM-fi-seez) are joints in which thin plates of hyaline cartilage separate a disc of fibrocartilage from the bones. Examples include the vertebral joints and the pubic symphysis.

Freely Movable Joints (Diarthroses)

Freely movable joints are called **diarthroses** (DIGH-ar-THROH-seez). They are also referred to as **synovial** (si-NOH-vee-al) **joints** because each joint is surrounded by an articular capsule with a synovial membrane lining that secretes a lubricant known as synovial fluid (**Figure 4.30**). There are six different types of diarthroses, with each structured to permit different types of motion (**Figure 4.31** on the next page).

At **gliding joints** the articulating bone surfaces are nearly flat, and the only movement permitted is gliding.

In **hinge joints** one articulating bone surface is convex (curved outward), and the other is concave (curved inward). Strong ligaments restrict movement to a planar, hingelike motion, similar to the hinge on a door.

Pivot joints permit rotation around only one axis. (Think about moving around your stationary pivot foot in basketball).

At **condyloid** (KAHN-di-loyd) **joints** one articulating bone surface is an oval, convex shape, and the other is a reciprocally shaped concave surface. Flexion, extension, abduction, adduction, and circumduction are permitted.

Saddle joints are so named because their articulating bone surfaces are both shaped like the seat of a riding saddle. Movement capability is the same as that of the condyloid joint but with greater range of movement allowed.

Ball-and-socket joints are the most freely movable joints in the body. In these joints the surfaces of the articulating bones are reciprocally convex and concave, with one bone end shaped like a "ball" and the other like a "socket."

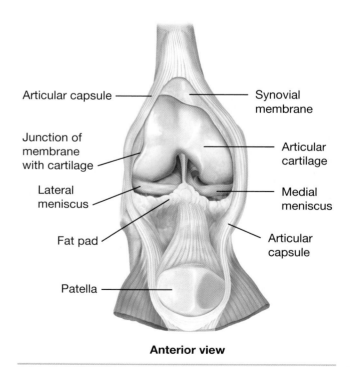

Figure 4.30 Anterior view of the knee, which is a synovial joint.

A. Gliding joint (intercarpal)

Carpal bones

B. Hinge joint (humeroulnar)

Humerus

Ulna

C. Pivot joint (radioulnar)

Radius — Ulna

D. Condylar joint (metacarpophalangeal)

Phalanx

Metacarpal bone

E. Saddle joint (trapeziometacarpal)

Metacarpal bone

Carpal bone

Animation

F. Ball-and-socket joint (humeroscapular)

Head of humerus   Scapula

Figure 4.31 Examples of the six different types of freely movable joints (diarthroses). *Which of these six types of joints is the most freely movable?*

Rotation in all three planes of movement is permitted. In cases where the joint socket is relatively shallow, such as in the shoulder, a large range of motion is permitted but at the sacrifice of joint stability. Alternatively, the deep socket of the hip joint maximizes stability but allows much less of a range of motion than at the shoulder.

Two structures often associated with diarthrodial joints are bursae and tendon sheaths. **Bursae** (BER-see) are small capsules lined with synovial membranes and filled with synovial fluid that cushion the structures they separate. Most bursae separate tendons from bone, reducing the friction on the tendons during joint motion.

Tendon sheaths are double-layered synovial structures surrounding tendons subject to friction because they are close to bones. These sheaths secrete synovial fluid to promote free motion of the tendon during joint movement.

Many long muscle tendons crossing the wrist and finger joints are protected by tendon sheaths.

Articular Tissues

The joints of any mechanical device must be properly lubricated if the movable parts are to move freely and not wear against each other. In the human body, as you learned earlier in this chapter, articular cartilage covers the ends of bones at diarthrodial joints and provides a protective lubrication. Articular cartilage cushions the joint and reduces friction and wear.

At some joints, **articular fibrocartilage**, shaped like a disc or a partial disc called a *meniscus*, is also present between the articulating bones. The intervertebral discs and the menisci of the knee are examples. These discs and menisci help to distribute forces evenly over the joint surfaces and absorb shock at the joint.

Tendons, which connect muscles to bones, and **ligaments**, which connect bones to other bones, are also present at the diarthrodial joints. Composed of collagen and elastic fibers, these tissues are slightly elastic and will return to their original length after being stretched, unless overstretched to the point of injury. The tendons and ligaments crossing a joint play an important role in joint stability. The hip joints, in particular, are crossed by a number of large, strong tendons and ligaments.

Lesson 4.4 Review and Assessment

Mini Glossary
Make sure that you know the meaning of each key term.

 Build vocabulary with e-flash cards and games

amphiarthrosis   joint type that permits only slight motions

articular fibrocartilage   tissue shaped like a disc or partial disc called a *meniscus* that provides cushioning at a joint

ball-and-socket joint   synovial joint formed between one bone end shaped roughly like a ball and the receiving bone reciprocally shaped like a socket

bursae   small capsules lined with synovial membranes and filled with synovial fluid; they cushion the structures they separate

condyloid joint   type of diarthrosis in which one articulating bone surface is an oval, convex shape, and the other is a reciprocally shaped concave surface

diarthrosis   freely movable joints; also known as *synovial joints*

gliding joint   type of diarthrosis that allows only sliding motion of the articulating bones

hinge joint   type of diarthrosis that allows only hingelike movements in forward and backward directions

ligaments   bands composed of collagen and elastic fibers that connect bones to other bones

pivot joint   type of diarthrosis that permits rotation around only one axis

saddle joint   type of diarthrosis in which the articulating bone surfaces are both shaped like the seat of a riding saddle

symphysis   type of amphiarthrosis joint in which a thin plate of hyaline cartilage separates a disc of fibrocartilage from the bones

synarthrosis   fibrous joint that can absorb shock, but permits little or no movement of the articulating bones

synchondrosis   type of amphiarthrosis joint in which the articulating bones are held together by a thin layer of hyaline cartilage

syndesmosis   joint at which dense, fibrous tissue binds the bones together, permitting extremely limited movement

synovial joint   a diarthrodial joint

tendon   tissue band composed of collagen and elastic fibers that connects a muscle to a bone

tendon sheaths   double-layered synovial structures surrounding tendons subject to friction given their position close to bones; secrete synovial fluid to promote free motion of the tendons during joint movement

Know and Understand

 Assess

1. What does it mean to say that bones articulate with each other?
2. Give two examples of immovable joints and where they are found in the body.
3. Give two examples of slightly movable joints and where they are found in the body.
4. Give six examples of freely movable joints and where they are found in the body.

Analyze and Apply

5. Why is it important to have a layer of cartilage between bones that articulate with each other?

6. Why do we need joints that permit little to no movement in our skeletons?
7. What happens when articular cartilage begins to erode from excessive wear and stress on a joint?

In the Lab

8. Obtain (or draw) a picture of a skeleton. Label the areas on the skeleton where these types of joints are located: sutures, syndesmoses, synchondroses, symphyses, gliding, hinge, pivot, condyloid, saddle, and ball-and-socket. Be prepared to explain to the class the kind of movement that each type of joint allows.

Common Injuries and Disorders of the Skeletal System

Lesson Objectives

1. Identify the different types of bone and epiphyseal injuries, and in each case explain the types of forces that can cause these injuries.
2. Discuss osteoporosis, including contributing factors, groups at risk, consequences, and prevention strategies.
3. Describe the common types of joint injuries, including the structures affected and symptoms.
4. Explain what is involved with arthritis and describe specific types of arthritis, including symptoms.

Key Terms

E-Flash Cards

amenorrhea
anorexia nervosa
apophysis
arthritis
bulimia nervosa
bursitis
dislocation
female athlete triad

fracture
osteoarthritis
osteopenia
osteoporosis
rheumatoid arthritis
sprain
stress fracture

Common Bone Injuries

Considering all of the important functions performed by bone, bone health is a vital part of general health. Bone health can be diminished by injuries and pathologies.

Fractures

A **fracture** is a break or a crack in a bone. The nature of a fracture depends on the size, direction, and duration of the injurious force, as well as the health and maturity of the bone.

Fractures are classified as *simple* when the bone ends remain within the surrounding soft tissues, and *compound* when one or both bone ends protrude from the skin. When the bone is splintered, the fracture is classified as *comminuted*. See **Figure 4.32**.

Avulsions are fractures caused when a tendon or ligament pulls away from its attachment to a bone, taking a small chip of bone with it. Explosive throwing and jumping movements may cause avulsion fractures of the medial epicondyle (EHP-i-KAHN-dighl) of the humerus and the calcaneus.

Forceful bending and twisting movements can produce spiral fractures of the long bones. A common example occurs during downhill skiing. When a ski is planted in one direction, and the skier rotates while falling in a different direction, a spiral fracture of the tibia can result.

The bones of children contain relatively larger amounts of collagen than do the bones of adults. For this reason, children's bones are more flexible and are generally less likely to fracture than adult bones. Consequently, greenstick fractures, or incomplete fractures, are more common in children than in adults. A greenstick fracture is an incomplete fracture caused when

A. A *greenstick fracture* is incomplete. The break occurs on the convex surface of the bend in the bone.

B. A *stress fracture* involves an incomplete break.

C. A *comminuted fracture* is complete and splinters the bone.

D. A *spiral fracture* is caused by twisting a bone excessively.

Figure 4.32 Types of fractures.

a bone bends or twists but does not break all the way through.

Stress fractures are tiny, painful cracks in bone that result from overuse. Under normal circumstances, bone responds to stress-related injury by remodeling. Osteoclasts resorb the damaged tissue, and then osteoblasts deposit new bone at the site, resulting in repair of the injury. However, when repeated overuse continues, the remodeling process cannot keep up with the damage being done by the overuse. When this happens, the condition progresses to a stress fracture. Runners are prone to stress fractures, particularly in the tibia and the metatarsals.

Epiphyseal Injuries

Epiphyseal injuries include injuries to the epiphyseal plate (growth plate), articular cartilage, and the apophysis. An **apophysis** (a-PAHF-i-sis) is a site where a tendon attaches

to a bone. Both acute and overuse-related injuries can damage the growth plate, potentially resulting in premature closure of the epiphyseal junction and termination of bone growth.

Osteochondrosis (AHS-tee-oh-kahn-DROH-sis), also known as *Osgood-Schlatter disease*, is another form of bone injury. The powerful quadriceps muscle group on the front of the thigh attaches distally to the upper tibia. When the quadriceps is used a lot in sports activities during the adolescent growth spurt, the area of the tibia around the attachment site becomes irritated or swollen, causing pain. The condition is believed to be caused by overuse injuries before the area has finished growing.

Osteochondrosis is common in adolescents who play soccer, basketball, and volleyball, and who participate in gymnastics, with more boys affected than girls. The primary symptom is a painful region of swelling at the muscle attachment site, which can occur on one or both legs. The pain worsens with physical activity.

 Check Your Understanding

1. List and describe these different types of fractures: simple, compound, comminuted, avulsion, spiral, greenstick, and stress.
2. Explain osteochondrosis.
3. Why is it important for children to avoid activities that could cause damage to an epiphyseal plate?

Osteoporosis

Osteoporosis (AHS-tee-oh-poh-ROH-sis) is a condition in which bone mineralization and strength are so abnormally low that regular, daily activities can result in painful fractures. With its honeycomb structure, trabecular bone is most commonly the site of osteoporotic fractures (**Figure 4.33** on the next page).

Age-Related Osteoporosis

Osteoporosis occurs in most elderly individuals, with earlier onset in women. The

A.   Healthy bone

B.   Diseased bone

Figure 4.33 Compare the normal trabecular bone (A) with the brittle, degraded bone (B) characteristic of osteoporosis. The yellowish, underlying tissue in B is visible because the surface of the bone (orange colored) has worn away. As the bone becomes more brittle, it is more likely to fracture. *Which groups of people are more likely to suffer from osteoporosis?*

condition begins as **osteopenia** (AHS-tee-oh-PEE-nee-a), reduced bone mass without the presence of a fracture. The osteopenia often progresses to osteoporosis, with fractures present. Although once regarded as primarily a health issue for women, with the increasing age of the population, osteoporosis is now also becoming a concern for older men.

With type I osteoporosis, also known as *postmenopausal osteoporosis*, fractures usually begin to occur about 15 years postmenopause; the femoral neck, vertebrae, and wrist bones are the most common fracture sites. Type II osteoporosis, also called *age-associated osteoporosis*, affects most women and also affects men over 70 years old. After 60 years of age, the majority of fractures in both men and women are osteoporosis-related. In the elderly population fractures of the femoral neck, in particular, often trigger a downward health spiral that leads to death.

The most common symptom of osteoporosis, however, is back pain derived from crush-type fractures of the weakened trabecular bone of the vertebrae. These fractures can be caused by activities as simple as picking up a bag of groceries or a bag of trash. These vertebral crush fractures frequently cause reduction of body height and tend to accentuate the kyphotic curve in the thoracic region of the spine. This disabling deformity is known as *dowager's hump*.

The Female Athlete Triad

Unfortunately, osteoporosis is not confined to the elderly population. It can also occur in female athletes at the high school and collegiate levels who strive to maintain an excessively low body weight.

Striving for an extremely low weight can cause a dangerous condition known as the **female athlete triad**. This condition involves a combination of disordered eating, **amenorrhea** (ay-MEN-oh-REE-a)—having no period or menses—and osteoporosis. Because the triad can cause negative health consequences ranging from irreversible bone loss to death, friends, parents, coaches, and physicians need to be alert to the signs.

Female athletes participating in endurance or appearance-related sports are most likely to be affected by the female athlete triad. Disordered eating can take the form of anorexia nervosa or bulimia nervosa.

Symptoms of **anorexia nervosa** in girls and women include a body weight that is 15% or more below the minimal normal weight range, extreme fear of gaining weight, an unrealistic body image, and amenorrhea. **Bulimia nervosa** involves a minimum of two eating binges per week for at least three months; an associated feeling of lack of control; use of self-induced vomiting, laxatives, diuretics, strict dieting, or

WHAT RESEARCH TELLS US

...*about* Preventing Osteoporosis

Osteoporosis is not inevitable with advancing age. It is typically the result of a lifetime of habits that are erosive (causing erosion) to the skeletal system. Simply stated, it is easier to prevent osteoporosis than it is to treat it.

The single most important strategy for preventing or delaying the onset of osteoporosis is maximizing bone mass during childhood and adolescence. Weight-bearing exercise such as running, jumping, and even walking is particularly important prior to puberty because of the high level of growth hormone present during this period. Growth hormone makes exercise particularly effective in increasing bone density.

Diet also plays an important role in bone health. Physicians now recognize that a predisposition for osteoporosis can begin in childhood and adolescence when a poor diet interferes with bone mass development. Adequate dietary calcium is particularly important during the teenage years, but unfortunately the typical American girl falls below the recommended daily intake of 1,200 mg per day by 11 years of age. A modified diet or calcium supplementation can be critically important for the development of peak bone mass among adolescent females who have this dietary deficiency (**Figure 4.34**).

Tatiana Popova/Shutterstock.com

Figure 4.34 *Besides drinking milk, what can this girl do to prevent or delay the onset of osteoporosis?*

The role of vitamin D is also important, in that vitamin D enables bone to absorb calcium. In North America, more than 50% of women being treated for low bone density also have a vitamin D deficiency.

Other lifestyle factors also affect bone mineralization. Risk factors for developing osteoporosis include a sedentary lifestyle, weight loss or excessive thinness, and smoking tobacco.

To help prevent later development of osteoporosis, young women are encouraged to engage in regular physical activity and to avoid the lifestyle factors that negatively affect bone health.

Taking It Further

1. Make a list of activities that you can engage in now that will increase your chances of preventing or delaying the onset of osteoporosis. Share your list with classmates.

exercise to prevent weight gain; and an obsession with body image.

Although the incidence of osteoporosis among female athletes is unknown, the consequences of the female athlete triad are potentially tragic. Amenorrheic, premenopausal female athletes are known to have an elevated rate of stress fractures. More important, the loss of bone that occurs may be irreversible, and osteoporotic wedge fractures of the vertebrae can ruin posture for life.

Common Joint Injuries

The freely movable joints of the human body are subjected to significant wear over the course of a lifetime. Both acute and overuse injuries affect the joints.

Sprains

Sprains are injuries caused by abnormal motion of the articulating bones that result in overstretching or tearing of ligaments, tendons, or other connective tissues crossing a joint. The most common site of sprain is the ankle, and the most common mechanism is injury to the lateral ligaments.

Lateral ankle sprains occur frequently because the ankle is a major weight-bearing joint and because there is less ligamentous support on the lateral than on the medial side of the ankle.

Pain and swelling are the symptoms of joint sprains. Immediate treatment should include intermittent icing and elevation.

Dislocations

When one of the articulating bones is displaced from the joint socket, the injury is called a **dislocation** of that joint. Dislocations usually result from falls or forceful collisions.

Common dislocation sites are the shoulders, fingers, knees, elbows, and jaw. Signs and symptoms include visible joint deformity, pain, swelling, and some loss of movement capability.

Bursitis

Bursitis is the inflammation of one or more bursae, the fluid-filled sacs that provide cushioning of the moving tissues around a joint. Bursitis is an overuse injury that produces irritation and inflammation of the bursae due to friction. For example, runners who overtrain may experience inflammation of the bursa between the Achilles tendon and the calcaneus. Symptoms of bursitis include pain and sometimes swelling.

 ### Check Your Understanding

1. How does osteoporosis differ from osteopenia?
2. Which structures are affected when a joint is sprained?
3. What types of actions may result in dislocations?
4. What are the causes and symptoms of bursitis?

Arthritis

Arthritis is a common pathology associated with aging. It is characterized by joint inflammation accompanied by pain, stiffness, and sometimes swelling. Arthritis is not a single condition but a large family of pathologies. Over one hundred different types of arthritis have been identified.

Rheumatoid Arthritis

Rheumatoid arthritis is an autoimmune disorder in which the body's own immune system attacks healthy joint tissues (**Figure 4.35**). It is the most debilitating and painful form of arthritis. Rheumatoid arthritis is more common in adults but occasionally occurs in children (*juvenile rheumatoid arthritis*).

Symptoms of rheumatoid arthritis include inflammation and thickening of the synovial membranes and breakdown of the articular cartilage. The result is extremely limited joint motion and, in extreme cases, complete fusing of the articulating bones. Associated symptoms can include anemia, fatigue, and muscular atrophy.

Osteoarthritis

Arthritis also takes a noninflammatory form as **osteoarthritis**, a degenerative disease of articular cartilage. Onset of osteoarthritis is characterized by progressive roughening of the normally smooth joint cartilage, with the cartilage eventually completely wearing away. Pain, swelling, range-of-motion restriction, and stiffness are all symptoms, with the pain typically relieved by rest and joint stiffness improved by activity.

Laurin Rinder/Shutterstock.com

Figure 4.35 This person's hands have been disfigured by rheumatoid arthritis. Most patients take medication for the intense pain.

Lesson 4.5 Review and Assessment

Mini Glossary
Make sure that you know the meaning of each key term.

Build vocabulary with
e-flash cards and games

amenorrhea   absence of a menstrual period in women of reproductive age

anorexia nervosa   condition characterized by body weight 15% or more below the minimal normal weight range, extreme fear of gaining weight, an unrealistic body image, and amenorrhea

apophysis   site at which a tendon attaches to bone

arthritis   family of more than 100 common pathologies associated with aging, characterized by joint inflammation accompanied by pain, stiffness, and sometimes swelling

bulimia nervosa   disordered eating that involves a minimum of two eating binges a week for at least three months; an associated feeling

of lack of control; use of self-induced vomiting, laxatives, diuretics, strict dieting, or exercise to prevent weight gain; and an obsession with body image

bursitis   inflammation of one or more bursae

dislocation   injury that involves displacement of a bone from its joint socket

female athlete triad   a combination of disordered eating, amenorrhea, and osteoporosis

fracture   any break or disruption of continuity in a bone

osteoarthritis   degenerative disease of articular cartilage, characterized by pain, swelling, range-of-motion restriction, and stiffness

osteopenia   reduced bone mass without the presence of a fracture

osteoporosis   condition in which bone mineralization and strength are so abnormally low that regular, daily activities can result in painful fractures

rheumatoid arthritis   autoimmune disorder in which the body's own immune system attacks healthy joint tissues; the most debilitating and painful form of arthritis

sprain   injuries caused by abnormal motion of the articulating bones that result in overstretching or tearing of ligaments, tendons, or other connective tissues crossing a joint

stress fracture   tiny, painful crack in bone that results from overuse

Know and Understand

Assess

1. What is an avulsion?

2. At what point in a person's life is osteochondrosis most likely to occur?

3. What is the most common symptom of osteoporosis?

4. Which joint in the skeleton is the most commonly sprained?

5. What happens to healthy joint tissue in a person with rheumatoid arthritis?

Analyze and Apply

6. Explain how the remodeling of a bone and a stress fracture are related.

7. Why are females who participate in certain sports more vulnerable to the condition known as the *female athlete triad*?

8. A 17-year-old soccer player has sustained several fractures to different parts of her body. When her bone density was tested, she was found to be on the low end of the normal range. What would you suggest that she do to increase her bone strength?

In the Lab

9. You are a healthcare worker, and you have a patient with one of the following conditions: osteoporosis, osteopenia, rheumatoid arthritis, bursitis, or osteoarthritis.

Decide which condition your patient has and then create a treatment plan for the patient. Your plan should include the following: description of the disorder; age groups typically affected by the disorder; medications that can be taken to ease pain and inflammation, if any; foods to add to the diet to help minimize the progression of the disorder; foods to omit from the diet; physical activities to add to the daily routine or to increase in the daily routine; and a workout schedule for each day of the week.

Create your treatment plan in the form of a presentation. Share the presentation with the class, as though the class were your patient. Ask for and answer any questions that your "patient" might have.

Career Corner
Anatomy and Physiology at Work

Orthopedics is a field of medical science that specializes in treating injuries, disorders, and diseases of the bones and joints. Many different health professionals, however, are involved in helping patients overcome skeletal injuries and improve the health of their bones and joints.

Physician

When bone and joint injuries or age-related conditions arise, which healthcare professionals team up to take care of these problems? The person injured should usually seek help first from a family physician, general practitioner, or medical professional who provides comprehensive health care for people of all ages.

Family physicians have either the MD (Doctor of Medicine) degree or the DO (Doctor of Osteopathic Medicine) degree. The family physician can examine the patient and, as appropriate, administer a series of tests to determine whether referral to an orthopedic surgeon is warranted for more specialized care (**Figure 4.36**).

Orthopedic surgeons have specialized training beyond the MD or DO degree in the care of bone and joint injuries and pathologies. The orthopedic surgeon most likely will want to see an X-ray and sometimes an MRI (magnetic resonance image) to determine whether surgery is warranted, and what other follow-up care may be appropriate.

Radiographer

Radiographers use imaging techniques, such as radiographs (X-rays) and MRI scans, to capture pictures of injured or pathological tissues. These professionals, also called *medical radiation technologists*, provide the images to doctors, who evaluate the images to determine the most effective treatment for the patient.

These technologists are trained in positioning patients to get the best kinds of images for evaluation (**Figure 4.37**). Radiographers may specialize in mammography, fluoroscopy, computed tomography, ultrasound, or MRI. The education required to become a radiologic

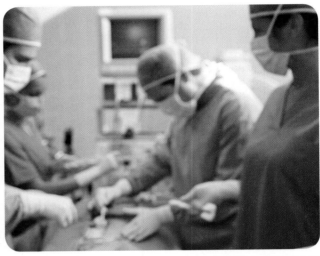

Wavebreakmedia/Shutterstock.com

Figure 4.36 In the case of a severe bone or joint injury, an orthopedic surgeon performs an operation to repair the damage.

technologist typically is a bachelor's degree that includes training in radiography.

Orthotist/Prosthetist

Sometimes the best way to treat an orthopedic injury is with a customized device. Such devices, called orthotics, include custom shoe inserts and leg braces. For more serious injuries, a patient's limb may need to be replaced with a prosthetic one. A prosthetic is a fabricated substitute developed to assist a damaged body part or replace one that is missing. A person who treats patients with orthotics or prosthetics is called an orthotist/prosthetist (OR-tha-tist/PRAHS-theh-tist), or O&P professional.

O&P professionals have a master's degree in orthotics and prosthetics, and they have passed a certification exam administered by the American Board for Certification in Orthotics, Prosthetics and Pedorthics (ABC). O&P professionals may specialize in both orthotics and prosthetics, or only one of these fields. To be certified in both fields, candidates must complete one year of residency in each specialty and pass the required ABC exams.

Orthotists and prosthetists meet with patients to evaluate their needs, measure patients for custom design and fitting of medical devices, and design their patients' devices and repair or update them as needed. They also instruct patients in the proper use and care of their devices. O&P professionals are employed in small, private offices or in larger medical facilities, and they often work in the shops where orthotics and prosthetics are made.

Planning for a Health-Related Career

Research the career of an orthopedic surgeon, a radiographer, or an orthotist/prosthetist. Alternatively, select a profession from the list of **Related Career Options**. Using the Internet or resources at your local library, find answers to questions such as the following:

1. What are the main tasks and responsibilities of the career you are researching?
2. What is the outlook for this career? Are workers in demand, or are jobs dwindling? For complete information, consult the current edition of the *Occupational Outlook Handbook*, published by the US Department of Labor. This handbook is available online or at your local library.
3. What special skills or talents are required? For example, do you need to be good at biology and chemistry? Do you need to enjoy interacting with other people?
4. What personality traits do you think are needed to be successful in this job? For example, a career as a surgeon requires directing other people. Are you comfortable with giving directions to others?
5. Does this career involve a great deal of routine, or are the day-to-day responsibilities varied?
6. Does the work require long hours, or is it a standard, "9-to-5" job?

7. What is the salary range for this job?
8. What do you think you would like about this career? Is there anything about it that you might dislike?

Related Career Options

- Family Practitioner
- Magnetic Resonance (MR) Technologist
- Orthotist/Prosthetist
- Physical Therapist
- Physician Assistant
- Podiatrist
- Surgical Nurse

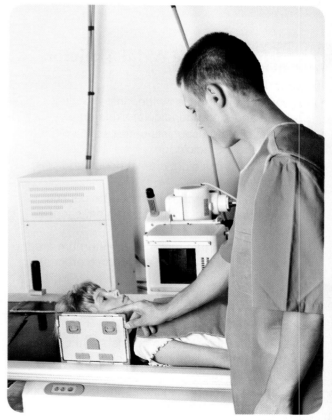

Poznyakov/Shutterstock.com

Figure 4.37 A radiographer takes an X-ray of his young patient. *Do you think this is an occupation you would enjoy? How much education and training do you think would be required?*

Chapter Summaries

Lesson 4.1 **Bone as a Living Tissue**

Build vocabulary with e-flash cards and games

Key Points

- The human skeleton contains 206 bones.
- The five functions of the skeletal system are support, protection, movement, storage, and blood cell formation.
- The four categories (by shape) of bones are long bones, short bones, flat bones, and irregular bones.
- Remodeling of bones continues throughout life to keep bones strong.

Key Terms

articular cartilage	ossification
bone marrow	osteoblasts
cortical bone	osteoclasts
diaphysis	osteocytes
epiphyseal plate	osteon
epiphysis	perforating (Volkmann's) canals
Haversian canals	periosteum
Haversian system	remodeling
hematopoiesis	trabecular bone
lacunae	
medullary cavity	

Lesson 4.2 **The Axial Skeleton**

Key Points

- The human skeleton is divided into the axial skeleton and the appendicular skeleton.
- The axial skeleton consists of the skull, spinal column, and thoracic cage.
- The skull contains eight cranial bones and fourteen facial bones.
- The five sections of the spine are the cervical region, thoracic region, lumbar region, sacrum, and coccyx.
- The three bones that make up the sternum are the manubrium, the body, and the xiphoid process.

Key Terms

atlas	mandible
axial skeleton	maxillary bones
axis	sacrum
cervical region	skull
coccyx	sternum
cranium	sutures
facial bones	thoracic cage
fontanel	thoracic region
intervertebral discs	vertebra
lumbar region	

Lesson 4.3 **The Appendicular Skeleton**

Key Points

- The appendicular skeleton consists of the shoulder complex, arms, wrists, hands, pelvic girdle, legs, ankles, and feet.
- The shoulder complex includes the left and right clavicles and the left and right scapula.
- The pelvic girdle consists of two coxal bones and the sacrum.

Key Terms

appendicular skeleton	pelvis
carpal bones	phalanges
clavicle	radius
femur	scapula
fibula	shoulder complex
humerus	shoulder girdle
lower extremity	tarsals
metacarpals	tibia
metatarsals	ulna
patella	upper extremity

Lesson 4.4 Joints

Key Points
- The three main categories of joints, with regard to function, are the immovable joints, the slightly movable joints, and the freely movable joints.
- The immovable joints are called *synarthroses*.
- The slightly movable joints are called *amphiarthroses*.
- The freely movable joints are called *diarthroses*, and they consist of gliding, hinge, pivot, condyloid, saddle, and ball-and-socket joints.

Key Terms
amphiarthrosis
articular fibrocartilage
ball-and-socket joint
bursae
condyloid joint
diarthrosis
gliding joint
hinge joint
ligament

pivot joint
saddle joint
symphysis
synarthrosis
synchondrosis
syndesmosis
synovial joint
tendon
tendon sheath

Lesson 4.5 Common Injuries and Disorders of the Skeletal System

Key Points
- Fractures are breaks in a bone, and they are classified as *simple*, *compound*, and *comminuted*.
- Osteoporosis is a condition, commonly seen in the elderly, in which bone mineralization and strength are critically low, often leading to fractures.
- The condition known as *female athlete triad* involves a combination of an eating disorder, amenorrhea, and osteoporosis.
- Sprains and dislocations are common joint injuries.

Key Terms
amenorrhea
anorexia nervosa
apophysis
arthritis
bulimia nervosa
bursitis
dislocation
female athlete triad

fracture
osteoarthritis
osteopenia
osteoporosis
rheumatoid arthritis
sprain
stress fracture

Chapter Assessments

Assess

Lesson 4.1

Bone as a Living Tissue

Learning Key Terms and Concepts

1. The five functions of the skeletal system are _____, _____, _____, _____, and _____.
2. The term for blood cell formation is:
   - A. osteocyte
   - B. hematopoiesis
   - C. osteogenesis
   - D. osteoblast
3. The strong, dense bone tissue is called _____.
   - A. trabecular bone
   - B. coxal bone
   - C. cortical bone
   - D. hard bone
4. The four shape categories of bones are _____, _____, _____, and _____.
5. The shaft, or middle, of a bone is called the _____; the ends of a bone are called the _____.
6. Specialized bone cells that break down bone are called _____.
   - A. osteocytes
   - B. osteoclasts
   - C. osteoblasts
   - D. none of the above
7. Specialized bone cells that build new bone are called _____.
   - A. osteocytes
   - B. osteoclasts
   - C. osteoblasts
   - D. all of the above

Thinking Critically

8. The microscopic structure of long bones can be compared to a city. Using the following terms, describe what each type of long bone could be compared to in your city (a building, streets running through the city, or a water tower, for example): Haversian canal, lacunae, lamellae, canaliculi. Draw a picture to illustrate.

Lesson 4.2

The Axial Skeleton

Learning Key Terms and Concepts

9. Which spinal region includes the vertebrae of the neck?
   - A. thoracic
   - B. lumbar
   - C. sacral
   - D. cervical
10. Which spinal region connects to the ribs?
   - A. thoracic
   - B. lumbar
   - C. sacral
   - D. cervical
11. Which condition causes a lateral (sideways) curvature of the spine?
   - A. lordosis
   - B. kyphosis
   - C. scoliosis
   - D. none of the above

12. Which of the following is part of the thoracic cage?
   A. the ribs
   B. the thoracic vertebrae
   C. the sternum
   D. all of the above

13. Which of the following is true about the false ribs?
   A. They do not attach directly to the sternum.
   B. They do not attach directly to the vertebrae.
   C. They do not attach directly to anything.
   D. They do not exist.

14. Which structures make up the axial skeleton?
   A. the appendages
   B. the head and trunk
   C. the thoracic cage and the legs
   D. none of the above

Thinking Critically

15. Given your knowledge of the intervertebral discs, what activities should a person avoid to promote disc health? Name at least two activities and explain why each should be avoided.

Lesson 4.3

The Appendicular Skeleton

Learning Key Terms and Concepts

16. Which structures are part of the appendicular skeleton?
   A. the head and trunk
   B. the spinal colum
   C. the arms and legs
   D. none of the above

17. Which bone is always on the "little finger" side of the forearm?
   A. humerus
   B. radius
   C. ulna
   D. tibia

18. What is the term for the prominent, upper edge of the hip bone?
   A. sacroiliac joint
   B. acetabulum
   C. ischium
   D. iliac crest

19. What is the longest, strongest bone in the body?
   A. sternum
   B. humerus
   C. femur
   D. tibia

20. Which of the following is the heel bone?
   A. talus
   B. femur
   C. patella
   D. calcaneus

21. The shoulder girdle consists of the right and left _____, and the right and left _____.

22. There are _____ bones in each wrist and hand.

23. Each coxal bone is formed by the fusion of the _____, _____, and the _____.

Thinking Critically

24. If a forensic scientist finds skeletal remains after a house fire, how will she determine whether the individual was a male or female?

Lesson 4.4

Joints

Learning Key Terms and Concepts

25. Which of the following are immovable joints?
   A. sutures of the skull
   B. gliding joints
   C. pivot joints
   D. hinge joints

26. Which of the following are functions of articular cartilage?
   A. cushions the joint
   B. reduces wear to the joint
   C. reduces friction at the joint
   D. all of the above

27. Another term for freely movable joints is _____.

28. _____ are small sacs filled with synovial fluid that cushion the structures they separate.

29. _____ connect muscle to bone, while _____ connect bone to bone.

Thinking Critically

30. Give reasons why you either would or would not want all of your joints to be ball-and-socket joints.

Lesson 4.5

Common Injuries and Disorders of the Skeletal System

Learning Key Terms and Concepts

31. Which term describes a fracture in which the ends of a bone protrude from the skin?
   A. comminuted
   B. compound
   C. simple
   D. avulsion

32. Which type of fracture is more common in children than in adults?
   A. compound
   B. avulsion
   C. greenstick
   D. simple

33. Injuries to which of the following can stop the growth of a long bone?
   A. intervertebral disc
   B. meniscus
   C. epiphyseal plate
   D. sutures

34. _____ fractures are tiny, painful cracks in a bone that result from overuse.

35. The site where a tendon attaches to a bone is known as the _____.

36. _____ is an autoimmune disorder in which the body's own immune system attacks healthy joint tissues.

Thinking Critically

37. A 10-year-old boy and his 42-year-old father were building a tree house when the branch they were standing on broke away from the tree. The father sustained two broken ribs, but the boy had only a few bruises. Explain.

Building Skills and Connecting Concepts

Analyzing & Evaluating Data

This astronaut is exercising on a special treadmill system in the International Space Station. Without this type of resistance training, he could lose 1% to 2% bone mass per month.

38. If the astronaut spends three months in space and never exercises, what percentage of his bone mass might he lose?

39. You read in this chapter that our bones account for about 15% of body weight. If this astronaut weighs 170 pounds, how much do his bones weigh?

40. If he fails to exercise for six months in space, how much weight might this astronaut lose in bone mass?

Communicating about Anatomy and Physiology

41. **Speaking and Listening** Divide into groups of four or five students. Each group should choose one of the following topics: anorexia nervosa, bursitis, dislocation, female athlete triad, fracture, osteoporosis, rheumatoid arthritis, sprain, or stress fracture.

    Using your textbook as a starting point, research your topic and prepare a report on causes and treatments. As a group, deliver your presentation to the rest of the class. Take notes while other students give their reports. Ask questions about any details that you would like clarified.

42. **Writing** Write an "osteostory" about a super hero who helps someone in distress. Be creative and find ways to mention the following bones in your story: skull, sternum, femur, humerus, tibia, calcaneus, tarsals, carpals, metatarsals, metacarpals, ribs, clavicle, scapula, mandible, and patella. Try to work into the story reasons for describing the locations of these bones in the body.

Lab Investigations

43. Build a skeleton using poster board or card stock, glue, toothpicks, colored pencils, markers, and your textbook.
    A. Construct a skeleton of an animal of your choice using toothpicks and glue. Your animal can be real or imaginary.
    B. Draw the outline for your animal and then use the toothpicks to make the bones of your animal's skeleton.
    C. When you are finished, use labels to identify the bones.
    D. Include a label for the name and species of your animal.

Include these bones in your skeleton:

carpals, cervical vertebrae, coxal bones, femur, fibula, humerus, lumbar vertebrae, mandible, maxilla, metacarpalsm metatarsals, patella, phalanges, radius, ribs, scapula, skull, sternum, tarsals, thoracic vertebrae, tibia, ulna

Expand your learning with additional online resources
- Supplemental Lab Activities
- Interactive Exercises
- Animations

Expand

www.g-wlearning.com/healthsciences

Which is most important for an athlete—muscular strength, power, or endurance?

Yeko Photo Studio/Shutterstock.com

The Muscular System

*M*uscle is the only human tissue capable of shortening, or contracting. This unique ability is what makes body movements possible.

Without muscle the powerful movements required in athletic performances would be impossible, as would the finely tuned, graceful movements needed to send a text message or play a musical instrument. Muscles also control the movements of our eyes, the movement of food through our digestive systems, and the beating of our hearts.

What enables muscle to be so versatile? In this chapter we will look at the different types, properties, and structures of muscle, and examine the effects of different kinds of physical training on skeletal muscle. We will also discuss some of the common injuries and disorders of muscles, how these problems tend to occur, and how their likelihood, in some cases, can be reduced.

Chapter 5 Lessons

Lesson 5.1
Muscle Tissue Categories and Functions

Lesson 5.2
Skeletal Muscle Actions

Lesson 5.3
The Major Skeletal Muscles

Lesson 5.4
Common Injuries and Disorders of Muscles

While studying, look for the online icon **to:**

- **Practice** with e-flash cards and vocabulary games
- **Review** with interactive art labeling
- **Assess** with online exercises
- **Expand** with interactive activities and animated videos
- **Listen** to pronunciations of key terms in the audio glossary

www.g-wlearning.com/healthsciences

Companion Website

Study on the Go

Use a mobile device to practice vocabulary terms, listen to pronunciations, and review with self-assessment quizzes.

www.m.g-wlearning.com

G-W Mobile

Muscle Tissue Categories and Functions

Before You Read

Try to answer the following questions before you read this lesson.

Why are some muscles controlled involuntarily?

When a skeletal muscle is stimulated to contract, what three types of actions can occur?

Are muscles irritable?

Lesson Objectives

1. Discuss the structural and functional characteristics of each of the three categories of muscle.
2. Describe the four behavioral characteristics of all muscle tissue.
3. Explain the roles of agonist and antagonist muscles.

Key Terms

E-Flash Cards

agonist
antagonist
aponeurosis
concentric
contractility
eccentric
endomysium
epimysium

extensibility
fascicle
irritability
isometric
muscle fiber
perimysium
peristalsis
sarcolemma

Muscle Categories

The three major categories of muscle fibers are *skeletal*, *smooth*, and *cardiac*. In this section we will examine the important structural and functional differences among these three types of muscle fibers.

Skeletal Muscle

The skeletal muscles attach to bones and are largely responsible for body movements. Skeletal muscle is also known as *striated muscle* due to the prominent cross-stripes, or striations, which can be seen when examining this tissue under a microscope (**Figure 5.1A**). A third name, *voluntary muscle*, is an appropriate name because this type of muscle is stimulated by consciously directed nerve activity.

An individual skeletal muscle cell is referred to as a **muscle fiber** because of its thread-like shape. Muscle fibers include many nuclei and vary considerably in length and diameter. Some fibers run the entire length of a muscle; others are much shorter.

The number of muscle fibers in a given person is genetically determined, and does not change as we age, except for occasional loss of fibers resulting from injury. Although fiber number doesn't change, the skeletal muscle fibers grow in length and diameter from birth to adulthood. Adults can increase their fiber diameter, and strength, by resistance training with just a few repetitions of heavy loads on a regular basis over a period of time.

As **Figure 5.2** shows, skeletal muscle is highly organized. The cell membrane of the muscle fiber is called the **sarcolemma** (SAR-koh-LEHM-a). Over the sarcolemma of each muscle fiber is a fine, protective sheath of connective

Nuclei

Cross-
striations

A. Skeletal muscle tissue. The skeletal muscles move the body.

Smooth
muscle
cells

Nuclei

B. Smooth muscle tissue. The smooth muscles move food through the digestive system and perform other important involuntary functions.

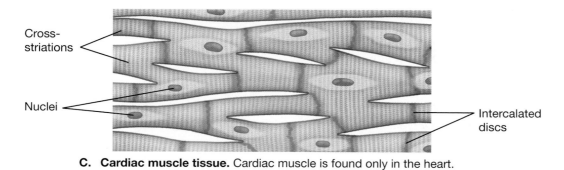

Cross-
striations

Nuclei

Intercalated
discs

C. Cardiac muscle tissue. Cardiac muscle is found only in the heart.

Figure 5.1 The three primary types of muscle tissue. *What are two additional names for skeletal muscle?*

tissue called an **endomysium** (EHN-doh-MIZ-ee-um). Groups of muscle fibers are bundled together by a strong fibrous membrane called a **perimysium** (PER-i-MIZ-ee-um) into a unit known as a **fascicle** (FAS-i-kuhl).

All of the fascicles in a muscle are enclosed by a thick, tough connective tissue called an **epimysium** (EHP-i-MIZ-ee-um). The epimysium connects at both ends of the muscle with either a cordlike tendon composed of extremely strong connective tissue or with a flat, sheetlike **aponeurosis** (AP-oh-noo-ROH-sis).

Tendons and aponeuroses directly connect each muscle to a bone, cartilage, or other connective tissue. Recall from chapter 4 that

tendons differ from ligaments in that ligaments connect bone to bone.

Smooth Muscle

In contrast to skeletal muscle fibers, smooth muscle cells are small, spindle-shaped, and nonstriated. They are involuntary (not under conscious control), and they have a single nucleus (**Figure 5.1B**). Also known as *visceral muscle*, this type of muscle is found in the walls of many internal organs such as the stomach, intestines, urinary bladder, and respiratory passages.

Smooth muscle cells are arranged in layers, with one layer running lengthwise and the other

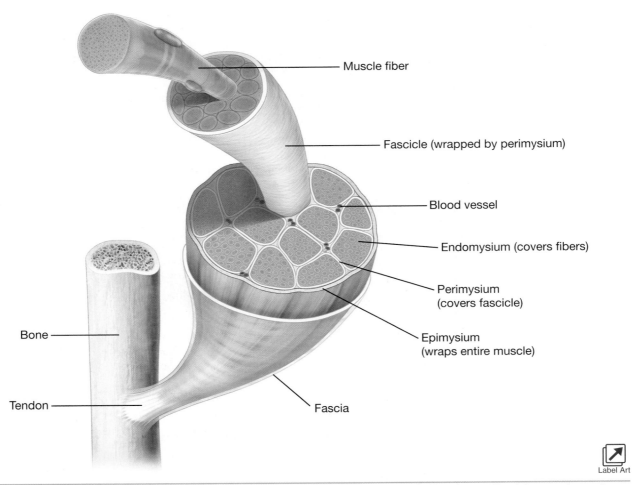

Label Art

Figure 5.2 The organization of skeletal muscle. The sarcolemma (membrane of muscle fiber) is not shown in this view. *What is the benefit of increasing the diameter of skeletal muscles through repeated lifting?*

surrounding the organ in which the muscles are contained. The coordinated, alternate contracting and relaxing of these layers changes the size and shape of the organ and can aid in moving the contents of the organ. Moving food through the digestive system, emptying the bladder, and changing the diameter of the blood vessels are examples of the important functions of these muscles. During digestion, food is propelled along by a wave of symmetrical squeezing of the walls of the digestive tract. This process is called **peristalsis**, which you will learn more about in chapter 13.

The autonomic (automatic) nervous system controls smooth muscle activity. Unlike the skeletal muscles, smooth muscles can sustain contraction for long periods of time without the muscles becoming fatigued.

Cardiac Muscle

As the name suggests, cardiac muscle is located solely in the walls of the heart. Cardiac muscle cells are branched, cross-striated, and involuntary—under the control of the autonomic nervous system (**Figure 5.1C**). Cardiac cells are arranged in an interconnected network of figure-eight or spiral-shaped bundles that join together at structures called *intercalated* (in-TER-kah-lay-tehd) *discs*. This arrangement enables simultaneous contraction of neighboring cells to produce the heartbeat.

The table in **Figure 5.3** summarizes the major features of the three categories of muscle tissue. Although all three types are important and, in fact, essential for human life, we will focus primarily on the skeletal muscles in this chapter.

Figure 5.3 Muscle Categories

Characteristic	Skeletal	Smooth	Cardiac
Cell structure	varying lengths, thread-shaped, striated	short, spindle-shaped, no striations	branching interconnected chains, striated
Nucleus	multinucleate	one nucleus	one nucleus
Control	voluntary	involuntary	involuntary
Location	most attach to bones; some facial muscles attach to skin	walls of internal organs other than the heart	walls of the heart

✔ Check Your Understanding

1. What is the difference between voluntary and involuntary muscles?
2. Categorize each muscle type as voluntary or involuntary.
3. What are the three layers of tissue that run the length of a skeletal muscle?

Muscle Functions

Despite the different properties of the three types of muscle, certain behavioral characteristics are common to all muscle tissue. In the case of skeletal muscles, there are also certain functional roles that muscles can play in contributing to different movements of the body.

Behavioral Properties

All muscle tissues have four behavioral characteristics in common: irritability, extensibility, elasticity, and contractility. Two of these—**extensibility**, the ability to be stretched, and elasticity, the ability to return to normal length after a stretch—are common not just to muscle, but to many types of biological tissues. For example, when a muscle group such as the hamstrings (on the posterior side of the thigh) is stretched over a period of time, the muscles lengthen, and the range of motion at the hip increases, making it easier to touch the toes. The stretched muscles do not return to resting length immediately, but shorten over a period of time.

Another behavioral characteristic common to all muscle is **irritability**, or the ability to respond to a stimulus. Muscles are routinely stimulated by signals from the nerves that supply them. Muscles can also be irritated by a mechanical stimulus, such as an external blow to a muscle. The response to all forms of stimuli is muscle contraction.

As mentioned in the chapter introduction, **contractility**, the ability to contract or shorten, is the one behavioral characteristic unique to muscle tissue. Most muscles have a tendon attaching to a bone at one end and a tendon attaching to another bone at the other end. When a muscle contracts, it pulls on the bones at the attachment sites. This pulling force is called a *tensile force*, or tension. The amount of tension developed is constant throughout the muscle, tendons, and attachment sites.

Tension and Types of Skeletal Muscle Contraction

Although we commonly use the term *contraction* (which implies *shortening*) to mean that tension has developed in a muscle, muscles do not always shorten when they develop tension. When a skeletal muscle develops tension, one of three actions can happen: the muscle can shorten, remain the same length, or actually lengthen. Let's look at the familiar large muscle groups, the biceps and triceps, on the anterior and posterior sides of your upper arm, to see examples of these three different types of tension.

A. Concentric contraction

Tension in biceps (agonist)

Triceps relaxed (antagonist)

B. Eccentric contraction

Tension in biceps

Triceps relaxed

C. Isometric contractions

Tension in triceps

Tension in biceps

Animation

Figure 5.4 A—In this depiction of concentric contraction, the agonist biceps contracts and the antagonist triceps relaxes. B—The biceps is eccentrically contracting (lengthening) while serving as a brake to control the downward motion of the weight. C—Isometric contractions involve both the biceps and triceps developing tension, but neither muscle shortens, and there is no motion. *If you push against an immovable object, such as a wall, as hard as you can, do your muscles contract? If so, what kind of contraction occurs?*

When the biceps muscle develops tension and shortens, your hand moves up toward your shoulder (**Figure 5.4A**). This is called a **concentric** (kun-SEHN-trik), or shortening, contraction of the biceps.

In the example just described, the biceps is performing the role of **agonist** (AG-un-ist), or prime mover, and the opposing muscle group, the triceps, is playing the role of **antagonist** (an-TAG-un-ist). The antagonist muscles may be completely relaxed or may develop a slight amount of tension, depending on the requirements of the movement.

You might wonder if a muscle can lengthen while developing tension, and if so, how it can lengthen. Suppose someone were to place in your hands a very heavy weight that was too heavy for you to hold in position. At first, your biceps would develop tension in an effort to hold the weight in place. But if the weight were too heavy to manage, causing you to lower the weight, your biceps would lengthen. This type of action is known as an **eccentric** (ehk-SEHN-trik), or lengthening, contraction (**Figure 5.4B**). In this case

the force of gravity (not the triceps) acting on the weight causes the weight to lower.

In a third scenario (**Figure 5.4C**) you "flex" the muscles in your arm, developing tension in both the biceps and triceps, but there is no movement. This is called an **isometric** (IGH-soh-MEHT-rik) contraction of both the biceps and triceps. With an isometric contraction no change in muscle length occurs.

It is the versatility of the arrangements of human muscles in agonist and antagonist pairs around joints that enables the different movements of the human body. These versatile arrangements also help to stabilize joints and maintain body posture.

The Production of Heat

We all know that vigorous exercise is typically accompanied by an increase in body temperature and sweating. Do you know why this happens? It happens because the working muscles generate heat.

But even when we are not exercising, the muscles, typically comprising at least 40% of body mass, generate heat, and this heat helps maintain normal body temperature.

How does this happen? Muscles require energy in the form of adenosine triphosphate (ATP) to function. You may recall from your study of chapter 2 that ATP is generated within muscle cells. The ATP is then released to provide energy when the muscle is stimulated, generating heat in the process.

 Check Your Understanding

1. Explain contractility and how it creates movement.
2. When you are in the process of moving from a standing to a sitting position, what type of contraction are your quadricep (page 180) muscles experiencing?
3. What chemical substance in the body provides energy for muscles?

Lesson 5.1 Review and Assessment

Mini Glossary   Make sure that you know the meaning of each key term.

 Build vocabulary with e-flash cards and games

agonist   role played by a skeletal muscle to cause a movement

antagonist   role played by a skeletal muscle acting to slow or stop a movement

aponeurosis   a flat, sheetlike fibrous tissue that connects muscle or bone to other tissues

concentric   a type of contraction that results in shortening of a muscle

contractility   the ability to contract or shorten

eccentric   contraction accompanied by lengthening of a muscle

endomysium   a fine, protective sheath of connective tissue around a skeletal muscle fiber

epimysium   the outermost sheath of connective tissue that surrounds a skeletal muscle

extensibility   the ability to be stretched

fascicle   a bundle of muscle fibers

irritability   the ability to respond to a stimulus

isometric   a type of contraction that involves no change in muscle length

muscle fiber   an individual skeletal muscle cell

perimysium   a connective tissue sheath that envelops each primary bundle of muscle fibers

peristalsis   a wave of symmetrical squeezing of the digestive tract walls that occurs during digestion

sarcolemma   the delicate membrane surrounding each striated muscle fiber

Know and Understand

 Assess

1. Starting with a muscle fiber and working from the inside out, name each part of the skeletal muscle structure.
2. Describe the role of each type of muscle tissue (cardiac, smooth, and skeletal).
3. Explain the difference between irritability and contractility.
4. What is the difference between extensibility and elasticity?

Analyze and Apply

5. Give three examples of how you use isometric contractions during a typical day.
6. Compare and contrast the three types of muscles.

7. What do you think would happen if your antagonist muscles no longer functioned?

In the Lab

8. Using spaghetti and plastic wrap, create a muscle that includes muscle fibers, fascicles, endomysium, perimysium, and the epimysium. Work in groups and verbally describe which part of the muscle you are constructing as you assemble it.
9. Do a full push-up (up then down). Determine when the triceps experienced concentric contractions and when they experienced eccentric contractions.
10. Dissect a chicken leg and identify the muscle, tendon, aponeurosis, and epimysium.

Skeletal Muscle Actions

Before You Read

Try to answer the following questions before you read this lesson.

Do sprinters and distance runners have different types of skeletal muscle fibers?

What factors influence how rapidly a muscle fatigues?

Lesson Objectives

1. Describe a motor unit and explain the functional differences between motor units that contain large and small numbers of muscle fibers.

2. Explain how a nerve impulse generates an action potential in a muscle fiber.

3. Explain how muscle contraction occurs at the level of the sarcomere.

4. Describe the differences between slow-twitch and fast-twitch skeletal muscle fibers.

5. Discuss the concepts of muscular strength, power, and endurance.

Key Terms

E-Flash Cards

acetylcholine	motor unit
action potential	neuromuscular junction
all-or-none law	parallel
axon	pennate
axon terminals	sarcomeres
cross bridges	slow-twitch
fast-twitch	synaptic cleft
motor neuron	tetanus

The development of tension in a skeletal muscle is influenced by a number of variables. Among these variables are signals from the nervous system, the properties of the muscle fibers, and the arrangement of fibers within the muscle. This lesson describes the effects of these influences. You will also learn in this lesson how muscle actions contribute to muscular strength, power, and endurance.

The Motor Unit

Muscle tissue is not able to develop tension unless stimulated by one or more nerves. Because of the dependent relationship of the muscular system on the nervous system, the two are often referred to collectively as the *neuromuscular system*.

A nerve that stimulates skeletal muscle, which is under voluntary control, is known as a **motor neuron**. A single motor neuron and all of the muscle cells that it stimulates is known as a **motor unit** (**Figure 5.5**). The motor unit is considered to be the functional unit of the neuromuscular system.

One motor neuron supplying impulses to a muscle may connect to anywhere between 100 to nearly 2,000 skeletal muscle fibers, depending on the size and function of the muscle. The small muscles responsible for finely tuned movements, such as those in the eyes and fingers, have small motor units with few fibers per motor unit. Large, powerful muscles, such as those surrounding the hips, have large motor units with many fibers. Motor units are typically contained within a portion of a muscle, but may also be interspersed with the muscle cells of other motor units.

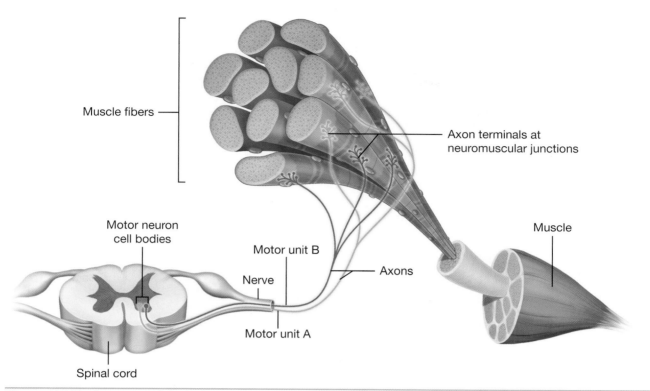

Figure 5.5 Each motor unit includes a motor neuron and all the muscle fibers it activates. *How does a motor neuron activate muscle fibers?*

Generating Action Potentials

How does the motor neuron communicate with the muscle cells in the motor unit to stimulate them? As **Figure 5.5** shows, a long, thin fiber called an **axon** connects the motor neuron cell body with the muscle fibers included in the motor unit. Close to the fibers, the axon branches into **axon terminals** which in turn branch out to individual muscle fibers. The link between each axon terminal and muscle fiber is called the **neuromuscular junction**. The axon terminal and fiber are separated by a tiny gap known as the **synaptic cleft**, which is filled with interstitial fluid (**Figure 5.6** on the next page).

When a nerve impulse reaches the end of an axon terminal, a chemical called a *neurotransmitter* discharges and diffuses across the synaptic cleft to attach to receptors on the muscle fiber sarcolemma. The neurotransmitter that stimulates muscle is called **acetylcholine** (a-SEE-til-KOH-leen).

The effect of acetylcholine is to make the sarcolemma temporarily permeable. Channels open that allow positive sodium ions (Na+) to rapidly invade the fiber at the same time that positive potassium ions (K+) rush out of the fiber. Because more Na+ enters than K+ exits, the net effect is the creation of a positive charge inside the muscle fiber.

This reversal of electrical charge is known as *depolarization*. Depolarization triggers the opening of additional channels in the fiber membrane that allow only entry of additional Na+. This flood of positive ions into the fiber generates an electrical charge called an **action potential**.

Contractions of the Sarcomeres

Glucose stored in the form of glycogen within the muscle cell provides the energy for creating the action potential. Phosphocreatine within the cell enables the transfer of energy to the protein filaments actin and myosin. Actin and myosin are contractile proteins that reside in functional units called **sarcomeres** (SAR-koh-mairz) inside the muscle fiber. The release of calcium ions (Ca++) triggers the sliding of

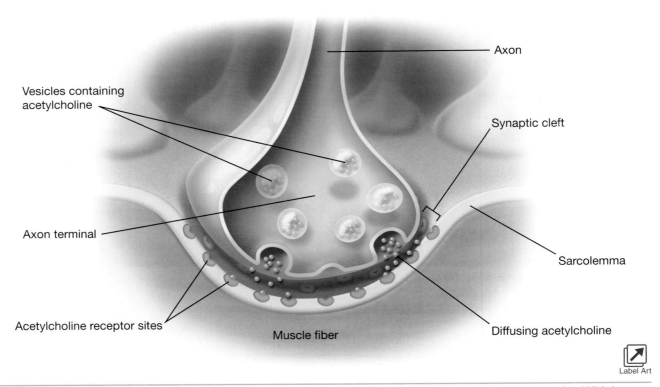

Axon

Vesicles containing acetylcholine

Synaptic cleft

Axon terminal

Sarcolemma

Acetylcholine receptor sites

Muscle fiber

Diffusing acetylcholine

Label Art

Figure 5.6 The neuromuscular junction, the site at which nerve impulses are transmitted to muscle. *Which chemical labeled in this drawing is a neurotransmitter?*

the actin filaments over the myosin filaments, resulting in a contraction of the sarcomere (**Figure 5.7**).

What causes the actin filaments to slide over the myosin filaments? Notice in **Figure 5.7** that the myosin filaments are encircled by small protrusions called *heads*. When the sarcomere is activated by an action potential, these heads attach to receptor sites on the actin filaments, forming **cross bridges**. The cross bridges contract, pulling the actin filaments toward the center of the sarcomere. During the process of sarcomere contraction, these cross bridges attach, pull, and release multiple times. The Ca++ ions released with the arrival of the action potential enable the attachments of the myosin heads to the actin filaments.

The neuromuscular system has the ability to produce slow, gentle movements as well as fast, forceful movements. This ability to produce different kinds of movements and force variance is accomplished by regulating the number and frequency of action potentials. Only a small number of action potentials are needed for

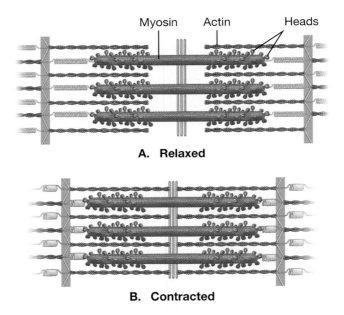

Myosin   Actin   Heads

A. Relaxed

B. Contracted

Figure 5.7 The sarcomere is the contractile unit of muscle. When the muscle is stimulated, the actin filaments slide together, producing contraction of the sarcomere.

slow, gentle movements, while fast or forceful movements require a large number of action potentials, released rapidly.

Maximum Tension and Return to Relaxation

When receiving an action potential, a given motor unit always develops maximum tension, a physiological principle known as the **all-or-none law**. But because each whole muscle includes multiple motor units, simultaneous activation of many motor units is required for the muscle to develop maximum tension. The diagram in **Figure 5.8** displays the relationship between number and frequency of action potentials and the development of tension in the muscle. With high-frequency stimulation, the muscle develops a sustained, maximal level of tension called **tetanus**.

Almost all skeletal motor units develop tension in a twitch-like fashion, generating maximum tension very briefly and then immediately relaxing. After the action potential has traveled the length of the muscle fiber, chemical processes return the fiber to its resting state. Sodium ions diffuse back out of the cell into the interstitial fluid, and calcium ions return to storage sites within the cell. The actin filaments slide back to their original positions as the cross bridges release them, and the muscle fiber returns to a state of relaxation.

Check Your Understanding

1. What structures make up a motor unit?
2. Describe the neuromuscular junction.
3. What is an action potential?
4. Why do you want a small motor unit for fine motor skills?
5. Explain the all-or-none law.
6. How do muscles relax?

Skeletal Fiber Types

Why are some athletes especially good at events or tasks that require endurance, whereas others excel at activities that require explosive strength or speed? The answer may have something to do with the ways in which these individuals train, but that is only a small part of the explanation. In fact, a big part of why certain people are better at particular activities and sports may relate to the characteristics of their skeletal muscle fibers.

Skeletal muscle fibers may be divided into two umbrella categories—**slow-twitch** (Type I) and **fast-twitch** (Type II). As the names suggest,

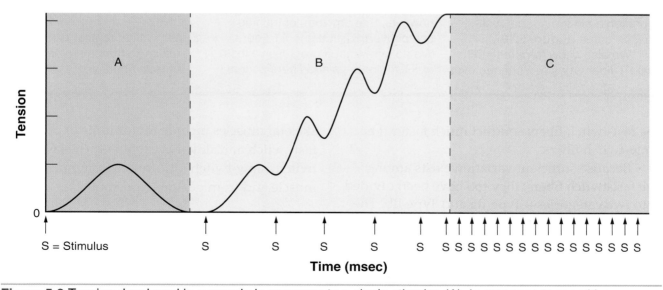

Figure 5.8 Tension developed in a muscle in response to a single stimulus (A), in response to repetitive stimulation (B), and in response to high-frequency stimulation, or tetanus (C). *Do you think this graph represents the activation of one or many motor units? Explain.*

WHAT RESEARCH TELLS US

...*about* Fast- and Slow-Twitch Muscles

Researchers have taken muscle biopsies (small, needle-sized plugs of muscle tissue) from elite athletes in a variety of sports. They have found that individuals specializing in events that require explosive strength or speed have unusually high proportions of fast-twitch (FT) fibers, and that elite endurance athletes tend to have very high proportions of slow-twitch (ST) fibers.

It may be the case that many of those who are able to achieve athletic success at the highest levels are simply born with high percentages of either FT or ST fibers. Once these individuals have experienced success in a particular sport or event, it is likely that they gravitate toward that sport or event (**Figure 5.9**).

Of course, certain individuals within the general population of untrained people also have high percentages of FT or ST muscles. The distribution of FT/ST ratios among the general population is represented in the normal, bell-shaped curve (**Figure 5.10**).

We also know from research that FT-fiber types can change over

Rena Schild/Shutterstock.com

Figure 5.9 Elite sprint cyclists tend to have high percentages of fast-twitch muscle fibers. *Aside from sprint cycling, what are some sports in which athletes with high percentages of fast-twitch muscle fibers would be particularly successful?*

time. FT fibers can be converted to ST fibers with years of endurance training. No evidence exists, however, that any form of training can convert ST fibers to FT fibers. We do know that a progressive loss of FT motor units and fibers occurs

Figure 5.10 The percentages of fast-twitch (FT) and slow-twitch (ST) fibers in the general population are normally distributed.

as we age, although this loss can be minimized by regular, high-intensity exercise throughout life.

Taking It Further

1. Why do FT muscle fibers affect strength and speed? Why do ST muscle fibers provide increased endurance?

2. Why might regular exercise minimize the natural loss of FT muscle fibers with age?

the fast-twitch fibers contract much faster than slow-twitch fibers.

Because sufficient variation exists among the fast-twitch fibers, they too have been divided into two categories—Type IIa and Type IIb. The Type IIa fibers are intermediate in contraction speed between the slow-twitch fibers and the classic fast-twitch fibers, which are Type IIb. The Type IIb fibers contract very rapidly, in about one-seventh the time required for slow-twitch fibers to contract. As a result, the Type IIb fibers also fatigue rapidly. Although all of the muscle fibers in a motor unit are of the same type, most

skeletal muscles include motor units of both fast-twitch and slow-twitch fibers. The fast-twitch/slow-twitch ratio varies from muscle to muscle and from person to person.

Fiber Architecture

Another factor that affects the ways in which skeletal muscles function is fiber architecture. Fiber architecture refers to the ways in which fibers are arranged within the muscle. The two major categories of muscle fiber arrangement are **parallel** and **pennate**.

Parallel Fiber Architecture

With parallel fiber architecture, the fibers run largely parallel to each other along the length of the muscle. As **Figure 5.11** shows, these parallel fiber arrangements may result in muscle shapes that are fusiform (wide in the middle and tapering on both ends), bundled, or triangular. Examples of muscles with this type of architecture are the biceps brachii (fusiform), rectus abdominis (bundled), and pectoralis major (triangular).

The individual fibers in the parallel architecture typically do not run the entire length of the muscle. Instead, the individual parallel fibers have interconnections with neighboring fibers. These interconnections promote contraction when the muscle is stimulated. This fiber arrangement enables shortening of the muscle and the ability to move body segments through large ranges of motion.

Fusiform   Bundled   Triangular

A. Parallel fiber arrangements

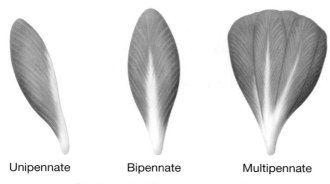

Unipennate   Bipennate   Multipennate

B. Pennate fiber arrangements

Figure 5.11 Fibers within a muscle may be arranged so that they are largely parallel or pennate (feathered). *Can you identify a muscle with parallel fiber arrangement? With pennate fiber arrangement?*

Pennate Fiber Architecture

In a pennate fiber arrangement, each fiber attaches obliquely to a central tendon, and sometimes attaches to more than one tendon. As **Figure 5.11** shows,

- fibers that are aligned in one direction to a central tendon are *unipennate*;
- fibers that attach to a central tendon are *bipennate*; and
- fibers that attach to a central tendon in more than two directions are referred to as *multipennate*.

Certain muscles of the hand are unipennate, the rectus femoris (a member of the quadriceps group in the thigh) is bipennate, and the deltoid is multipennate.

With a pennate fiber arrangement, the muscle does not shorten as much upon contraction as a muscle with a parallel fiber arrangement. However, the pennate arrangement makes it possible to pack more fibers into the muscle. This means that the muscle can generate more force.

> **Check Your Understanding**
>
> 1. What is the difference between fast-twitch and slow-twitch fibers?
> 2. Which fiber type helps a sprinter get out of the blocks fast?
> 3. Why can pennate-arranged fibers generate more force than parallel-arranged fibers?

Muscular Strength, Power, and Endurance

In everyday conversation we sometimes use *strength* and *power* interchangeably. However, as we will discuss in this section of the lesson, muscular strength and power are quite different concepts. We will examine what it means to have muscle fatigue, along with the related concept of muscular endurance, which is a little more complicated.

Muscular Strength

It may be tempting to think that muscular strength is the amount of force a given muscle can produce. It is impossible, however, to measure muscle force directly without penetrating the body. So to avoid invasive procedures, we use external measures (such as the amount of resistance a person can move) to establish an indirect measure of muscle strength.

Remember that most joints in the human body are crossed by more than just one muscle. Additionally, many exercises involve more than one joint. This means that an index-of-strength measure such as maximum bench press actually assesses the collective work of several muscles that cross the shoulder and elbow (**Figure 5.12**). The main muscles that work during execution

Figure 5.12 The amount of weight being lifted is an indirect measure of this person's muscular strength. *What would be a more precise, direct method of measuring his strength?*

of a bench press include the pectoralis major, pectoralis minor, anterior deltoid, and triceps brachii.

A more precise assessment of the strength of a muscle group at a given joint is the amount of torque (TORK), or rotary force, that the muscles can generate. Torque is the product of the size of a force and the perpendicular distance of that force from an axis of rotation. For the joint shown in **Figure 5.13**, the torque produced by a muscle is the product of muscle force and the perpendicular distance from the muscle attachment to the center of rotation at the joint.

The more torque a muscle generates at a joint, the greater the tendency for movement of the bones at the joint. Machines called *dynamometers* measure joint torques. Measures of joint torque, which we use as a measure of strength, are based solely on the resistance moved or matched. The speed with which a resistance is moved is not relevant to the strength measurement.

Muscular Power

The variable that does involve speed is muscular power. Mechanical power is defined as force multiplied by velocity (force × velocity). Muscular power, then, has been defined specifically as muscle force multiplied by muscle-shortening velocity during contraction. Notice, however, that neither muscle force nor shortening velocity can be measured from outside the body. Research dynamometers have the ability to generate estimates of muscular power based on the resistance moved and movement speed.

Like muscular strength, muscular power is typically generated by several different muscles working collectively. Sprinting, along with the jumping and throwing events in track and field, are good examples of activities that require muscular power. Because force production and movement speed contribute equally to muscular power, the sprinter with the greatest leg strength may not necessarily be the fastest.

Muscular Endurance

Muscular endurance is the ability of a muscle to produce tension over a period of

Figure 5.13 Calculating Muscle Force

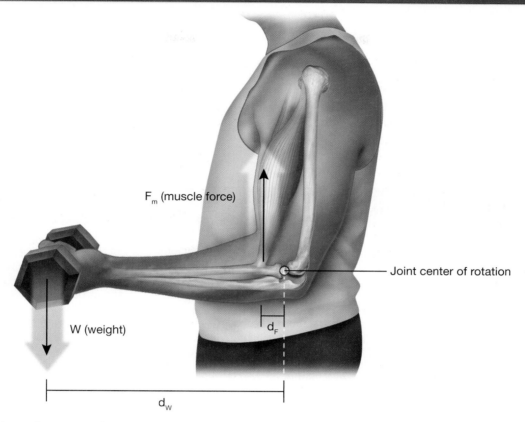

F_m (muscle force)

Joint center of rotation

d_F

W (weight)

d_W

Do you know how much force your muscle must generate to hold a five-pound weight in the position shown in the illustration? Let's see if we can calculate the amount of force needed.

To hold the weight in this position, the torque at the elbow joint *generated by the muscle* (muscle torque) must balance the torque *produced by the weight* (weight torque) at the elbow.

As you know from reading this lesson, muscle torque is the product of muscle force and the perpendicular distance of that force from the center of rotation at the joint. We can state this in a formula as

$$T_m = F_m \times d_F$$

where T_m = muscle torque, F_m = muscle force, and d_F = the perpendicular distance.

Weight torque is the product of the weight and the perpendicular distance of that weight from the center of rotation at the joint. This formula can be stated as

$$T_W = W \times d_W$$

where T_W = weight torque, W = weight, and d_W = the perpendicular distance.

Let's suppose that the weight in the illustration is 5 pounds, and that it is being held at a distance (d_W) of 12 inches from the center of the joint. The distance of the muscle attachment from the joint center (d_F) is 1 inch. How much force must the muscle produce to support the weight?

$$T_m = T_W$$
$$F_m \times d_F = W \times d_W$$
$$F_m \times 1'' = 5 \text{ lb} \times 12''$$
$$F_m = 60 \text{ lb}$$

Are you surprised? To support just 5 pounds in the hand, the muscle must generate 60 pounds of force. What can we learn from this? Because muscles attach so closely to joints, the human musculoskeletal system is designed more for movement speed than for strength.

Now you try: Suppose that the weight (W) in this picture is 10 pounds, the d_W is 15 inches, and the d_F is 1 inch. What is the F_m?

time. The tension may be constant (for example, when a gymnast holds a motionless handstand), or it may vary cyclically (for example, during running, cycling, or rowing). Generally, the longer the physical activity is maintained, the greater the required muscular endurance. Because the force and speed requirements of different movements can vary significantly, the definition of muscular endurance is specific to each physical activity.

In general, muscle fatigue can be thought of as the opposite of muscular endurance. The faster a muscle fatigues, the less endurance it has. A variety of factors affect the rate at which a muscle fatigues, including the nature of the work or exercise being done, how often the muscle is used, the muscle fiber composition of the muscle, and the temperature and humidity of the environment.

 Check Your Understanding

1. What is measured to determine muscular strength?
2. What is measured to determine muscular power?
3. Is the strongest athlete the fastest? Why or why not?
4. What is muscular endurance?
5. What influences muscular endurance?

Lesson 5.2 Review and Assessment

Mini Glossary   Make sure that you know the meaning of each key term.

 Build vocabulary with e-flash cards and games

acetylcholine a neurotransmitter chemical that stimulates muscle

action potential the electric charge produced in nerve or muscle fiber by stimulation

all-or-none law the rule stating that the fibers in a given motor unit always develop maximum tension when stimulated

axon a long, thin fiber connected to the motor neuron cell body

axon terminals offshoots of the axon that branch out to connect with individual muscle fibers

cross bridges connections between the heads of myosin filaments and receptor sites on the actin filaments

fast-twitch type of muscle that contracts quickly

motor neuron a nerve that stimulates skeletal muscle tissue

motor unit a single motor neuron and all of the muscle fibers that it stimulates

neuromuscular junction the link between an axon terminal and a muscle fiber

parallel a type of muscle fiber arrangement in which fibers run largely parallel to each other along the length of the muscle

pennate a type of muscle fiber arrangement in which each fiber attaches obliquely to a central tendon

sarcomeres units composed of actin and myosin that contract inside the muscle fiber

slow-twitch type of muscle that contracts slowly and is fatigue resistant

synaptic cleft the tiny gap that separates the axon terminal and muscle fiber

tetanus a sustained, maximal level of muscle tension that occurs with high-frequency stimulation

Know and Understand

 Assess

1. Explain the role of acetylcholine in muscle contractions.
2. Describe the parts of a motor unit.
3. Discuss the differences between a large and small motor unit and their functions.
4. Describe parallel and pennate fiber patterns.

Analyze and Apply

5. Which fiber types do you think contribute to each of the following: muscular strength, power, and endurance? Explain your reasoning.
6. What would happen if you had no Na+ in your body? no Ca++?

7. Why do temperature and humidity increase the rate of muscle fatigue?
8. Do you think a soccer player has more fast-twitch or slow-twitch muscle fibers? Why?

In the Lab

9. Try an experiment. Get into and then hold a squatting position for as long as you can while a partner times you. Allow five minutes to rest; then continually move into and out of a squatting position for as long as possible, again with your partner timing you. Did you fatigue more quickly holding a squatting position or while moving up and down in a squatting motion? Why? Now reverse roles with your partner.

The Major Skeletal Muscles

Before You Read

Try to answer the following questions before you read this lesson.

What muscles are responsible for breathing?

What important functions do the neck and trunk muscles contribute beyond movement capabilities?

What are the primary functions of the lower limb?

Lesson Objectives

1. Describe and give examples of the types of body motions that occur in the sagittal, frontal, and transverse planes.

2. Identify the locations and functions of the muscles of the head and neck.

3. Identify the locations and functions of the trunk muscles.

4. Identify the locations and functions of the muscles of the upper limb.

5. Identify the locations and functions of the muscles of the lower limb.

Key Terms

E-Flash Cards

abduction	lateral rotation
adduction	medial rotation
circumduction	opposition
dorsiflexion	origin
eversion	plantar flexion
extension	pronation
flexion	radial deviation
hyperextension	supination
insertion	ulnar deviation
inversion	

There are more than 650 skeletal muscles in the human body. In this lesson we will present only the most important muscles from the standpoint of functional movement. Almost all of these muscles are arranged in agonist-antagonist pairs, causing opposing actions at one or more joints.

Directional Motions

To understand the functional movement of muscles, you need to learn a new concept about muscle attachments. It will also be helpful to review some directional terms that you learned in chapter 1.

Skeletal muscles attach at either end of the muscle; the most common attachments are tendon connections to bone. The end of a muscle that attaches to a relatively fixed structure is called the **origin**. The end of a muscle that attaches to a bone that typically moves when the muscle contracts is called the **insertion**.

For an example of origin and insertion, let's look at the brachialis muscle, which crosses the anterior side of the elbow. Its origin is on the humerus, and its insertion is on the ulna in the forearm. When the brachialis contracts, the forearm (ulna) is pulled toward the upper arm, while the upper arm (humerus) remains stationary.

Remember—when stimulated to develop tension, muscles can only pull. They are incapable of pushing.

In addition, remember from chapter 1 that to describe the human body and its movements, we refer to three major planes that pass through the center of the body:

- The *sagittal* plane is in line with forward and backward motions;
- The *frontal* plane is in line with sideways movement; and

- Rotational movements occur in the *transverse* plane.

As we learned in chapter 1, the frame of reference for all movement is the anatomical position. In this position the human body is erect with the hands at the sides and the palms facing forward.

✔ Check Your Understanding

1. Which end of the muscle typically moves?
2. Define anatomical position.
3. What are the three major anatomical planes?

Sagittal Plane Movements

The primary sagittal plane (forward/backward) movements are **flexion** (FLEHK-shun), **extension**, and **hyperextension** (**Figure 5.14**). Flexion describes forward-bending motion of the head, trunk, upper arm, forearm, hand, and hip; and backward motion of the lower leg at the knee. In flexion movements, body surfaces are coming together. Extension returns body segments from a position of flexion to anatomical position. Hyperextension continues the extension motion past anatomical position.

Two movements of the foot also occur primarily in the sagittal (SAJ-i-tal) plane. Bringing the top of the foot toward the lower leg is called **dorsiflexion** (DOR-si-FLEHK-shun), and moving the foot in the opposite direction away from the lower leg is called **plantar flexion** (**Figure 5.14**).

Memory Tip
Planting the ball of the foot is the motion involved in *plantar* flexion.

Frontal Plane Movements

Common movements in the frontal plane include **abduction** and **adduction** (**Figure 5.14**). Movements at the shoulder and hip that take the arm and leg away from the midline of the body are called *abduction*. Oppositely directed movements that bring the arm and leg closer to the midline of the body are called *adduction*.

Memory Tip
Just as *abduct* means "to take away," abduction takes a body segment away from the body. Just as *add* means "to bring back," adduction returns a body segment closer to the body.

Movements of the foot that occur mainly in the frontal plane are **inversion** and **eversion**. Rolling the sole of the foot inward is inversion, while rolling the sole of the foot outward is eversion (**Figure 5.14**).

Frontal plane movements of the hand at the wrist are called **radial deviation** and **ulnar deviation**. Recall from chapter 4 that the forearm has two bones—the radius and the ulna. The radius is on the thumb side of the hand, and the ulna is on the "little finger" side of the arm. From anatomical position, with the palms facing forward, abduction of the hand toward the thumb is called *radial deviation*, and adduction of the hand toward the little finger is called *ulnar deviation* (**Figure 5.14**).

Trunk and neck motions away from anatomical position in the frontal plane are called *lateral flexion* and *side bending*. Return from a position of lateral flexion to anatomical position is called *lateral extension*.

Transverse Plane Movements

Transverse plane movements mostly involve rotation around the long axis of a body segment. When the head or trunk rotate from side to side, the movement is simply called *left* or *right rotation*. Rotation of an arm or a leg in the transverse plane is called **medial rotation** if the rotation is directed medially, or inward, and **lateral rotation** if the movement is directed laterally, or outward (**Figure 5.14**). The special terms used for rotation of the forearm are **pronation** for medial (palm down) rotation and **supination** (SOO-pi-NAY-shun) for lateral (palm up) rotation (**Figure 5.14**).

Dorsiflexion

Plantar flexion

A. Sagittal plane movements

Flexion

Extension

Hyperextension

Adduction

Abduction

Inversion

Eversion

Radial deviation

Ulnar deviation

B. Frontal plane movements

Lateral rotation

Medial rotation

Pronation

Supination

C. Transverse plane movements

Circumduction

D. Multi-plane movement

Figure 5.14 Directional movement terminology.

Multiplanar Movements

A few movements of body segments do not fall within a single plane. If you have ever purchased running shoes, you may have heard the terms *pronation* and *supination* used to describe motions of the foot occurring specifically at the subtalar joint (where the heel and ankle bones meet). Pronation at the subtalar joint is a combination of eversion, abduction, and dorsiflexion. Supination at this joint includes inversion, adduction, and plantar flexion. Moving a finger, arm, or leg in a rotational manner such that the end of the segment traces a circle is called **circumduction** (SER-kum-DUK-shun), which you can see in **Figure 5.14**. And, finally, touching any of your four fingers to the thumb is known as **opposition**. Having an opposable thumb gives us the all-important ability to grasp objects.

Check Your Understanding

1. In what direction are movements guided on the sagittal plane?
2. What special movements occur on the frontal plane at the hand? the foot?
3. What is the difference between pronation and supination of the hand and the foot?
4. Describe circumduction.
5. Define medial and lateral rotation.

Head and Neck Muscles

The muscles of the head and neck can be divided into three groups: facial muscles, chewing muscles, and neck muscles. The difference between facial muscles and most other muscles is that facial muscle insertions connect them to other muscles or skin. When these muscles contract, pulling on the skin, they produce an array of facial expressions.

With the exception of the orbicularis oris, which encircles the mouth, and the sheetlike platysma on the front and sides of the neck, all of the other head and neck muscles are paired—one on the right and one on the left. The head and neck muscles are displayed in **Figure 5.15**, and

their locations and functions are summarized in **Figure 5.16**.

Trunk Muscles

The trunk muscles provide stability for the vertebral column. They are also responsible for maintaining upright posture. American football players train to strengthen the neck and trunk muscles in an effort to maximize spinal stability and minimize risk of injury to the delicate spinal cord and internal organs (**Figure 5.17**). Conversely, female gymnasts train to enhance the flexibility of the spine and are capable of extraordinary spinal hyperextension, especially during balance-beam and floor-exercise routines.

Collectively, the trunk muscles enable flexion, extension, hyperextension, lateral flexion, and rotation of the head and trunk. From a functional perspective, the anterior abdominal muscles also assist with urination, defecation, forced expiration during breathing, and childbirth. The all-important diaphragm muscle regulates breathing. The trunk muscles also

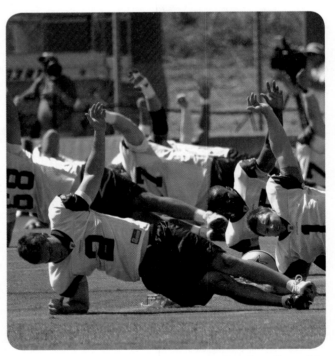

Arthur Eugene Preston/Shutterstock, Inc.

Figure 5.17 Football players conditioning. *Why is it critically important for football players to strengthen their neck and trunk muscles?*

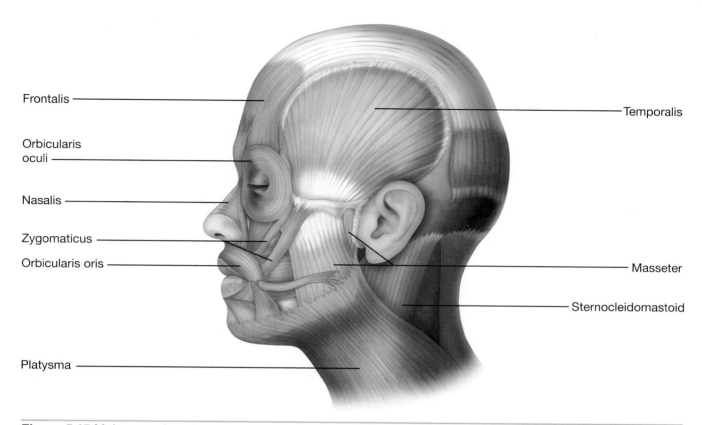

Figure 5.15 Major muscles of the head and neck. *Which muscle is referred to as the "smiling" muscle?*

Figure 5.16 Muscles of the Head and Neck		
Muscle	**Location**	**Primary Functions**
Facial Muscles		
Frontalis	forehead; connects cranium to skin above eyebrows	raises eyebrows, wrinkles forehead
Orbicularis oculi	encircles the eyes	closes eyes, enables squinting
Nasalis	nose	modifies size of nostrils
Orbicularis oris	encircles mouth	closes lips, produces kissing motion
Zygomaticus	connects cheekbones to corners of mouth	the "smiling" muscle
Platysma	front and sides of neck	pulls corners of mouth down, opens mouth wide
Chewing Muscles		
Masseter	connects zygomatic bone to mandible	closes the jaw
Temporalis	fan-shaped muscle over temporal bone	assists masseter with closing jaw
Neck Muscles		
Sternocleidomastoid	sides of neck	flexion of head, rotation of head toward opposite side of contraction

serve as a protective sheath for the organs of the thoracic and abdominal cavities. The locations and primary functions of the major muscles of the anterior and posterior trunk are summarized in the table in **Figure 5.18**. These muscles are showin in **Figure 5.19**.

Upper Limb Muscles

Because the shoulder is a ball-and-socket joint and the most freely movable joint in the human body, the movement capabilities of the upper limb are impressive. This large range of motion is achieved because the bone structure of the glenohumeral (GLEH-noh-HYOO-mer-al) joint provides little to no stability, rendering it susceptible to dislocation. Therefore, it is up to the large, powerful muscles surrounding the shoulder to maintain the stability and integrity of the joint.

The arm muscles enable strong, controlled movements in sports such as gymnastics, rowing, and archery, as well as fast, powerful movements in weightlifting, boxing, and throwing. The dexterity of the finger muscles enables precise movements, such as typing, texting, knitting, and playing musical instruments.

The joints of the upper limb include those of the shoulder, elbow, wrist, and fingers. In this lesson we include information about the major muscles that cross the shoulder and elbow joints. Because there are nine muscles that cross the wrist and ten muscles within the hand (some

Figure 5.18 Muscles of the Trunk

Muscle	Location	Primary Functions
Anterior Muscles		
Pectoralis major	upper chest; connects sternum, shoulder girdle, and upper ribs to proximal humerus	adduction and flexion of arm
Rectus abdominis	center front of abdomen; connects ribs to pubic crest	flexion and lateral flexion of trunk
External oblique	front of abdomen; connects lower eight ribs to anterior iliac crest	flexion, lateral flexion, and rotation to opposite side of trunk
Internal oblique	front of abdomen beneath the external obliques;connects lower four ribs with the iliac crest	flexion, lateral flexion, and rotation to same side of trunk
Posterior Muscles		
Trapezius	upper back and neck; connects skull and thoracic vertebrae to clavicle and scapula	extension and hyperextension of head
Erector spinae	length of vertebral column; connects adjacent vertebrae	extension, lateral flexion, and rotation to opposite side of vertebral column
Muscles for Breathing		
Diaphragm	dome-shaped muscle separating thoracic and abdominal cavities	enlarges thoracic cavity for inhalation
Internal intercostals	connect the ribs; located between them	decrease thoracic cavity during forced expiration
External intercostals	connect the ribs; located between them	help enlarge thoracic cavity for inhalation

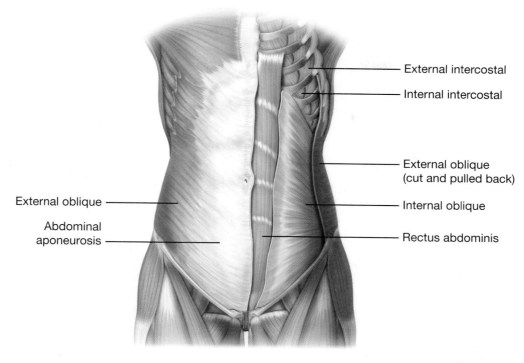

External intercostal

Internal intercostal

External oblique
(cut and pulled back)

Internal oblique

Rectus abdominis

External oblique

Abdominal
aponeurosis

A. Anterior view

Trapezius

Erector spinae muscle group

B. Posterior view

Label Art

Figure 5.19 Major muscles of the trunk. *What are some basic functions that the muscles of the trunk assist with, in addition to movement of the trunk and the head and protection of the organs?*

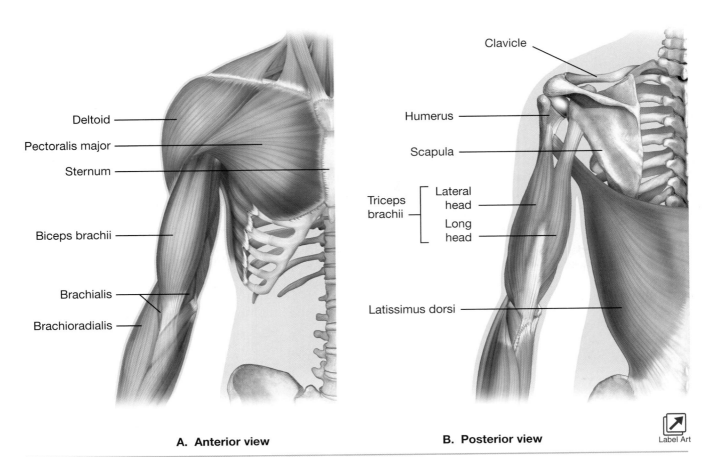

A. Anterior view   B. Posterior view

Label Art

Figure 5.20 Muscles of the upper limb.

Figure 5.21 **Muscles of the Upper Limb**		
Muscle	**Location**	**Primary Functions**
Shoulder Muscles		
Pectoralis major	upper chest; connects sternum, shoulder girdle, and upper ribs to proximal humerus	adduction and flexion of arm
Deltoid	covers external shoulder; connects scapula and clavicle to humerus	abduction, flexion, extension, and rotation of arm
Latissimus dorsi	midback and lower back; connects lower vertebral column and lower ribs to the humerus	extension, adduction, and medial rotation of arm
Elbow Muscles		
Biceps brachii	anterior arm; connects scapula to radius	flexion, and assists with supination of forearm
Brachialis	connects upper arm to forearm (humerus to ulna)	flexion of forearm
Brachioradialis	connects upper arm to forearm (humerus to radius)	flexion of forearm
Triceps brachii	posterior arm; connects scapula and humerus to ulna	extension of forearm

of which branch out to several of the fingers) these are not discussed. **Figure 5.20** lists the major muscles of the upper limb, and **Figure 5.21** summarizes their locations and functions.

Lower Limb Muscles

While the structure of the upper limb lends itself well to activities that involve large ranges of motion, the lower limb is well designed for its primary jobs of standing and walking. Running, jumping, kicking, climbing, skipping, hopping, and dancing are just a few of the additional capabilities of the lower limb.

The lower limb includes the joints of the hip, knee, and ankle, along with numerous joints in the foot. In this lesson we include the major muscles of the hip, knee, and ankle, but we omit a number of small muscles that play assistive roles. The table in **Figure 5.22** outlines the locations and primary functions of the major muscles of the lower limb. **Figure 5.23** on the next page shows these muscles.

Notice in **Figures 5.22** and **5.23** the two muscle groups on the anterior side and posterior side of the thigh. The anterior group, the quadriceps, includes the rectus femoris, vastus lateralis, vastus medialis, and vastus intermedius, which lies under the rectus femoris. These four muscles are often referred to as a group because they all attach to the patellar tendon.

Figure 5.22 Muscles of the Lower Limb

Muscle	Location	Primary Functions
Hip Muscles		
Gluteus maximus	external buttocks; connects pelvis to femur	extension and lateral rotation of leg
Gluteus medius	directly under maximus; connects ilium of pelvis to femur	abduction and medial rotation of leg
Iliopsoas	anterior groin; connects ilium and lower vertebrae to femur	flexion of leg at hip
Adductor muscles	anterior-medial thigh	adduction and medial rotation of leg
Knee Muscles		
Quadriceps	anterior thigh; connects ilium and proximal femur to tibia	extension of leg at knee
Hamstrings	posterior thigh; connect ischium to tibia and fibula	flexion of leg at knee
Sartorius	long, straplike muscle that crosses anterior thigh obliquely; connects ilium to proximal tibia	assists with flexion, abduction, and lateral rotation of thigh
Ankle/Foot Muscles		
Gastrocnemius	prominent muscle on posterior calf; connects femur to calcaneus (heel bone) via Achilles tendon	plantar flexion of foot, flexion of leg at knee
Soleus	underlies gastrocnemius on posterior calf; connects fibula and tibia to calcaneus	plantar flexion of foot
Tibialis anterior	anterior lower leg; connects tibia to tarsal and metatarsal bones of foot	dorsiflexion and inversion of foot

A. Anterior view

B. Posterior view

Label Art

Figure 5.23 Major muscles of the lower limb. *Are your hamstring muscles part of an anterior or posterior muscle group?*

The posterior group, the hamstrings, includes the biceps femoris, semimembranosus (SEHM-ee-MEHM-bray-NOH-suhs), and semitendinosus (SEHM-ee-TEHN-di-NOH-suhs). What these muscles have in common, besides their general location, is strong, stringlike tendons that can be felt on either side of the back of the knee. The name *hamstrings* comes from the fact that hams consist of thigh and hip muscles, and butchers use the tendons of these muscles to hang the hams for smoking.

 Check Your Understanding

1. How do the attachments for facial muscles differ from the attachments for other muscles?
2. Which muscles help with posture?
3. What is sacrificed at the shoulder to allow greater range of motion?
4. For which two primary functions is the lower limb designed?

Lesson 5.3 Review and Assessment

Mini Glossary   Make sure that you know the meaning of each key term.

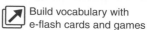 Build vocabulary with e-flash cards and games

abduction   movement of a body segment away from the body in the frontal plane

adduction   movement of a body segment closer to the body in the frontal plane

circumduction   rotational movement of a body segment such that the end of the segment traces a circle

dorsiflexion   movement of the top of the foot toward the lower leg

eversion   movement in which the sole of the foot is rolled outward

extension   movement that returns a body segment to anatomical position in the sagittal plane

flexion   forward movement of a body segment away from anatomical position in the sagittal plane

hyperextension   backward movement of a body segment past anatomical position in the sagittal plane

insertion   muscle attachment to a bone that tends to move when the muscle contracts

inversion   movement in which the sole of the foot is rolled inward

lateral rotation   outward (lateral) movement of a body segment in the transverse plane

medial rotation   inward (medial) movement of a body segment in the transverse plane

opposition   touching any of your four fingers to your thumb; this movement enables grasping of objects

origin   muscle attachment to a relatively fixed structure

plantar flexion   downward motion of the foot away from the lower leg

pronation   medial rotation of the forearm (palm down)

radial deviation   rotation of the hand toward the thumb

supination   lateral rotation of the forearm (palm up)

ulnar deviation   rotation of the hand toward the little finger

Know and Understand

 Assess

1. What are the directions of movement for the sagittal, frontal, and transverse planes?
2. Describe hyperextension.
3. Describe the difference between abduction and adduction.
4. Using the drawings and tables in this lesson, identify the agonist/antagonist pairs for abduction/adduction of the hip and plantar flexion/dorsiflexion of the ankle.

Analyze and Apply

5. What type of motor units do you think the forearm and hands have? Why?
6. Compare and contrast inversion and eversion of the foot and supination and pronation of the hand.

7. Which joints in the upper and lower limbs can perform flexion and extension?

In the Lab

8. Try writing the answers to one of the questions at the left without using your thumb. Why is opposition important?
9. What position are you in if all of your joints that can perform flexion do so at the same time?
10. In a push-up, what movements are happening at the shoulder and elbow when you are moving up? Which muscles are performing these movements? What movements occur when you move down? Which muscles cause these movements?

Common Injuries and Disorders of Muscles

Before You Read

Try to answer the following questions before you read this lesson.

What causes muscle cramps?

Which individuals are at greatest risk for developing low back pain?

Lesson Objectives

1. Explain the differences between a muscle sprain, a contusion, and a cramp.
2. Discuss the differences between tendinitis and tendinosis.
3. Explain the causes of common muscular injuries that occur during participation in different sports.
4. Describe the causes and symptoms of whiplash injuries and hernias.
5. Describe the risk factors for low back pain and explain what strategies can be used to avoid it.

Key Terms

E-Flash Cards

contusion
delayed-onset muscle
 soreness (DOMS)
hernia
muscle cramps
muscle strain

muscular dystrophy
 (MD)
myositis ossificans
shin splints
tendinitis
tendinosis

Although common, most muscle injuries are relatively minor. Fortunately, the healthy human body has considerable ability to self-repair a variety of injuries, such as those to muscles. In this lesson you will learn about some of the common muscle injuries and disorders.

Strains

A **muscle strain** happens when a muscle is stretched beyond its usual limits. Someone who has a large degree of flexibility at a particular joint is at much lower risk of straining those muscles than someone with extremely "tight" muscles crossing that same joint.

Another factor in muscle strains is the speed with which the muscles are stretched. Many strains to the hamstrings, for example, result from participating in activities in which the individual is running, accelerating, and changing direction all at the same time. When the muscle group is overstretched, a strain results.

Strains are classified as *Grade I, II,* or *III:*

- With a grade I (mild) strain, you would feel a tightness in the muscle the day after the injury, but nothing more.
- Grade II (moderate) strains produce pain caused by a partial tear in the muscle. Associated weakness and temporary loss of function may also occur.
- With a grade III (severe) strain, the damage and symptoms are significantly greater than

Memory Tip
The terms *strain* (to muscles or tendons) and *sprain* (to a ligament at a joint) are very similar. Remember that <u>T</u>ight muscles and <u>T</u>endons get s<u>T</u>rains.

those accompanying grades I and II strains. Grade III strains involve a tearing of the muscle, loss of function, internal bleeding, and swelling.

Strains of the hamstrings are a frequent problem for athletes because these injuries are slow to heal and tend to recur. One-third of all hamstring strains will recur within the first year of returning to a sport or an activity.

Contusions

A **contusion** is a bruise or bleeding within a muscle, resulting from an impact. When an already injured muscle is repeatedly struck, a more serious condition, called **myositis ossificans** (migh-oh-SIGH-tis ah-SIF-i-kanz), can develop.

Myositis ossificans involves the formation of a calcium mass within the muscle over a period of three to four weeks. After six or seven weeks the mass usually begins to dissolve and is resorbed by the body. In some cases a bony lesion can remain in the muscle.

Cramps

Muscle cramps involve moderate to severe muscle spasms that cause pain. The cause of cramps is unknown; in fact, there may be numerous causes. Some of the possible causes include an electrolyte imbalance; deficiency in calcium, magnesium, or potassium; and dehydration.

Delayed-Onset Muscle Soreness

Muscle soreness is common and typically arises shortly after unaccustomed activity. **Delayed-onset muscle soreness (DOMS)** follows participation in a particularly long or strenuous activity, with the soreness beginning 24 to 72 hours after the activity. DOMS involves multiple, microscopic tears in the muscle tissue and causes inflammation, pain, swelling, and stiffness.

Check Your Understanding

1. Describe the differences among the three classifications of muscle strains.
2. Why are athletes more likely than others to have problems with strains?
3. What is the difference between cramps and DOMS?
4. What causes contusions? Give an example.
5. What are possible causes of cramps?

Tendinitis and Tendinosis

Tendons are the bands of tough, fibrous connective tissue that connect muscles to bones. **Tendinitis** is inflammation of a tendon, usually accompanied by pain and swelling.

Both acute and overuse injuries can cause tendinitis. The condition can also occur with aging, as the tendon wears and elasticity decreases. Diseases such as diabetes and rheumatoid arthritis can also promote the development of tendinitis. Tendinitis can occur in any part of the body, but common sites involving injury include the shoulder, elbow, wrist, and the Achilles tendon of the heel.

Treatment of tendinitis includes rest and application of heat or cold. Pain relievers such as aspirin and ibuprofen can reduce pain and inflammation. In severe cases, steroid injections into the tendon can help control pain. Once the pain is reduced, physical therapy to stretch and strengthen both muscle and tendon promotes healing and can help prevent reinjury.

If untreated, chronic tendinitis can progress to **tendinosis**. Tendinosis, or degeneration of a tendon, is believed to be caused by microtears in the tendon connective tissue that decrease the tendon's strength. This weakened condition increases the likelihood that the tendon will rupture.

Although the condition is painful, no inflammation is present, unlike with tendinitis. Once tendinosis has developed, recovery takes months to years of minimal use. In many cases physical therapy can help.

Rotational Injuries of the Shoulder

Repetition of forceful overhead motions at the shoulder (as in throwing and spiking in volleyball and serving in tennis) can lead to inflammation or tears of the muscles and muscle tendons surrounding the shoulder (**Figure 5.24**). A similar condition among competitive swimmers is known as *swimmer's shoulder*.

Improper motion mechanics increases the likelihood of these types of shoulder injuries. The symptoms are pain and stiffness with overhead or rapid movements. If not treated, the pain can become constant. Treatment includes application of ice, rest, and, when necessary, surgical repair.

Overuse Injuries of the Elbow

Epicondylitis (EHP-ih-kahn-di-LIGH-tis) involves inflammation and sometimes

Val Thoermer/Shutterstock.com

Figure 5.24 Sports such as volleyball can sometimes lead to overuse injuries of the shoulder muscles. *What other activities can cause injuries to the shoulder muscles?*

microtearing of the muscle tendons that cross the lateral and medial sides of the elbow. If unchecked, the condition can worsen, leading to swelling and then scarring of the tendons near the elbow. Lateral epicondylitis, which is reported in 30%–40% of tennis players, is known as *tennis elbow*, although it also occurs in activities such as swimming, fencing, and repetitious hammering. Medial epicondylitis, known as *Little Leaguer's elbow*, can result from repeated throwing, especially with improper pitching mechanics. Both lateral and medial epicondylitis commonly occur among amateur golfers.

Memory Tip
The suffix *-itis* means "inflammation." You will learn about numerous conditions that involve inflammation of a part of the body. The names for all of those conditions contain the *-itis* suffix.

Shin Splints

The term **shin splint** is often used to describe pain localized to the medial lower leg. The condition is an overuse injury that typically arises from running or dancing—particularly running on a hard surface or uphill. The cause of the pain is believed to be microdamage to the muscle tendons that attach to the tibia or inflammation of the periosteum of the tibia. The muscles potentially involved include the soleus, tibialis anterior, and extensor digitorum.

Whiplash Injuries

Whiplash injuries to the neck are fairly common, often resulting from automobile accidents in which the victim's car was rear-ended. Such injuries result from abnormal motion of the cervical vertebrae, accompanied by rapid, forceful contractions of the neck muscles as the neuromuscular system attempts to stabilize and protect the spine. Symptoms can include neck muscle pain; pain or numbness extending down to the shoulders, arms, and even the hands; as well as headache.

WHAT RESEARCH TELLS US

...*about* Low Back Pain (LBP)

Low back pain (LBP) is a major health problem. Approximately 80%–85% of people experience it at some time during their lives.

In addition, back injuries are the most common and most expensive of all worker's compensation claims. Second only to the common cold in causing absences from work, the incidence of LBP has steadily increased in the US for the past 15 years. This is likely due, in part, to the increasing proportion of overweight and obese individuals. LBP is significantly associated with excess weight in both men and women of all ages.

Nearly 30% of children in the US also experience LBP. The likelihood that children will experience LBP increases with age. By age 16, the percentage of children with LBP is similar to that of adults. Children who are more physically active tend to incur LBP more often than sedentary children.

Athletes of all ages have a much higher incidence of LBP than nonathletes. In fact, more than 9% of college athletes receive treatment for LBP. Gymnasts (particularly those who are female) have much higher incidences of LBP. Studies show that as many as 85% of competitive gymnasts experience this health problem (**Figure 5.25**).

What causes LBP? Although injuries and certain disorders may cause LBP, 60% of LBP is of unknown origin. Low back muscle strains, resulting in soreness and stiffness, can be one source of LBP. In almost all cases of LBP,

Sergej Khakimullin/Shutterstock.com

Figure 5.25 Repeated, extreme lumbar hyperextension increases the likelihood that female gymnasts will develop low back pain.

the low back muscles are sore and painful.

In some cases this pain is caused by muscle injury. In many cases, however, this pain may be due to what is called a *sympathetic contraction* of the low back muscles. This means that the muscles involuntarily contract as the body attempts to stabilize an underlying injury of the spinal column.

Fortunately, most LBP is self-limiting—75% of patients are back to normal within three weeks. Approximately 90% have recovered within two months, with or without medical treatment.

What can you do to avoid developing LBP? Known risk factors for LBP include the following:

- sitting for prolonged periods;
- standing for long periods in an unchanging position;
- working in an unnatural posture;
- working with one hand;
- encountering sudden or unexpected motions; and
- performing heavy manual labor.

Taller and heavier individuals are at increased risk for developing LBP. Cigarette smoking is also associated with increased risk of LBP, most likely because habitual smoking can contribute to degeneration of the intervertebral discs.

Taking It Further

1. Why do you think LBP is so common? Based on what you have read about LBP, do you think a higher or lower percentage of people will have LBP in the future? Explain your reasoning.

2. What do you think *self-limiting* means? Do some research, write a definition, and then give some examples of self-limiting behavior.

3. Conduct a survey among people you know to find out who has and who has not experienced LBP. Include males and females, athletes and nonathletes, and people of various ages in your survey. What conclusions can you draw from your survey about the occurrence of LBP?

Muscular Dystrophy

Muscular dystrophy (MD) is a group of similar, inherited disorders characterized by progressively worsening muscle weakness and loss of muscle tissue. Depending on the specific type, the onset of MD may occur during either childhood or adulthood, and the symptoms vary.

Some forms of MD affect only certain muscle groups, whereas other forms affect all of the muscles. The more severe types of MD begin in childhood; symptoms may include intellectual disability, delayed development of motor skills, frequent falling, drooling, and drooping of the eyelids. Some forms of MD also affect the heart muscle, resulting in an irregular heartbeat.

There are no known cures for the various muscular dystrophies; the goal of treatment is to control symptoms (**Figure 5.26**). Some types of muscular dystrophy lead to a shortened life; others cause little disability, allowing for a normal lifespan.

Check Your Understanding

1. What is the role of the neuromuscular system in whiplash injuries?
2. What causes swimmer's shoulder?
3. What is the difference between tennis elbow and Little Leaguer's elbow?
4. What are the characteristics of MD?
5. What are the different forms that MD may take?

Hernia

A **hernia** is a balloon-like section of the abdominal cavity lining that protrudes through a hole or weakened section of the muscles in the abdomen. A hernia can be caused by heavy lifting or by any activity or medical problem that increases pressure inside the abdominal cavity. In

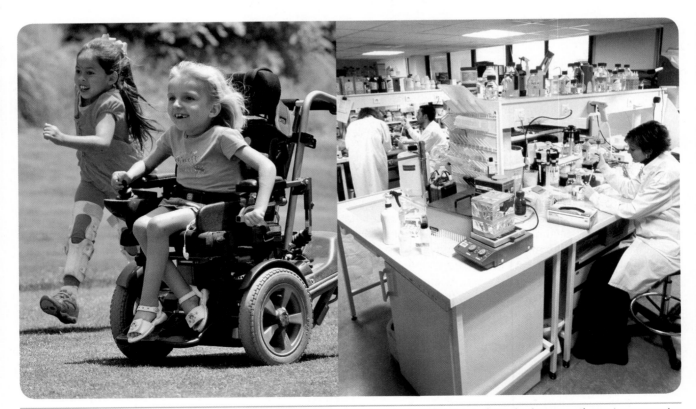

Figure 5.26 Two young girls, both with rare forms of muscular dystrophy, have fun playing together at an event to benefit the Muscular Dystrophy Association (MDA). We currently have no cures for the various forms of muscular dystrophy but hopefully research conducted in genetics labs such as the one shown here will lead to methods and treatments that reduce the effects of or eliminate the disease. *Have you donated to a campaign to raise money for muscular dystrophy research?*

most cases, however, no specific cause is evident. Some hernias are present at birth, and some occur in infants and children. A hernia that is present at birth may not become noticeable until later in life.

Most hernias produce no symptoms, although some are accompanied by discomfort or pain that intensifies with heavy lifting or other activities that produce abdominal strain. A large hernia may "strangulate," or cut off the blood supply to the tissue inside the hernia. A strangulated hernia requires immediate surgery.

Small hernias that cause no symptoms do not necessarily require treatment. Larger hernias and those that cause discomfort can be permanently remedied with surgery.

Lesson 5.4 Review and Assessment

Mini Glossary
Make sure that you know the meaning of each key term.

Build vocabulary with
e-flash cards and games

contusion   the bruises or bleeding within a muscle that result from an impact

delayed-onset muscle soreness (DOMS)   muscle pain that follows participation in a particularly long or strenuous activity, begins 24–73 hours later, and involves multiple, microscopic tears in the muscle tissue that cause inflammation, pain, swelling, and stiffness

hernia   a balloon-like section of the lining of the abdominal cavity

that protrudes through a hole or weakened section of the muscles in the abdomen

muscle cramps   moderate to severe muscle spasms that cause pain

muscle strain   an injury that occurs when a muscle is stretched beyond the limits to which it is accustomed

muscular dystrophy (MD)   a group of similar, inherited disorders characterized by progressively worsening muscle weakness and loss of muscle tissue

myositis ossificans   a condition in which a calcium mass forms within a muscle three to four weeks after a muscle injury

shin splint   the name for pain localized to the anterior lower leg

tendinitis   inflammation of a tendon, usually accompanied by pain and swelling

tendinosis   degeneration of a tendon believed to be caused by microtears in the tendon connective tissue

Know and Understand

Assess

1. What causes a muscle strain?
2. What can you do to increase your chances of avoiding muscle strains?
3. What is myositis ossificans? What problems can it cause?
4. What do shoulder, elbow, and shin injuries have in common?
5. What is the main cause of DOMS?
6. Why is it important to treat chronic tendinitis?
7. What is believed to be the main cause of shin splints?
8. Name an activity often associated with hernias.

Analyze and Apply

9. If obesity is a major cause of LBP, why would gymnasts experience this health problem?
10. How do poor mechanics contribute to overuse injuries such as swimmer's shoulder and tennis elbow? Describe and analyze the effect of torque in these injuries.

11. What types of muscle can be affected by muscular dystrophy?

In the Lab

12. Interview a physical therapist or an athletic trainer. Ask the person to describe a typical day at work. Here are some questions you might ask:
   • What is the work environment like?
   • What are the job duties?
   • What kinds of injuries are dealt with?
   • What other types of professionals does he or she work with?

   Report your findings to the class, giving reasons why you would or would not want to pursue a career similar to that of the person you interviewed. You may want to incorporate additional research from the Career Corner activity on the next two pages into your report.

13. Research shin-splint taping. Determine its purpose and how it helps the athlete.

Career Corner
Anatomy and Physiology at Work

Many challenging and rewarding careers involve treating and rehabilitating the muscles of the body. We will discuss two career options below.

Physical Therapist

Physicians often prescribe physical therapy for patients with muscle injuries. Frequently employed in physical therapy clinics, physical therapists and related professionals treat each patient's condition with appropriate exercise, stretching, and other therapeutic protocols (**Figure 5.27**). Treatment at a physical therapy clinic can last from a few visits to a series of visits over a period of months, depending on the severity of the condition being treated.

Prescribed exercise and stretching regimens are typically progressive in nature, beginning with a relatively easy routine that grows increasingly challenging. All patient activity in the clinic is closely supervised by a physical therapist to ensure that all movements are carried out in the correct directions and through appropriate ranges of motion.

The academic degree that physical therapists must earn is the DPT, or Doctor of Physical Therapy. Nationwide, entry into DPT programs is highly competitive. To qualify, students must possess a bachelor's degree and must also have completed prerequisite courses in biology, chemistry, physics, calculus, and human anatomy and physiology, to name just a few. When applying to a DPT program, candidates must provide documentation showing that they have a substantial amount of experience (paid or unpaid) assisting patients in a physical therapy clinic. This documentation ensures that applicants are appropriately familiar with the field of physical therapy. Most DPT programs take approximately three years to complete and require supervised clinical rotations as well as academic coursework. Physical therapists are employed by schools and universities, as well as in hospitals and other clinical environments.

Tyler Olson/Shutterstock.com

Figure 5.27 A physical therapist works with a patient to rehabilitate her knee after surgery. *Why do all physical-therapy patient activities need to be closely monitored by the physical therapist?*

Athletic Trainer

If an injury is related to a sport played at the high school or collegiate level, the first professional to examine the patient will likely be an expert in athletic training (**Figure 5.28**). Athletic trainers are knowledgeable first responders who are trained to apply advanced first aid, as well as to know when immediate referral to emergency care, a physician, or a specialist is necessary.

Athletic trainers are also well qualified to administer rehabilitative treatments when appropriate, typically after the injured athlete has been seen by a physician. Athletic trainers work with active individuals of all ages and physical abilities in industrial settings, gyms, fitness centers, youth athletic leagues, the Special Olympics, and anywhere that people are active.

To become an ATC, or Certified Athletic Trainer, students must complete a bachelor's degree in athletic training and then pass a national certification examination. Programs of study in athletic training include a number of basic science courses, human anatomy and physiology, and in-depth lecture/laboratory courses that cover prevention and treatment of athletic injuries to all parts of the body. Athletic trainers are employed in high schools, colleges and universities, hospitals, and clinics.

Planning for a Health-Related Career

Do some research on career opportunities for physical therapists or athletic trainers. Keep in mind the different levels of education and certifications that are required.

You may want to select a profession from the list of **Related Career Options**. Using the Internet or resources at your local library, find answers to the following questions:

1. What are the main tasks and responsibilities of an athletic trainer or a physical therapist?
2. What is the outlook for these careers? Are workers in demand, or are jobs dwindling? For complete information, consult the current edition of the *Occupational Outlook Handbook*, published by the US Department of Labor. This handbook is available online or at your local library.
3. What special skills or talents are required? For example, do you need to be capable of lifting? Are you comfortable looking at injuries that may be severe?
4. What personality traits do you think are needed to be successful in these jobs? For

instance, both athletic trainers and physical therapist must work closely with their patients. Do you enjoy working with others?
5. Do these careers involve a great deal of routine, or are the day-to-day responsibilities varied?
6. Does the work require long hours, or are these standard, "9-to-5" jobs?
7. What is the salary range for these jobs?
8. What do you think you would like about each career? Is there anything about them that you might dislike?

Related Career Options

- Athletic Trainer
- Massage Therapist
- Occupational Therapist
- Physical Therapist Assistant
- Recreational Therapist
- Rehabilitation Counselor

Aspen Photo/Shutterstock.com

Figure 5.28 Athletic trainers work with student athletes to prevent, treat, and rehabilitate injuries.

Chapter Summaries

Lesson 5.1 — Muscle Tissue Categories and Functions

 Build vocabulary with e-flash cards and games

Key Points
- The three major categories of muscle fibers are *smooth*, *cardiac*, and *skeletal* (striated), each with a different function.
- Muscles are either voluntary or involuntary.
- Muscles have four common behavioral characteristics: extensibility, elasticity, irritability, and contractility.
- Skeletal muscles work in an agonist/antagonist relationship and can experience concentric, eccentric, or isometric contractions.

Key Terms

agonist	extensibility
antagonist	fascicle
aponeurosis	irritability
concentric	isometric
contractility	muscle fiber
eccentric	perimysium
endomysium	peristalsis
epimysium	sarcolemma

Lesson 5.2 — Skeletal Muscle Actions

Key Points
- The muscular and nervous systems work together and are known as the *neuromuscular system*.
- The motor unit is the functional unit of the neuromuscular system and is made up of the neuron and the muscle fibers that the neuron stimulates. The location at which the neurons and the fibers come together is known as the *neuromuscular junction*.
- Skeletal muscle fibers are divided into fast-twitch fibers, which are powerful and fatigue quickly, or slow-twitch fibers, which are fatigue resistant.
- Muscular strength is determined by measuring torque, muscular power is defined as force × velocity, and muscular endurance is how long a muscle fiber can continuously contract before it fatigues.

Key Terms

acetylcholine	motor unit
action potential	neuromuscular junction
all-or-none law	parallel
axon	pennate
axon terminals	sarcomeres
cross bridges	slow-twitch
fast-twitch	synaptic cleft
motor neuron	tetanus

Lesson 5.3 — The Major Skeletal Muscles

Key Points
- Muscles are attached to bone via the origin and insertion.
- The sagittal plane movements are forward and backward actions.
- The frontal plane movements take the body part toward or away from the midline of the body.

Key Terms

abduction	flexion
adduction	hyperextension
circumduction	insertion
dorsiflexion	inversion
eversion	lateral rotation
extension	medial rotation

- Transverse plane movements are actions that move side to side or rotate around a longitudinal axis.
- The upper limb sacrifices stability for increased range of motion when compared with the lower limb.

opposition
origin
plantar flexion
pronation

radial deviation
supination
ulnar deviation

Lesson 5.4 Common Injuries and Disorders of Muscles

Key Points

- Strains are injuries that occur when muscles are stretched beyond their limits.
- Contusions are caused by impact; severe contusions can result in myositis ossificans.
- Possible causes of cramps are dehydration, mineral deficiency, and electrolyte imbalance.
- Delayed-onset muscle soreness is brought on by long, strenuous activity resulting in inflammation, pain, swelling, and stiffness.
- Many muscle injuries, such as DOMS, strains, rotational injuries, and shin splints, result from muscle overuse.
- Low back pain (LBP) can be caused by obesity, muscle strain, muscle overuse, or an issue with the spinal column.
- Muscular dystrophy (MD) is a neuromuscular disease that results in progressively worsening muscle weakness and atrophy.

Key Terms

contusion
delayed-onset muscle
  soreness (DOMS)
hernia
muscle cramps
muscle strain

muscular dystrophy (MD)
myositis ossificans
shin splint
tendinitis
tendinosis

Chapter Assessments

Lesson 5.1

Muscle Tissue Categories and Functions

Learning Key Terms and Concepts

1. The individual skeletal muscle cell is referred to as a(n) _____.
2. The three layers of muscle tissue, from the inside out, are _____, _____, and _____.
3. Skeletal muscle is connected to bone by either _____ or aponeuroses.
4. _____ muscle is found in organs and blood vessels.
5. The heart is made up of _____ muscle cells.
6. The ability of a muscle and other tissue to be stretched is the behavioral characteristic known as _____.
   - A. extensibility
   - B. elasticity
   - C. irritability
   - D. contractility
7. The ability of a muscle to respond to stimuli is the behavioral characteristic known as _____.
   - A. extensibility
   - B. elasticity
   - C. irritability
   - D. contractility

Thinking Critically

8. Discuss in depth the differences between concentric, isometric, and eccentric contractions and provide examples of how each one is used in daily life.
9. What do you think would be the pros and cons of body organs being made up exclusively of voluntary muscle (no involuntary muscle)? Provide specific examples and some pros and some cons for each.
10. Describe the structure of skeletal muscle. What different parts make up what we typically think of as a muscle?

Lesson 5.2

Skeletal Muscle Actions

Learning Key Terms and Concepts

11. A nerve that stimulates skeletal muscle is called a(n) _____.
12. The functional unit of the neuromuscular system is the _____.

13. A(n) _____ is an electrical charge that creates tension within a muscle fiber.

14. _____ twitch muscle fibers contract powerfully but fatigue quickly.

Thinking Critically

15. Discuss muscle fiber arrangements that contribute to the force a muscle can generate.

16. How do you think slow-twitch muscle fibers are usually arranged? Give reasons for your answer.

17. Who generates more power: an olympic weight lifter who must lift 400 pounds from the ground to a position over his head very rapidly, or a power lifter who must squat down and stand up with 800 pounds on his back? Defend your answer.

18. Discuss how torque is used to measure the strength of a muscle group at a specific joint.

Lesson 5.3
The Major Skeletal Muscles

Learning Key Terms and Concepts

Instructions: Write the **letter** of the name of the **muscle** on your answer sheet next to the corresponding number.

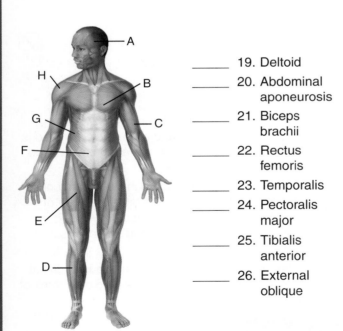

_____ 19. Deltoid

_____ 20. Abdominal aponeurosis

_____ 21. Biceps brachii

_____ 22. Rectus femoris

_____ 23. Temporalis

_____ 24. Pectoralis major

_____ 25. Tibialis anterior

_____ 26. External oblique

Thinking Critically

27. Compare and contrast the sagittal and frontal planes. Be sure to discuss the movements that occur in each plane.

28. In circumduction, which planes does the limb move through and what actions do you think are being utilized to make the conical/circular motion?

29. Do agonists and antagonists have to perform their actions in the same plane? Why?

Lesson 5.4
Common Injuries and Disorders of Muscles

Learning Key Terms and Concepts

30. A muscle strain is classified as _____, _____, or _____.

31. A(n) _____ is a bruise or bleeding within a muscle.

32. A complication that can arise from a contusion is _____.
   A. sarcolemma
   B. myositis ossificans
   C. neuroma
   D. spondylosis

33. Which of the following may be a cause of cramps?
   A. electrolyte imbalance
   B. dehydration
   C. deficiency in minerals such as calcium or potassium
   D. all of the above

34. The role of the neuromuscular system in a whiplash injury is _____.
   A. an inhibitory response that causes the muscles to relax and the head to move freely
   B. a strong, fast series of contractions that attempt to stabilize the head
   C. not present because the movement is so intense that muscles don't have time to contract
   D. dependent upon whether the movement is mediolateral or anteroposterior

35. Lateral epicondylitis is also known as _____.
   A. Little Leaguer's elbow
   B. Swimmer's shoulder
   C. Jumper's knee
   D. Tennis elbow

Thinking Critically

36. If being active is considered healthy, why do you think active people and athletes have a significantly higher incidence of LBP than inactive, sedentary people?

37. Compare and contrast the responsibilities of physical therapists and athletic trainers. How are they similar? How are they different? Which job seems more appealing to you and why?

Building Skills and Connecting Concepts

Analyzing and Evaluating Data

Use the bar graph to answer the following questions.

38. Which sport involves the most muscle strains?

39. Which sport involves the most muscle contusions?

40. What percentage of swimming injuries is attributed to muscle strains?

41. What is the approximate ratio of muscle contusions in figure skating to muscle contusions in baseball?

42. Compare the total number of swimming injuries with the total number of figure skating injuries.

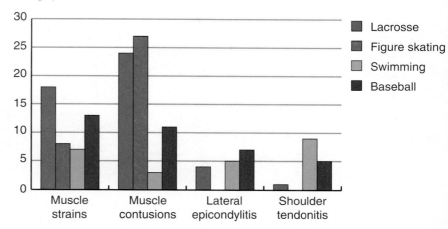

Communicating about Anatomy and Physiology

43. **Listening** In small groups discuss with your classmates—in basic, everyday language—your knowledge and awareness of your muscles as you go about your daily routine. Conduct this discussion as though you had never read this chapter. Take notes on the observations expressed. Then review the points discussed, factoring in your new knowledge of muscles. Develop a summary of what you have learned about muscles and present it to the class, using the terms that you have learned about the muscular system in this chapter.

44. **Speaking** Pick a figure in this chapter, such as Figure 5.1, 5.4, or 5.6. Working with a partner, tell and then retell the important information being conveyed by that figure. Through your collaboration, develop what you and your partner believe is the most interesting verbal description of the importance of the chosen figure. Present your narration to the class.

Lab Investigations

45. Do a push-up starting in the "up" position. Go down. Which muscles are experiencing concentric contractions? Which muscles are experiencing eccentric contractions? Which muscles are experiencing isometric contractions? Which plane(s) is the shoulder moving through? What actions are occurring at the shoulder, elbow, and wrist? Record your observations and then compare them with those of your classmates in a class discussion.

46. Make a working model of a joint that includes both the agonist and the antagonist muscles. Write a brief explanation of how they work together to produce movement.

47. Try to switch the common (what we think of as normal) origin and insertion points of as many muscles as you can. Focus on the most frequent, everyday movements. Make a list and describe what you did to switch them. Hint: Compare origin and insertion points when doing straight-leg sit-ups and straight-leg leg lifts.

Expand your learning with additional online resources
- Supplemental Lab Activities
- Interactive Exercises
- Animations

www.g-wlearning.com/healthsciences

Did you know that the human brain runs on electricity?

The Nervous System

*T*o understand the nervous system, start by thinking of your body as a biological machine that runs on electricity. In fact, this is true; your body does run on electricity! Your brain is the control center of your biological machine and sends and receives electrical impulses, or signals, throughout your body. The sophisticated communication system that delivers these electrical signals to and from the brain is your nervous system.

With all this electrical activity going on, why don't our bodies light up? The answer is that the electrical charges within our bodies are very tiny. In the eighteenth century, Italian scientist Luigi Galvani discovered that muscle produces a detectable electric current, or voltage, when developing tension. But it was not until the twentieth century that technology became sophisticated enough to detect and record the extremely small electrical charges that move through the nervous system.

The activities performed by the nervous system are crucial. What enables the nervous system to perform these various functions so efficiently? In this chapter, we will take a look at the different anatomical structures and the functions of the nervous system. We will also discuss some of the common injuries and disorders of the nervous system, along with their symptoms and treatments.

Chapter 6 Lessons

Lesson 6.1
Overview of the Nervous System

Lesson 6.2
Transmission of Nerve Impulses

Lesson 6.3
Functional Anatomy of the Central Nervous System

Lesson 6.4
Functional Anatomy of the Peripheral Nervous System

Lesson 6.5
Injuries and Disorders of the Nervous System

While studying, look for the online icon to:

- **Practice** with e-flash cards and vocabulary games
- **Review** with interactive art labeling
- **Assess** with online exercises
- **Expand** with interactive activities and animated videos
- **Listen** to pronunciations of key terms in the audio glossary

www.g-wlearning.com/healthsciences

Companion Website

Study on the Go

Use a mobile device to practice vocabulary terms, listen to pronunciations, and review with self-assessment quizzes.

www.m.g-wlearning.com

G-W Mobile

Overview of the Nervous System

Before You Read

Try to answer the following questions before you read this lesson.

Why are some body functions under involuntary control?

Why is the myelin sheath around nerve axons so important?

Lesson Objectives

1. Differentiate between the central nervous system and peripheral nervous system, and explain the function of each.
2. Explain the differences between afferent and efferent nerves.
3. Describe the functions of the somatic and autonomic branches of the nervous system.
4. Identify the general role of the glial cells.
5. Describe the anatomical structure of a typical neuron.

Key Terms

E-Flash Cards

afferent nerves
autonomic nervous system
cell body
central nervous system (CNS)
dendrites
efferent nerves

myelin sheath
neurilemma
neuroglia
nodes of Ranvier
peripheral nervous system (PNS)
somatic nervous system
synapse

Our nervous system is amazing in its ability to simultaneously direct a whole host of different functions. The nervous system not only controls voluntary movement by activating skeletal muscle, but it also directs the involuntary functions of smooth muscle in internal organs and cardiac muscle in the heart. By automatically controlling the functions of smooth muscle and cardiac muscle, the nervous system ensures that these life functions are able to occur without conscious thought.

At the same time that your heart is beating and your last meal is making its way through your digestive tract, you may be talking to a friend, walking to a class, or even reading this book. Our senses—the ability to see, hear, smell, taste, feel pressure, and feel pain—are all dependent on sensory electrical input from specialized receptors.

For the purpose of discussion, the nervous system is organized into structural and functional subdivisions. This organization makes it easier to learn about the activities directed by the various parts of the nervous system, and how these parts interact.

Organization of the Nervous System

There are two major divisions of the human body's nervous system: the central nervous system and the peripheral nervous system. There are further subdivisions of the peripheral nervous system. Figure 6.1 illustrates these major divisions and subdivisions.

First, let's look at the organization of the nervous system. We will examine the structure and function of the two major divisions of the nervous system in greater detail later in the chapter.

Figure 6.1 This diagram represents the organization of the nervous system and summarizes the relationships among the subdivisions. *If you were asked to put the word voluntary into one of the six boxes above and involuntary into another one of the boxes, where would you put each word?*

Two Major Divisions

The **central nervous system (CNS)** includes the brain and spinal cord. The CNS directs the activity of the entire nervous system. Injuries to either the brain or the spinal cord have serious consequences and can be life threatening. Fortunately, these delicate structures are well protected inside the skull and vertebral column.

The parts of the nervous system other than the brain and spinal cord make up what is called the **peripheral nervous system (PNS)**. For example, the PNS includes spinal nerves that transmit information to and from the spinal cord and cranial nerves that transmit information to and from the brain. The PNS also includes specialized nerve endings called *sensory receptors*, which respond to stimuli such as pressure, pain, or temperature.

Nerves that transmit impulses from the sensory receptors in the skin, muscles, and joints to the CNS are known as **afferent** (sensory) **nerves**. Those that carry impulses from the CNS out to the muscles and glands are **efferent** (motor) **nerves**.

Memory Tip

Afferent nerves tell the body how it is being *affected* by stimuli such as light, heat, and pressure.

Efferent nerves stimulate muscles to produce *effort*.

The Efferent Nerves

There are two functional subdivisions of the efferent, or motor, nerves. The **somatic** (voluntary) **nervous system** stimulates our skeletal muscles, causing them to develop tension. The **autonomic** (involuntary) **nervous system** controls the cardiac muscle of the heart and the smooth muscles of the internal organs. The autonomic nervous system prompts the heart to beat faster when we exercise and causes the smooth muscle activities that move food through the digestive system.

Thanks to our autonomic nervous system, we do not have to think about everyday body functions that sustain life. And under certain circumstances, such as when we inadvertently touch a hot surface, the efferent neurons can trigger involuntary action of the skeletal muscles through a reflex arc. The autonomic nervous system includes *sympathetic* and *parasympathetic* branches, which you will learn about in Lesson 6.4.

Becoming aware of these various subdivisions of the nervous system will help you learn and understand the different functional capabilities of the nervous system. Keep in mind, however, that the nervous system as a whole is a single, remarkably coordinated, functioning unit.

> ✓ **Check Your Understanding**
>
> 1. Which structures make up the central nervous system (CNS)?
> 2. Which structures make up the peripheral nervous system (PNS)?
> 3. Which function is the somatic nervous system responsible for?
> 4. Which functions is the autonomic nervous system responsible for?

Nervous Tissues

Two categories of tissues exist within the nervous system. These include specialized supporting cells called *neuroglia* and *neurons*.

Neuroglia

The **neuroglia** (ner-ROHG-lee-a), also known as *glial* (GLIGH-al) *cells*, are a category of specialized cells that perform support functions (**Figure 6.2**). Within the CNS are four types of glial cells:

- *Astrocytes* (AS-troh-sights) are positioned between neurons and capillaries. Astrocytes link the nutrient-supplying capillaries to neurons and control the chemical environment to protect the neurons from any harmful substances in the blood. The astrocytes are so numerous that they account for nearly half of all neural tissue.
- *Microglia* (migh-KROHG-lee-a) absorb and dispose of dead cells and bacteria.

- *Ependymal* (eh-PEHN-di-mal) *cells* form a protective covering around the spinal cord and central cavities within the brain.
- *Oligodendrocytes* (AHL-i-goh-DEHN-droh-sights) wrap around nerve fibers and produce a fatty insulating material called *myelin*.

The PNS includes two forms of glial cells:

- *Schwann* (shwahn) *cells* form the fatty myelin sheaths around nerve fibers in the PNS.
- *Satellite cells* serve as cushioning support cells.

Neurons

The glial cells provide support and protection for the nervous system, but it is the neurons that transmit information in the form of nerve impulses throughout the body. A typical neuron, or nerve cell, consists of a cell body surrounded by branching dendrites. The typical neuron also has a long, tail-like projection called an *axon* (**Figure 6.3**).

The **cell body** includes a nucleus and mitochondria, like all cell bodies, as described in chapter 2. The **dendrites** (DEHN-drights) collect stimuli and transport them to the cell body. Axons (AK-sahns) transmit impulses away from the cell body.

Within the PNS, the Schwann cells wrap around the axon, covering most of it with a fatty **myelin** (MIGH-eh-lin) **sheath**. The myelin sheaths serve an important purpose: insulating the axon fibers, which increases the rate of neural impulse transmission.

The external covering of the Schwann cell, outside the myelin sheath, is called the **neurilemma** (NOO-ri-LEHM-a). The uninsulated gaps, where the axon is exposed between the Schwann cells, are known as the **nodes of Ranvier** (rahn-vee-AY). The myelin sheaths are white, giving rise to the term *white matter* to describe tracts of myelinated fibers within the CNS. *Gray matter* is the term for unmyelinated nerve fibers.

At the terminal end of each axon, there can be up to thousands of axon terminals that connect with other neurons or muscles (**Figure 6.3**). The axon terminals are filled with

A. CNS Glial Cells

Capillary

Astrocyte
(support)

Neuron cell bodies

Central canal
of spine

Ependymal cells
(line canal or cavity)

Microglia
(remove debris)

Myelinated axons

Oligodendrocyte
(produces myelin)

Satellite cells

Cell body of neuron

Schwann cells
(forming myelin sheath)

Nerve fiber

Nodes of Ranvier

B. PNS Glial Cells

Label Art

Figure 6.2 The glial cells of the central nervous system and peripheral nervous system. *Write one sentence summarizing in general terms the functions of the six types of glial cells.*

tiny sacs, or vesicles, that contain chemical messengers called *neurotransmitters* (**Figure 6.6**).

Axon terminals do not actually touch the other neuron or muscle, but are separated by a microscopic gap called the *synaptic cleft*. This intersection, including the synaptic cleft, is known as the **synapse** (SIN-aps). A synapse between an axon terminal and a muscle fiber is called the *neuromuscular junction*, as you learned in chapter 5.

When classified by their function, there are three types of neurons:

- *Sensory* (afferent) *neurons* carry impulses from the skin and organs to the spinal cord and brain, providing information about the external and internal environments.

- *Motor* (efferent) *neurons* transmit impulses from the brain and spinal cord to the muscles and glands, directing body actions.
- Neurons that form bridges to transmit impulses between other neurons are *interneurons* (inter-NOO-rahnz), or *association neurons*.

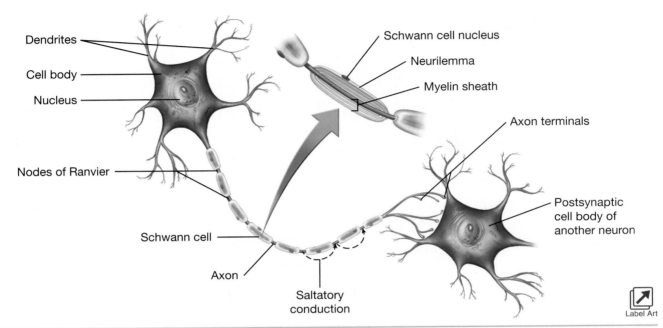

Figure 6.3 A typical neuron. *Why do neural impulses travel faster through myelinated axons than through nonmyelinated axons?*

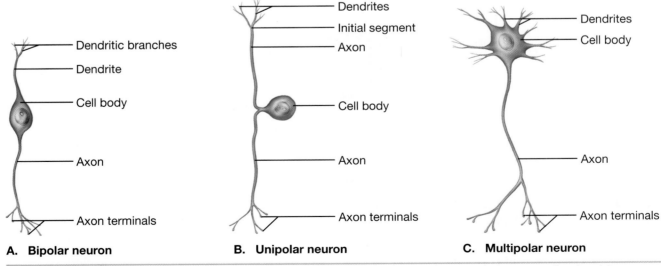

A. Bipolar neuron   **B. Unipolar neuron**   **C. Multipolar neuron**

Figure 6.4 Different neuron structures. A—Bipolar neurons have two processes: an axon and a dendrite. B—Unipolar neurons have a single axon process, with the cell body in the middle and to the side. C—Multipolar neurons have a single axon and multiple dendrites.

As shown in **Figure 6.4**, there are also three different neuron structures:

- *Bipolar neurons* have one axon and one dendrite. These are sensory processing cells found in the eyes and nose.
- *Unipolar neurons* have a single axon with dendrites on the peripheral end and axon terminals on the central end. The peripheral process carries impulses to the cell body, while the central process carries impulses to the central nervous system. Some of the sensory neurons in the PNS are unipolar.

- *Multipolar neurons* have one axon and multiple dendrites. All motor neurons and interneurons are multipolar.

 Check Your Understanding

1. List the four types of glial cells in the CNS and state their functions.
2. List the two types of glial cells in the PNS and state their functions.
3. What is the purpose of a myelin sheath?

Lesson 6.1 Review and Assessment

Mini Glossary   Make sure that you know the meaning of each key term.

 Build vocabulary with e-flash cards and games

afferent nerves   sensory transmitters that send impulses from receptors in the skin, muscles, and joints to the central nervous system

autonomic nervous system   branch of the nervous system that controls involuntary body functions

cell body   part of an axon that contains a nucleus

central nervous system (CNS)   the brain and spinal cord

dendrites   branches of a neuron that collect stimuli and transport them to the cell body

efferent nerves   motor transmitters that carry impulses from the central nervous system out to the muscles and glands

myelin sheath   the fatty bands of insulation surrounding axon fibers

neurilemma   the thin, membranous sheath enveloping a nerve fiber

neuroglia   non-neural tissue that forms the interstitial or supporting elements of the CNS; also known as *glial cells*

nodes of Ranvier   the uninsulated gaps in the myelin sheath of a nerve fiber where the axon is exposed

peripheral nervous system (PNS)   all parts of the nervous system external to the brain and spinal cord

somatic nervous system   branch of the nervous system that stimulates the skeletal muscles

synapse   the intersection between a neuron and another neuron, a muscle, a gland, or a sensory receptor

Know and Understand

 Assess

1. Explain how the nervous system is organized, including subdivisions of each component.
2. What is a sensory receptor?
3. Which nerves—the afferent nerves or efferent nerves—are also referred to as motor nerves? Why are they called motor nerves?
4. List the three parts of a typical neuron and state the function of each part.
5. What do the tiny sacs inside axon terminals contain?
6. What are the two ways of classifying neurons?
7. Explain the difference between bipolar, unipolar, and multipolar neurons.

Analyze and Apply

8. Describe a synapse. In your description use at least three terms that you learned in this lesson.
9. Explain the negative effects on a neuron when the myelin sheath is damaged or destroyed by a demyelinating disorder.

In the Lab

10. Using clay, or a substitute material, create a model of a typical neuron as described in the lesson. Include all of the different parts mentioned. Label the parts and list the functions of those parts.

Transmission of Nerve Impulses

Before You Read

Try to answer the following questions before you read this lesson.

How fast do nerve impulses travel?

How can muscles contract without the brain being involved?

Lesson Objectives

1. Define *action potential* and explain how action potentials are generated.
2. Explain the factors that influence the speed of neural impulse transmission.
3. Describe how impulses are transmitted across the synapse.
4. Discuss the roles played by neurotransmitters.
5. Describe the three types of reflexes and explain how they work.

Key Terms

E-Flash Cards

autonomic reflexes
conductivity
depolarized
nerve impulse
polarized

reflexes
refractory period
repolarization
saltatory conduction
somatic reflexes

Neurons have one behavioral property in common with muscle: irritability (the ability to respond to a stimulus). Neurons, however, have an aspect of irritability that muscles do not have: the ability to convert a stimulus into a nerve impulse. **Conductivity**, the other behavioral property of neurons, is the ability to transmit nerve impulses.

What, exactly, is a nerve impulse? It is a tiny electrical charge that transmits information between neurons. In this lesson we will explore the processes by which nerve impulses are created and spread throughout the nervous system.

Action Potentials

When a neuron is inactive or at rest, there are potassium (K+) ions inside the cell and sodium (Na+) ions outside the cell membrane. The overall distribution of ions is such that the inside of the membrane is more negatively charged than the outside. Because of this difference in electrical charge, the cell membrane is said to be **polarized**.

Many different stimuli can activate a neuron. A bright light in the eyes, a bitter taste on the tongue, or the reception of neurotransmitter chemicals from another neuron are possible stimuli. In all cases, if the stimulus exceeds a critical voltage, hundreds of gated sodium channels in the cell membrane briefly open. This allows the sodium ions outside the cell to rapidly diffuse into the neuron. As a result, the electrical charge inside the membrane becomes more positive and the neuron membrane is **depolarized**.

The depolarization of the neuron membrane opens more gated ion channels along the membrane, generating a wave of depolarization through the neuron. This electrical charge is known as a **nerve impulse**, or *action potential*, and it executes in an *all-or-none* fashion. This means that the electrical charge of the action potential is always the same size, and once initiated, it always travels the full length of the axon.

Following the discharge of the action potential, the membrane becomes permeable to (or accepting of) potassium ions, which rapidly diffuse out of the cell. This begins the process of restoring the membrane to its original, polarized resting state, a process called **repolarization**. Until the cell membrane is repolarized, it cannot respond to another stimulus. The time between the completion of the action potential and repolarization is called the **refractory** (ree-FRAK-toh-ree) **period**. During the refractory period the neuron is temporarily "fatigued."

Impulse Transmission

Two factors—the presence or absence of a myelin sheath and the diameter of the axon—have a major impact on the speed at which a nerve impulse travels. Because the fatty myelin sheath is an electrical insulator, action potentials in a myelinated axon "jump over" the myelinated regions of the axon. Depolarization occurs only at the nodes of Ranvier, where the axon is exposed (**Figure 6.3**). This process, known as **saltatory** (SAWL-ta-TOH-ree) **conduction**, results in significantly faster impulse transmission than is possible in nonmyelinated axons.

Impulse conduction is much faster in nonmyelinated axons with larger diameters than in those with smaller diameters. The larger the axon, the greater the number of ions there will be to conduct current. This is somewhat like a large-diameter pipe versus a small-diameter pipe when transferring water from one place to another. The water moves through the large-diameter pipe faster than it does through the pipe with a small diameter.

A third factor influencing conduction speed is body temperature. Warmer temperatures increase ion diffusion rates, whereas local cooling, which occurs when holding an ice cube, for example, decreases ion diffusion rates.

So how fast do nerve impulses travel? As is clear from our recent discussion, the type and size of the nerve axon have much to do with this. Impulses that signal limb position to the brain travel extremely fast—up to 119 m/s (meters per second). Information or impulses from the objects that we touch travel more slowly, at around 76 m/s (**Figure 6.5**). By contrast, the sensation of pain moves more slowly, at less than 1 m/s. Thought signals, which are happening right now as you are reading, transmit at 20–30 m/s. For a nerve to transmit impulses at speeds greater than 1 m/s, it must have a myelinated axon.

 Check Your Understanding

1. What is meant when a cell membrane is said to be polarized?
2. Do action potentials occur when neuron cell membranes are polarized or depolarized?
3. What two factors influence the speed at which a nerve impulse travels?

Transmission at Synapses

Communication between some cells occurs through direct transfer of electrical charges at *electrical synapses* within specialized sites called *gap junctions*. The intercalated discs between cardiac muscle fibers, for example, serve as gap junctions.

Maridav/Shutterstock.com

Figure 6.5 Although it may seem as though we feel pain instantly, nerve impulses communicating pain travel more slowly than other nerve impulses.

Communication between neurons, however, occurs at the synapse. Because the action potential is electrical, and what occurs at the synapse is chemical, transmission of nerve impulses is an *electrochemical event*.

When an action potential reaches an axon terminal, the terminal depolarizes, calcium gates open, and calcium (Ca++) ions flow into the terminal. The axon terminal is filled with tiny vesicles containing neurotransmitter (NOO-roh-TRANS-mit-er) chemicals (**Figure 6.6**). The influx of calcium causes these vesicles to join to the cell membrane adjacent to the synaptic cleft. Pores then form in the membrane, allowing the neurotransmitter to diffuse across the synapse to receptors on the membrane of the joining neuron or muscle fiber.

Neurotransmitters can have an excitatory effect or an inhibitory effect on the receiving cell. An example of an excitatory neurotransmitter is acetylcholine (a-SEE-til-KOH-leen), the chemical that activates muscle fibers. Endorphins are neurotransmitters released to inhibit nerve cells from discharging more pain signals.

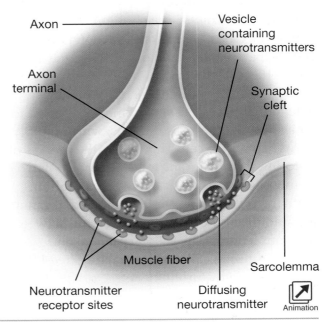

Figure 6.6 The synapse is the site at which the neurotransmitter is released from the nerve axon terminal. The neurotransmitter then diffuses across the synaptic cleft to receptor sites on the next nerve cell body, or to a muscle fiber, as shown here. *What two decidedly different effects can neurotransmitters have on the receiving cells?*

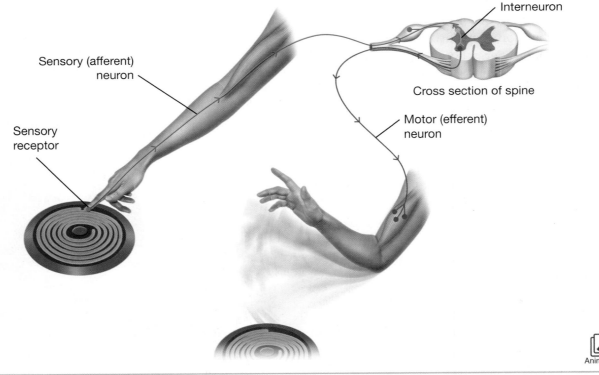

Figure 6.7 A sensory receptor is stimulated by a hot surface, sending an afferent signal to the spinal cord. The signal is then transferred by an interneuron directly to a motor neuron, stimulating quick removal of the hand from the hot surface.

The final step in communication between nerves at a synapse is the removal of the neurotransmitter, usually by an enzyme, to prevent ongoing stimulation of the receptor cell. Acetylcholine, for example, is deactivated by the enzyme acetylcholinesterase (a-SEE-til-KOH-leen-EHS-ter-ays).

Reflexes

Reflexes are simple, rapid, involuntary, programmed responses to stimuli. The transmission of impulses follows a reflex arc that includes both PNS and CNS structures (**Figure 6.7**). There are two categories of reflexes.

WHAT RESEARCH TELLS US

...*about* Measuring Nerve Impulses

How do scientists and clinicians measure the speed and function of nerve impulses? One common method is the use of a nerve conduction velocity (NCV) test.

Conducting and Interpreting NCV Tests

The NCV test begins with the attachment of three small, flat, disc-shaped electrodes to the skin. The electrodes are attached over the nerve being studied and over the muscle supplied by the nerve. The third electrode is attached over a bony site, such as the elbow or ankle, to serve as an electrical ground.

The technician then administers short, tiny electrical pulses to the nerve through the first electrode and records the time it takes for the muscle to contract (as sensed by the second electrode). Computer software calculates the NCV as the distance between the stimulating and sensing electrodes divided by the elapsed time between stimulation and contraction.

Placing stimulating electrodes at two or more different locations along the same nerve makes it possible to determine the NCV across different segments of the nerve. To test for sensory neuron function, the stimulating electrode is placed over a region of sensory receptors such as a fingertip. The recording electrode is then placed at a distance up the limb.

How are the results of a clinical NCV test interpreted? An NCV that is significantly slower than normal suggests that damage to the myelin sheath is likely. Alternatively, if NCV is slowed but close to the normal range, damage to the axons of the involved neurons is suspected. Evaluation of the overall pattern of responses can serve as a diagnostic tool in helping a clinician determine the likely pathology involved in an abnormal NCV.

Microneurography

Scientists have used a similar but more sophisticated procedure called *microneurography* (MIGH-kroh-noo-RAHG-ra-fee) to record electrical activity from single sensory fibers. **Figure 6.8** shows that the technique involves the direct insertion of fine-tipped needle electrodes into the nerve being studied.

Through the use of microneurography we have developed our current understanding of the sympathetic nervous system. Topics studied include various reflexes, interactions within the sympathetic nervous system, metabolism, hormones, and the effects of drugs or anesthesia during operative procedures. Sympathetic

Figure 6.8 Microneurography is a technique involving insertion of fine wire electrodes into a nerve for direct recording of electrical impulse activity.

recordings have also been used to study the effects of performance at high altitudes, as well as in space.

Taking It Further

1. Working with a partner, research nerve damage further. Develop a report for the class on the more common causes.

2. Investigate and report to the class on technologies, in addition to NCV tests, that are used for diagnostic and therapeutic purposes to treat nerve disorders.

Somatic reflexes are those that involve stimulation of skeletal muscles. For example, have you ever withdrawn your hand quickly from something hot, even before you realized that it was hot? If so, you were experiencing a somatic reflex. In such a situation the motion of your hand occurs so quickly because a motor nerve has been directly stimulated by a sensory neuron, by way of an interneuron in the spinal cord. The signal between neurons is so fast because it did not have to travel to the brain and back.

Autonomic reflexes are those that send involuntary stimuli to the cardiac muscle of the heart and the smooth muscle of internal organs.

Digestion, elimination, sweating, and blood pressure are all activities that are regulated by autonomic reflexes.

Check Your Understanding

1. Why is the transmission of nerve impulses often referred to as an electrochemical event?
2. Give an example of both an excitatory neurotransmitter and an inhibitory neurotransmitter.
3. What are the two types of reflexes discussed in this lesson?

Lesson 6.2 Review and Assessment

Mini Glossary
Make sure that you know the meaning of each key term.

 Build vocabulary with e-flash cards and games

autonomic reflexes involuntary stimuli transmitted to cardiac and smooth muscle

conductivity the ability of a neuron to transmit a nerve impulse

depolarized a condition in which the inside of a cell membrane is more positively charged than the outside

nerve impulse electrical charge that travels along a nerve fiber when stimulated

polarized a condition that occurs when the inside of a cell membrane is more negatively charged than the outside

reflexes simple, rapid, involuntary, programmed responses to stimuli

refractory period the time between the completion of the action potential and repolarization

repolarization the reestablishment of a polarized state in a cell after depolarization

saltatory conduction the rapid skipping of an action potential from node to node on myelinated neurons

somatic reflexes involuntary stimuli transmitted to skeletal muscles from neural arcs in the spinal cord

Know and Understand

 Assess

1. Name two behavioral properties of a nerve impulse.
2. Describe a neuron at rest compared to a neuron activated by a stimulus.
3. What has to happen before a cell membrane can respond to a second stimulus?
4. Do myelin sheaths slow down or speed up nerve impulses?
5. How does body temperature affect the conduction speed of an electrical impulse?
6. What are the two categories of reflexes? Name a body part that would be affected by each of the two types.

Analyze and Apply

7. How would submerging a person in a tub of cold water affect the conduction speeds of the person's nerve impulses?

8. Is conduction of nerve impulses always faster in axons with a larger diameter, compared to axons with a smaller diameter? Explain.
9. Aside from touching a hot surface, in what other circumstances might a sensory receptor bypass the brain and stimulate an interneuron to instigate quick action?

In the Lab

10. Using a toothpick and a piece of ice, test a fellow student's sensory impulse reaction. Gently poke the student's ventral forearm (the part of the forearm closer to the wrist) with the toothpick and note the length of time it takes for your partner to sense pain. Then place a piece of ice on the same spot on the student's ventral forearm for one minute. Remove the ice and again gently poke the forearm. Note the length of time and amount of pressure required before the student senses pain. Explain your results.

Functional Anatomy of the Central Nervous System

Before You Read

Try to answer the following questions before you read this lesson.

Is brain size related to intelligence?

Which functions do the left brain and right brain control?

Which brain structure functions particularly well in athletes?

Lesson Objectives

1. Identify the four lobes of the brain and their functions.
2. Describe the location, structures, and functions of the diencephalon, or interbrain.
3. Describe the location, structures, and functions of the brain stem.
4. Explain the role of the cerebellum.
5. Identify the membranes that comprise the meninges and explain their purposes.
6. Describe how the capillaries in the brain are different from other capillaries and explain why this is important.
7. Identify the location and functions of the spinal cord.

Key Terms

E-Flash Cards

cerebellum	midbrain
cerebrum	occipital lobes
diencephalon	parietal lobes
epithalamus	pons
fissures	primary motor cortex
frontal lobes	primary somatic
hypothalamus	sensory cortex
lobes	spinal cord
medulla oblongata	temporal lobes
meninges	thalamus

The central nervous system includes numerous anatomical structures with specialized functions. Using sophisticated imaging techniques, scientists have been able to identify which structures control or contribute to physiological processes and actions.

The Brain

As you might expect, given its all-important role in directing the activity of the entire nervous system, the brain is structurally and functionally complex. The adult human brain weighs between 2¼ and 3¼ pounds and contains approximately 100 billion neurons and even more glial cells. Recent research indicates that the size of a person's brain does have some relationship to intelligence; about 6.7% of individual variation in intelligence is attributed to brain size. The four major anatomic regions of the brain are the cerebrum, diencephalon, brain stem, and cerebellum.

Cerebrum

The left and right *cerebral* (seh-REE-bral) *hemispheres* are collectively referred to as the **cerebrum** (seh-REE-brum), which makes up the largest portion of the brain. The outer surface of the cerebrum, the *cerebral cortex*, is composed of nonmyelinated gray matter. The internal tissue is myelinated white matter, with small, interspersed regions of gray matter called *basal nuclei*.

As you can see in **Figure 6.9** on the next page, the surface of the brain is not smooth; instead, it is convoluted. Each of the curved, raised areas is called a *gyrus* (JIGH-rus), and each of the grooves between the gyri is called a *sulcus* (SUL-kus). Together, these structures are referred

Left cerebral
hemisphere

Longitudinal
fissure

Right cerebral
hemisphere

Lateral sulcus

Alex Mit/Shutterstock.com

A.   Exterior view of the brain

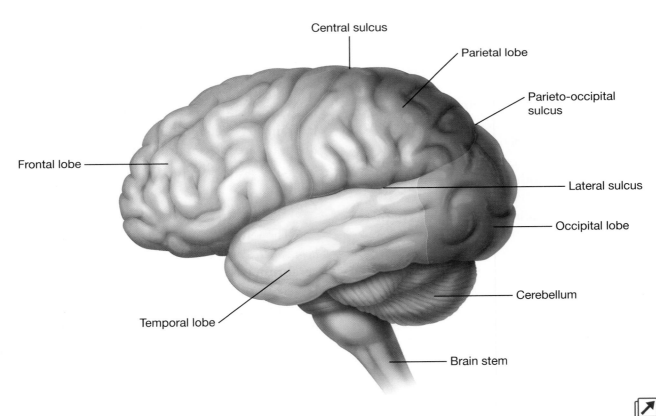

Central sulcus

Parietal lobe

Parieto-occipital
sulcus

Frontal lobe

Lateral sulcus

Occipital lobe

Cerebellum

Temporal lobe

Brain stem

B.   Lobes of the brain

Label Art

Figure 6.9 A—The hemispheres of the cerebrum. B—The four lobes of the cerebrum (shown in contrasting colors) are separated by indentations called sulci.

to as *convolutions*. No two brains look exactly alike in their pattern of convolutions. However, the major sulci are arranged in the same pattern in all human brains.

The sulci divide the brain into four regions called **lobes**. The four lobes of the brain are the frontal, parietal, occipital, and temporal.

Like the sulci, **fissures** are uniformly positioned, deep grooves in the brain. The longitudinal fissure runs the length of the brain and divides it into left and right hemispheres. As a result, the lobes are paired on the left and right sides of the body. Neural communications to and from the right side of the body are controlled by the left brain, and communications with the left side of the body are controlled by the right brain.

The **frontal lobes**, located behind the forehead in the most anterior portion of the brain, are sectioned off from the rest of the brain by the central sulcus (**Figure 6.9B**). Just anterior to the central sulcus is the **primary motor cortex**, which sends neural impulses to the skeletal muscles to initiate and control the development of muscle tension and movement of our body parts.

As **Figure 6.10** shows, scientists have mapped the primary motor cortex so that we know which body parts are controlled in each region of the cortex. Notice that relatively small regions of the cortex control major body segments, such as the trunk, pelvis, thigh, and arm. Much larger regions of the cortex are allocated for control of smaller body segments, such as the hands, lips, and tongue.

Why is this the case? If you think about it, the body parts associated with larger areas of the motor cortex are the ones capable of the more fine-tuned movements. Such movements require the activation of more nerves.

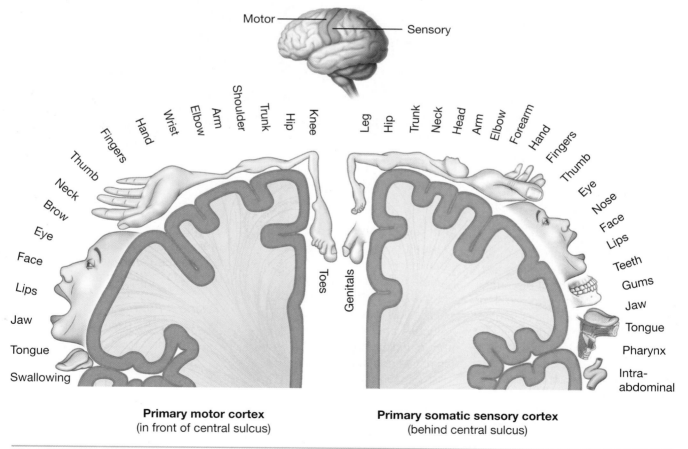

Primary motor cortex
(in front of central sulcus)

Primary somatic sensory cortex
(behind central sulcus)

Figure 6.10 The primary motor and somatic sensory cortexes, with mapped regions of motor output and sensory input depicted. *Why do smaller areas of the body, such as the fingers or lips, require more nerves than larger areas, such as the shoulder or trunk?*

WHAT RESEARCH TELLS US

...*about* **Studying the Brain**

An increasing variety of approaches is available for studying the functional roles of different parts of the central nervous system. As technology advances, more sophisticated techniques emerge.

fMRI Scans

One procedure extremely useful for both scientific and clinical evaluation of the brain is called *functional magnetic resonance imaging (fMRI)*. This technology creates images of changes in blood flow to activated brain structures. This is made possible by the slightly different magnetic properties of oxygenated and deoxygenated blood. The images show which brain structures are activated and the amount of time they are activated during performance of different tasks. The individual undergoing the brain scan is presented with certain tasks that can cause activation (increased blood flow) to the regions of the brain responsible for perception, thought, and a stimulated motor action, such as raising an arm or smiling (**Figure 6.11**).

Increasingly, physicians are using fMRI to diagnose disorders and diseases of the brain. With a fine sensitivity to changes in blood flow, fMRI is particularly useful for evaluating patients who may have suffered a stroke. Early diagnosis of stroke is important because treatment can be significantly more effective the earlier it is given.

PET Scans

Another approach for studying brain function involves positron

Figure 6.11 Functional magnetic resonance imaging (fMRI) scans of the brain show different areas of activation.

emission tomography (toh-MAHG-ra-fee), or PET. This procedure tracks the locations of radioactively labeled chemicals in the bloodstream. PET scans can show blood flow, oxygen absorption, and glucose absorption in the active brain, indicating where the brain is active and inactive. Although fMRI has largely replaced PET for the study of brain activation patterns, PET scans still provide the advantage of showing where particular neurotransmitters are concentrated in the brain. PET scans are also still widely used

in diagnosing various forms of brain disease because they can be analyzed and interpreted more quickly than fMRI scans.

Taking It Further

1. How is an fMRI used to help diagnose disease and disorders?

2. Why is the blood-flow pattern to the brain a revealing factor in the diagnosis of a particular brain disease or disorder?

3. In what situations might a doctor prefer to use an fMRI or PET scan?

The left frontal lobe also includes *Broca's area*, which controls the tongue and lip movements required for speech. Damage to this area in stroke patients produces difficulty with speaking. The *association cortex* on the most anterior portion of the frontal lobe is believed to be responsible for intellect.

The **parietal** (pa-RIGH-eh-tal) **lobes** are immediately posterior to the frontal lobes. The parietal lobes include the **primary somatic sensory cortex**, which interprets sensory impulses received from the skin, internal organs, muscles, and joints. The display of body parts in the somatic sensory part of **Figure 6.10** represents the density, or amount, of sensory neural input received from different parts of the body. Notice that the fingertips and lips, in particular, have a lot of sensory receptors. This is why they occupy large portions of the sensory cortex.

The **occipital** (ahk-SIP-i-tal) **lobes**, posterior to the parietal lobes, are responsible for vision. The lateral sulci divide the **temporal** (TEHM-poh-ral) **lobes**, the most inferior lobes, from the frontal and parietal lobes above them. The temporal lobes are involved in speech, hearing, vision, memory, and emotion. The region responsible for speech is located at the intersection of the occipital, temporal, and parietal lobes.

Check Your Understanding

1. List the four major anatomic regions of the brain.
2. Describe the relationship between gyri and sulci.
3. List the four lobes of the brain and state their locations.
4. List the function(s) of each lobe.

Diencephalon

The **diencephalon** (DIGH-ehn-SEHF-a-lahn), also known as the *interbrain*, is located deep inside the brain, enclosed by the cerebral hemispheres (**Figure 6.12**). It includes several important structures—the thalamus, hypothalamus, and epithalamus.

- The **thalamus** (THAL-a-mus) serves as a relay station for communicating both sensory and motor information between the body and the cerebral cortex. It also plays a major role in regulating the body's states of arousal, including sleep, wakefulness, and high-alert consciousness.
- Only about the size of a pearl, the **hypothalamus** (HIGH-poh-THAL-a-mus) is a key part of the autonomic nervous system, regulating such functions as metabolism, heart rate, blood pressure, thirst, hunger, energy level, and body temperature. The centers for sex, pain, and pleasure also lie within the hypothalamus.
- The **epithalamus** (EHP-i-THAL-a-mus) includes the pineal gland and regulates the sleep-cycle hormones that it secretes.

Brain Stem

Approximately the size of a thumb, the brain stem is shaped somewhat like a stem and includes three structures: the midbrain, pons, and medulla oblongata (**Figure 6.12**).

- The **midbrain** on the superior end of the brain stem serves as a relay station for sensory and motor impulses. Specifically, it relays information concerning vision, hearing, motor activity, sleep and wake cycles, arousal (alertness), and temperature regulation.
- The **pons** (pahnz), located immediately below the midbrain, plays a role in regulating breathing.
- Inferior to the pons, the **medulla oblongata** (meh-DOOL-a AHB-lawn-gah-tah) regulates heart rate, blood pressure, and breathing, and controls the reflexes for coughing, sneezing, and vomiting.

The *reticular* (reh-TIK-yoo-lar) *formation* is a collection of gray matter that extends the length of the brain stem. The reticular formation regulates waking from slumber, as well as heightened states of awareness. Individuals with severe brain injuries can continue to live as long as the brain stem remains functional and they receive sufficient hydration and nutrition.

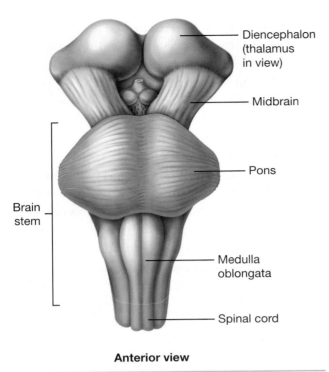

Anterior view

Figure 6.12 The diencephalon includes the thalamus (exterior), and the hypothalamus and epithalamus (both interior). The brain stem includes the midbrain, pons, and medulla oblongata. *Which area of the brain identified above controls your sneezing reflex?*

Cerebellum

The **cerebellum** (SER-eh-BEHL-um), found below the occipital lobe, looks similar to the cerebrum with its outer gray cortex, convolutions, and dual hemispheres (**Figure 6.9**). The cerebellum serves the important role of coordinating body movements, including balance.

To coordinate body movements and balance, the cerebellum receives input from the eyes, inner ears, and sensory receptors throughout the body. It also continuously monitors body segment positions and motions. If the body's positions and motions are not what the cerebellum intended them to be, it sends out signals to make adjustments.

The primary functions of the different structures of the brain are summarized in **Figure 6.13**.

Meninges

Three protective membranes, the **meninges** (meh-NIN-jeez), surround the brain and spinal

cord (**Figure 6.14**). The outer membrane, the *dura mater* (DOO-rah MAY-ter), meaning "hard mother," is a tough, double-layered membrane that lies beneath the skull and surrounds the brain. The inner layer of the dura mater continues down to enclose the spinal cord.

The middle membrane, the *arachnoid mater*, is composed of weblike tissue. Beneath this membrane is the subarachnoid space, filled with cerebrospinal (seh-REE-broh-SPIGH-nal) fluid, which cushions the brain and spinal cord.

The innermost layer of the meninges attaches directly to the surface of the brain and spinal cord. This layer is the delicate *pia mater* (PIGH-ah MAY-ter), meaning "gentle mother."

Blood-Brain Barrier

A rich network of blood vessels supplies the brain. Like all tissues of the body, the brain depends on a circulating blood supply to provide nutrients and carry away the waste products of cell metabolism. At any given time, roughly 20%–25% of the blood in your body is circulating in the region of the brain.

The capillaries supplying the brain, however, are different from other capillaries in the body. Specifically, they are impermeable to many substances that freely diffuse through the walls of capillaries in other body regions. This property of impermeability has given rise to the term *blood-brain barrier*.

The blood-brain barrier protects the brain against surges in concentrations of hormones, ions, and some nutrients. Substances allowed to pass through the capillaries include water, glucose, and essential amino acids. Other substances that can penetrate the blood-brain barrier are blood-borne alcohol, nicotine, fats, respiratory gases, and anesthetics.

Spinal Cord

The **spinal cord** extends from the brain stem down to the beginning of the lumbar region of the spine. It serves as a major pathway for relaying sensory impulses to the brain and motor impulses from the brain. It also provides the

Figure 6.13 Functions of the Brain

Part of Brain	Primary Functions
Cerebral Lobes	
Frontal lobe	memory, intelligence, behavior, emotions, motor function, smell
Parietal lobe	somatic sensations (pain, touch, hot/cold), speech
Occipital lobe	vision, speech
Temporal lobe	hearing, smell, memory, speech
Diencephalon	
Thalamus	relays sensory impulses up to the sensory cortex
Hypothalamus	autonomic center regulating metabolism, heart rate, blood pressure, thirst, hunger, energy level, and body temperature
Epithalamus	regulates hormones secreted by pineal gland
Brain Stem	
Midbrain	relays sensory and motor impulses
Pons	assists with regulation of breathing
Medulla oblongata	regulates heart rate, blood pressure, and breathing, and controls the reflexes of coughing, sneezing, and vomiting
Reticular formation	regulates waking from slumber and heightened states of awareness
Cerebellum	coordinates body movements and balance

Figure 6.14 The three meninges (the protective linings of the brain and spinal cord) include the double-layered dura mater, the arachnoid mater, and the pia mater. *How do each of the meninges contribute to the protection of the brain and spinal cord?*

neural connections involved in reflex arcs. Like the brain, the spine is surrounded and protected by the three meninges and cerebrospinal fluid.

When viewed in cross section, the exterior of the spinal cord is myelinated white matter, with butterfly-shaped gray matter, composed of neuron cell bodies and interneurons (inter-NOO-rahnz), located centrally (**Figure 6.15**). The regions of the white and gray matter in the spinal cord are named after their locations—ventral (anterior), lateral, or dorsal (posterior). The dorsal columns of white matter carry sensory impulses to the brain, while the lateral and ventral columns transmit both sensory and motor impulses. The dorsal, lateral, and ventral projections of gray matter are called *horns*.

Figure 6.15 also shows the formations of the spinal nerves. These will be discussed in the next lesson.

✓ Check Your Understanding

1. Name the three structures that make up the diencephalon and state their functions.
2. Name the three structures that make up the brain stem and state the function of each.
3. Where is the cerebellum located and what is its function?
4. What are the three regions of white and gray matter in the spinal cord?

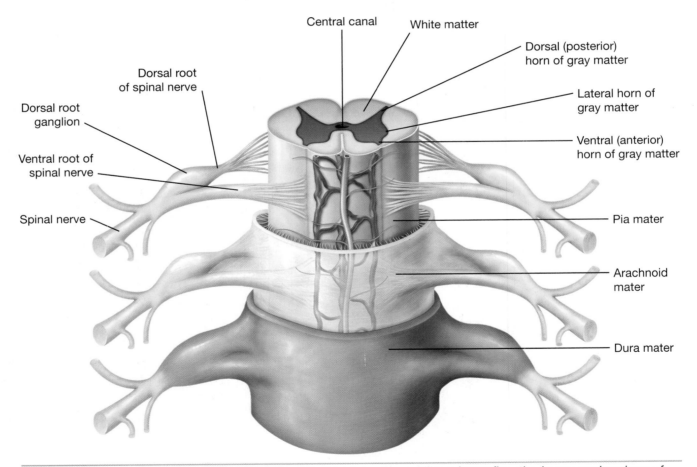

Figure 6.15 Layers and regions of the spinal cord. *Which is shaped like a butterfly—the layers and regions of the spinal cord, the gray matter, or the white matter?*

Lesson 6.3 Review and Assessment

Mini Glossary   Make sure that you know the meaning of each key term.

Build vocabulary with
e-flash cards and games

cerebellum   section of the brain that coordinates body movements, including balance

cerebrum   the largest part of the brain, consisting of the left and right hemispheres

diencephalon   area of the brain that includes the epithalamus, thalamus, metathalamus, and hypothalamus; also known as the interbrain

epithalamus   the uppermost portion of the diencephalon, which includes the pineal gland and regulates sleep-cycle hormones

fissures   the uniformly positioned, deep grooves in the brain

frontal lobes   sections of the brain located behind the forehead

hypothalamus   a portion of the diencephalon, which regulates functions such as metabolism, heart rate, and blood pressure

lobes   the name for the four regions of the brain—frontal, parietal, occipital, and temporal

medulla oblongata   the lower portion of the brain stem, which regulates heart rate, blood pressure, and breathing, and controls several reflexes

meninges   three protective membranes that surround the brain and spinal cord

midbrain   relay station for sensory and motor impulses; located on the superior end of the brain stem

occipital lobes   sections of the brain located behind the parietal lobes; integrate sensory information from the skin, internal organs, muscles, and joints

parietal lobes   sections of the brain located behind the frontal lobes; integrate sensory information from the skin, internal organs, muscles, and joints

pons   the section of the brain that plays a role in regulating breathing

primary motor cortex   outer region of the brain in the frontal lobes that sends neural impulses to the skeletal muscles

primary somatic sensory cortex outer region of the brain in the parietal lobes that interprets sensory impulses received from the skin, internal organs, muscles, and joints

spinal cord   a column of nerve tissue that extends from the brain stem to the beginning of the lumbar region of the spine

temporal lobes   the most inferior portions of the brain; responsible for speech, hearing, vision, memory, and emotion

thalamus   the largest portion of the diencephalon, which communicates sensory and motor information between the body and the cerebral cortex

Know and Understand

Assess

1. Is the brain divided into four lobes and two hemispheres or two lobes and four hemispheres?

2. What is the difference between gray matter and white matter in the brain? Where is each found?

3. Explain why someone might say that the brain is *convoluted*.

4. Are major body segments, such as the trunk and pelvis, controlled by large or small regions of the brain's primary motor cortex?

5. What area of the brain has probably been damaged if a stroke patient has difficulty speaking?

6. Like the brain, the spinal cord has gray and white matter. Identify the responsibility of both the gray and white matter when found in the spinal cord.

Analyze and Apply

7. Compare and contrast the three protective membranes surrounding the brain and spinal cord. Discuss their structures and functions.

8. Why are the capillaries in the brain different from the capillaries in other parts of the body?

9. Which general area of the brain—the anterior or posterior region—is associated with more sophisticated functions? Explain.

In the Lab

10. Obtain a model or picture of a human brain. Color-code the different lobes and structures on the model or picture and then list the function(s) and body processes that each area controls.

Functional Anatomy of the Peripheral Nervous System

Lesson Objectives

1. Describe the basic structure of a nerve.
2. Identify the twelve cranial nerves and the purpose of each.
3. Explain the organization of the spinal nerves, the dorsal and ventral rami, and the plexuses.
4. Describe the location, structure, and function of ganglions.
5. Differentiate between the functions of the sympathetic and parasympathetic nervous systems.

Key Terms

E-Flash Cards

cranial nerves
craniosacral division
dorsal ramus
endoneurium
epineurium
ganglion
norepinephrine
paravertebral ganglia

perineurium
plexuses
postganglionic neuron
preganglionic neuron
spinal nerves
thoracolumbar division
ventral ramus

The peripheral nervous system (PNS) transmits information to the CNS and carries instructions from the CNS. It achieves these functions through a network of nerves outside of the CNS.

Nerve Structure

Each nerve consists of a collection of axons (nerve fibers) and nutrient-supplying blood vessels, all bundled in a series of protective sheaths of connective tissue. As shown in **Figure 6.16**, each axon is covered by a fine **endoneurium** (EHN-doh-NOO-ree-um). In myelinated axons, the endoneurium surrounds the myelin sheath as well as the nodes of Ranvier.

Groups of these sheathed fibers are bundled into fascicles surrounded by a protective **perineurium** (PER-i-NOO-ree-um). Finally, groups of fascicles and blood vessels are encased in a tough **epineurium** (EHP-i-NOO-ree-um). This structural arrangement provides a cordlike strength that helps the nerve resist injury.

Cranial Nerves

Twelve pairs of **cranial nerves** relay impulses to and from the left and right sides of the brain. These pairs are referred to by both a name and a number (**Figure 6.18**). The functions of the cranial nerves are summarized in **Figure 6.17**. The names of these nerves indicate their functions.

Some of these nerves contain only afferent (sensory) fibers, some contain only efferent (motor) fibers, and others—the *mixed nerves*—carry both kinds of impulses. All but the first two cranial nerves emanate from the brain stem.

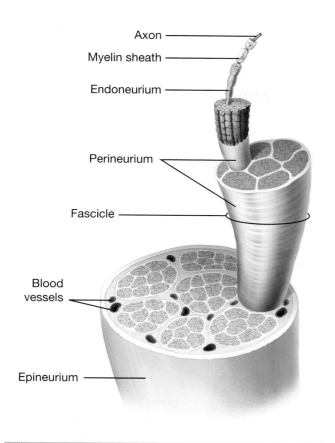

Axon
Myelin sheath
Endoneurium
Perineurium
Fascicle
Blood vessels
Epineurium

Figure 6.16 Structure of a nerve showing the protective, fibrous tissue sheaths. *How does the structure of a nerve help to protect it from injury?*

Spinal Nerves and Nerve Plexuses

Thirty-one pairs of **spinal nerves** branch out from the left and right sides of the spinal cord. Each pair is named for the vertebral level from which it originates. As you learned in chapter 4, the vertebral levels include the cervical, thoracic, and lumbar regions, as well as the sacrum. All of the spinal nerves are mixed nerves, carrying both afferent and efferent information.

The spinal nerve cell bodies are located within the gray matter of the spinal cord. The axons of spinal nerve cells extend out of the spinal cord and eventually connect with muscles. As shown earlier in **Figure 6.15**, dorsal (posterior) and ventral (anterior) spinal nerve roots unite to form the left and right spinal nerves that exit at each spinal level.

The spinal nerves are only about one-half inch long, immediately dividing into a **dorsal ramus** (DOR-sal RAY-mus) and **ventral ramus** (VEHN-tral RAY-mus) (**Figure 6.19**). The dorsal and ventral rami carry nerve impulses to the muscle and skin of the trunk.

Figure 6.17	Functions of the Cranial Nerves		
Nerve	**#**	**System**	**Function**
Olfactory	I	sensory	smell
Optic	II	sensory	sight
Oculomotor	III	both	eye movements
Trochlear	IV	both	eye movements
Trigeminal	V	both	facial sensation, jaw motion
Abducens	VI	both	eye movements
Facial	VII	both	facial movements, taste
Vestibulocochlear	VIII	sensory	hearing, balance
Glossopharyngeal	IX	both	throat muscle movements, taste
Vagus	X	both	autonomic control of heart, lungs, digestion, taste, communication between brain and organs
Accessory	XI	mostly motor	trapezius movements, sternocleidomastoid movements
Hypoglossal	XII	both	tongue muscle movements, tongue sensation

CNS Connection

- ☐ Cerebrum
- ☐ Diencephalon
- ☐ Midbrain
- ☐ Pons
- ☐ Medulla oblongata

Facial — VII

Olfactory — I

Trigeminal — V

Optic — II

Oculomotor — III

Trochlear — IV

Vestibulocochlear — VIII

Abducens — VI

Hypoglossal — XII

Glossopharyngeal — IX

Vagus — X

Accessory — XI

Figure 6.18 The cranial nerves. *Name at least two organs that receive impulses from the vagus nerve.*

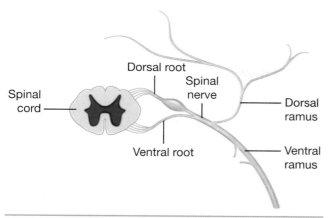

Figure 6.19 The spinal nerves, formed from dorsal and ventral roots, immediately branch into dorsal and ventral rami. *What motor impulses do the dorsal and ventral rami transmit? What sensory nerve impulses do they transmit?*

All of the rami are mixed nerves, carrying both afferent and efferent signals.

- The small dorsal rami transmit motor impulses to the posterior trunk muscles and relay sensory impulses from the skin of the back.
- The ventral rami in the thoracic region of the spine (T_1–T_{12}) become the intercostal nerves (running between the ribs). They communicate with the muscles and skin of the anterior and lateral trunk.
- The ventral rami in the cervical and lumbar regions branch out to form complex interconnections of nerves called **plexuses**. Most of the major efferent nerves in the neck, arms, and legs originate in the plexuses.

The four plexuses in the body are summarized in **Figure 6.20** on the next page. To see how the major nerves branch out from the lower three plexuses, refer to **Figure 6.21**. **Figure 6.21** shows that other large nerves branch out from the plexuses listed in **Figure 6.20**.

Autonomic Nervous System

As described in the first lesson of this chapter, the peripheral nervous system has two divisions—the somatic nervous system and the autonomic, or involuntary, nervous system. The somatic nervous system sends impulses to activate the skeletal muscles, whereas the autonomic nervous system is programmed by the CNS to activate the heart, smooth muscles, and glands.

Within the autonomic system, two nerves connect the CNS to the organs supplied. The cell body of the first nerve originates in the gray matter of the brain or spinal cord.

The autonomic cell bodies that originate in the spinal cord reside in the lateral horn. The axons of these nerves terminate with a synapse to a second neuron in an enlarged junction called a **ganglion** (GAYNG-glee-ahn). The second neuron then courses from the ganglion to the cardiac muscle, smooth muscle, or gland.

As you might suspect, the first neuron in the sequence just described is called the **preganglionic** (PREE-gayng-glee-AHN-ik) **neuron**. The second is called the **postganglionic** (POHST-gayng-glee-AHN-ik) **neuron**. Now let's look more closely at the two divisions of the autonomic nervous system. These are the sympathetic and parasympathetic divisions.

Sympathetic Nerves

The sympathetic nerves activate the fight-or-flight response by stimulating the adrenal gland to release epinephrine, also known as *adrenaline*. Supposedly in primitive times, when a person was confronted by a predator, the fight-or-flight response—characterized by increased heart and breathing rates and sweating—prepared the individual either to fight or run. In modern times the sympathetic response is physiologically the same, but it can be triggered by any type of situation that is perceived to be stressful. You will learn more about the fight-or-flight response in Chapter 8, *The Endocrine System*.

The preganglionic neurons in the sympathetic system arise from the spinal segments extending from T_1–L_2. For this reason, the sympathetic system is also called the **thoracolumbar** (THOH-rah-koh-LUM-bar) **division**. These neurons secrete acetylcholine to stimulate the postganglionic neurons in the **paravertebral ganglia** (pair-a-VER-teh-bral GAYNG-glee-a). The paravertebral ganglia are named after their location; they lie parallel to the spinal cord. The postganglionic neurons release the neurotransmitter **norepinephrine** (NOR-ehp-i-NEHF-rin).

Figure 6.20   Spinal Nerve Plexuses

Plexus	Spinal nerves	Exiting nerves	Region supplied
Cervical	C_1–C_5	phrenic	diaphragm, skin and muscles of neck and shoulder
Brachial	C_5–C_8 and T_1	axillary	skin and muscles of shoulder
		radial	skin and muscles of lateral and posterior arm and forearm
		median	skin and flexor muscles of forearm, some hand muscles
		musculocutaneous	skin of lateral forearm, elbow flexor muscles
		ulnar	skin of hand, flexor muscles of forearm, wrist and some hand muscles
Lumbar	L_1–L_4	femoral	skin of medial and anterior thigh, anterior thigh muscles
		obturator	skin and muscles of medial thigh and hip
		saphenous	skin of the medial thigh and medial lower leg
Sacral	L_4–L_5 and S_1–S_4	sciatic	two of the hamstrings (semimembranosus, semitendinosus), adductor magnus
		tibial	muscles of knee flexion, plantar flexion, and toe flexion; skin of the posterior lower leg and sole of the foot
		common fibular	biceps femoris, tibialis anterior, muscles of toe extension, skin of the anterior lower leg, superior surface of foot, and lateral side of foot
		superior and inferior gluteal	gluteal muscles
		posterior femoral cutaneous	skin of posterior thigh and posterior lower leg

Parasympathetic Nerves

In contrast to the sympathetic nervous system, the parasympathetic nervous system controls all of the automatic, day-in-and-day-out functions of the circulatory, respiratory, and digestive systems. For these reasons it is sometimes called the "resting and digesting system." In addition, after a fight-or-flight situation, the parasympathetic nervous system produces a calming effect that returns the body to a normal state.

Preganglionic parasympathetic neurons originate in one of two separate regions—the brain stem or the sacral (lowermost) region of the spinal cord. For this reason, the parasympathetic system is also known as the **craniosacral** (KRAY-nee-oh-SAY-kral) **division**. Activation of both preganglionic and postganglionic nerves in this system triggers the release of the neurotransmitter acetylcholine. Although acetylcholine stimulates skeletal muscle, it also inhibits activity in cardiac and smooth muscle.

Check Your Understanding

1. How many pairs of cranial nerves does the body have?
2. What kind of impulses do mixed nerves carry?
3. How many pairs of spinal nerves does the body have?
4. List the two divisions of the autonomic nervous system.
5. Which nerves—the sympathetic or the parasympathetic—activate the fight-or-flight response?

Axillary nerve

Musculocutaneous nerve

Radial nerve

Ulnar nerve

Radial nerve (superficial branch)

Median nerve

Femoral nerve

Obturator nerve

Saphenous nerve

Inferior gluteal nerve

Superior gluteal nerve

Sciatic nerve

Posterior femoral cutaneous nerve

Common fibular nerve

Tibial nerve

Label Art

A. Brachial plexus (anterior view)

B. Lumbar plexus (anterior view)

C. Sacral plexus (posterior view)

Figure 6.21 Major nerves emanate from the brachial, lumbar, and sacral plexuses. *The word plexus is derived from the Latin plectere, meaning "to braid." Why is this a fitting term for a group of nerves?*

Lesson 6.4 Review and Assessment

Mini Glossary   Make sure you that know the meaning of each key term.

Build vocabulary with
e-flash cards and games

cranial nerves   12 pairs of nerves that originate in the brain and relay impulses to and from the PNS

craniosacral division   the parasympathetic nervous system, in which nerves originate in the brain stem or sacral region of the spinal cord

dorsal ramus   the division of posterior spinal nerves that transmit motor impulses to the posterior trunk muscles and relay sensory impulses from the skin of the back

endoneurium   a delicate, connective tissue that surrounds each nerve fiber

epineurium   the tough outer covering of a nerve

ganglion   a mass of nervous tissue composed mostly of nerve-cell bodies

norepinephrine   a neurotransmitter released by postganglionic neurons in the sympathetic nervous system

paravertebral ganglia   mass of nerve cell bodies close to the spinal cord

perineurium   a protective sheath that surrounds a bundle of nerve fibers

plexuses   complex interconnections of nerves

postganglionic neuron   the second neuron in a series that transmits impulses from the CNS

preganglionic neuron   the first neuron in a series that transmits impulses from the CNS

spinal nerves   neural transmitters that branch from the left and right sides of the spinal cord

thoracolumbar division   the sympathetic system of nerves that lies near the thoracic and lumbar regions of the spine

ventral ramus   the anterior division of spinal nerves that communicate with the muscle and skin of the anterior and lateral trunk

Know and Understand

Assess

1. Explain the function of the peripheral nervous system.

2. What is the major purpose of the endoneurium, perineurium, and epineurium combined?

3. How would you describe cranial nerves in terms of sensory and motor fibers?

4. From where do the majority of cranial nerves emanate?

5. Are spinal nerves efferent, afferent, or mixed?

6. Which nervous system sends impulses to the heart—the somatic or the autonomic system?

7. Why is the parasympathetic nervous system also known as the *craniosacral division*?

8. Explain the difference between a preganglionic neuron and a postganglionic neuron.

Analyze and Apply

9. Explain how the structure of a nerve decreases the chances of nerve damage.

10. Describe the fight-or-flight response activated by sympathetic nerves and explain how it could be a lifesaver.

11. Neurons meet at junctions called *ganglions*. Explain the purpose of a ganglion and how these structures help transmit nerve impulses throughout the body.

12. Explain how the function of a cranial nerve might determine whether it is a sensory or motor fiber, or both.

In the Lab

13. Using clay, create a model of a nerve. Use different colors for the different parts of the nerve. Begin with a simpler structure, such as an axon, and continue until you have a more complex structure (complete nerve). Use the illustrations in this lesson to guide you in constructing your model.

Injuries and Disorders of the Nervous System

Before You Read

Try to answer the following questions before you read this lesson.

What are the important first steps to take—and actions not to take—when someone may have an injury to the brain or spinal cord?

What causes multiple sclerosis and what are the symptoms?

What are the symptoms of early and advanced Alzheimer's disease?

Lesson Objectives

1. Describe the symptoms and recovery strategies for someone who has suffered a traumatic brain injury.
2. Explain the causes and range of symptoms for cerebral palsy.
3. Explain the consequences of injuries at different levels of the spinal cord.
4. Describe some of the common diseases and disorders of the nervous system.

Key Terms

E-Flash Cards

Alzheimer's disease
cerebral palsy
dementia
epilepsy
meningitis

multiple sclerosis
paraplegia
Parkinson's disease
quadriplegia
traumatic brain injury

Given the critical roles played by the central nervous system, injuries and disorders of the CNS can have potentially serious consequences. Let's look at some of the more common injuries and disorders of the CNS.

Injuries to the Brain and Spinal Cord

The brain and spinal cord are well protected. They are encased, respectively, in the skull and vertebral column, and both are surrounded by the three meninges and cerebrospinal fluid. Unfortunately, violent injuries can still cause mild to severe damage to these CNS structures.

Traumatic Brain Injury

Traumatic brain injury (TBI) can occur during violent impacts to the head, particularly when the skull is pierced or fractured and bone fragments penetrate the brain. These injuries are classified as mild, moderate, or severe, with increasing levels of damage to the nervous system, particularly the cells and tissues of the brain.

With mild TBI, a person may remain conscious or may lose consciousness for a short time. Symptoms can include any of the following: headache, confusion, dizziness, disturbed vision, ringing in the ears, bad taste in the mouth, fatigue, abnormal sleep patterns, behavioral changes, and trouble with intellectual functions.

Symptoms of moderate to severe TBI include all of those listed above, and can also involve more serious symptoms such as prolonged headache, repeated nausea or vomiting, convulsions or seizures, inability to awaken from sleep, dilation of one or both pupils of the eyes, slurred speech, weakness or numbness in the extremities, loss of coordination, confusion, and agitation. Cases of moderate and severe TBI require immediate medical care, with the goal of preventing further brain injury. X-rays and imaging tests may be performed to help with assessment of the nature and extent of the damage. Maintaining proper blood pressure and flow of oxygenated blood to the brain and throughout the body are priorities. Furthermore, about 50% of severe TBI cases require surgical repair.

Case Study: Phineas Gage. A miraculous story of survival from a significant TBI is the case of Phineas Gage, a railroad construction foreman who was injured in 1848 at 25 years of age. Gage and his crew were blasting rock to make way for railroad construction outside the town of Cavendish, Vermont, when a 3½ foot iron rod was accidentally blasted through Gage's skull. The iron entered below the left cheekbone and exited through the top of the skull. The blast was of such force that the iron landed approximately 80 feet away.

Amazingly, within a few minutes Gage was able to speak, walk, and ride upright in a cart back to his home, where he received medical attention. Gage's recovery was slow, with advances and declines, including time spent in a coma due to brain swelling. Nevertheless, his physical recovery was complete.

Accounts of Gage's mental recovery vary, but they suggest that his personality was negatively altered. Gage survived for 12 years after the accident. He began to suffer a series of increasingly severe seizures that eventually resulted in his death. The case of Phineas Gage is still discussed in medical and neurology classes.

Treating and Preventing TBI. Today, follow-up care for TBI involves individualized rehabilitation programs that may include physical, occupational, and speech language therapies; psychiatry; and social support. The prognosis for those who have suffered from a traumatic brain injury varies greatly, with potential for lingering problems with intellectual functioning, sensation, and behavior. Serious head injuries can result in an unresponsive state or a coma.

Research is being conducted in scientific and clinical settings to achieve a clearer understanding of the biological effects of TBI. One goal of this research is to develop strategies and interventions that limit the brain damage that occurs during the first few days after a head injury. Another goal is to develop more effective therapies for facilitating recovery of function.

Cerebral Palsy

Cerebral palsy (CP) is a group of nervous system disorders caused by damage to the brain before or during birth (congenital defect), or in early infancy. Congenital defects that can cause CP include a brain that has an abnormal shape or structure, or damaged nerve cells and brain tissues. Infections such as rubella in the mother during pregnancy can produce CP. During the first two years, while the brain is still developing, several conditions—including brain infections, head injury, and impaired liver function—can cause CP. Sometimes, however, the cause is unknown.

The most common symptoms involve varying degrees of motor function impairment, but can also include hearing, seeing, and cognitive impairment. The degree of impairment may be barely noticeable or very severe (**Figure 6.22**). One or both sides of the body may be affected and the arms, legs, or both may be involved.

Martynova Anna/Shutterstock.com

Figure 6.22 Russian and British athletes with cerebral palsy play a game of soccer in preparation for the Paralympics.

WHAT RESEARCH TELLS US

...*about* Concussions

The most common form of traumatic brain injury is a concussion. Symptoms can include headache as well as problems with concentration, memory, judgment, balance, and coordination. Fortunately, these effects are usually temporary. Although a concussion can cause a loss of consciousness, most concussions do not. Thus, many people experience mild concussions without realizing it.

The most common cause of concussion is a blow to the head. However, concussions can also occur when the head and upper body are violently shaken. In fact, the word *concussion* comes from the Latin *concutere*, which means "to shake violently."

Concussions in Sports

Injuries that produce concussions are of particular concern for participants in American football, boxing, and soccer, although they also occur in other sports. According to the Centers for Disease Control, as many as 3.8 million sports- and recreation-related concussions occur in the United States each year. Concussions also result from car and bicycle accidents, work injuries, and falls.

Because all concussions injure the brain to some extent, it is crucial that these injuries have time to heal. Healing time is particularly important for athletes in contact sports, which involve higher risks of reinjury to the brain. For this reason, researchers are focusing attention on the consequences of repeated concussions.

Recent Research

A recent study shows that retired professional football players

Ken Durden/Shutterstock, Inc.

Figure 6.23 The NFL has implemented several new rules and regulations in an effort to prevent concussions.

appear to be at a higher risk of death from diseases of the brain, compared to the general US population. In the study, sponsored by the National Institute for Occupational Safety and Health (NIOSH), researchers examined the medical records of 3,439 former National Football League (NFL) players with an average age of 57. At the time of the analysis, only 10 percent of the participants had died, which is about half the death rate of men that age in the general population. The fact that relatively few had died indicates that the study participants were in better-than-average general health.

The medical records showed, however, that an NFL player's risk of death from Alzheimer's disease or amyotrophic lateral sclerosis (ALS), also known as Lou Gehrig's disease, was almost four times higher than in the general population. Furthermore, those players in "speed" positions—such as wide receiver, running back, and quarterback—accounted for most of the deaths from Alzheimer's disease and ALS. The researchers

emphasized that the data in this type of study do not establish a cause-effect relationship. They hypothesized, however, that the players in "speed" positions likely had experienced more high-speed collisions, and possibly repeated concussions, compared to the "non-speed" players.

NFL Takes Action

The NFL has donated $30 million to help establish the Sports and Health Research Program within the National Institutes of Health (NIH). This initiative provides funding for research on concussions and other common injuries in athletes across all sports, as well as members of the military.

The NFL also has taken steps to help prevent concussions, such as fining players for dangerous hits, notably helmet-to-helmet tackles. Rule changes at both the professional and collegiate levels now prevent players diagnosed with concussions from returning to play until they have been declared free of symptoms by a medical doctor.

Taking It Further

1. Working with a group of classmates, determine the standard operating procedure in athletic departments at local high schools and colleges for dealing with concussions. Are medical professionals involved in evaluating the severity of the concussion and determining when the athlete can resume practice and competitive events? What tests are used for the evaluations? Have rules been instituted to help prevent concussions? Report your findings to the class.

Several different types of cerebral palsy exist, with some individuals having mixed symptoms. The most common form is spastic CP, with symptoms that include

- very tight muscles and joints;
- muscle weakness; and
- gait (manner of walking) in which the arms are held close to the body with the elbows in flexion, the knees touch or cross, and the individual walks on tiptoes.

With other types of cerebral palsy, motor function degradation may include twisting or jerking movements; tremors; unsteady gait; impaired coordination; and excessive, floppy movements.

Sensory and cognitive symptoms may include learning disabilities or diminished intelligence; problems with speech; problems with hearing or sight; seizures; pain; and problems with swallowing and digestion.

Other symptoms may include slowed growth; drooling; breathing irregularities; and incontinence.

No cure for cerebral palsy exists, so the goal of treatment in moderate to severe cases is to promote quality of life and, when possible, independent living. In some cases, surgical intervention can improve gait, alleviate spasticity or pain, or restore joint range of motion.

Spinal Cord Injury

Fractures or displacements of the vertebrae can result in injury to the spinal cord. Such injuries most commonly occur during automobile accidents or participation in high-speed or contact sports. Although injuries to the spinal cord can occur at any level, these injuries most commonly develop in the cervical region because of the flexibility of the neck compared to that of the trunk.

A complete severing of the spinal cord produces permanent paralysis, with a total lack of sensory and motor function below the point of injury. The level of the spine at which the injury occurs is a major factor in determining the extent of injury:

- C_1–C_3—usually fatal
- C_1–C_4—**quadriplegia** (KWAH-dri-PLEE-jee-a), characterized by loss of function below the neck

- C_5–C_7—complete paralysis of the lower extremities, partial loss of function in the trunk and upper extremities
- T_1–L_5—**paraplegia** (PAIR-ah-PLEE-jee-ah), characterized by loss of function in the trunk and legs

Fortunately, most spinal cord injuries do not completely sever the spinal cord. In an *incomplete injury*, the ability of the spinal cord to transmit sensory and motor impulses is not completely lost. This allows some degree of sensory and/or motor function to remain below the point of injury. The prognosis in such cases is typically uncertain; some patients achieve nearly complete recovery, whereas others suffer complete paralysis.

Spinal cord injuries are medical emergencies. Immediate, aggressive treatment and follow-up rehabilitation can help minimize damage and preserve function. Because motion of a fractured or displaced vertebra can cause more damage to the spinal cord after the injury, it is critical that the head, neck, and trunk be immobilized before the victim is moved (**Figure 6.24**). In severe neck injuries of the spinal cord, breathing is affected in about one-third of the cases, and respiratory support is necessary. Surgery is often warranted to remove bone fragments or realign vertebrae to alleviate pressure on the spinal cord.

Ongoing research is aimed at developing techniques for repairing injured spinal cords.

Figure 6.24 It is critically important that the head, neck, and trunk are immobilized before transporting a patient with a potential spinal cord injury. *What might happen if a patient's head, neck, and truck are not immobilized after a potential spinal cord injury?*

Researchers are also working to advance our understanding of which rehabilitation approaches will be optimally successful at restoring lost function. Promising new rehabilitation techniques are helping patients with spinal cord injury become more mobile.

Check Your Understanding

1. Evaluate the causes of traumatic brain injury (TBI).
2. List the conditions that can cause cerebral palsy (CP).
3. What is the usual result of a spinal cord injury that occurs at each of the following levels? C_1–C_3; C_1–C_4; C_5–C_7; and T_1–L_5.

Common Diseases and Disorders of the CNS

In this section we will explore some of the common diseases and disorders that affect the central nervous system (CNS).

Meningitis

Meningitis (MEHN-in-JIGH-tis) is an inflammation of the meninges surrounding the brain and spinal cord. Swelling of these tissues, which is caused by an infection, often produces the signature symptoms of headache, fever, and a stiff neck.

Most infections that cause meningitis are viral, but bacterial and fungal infections can also lead to meningitis. Viral meningitis, the milder form, can resolve on its own. Bacterial meningitis is much more serious and potentially life threatening. Fortunately, bacterial meningitis can be treated with antibiotics. In either case, a person should seek immediate medical attention if meningitis is suspected.

Multiple Sclerosis

Multiple sclerosis (MS) is an autoimmune disease in which the body's own immune system causes inflammation that destroys the myelin sheath of nerve cell axons. This damage to the myelin sheath, which can occur in any part of the brain or spinal cord, impairs the ability of the affected nerves to transmit impulses. MS can occur at any age, but it is most commonly diagnosed between 20 and 40 years of age and occurs with greater frequency in women. The cause of MS is unknown.

An active attack of MS can last for days, weeks, or months. Periods during which the symptoms vanish or diminish are called *remissions*. Exposure to heat and stress can trigger or worsen attacks.

The symptoms of MS vary widely, depending on location within the CNS and severity of each episode.

- Impairments in motor function may include difficulties with balance, coordination, movement of the arms and legs, tremors, weakness, muscle spasms, and difficulty with speaking or swallowing.
- Sensory impairments may involve numbness, tingling, pain, double vision, uncontrollable eye movements, and loss of vision or hearing.
- Autonomic functions related to urination, defecation, and sexual function can also be affected.
- Associated cognitive issues may include decreased attention span, difficulty with reasoning, loss of memory, and depression.

There is no known cure for multiple sclerosis, so treatments are designed to help control symptoms and maintain quality of life. Exercise is often beneficial during the early stages. General recommendations for the MS patient include sufficient rest, sound nutrition, avoidance of hot temperatures, and minimization of stress. Although MS is a chronic condition, life expectancy can be normal. Many individuals with MS are able to continue functioning well in their jobs until retirement.

Epilepsy

Epilepsy (EHP-i-LEHP-see) is a group of brain disorders characterized by repeated seizures over time. A seizure is triggered by abnormal electrical activity in the brain that causes widely varying symptoms. Symptoms can range from changes in attention span or behavior to uncontrolled convulsions, depending on the type of epilepsy and area of the brain affected.

Epilepsy may be caused by a disease or injury that affects the brain, although in many cases the cause is unknown and genetics may play a role. Onset of epilepsy can happen at any age but occurs most frequently in infants and the elderly.

Epileptic seizures in a given individual are of a relatively consistent nature. Before a seizure, some people have an unusual sensation such as tingling, a strange smell, or an emotional change. This signal is referred to as an *aura*.

Epilepsy can be controlled with medication in most, but not all, people. Some types of epilepsy completely disappear after childhood. However, more than 30% of people with epilepsy are not able to control seizure incidence with medications. If epileptic seizures are caused by an observable problem, such as a tumor, abnormal blood vessels, or bleeding in the brain, surgery to address these issues may eliminate further seizures.

Parkinson's Disease

Parkinson's disease (PD) is one of the most common nervous system disorders among the elderly. It is characterized by tremors, difficulty with initiating movements—especially walking—and deficits in coordination. PD most often develops after the age of 50, although a genetic form of the disease may occur in younger adults. Men and women are equally affected.

PD is characterized by slow but progressive destruction of the brain cells responsible for production of the neurotransmitter dopamine, which plays a role in motor function. Without dopamine, the cells in the affected part of the brain cannot initiate nerve impulses, leading to progressive loss of muscle function. The cause of this condition is unknown.

The symptoms of PD tend to begin with a mild tremor of slight stiffness or weakness in one or both of the legs or feet. As brain cell destruction progresses, symptoms of motor

dysfunction affecting one or both sides of the body may include
- difficulty initiating and continuing movements;
- problems with balance and gait;
- stiff, painful muscles and tremors;
- slowed movement, including blinking;
- loss of fine motor control with hand movements;
- slowed speech, drooling, and difficulty swallowing;
- loss of facial expression; and
- stooped posture.

Autonomic and cognitive functions can also be impaired, as characterized by
- sweating and fluctuations in body temperature;
- fainting and inability to control blood pressure;
- constipation;
- confusion or dementia; and
- anxiety or depression.

Currently, no cure for PD exists; the goal of treatment is control of symptoms. If untreated, the disorder will progress, resulting in deterioration of all brain functions and early death. The medications prescribed for Parkinson's patients are designed to increase the levels of dopamine in the brain.

Dementia and Alzheimer's Disease

Dementia (deh-MEHN-shee-a) is a condition involving loss of function in two or more areas of cognition including memory, thinking, judgment, behavior, perception, and language. Dementia usually occurs after the age of 60, and risk increases with advancing age. Although forgetfulness is often the first sign of dementia, occasional forgetfulness alone does not qualify as dementia.

Dementia can be caused by disruption in the blood supply to the brain, as in stroke or related disorders. However, the single most common cause of dementia is Alzheimer's disease.

Alzheimer's disease (AD), or *senile dementia*, is a progressive loss of brain function with major consequences for memory, thinking, and behavior. In one form of the disease, called *early onset AD*, symptoms appear before 60 years of age. This type of AD tends to worsen quickly and is believed to involve genetic predisposition. The more common form, known as *late onset AD*, occurs after 60 years of age. The risk for developing Alzheimer's disease increases with advancing age. The cause of AD is currently unknown.

Early symptoms of AD may include difficulty with tasks that previously were routine; difficulty learning new ideas, concepts, or tasks; becoming lost in familiar territory; difficulty recalling the names of familiar objects; misplacing objects; a flat mood and loss of interest in activities; and personality changes and loss of social skills.

Worsening symptoms can include difficulty performing activities of daily living; progressive loss of short- and long-term memories; depression and agitation; delusions and aggressive behavior; inability to speak coherently; loss of judgment; and change in sleep patterns.

Advanced symptoms include the inability to understand language and recognize family members. Although no cure currently exists for Alzheimer's disease, medications can help to slow the worsening of symptoms.

 Check Your Understanding

1. Describe meningitis.
2. What happens to the body of a person with multiple sclerosis (MS)?
3. Describe Parkinson's disease.
4. Compare and contrast dementia and Alzheimer's disease.

Lesson 6.5 Review and Assessment

Mini Glossary   Make sure that you know the meaning of each key term.

 Build vocabulary with e-flash cards and games

Alzheimer's disease   condition involving a progressive loss of brain function with major consequences for memory, thinking, and behavior

cerebral palsy   a group of nervous system disorders resulting from brain damage before or during birth, or in early infancy

dementia   an organic brain disease involving loss of function in two or more areas of cognition

epilepsy   a group of brain disorders characterized by repeated seizures over time

meningitis   an infection-induced inflammation of the meninges surrounding the brain and spinal cord

multiple sclerosis   a chronic, slowly progressive disease of the central nervous system that destroys the myelin sheath of nerve cell axons

paraplegia   disorder characterized by loss of function in the lower trunk and legs

Parkinson's disease   a chronic nervous system disease characterized by a slowly spreading tremor, muscular weakness, and rigidity

quadriplegia   disorder characterized by loss of function below the neck

traumatic brain injury   mild or severe trauma that can result from a violent impact to the head

Know and Understand

Assess

1. Describe the body functions that may be affected in a person with cerebral palsy (CP).
2. What is meant by the term "incomplete injury" as it relates to a spinal cord injury?
3. What are the two types of meningitis and which is easier to treat?

Analyze and Apply

4. What autoimmune disease did you learn about in chapter 4? How are that disease and MS similar?

5. Explain what happens in the brain when a person has a seizure.

In the Lab

6. Do some research on images of brains. Find one brain image for each of the following: epilepsy, Alzheimer's disease, and dementia. Explain how the images are alike and how they are different. Point out specific areas in the brain in your explanations.

Career Corner
Anatomy and Physiology at Work

The nervous system is a complex organ system that plays an important role in your body's responses to numerous stimuli, both internal and external. That's quite a wide-ranging, significant role! Several careers are dedicated to the study of the nervous system, as well as to the diagnosis and treatment of neural disorders. We will explore two of these careers.

Neurologist

A neurologist (noo-RAHL-oh-jist) is a physician trained in the specialty field of neurology. Neurology involves the diagnosis and treatment of neurological injuries and diseases. A patient is typically referred to a neurologist by another physician who suspects that specialized treatment is needed.

Evaluation of a patient by a neurologist typically begins with a related medical history, followed by a physical examination that focuses on the nervous system. Components of the neurological examination may include assessment of the patient's cognitive function, muscular strength, sensation, reflexes, coordination, and gait. The neurologist may order diagnostic imaging studies when warranted (**Figure 6.25**).

Conditions commonly treated by neurologists include all of those discussed in this lesson. Treatment options vary by condition, and may include prescription of medications, referral for physical or occupational therapy, or referral to a surgeon.

Training to become a neurologist begins with four years of medical school, followed by a residency program or fellowship in pediatric or general neurology. The residency, which is usually four years, involves specific training. After residency, doctors may choose to pursue board certification through the American Board of Psychiatry and Neurology. Some neurologists voluntarily participate in additional training in a fellowship program to gain experience in a subspecialty area.

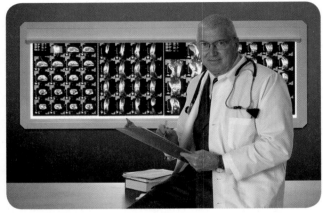

James Steidl/Shutterstock.com

Figure 6.25 A neurologist examines the MRI scans of a patient.

Neurosurgery is a different specialty that involves surgical treatment of neurological conditions. Training to be a neurosurgeon requires completion of four years of medical school followed by residency training under the supervision of neurosurgeons for an additional seven to eight years.

Neuroscientist

A scientist who specializes in research of the nervous system is called a neuroscientist. Neuroscientists usually work in a controlled laboratory environment. They conduct experiments to further our understanding of how the nervous system works. They also study the causes, treatment, and prevention of neurological diseases and disorders.

Some neuroscientists study topics such as the characteristics of the normal, aging nervous system and the characteristics of exceptionally well-functioning nervous systems, such as those of elite athletes. The graph in **Figure 6.26** provides an example of the kind of information these scientists gather and study. The graph shows the delay between the electrical stimulation of a muscle and the initiation of tension development in that muscle. This delay increases with aging, but is very short in both speed- and power-trained athletes. Neuroscientists and neurologists often collaborate on research projects—each bringing a different, specialized perspective to the work.

Becoming a neuroscientist requires a four-year bachelor's degree in an area of science, followed by a PhD in neuroscience. It typically takes four to six years to complete the PhD program. This education is often followed by an optional postdoctoral fellowship that lasts two to four years. A neuroscientist is typically employed as a university professor or research scientist. Neuroscientists working as researchers are often employed by a hospital or private company.

Planning for a Health-Related Career

Do some research on the career of a neurologist or neuroscientist. Note that both neurologists and neuroscientists may have dual careers. A neurologist, for example, may practice medicine and teach at a college or university. Likewise, a neuroscientist may teach in addition to performing research.

Alternatively, select a profession from the list of **Related Career Options**. Using the Internet or resources at your local library, find answers to the following questions:

1. What are the main tasks and responsibilities of a neurologist or neuroscientist?
2. What is the outlook for this career? Are workers in demand, or are jobs dwindling? For complete information, consult the current edition of the *Occupational Outlook Handbook*, published by the US Department of Labor. This handbook is available online or at your local library.
3. What special skills or talents are required? For example, do you enjoy research? Do you need to be good at problem solving—a skill that would be useful when developing a complicated diagnosis?

4. What personality traits do you think are necessary for success in the career you have chosen to research? For instance, neurologists must work closely with their patients. Do you enjoy working with others?
5. Does the work involve a great deal of routine, or are the day-to-day responsibilities varied?
6. Does the career require long hours, or is it a standard, "9-to-5" job?
7. What is the salary range for this job?
8. What do you think you would like about this career? Is there anything about it that you might dislike?

Related Career Options

- Neuroanatomist
- Neurochemist
- Neuroscience Nurse
- Neurosurgeon
- Pathologist
- Psychiatrist

Figure 6.26 This graph shows electrical activity (EMG) in a quadriceps muscle during tension development and the corresponding force output from the leg. Notice that the onset of electrical activity clearly precedes the onset of force production, demonstrating electromechanical delay (EMD). EMD has been found to be longer in elderly individuals and shorter in athletes, particularly those who specialize in speed and power events. Graph courtesy of Dr. Chris Knight, University of Delaware.

Chapter Summaries

Lesson 6.1 Overview of the Nervous System

⟶ Build vocabulary with e-flash cards and games

Key Points

- The structures within the nervous system are divided into two major divisions: the central nervous system and the peripheral nervous system.
- The CNS includes the brain and spinal cord.
- The PNS includes spinal nerves and cranial nerves.
- The two subdivisions of the efferent nerves are the somatic and autonomic nervous systems.
- The two types of tissue within the nervous system are neuroglia and neurons.

Key Terms

afferent nerves
autonomic nervous
    system
cell body
central nervous system
    (CNS)
dendrites
efferent nerves

myelin sheath
neurilemma
neuroglia
nodes of Ranvier
peripheral nervous
    system (PNS)
somatic nervous system
synapse

Lesson 6.2 Transmission of Nerve Impulses

Key Points

- Neurons have two main properties: irritability and conductivity.
- Stimuli bring about depolarization, which creates a nerve impulse, or action potential.
- Two major factors influence the speed at which a nerve impulse travels: the presence or absence of a myelin sheath and the diameter of the axon.
- Communication between nerve cells occurs at gap junctions; communication between neurons occurs at synapses.

Key Terms

autonomic reflexes
conductivity
depolarized
nerve impulse
polarized

reflexes
refractory period
repolarization
saltatory conduction
somatic reflexes

Lesson 6.3 Functional Anatomy of the Central Nervous System

Key Points

- The brain consists of four major anatomical regions: the cerebrum, diencephalon, brain stem, and cerebellum.
- The cerebrum consists of four main lobes: the frontal, parietal, occipital, and temporal lobes. Each controls different bodily functions.
- The meninges surround and protect the brain and spinal cord.
- The spinal cord serves as a major pathway for relaying sensory and motor impulses.

Key Terms

cerebellum
cerebrum
diencephalon
epithalamus
fissures
frontal lobes
hypothalamus
lobes
medulla oblongata
meninges

midbrain
occipital lobes
parietal lobes
pons
primary motor cortex
primary somatic sensory
    cortex
spinal cord
temporal lobes
thalamus

Lesson 6.4 Functional Anatomy of the Peripheral Nervous System

Key Points
- The structures of the PNS transmit information to the CNS.
- Twelve pairs of cranial nerves relay impulses to and from the right and left sides of the brain.
- Thirty-one pairs of spinal nerves branch out from the right and left sides of the spinal cord.
- The PNS has two subdivisions: the somatic nervous system and the autonomic nervous system.
- The sympathetic nerves activate the fight-or-flight response; the parasympathetic nerves control day-to-day functions.

Key Terms
cranial nerves
craniosacral division
dorsal ramus
endoneurium
epineurium
ganglion
norepinephrine
paravertebral ganglia

perineurium
plexuses
postganglionic neuron
preganglionic neuron
spinal nerves
thoracolumbar division
ventral ramus

Lesson 6.5 Injuries and Disorders of the Nervous System

Key Points
- The brain and spinal cord are well protected, but injuries do occur, and they can have serious consequences.
- The location of a spinal injury is a major factor in determining the extent of injury.
- Some common disorders and diseases of the CNS include meningitis, multiple sclerosis (MS), epilepsy, Parkinson's disease (PD), cerebral palsy (CP), dementia, and Alzheimer's disease.

Key Terms
Alzheimer's disease
cerebral palsy
dementia
epilepsy
meningitis

multiple sclerosis
paraplegia
Parkinson's disease
quadriplegia
traumatic brain injury

Chapter Assessments

Lesson 6.1
Overview of the Nervous System

Learning Key Terms and Concepts

1. The central nervous system (CNS) includes the _____ and the _____.
2. The peripheral nervous system (PNS) is made up of the _____ nerves and the _____ nerves.
3. Nerves that transmit impulses from sensory receptors to the CNS are known as _____.
4. Nerves that transmit impulses from the CNS to the muscles and glands are known as _____.
5. The two subdivisions of the efferent nerves are the _____ nervous system and the _____ nervous system.
6. The four types of glial cells in the CNS are _____, _____, _____, and _____.
7. The main function of an axon's myelin sheath is to _____.

Thinking Critically

8. Create a flowchart that shows the main components or structures of the nervous system and each of its subdivisions. List the functions and processes that each component controls.

Lesson 6.2
Transmission of Nerve Impulses

Learning Key Terms and Concepts

9. The two behavioral properties of a neuron are _____ and _____.
10. Because of the difference in electrical charge between the inside and outside of a resting cell, the cell membrane is said to be _____.
11. Some factors that can influence the speed of a nerve impulse are:
    A. body temperature
    B. diameter of the axon
    C. presence of a myelin sheath
    D. all of the above

12. Communication between cells occurs through direct transfer of electrical signals. The point at which this transfer occurs is called the _____.

13. A rapid, involuntary, programmed response to a stimulus is known as a(n) _____.

14. _____ reflexes send involuntary stimuli to the cardiac muscle of the heart and the smooth muscle of internal organs.

Thinking Critically

15. Recalling what you have learned about nerve impulses, how do you think each of the following substances affects conduction speeds: caffeine, sedatives, and energy drinks?

16. If a person has extremely low blood calcium levels, will that affect the transmission of electrical signals from one cell to another? Explain your answer.

Lesson 6.3

Functional Anatomy of the Central Nervous System

Learning Key Terms and Concepts

17. The adult human brain weighs approximately _____ pounds, and it contains about _____ neurons.

18. *True or False?* Recent evidence suggests that the size of a person's brain does have some relationship to intelligence.

19. Each curved, raised area of the brain is called a _____.
    A. sulcus   C. white matter
    B. gyrus   D. lobe

20. Each of the grooves between the gyri in the brain is called a(n) _____.

21. The four lobes of the brain are the _____, _____, _____, and _____.

22. The diencephalon is also called the _____.
    A. interbrain   C. left brain
    B. middle brain   D. outer brain

23. The three protective membranes that surround the brain are called the _____.

Thinking Critically

24. If one component or structure in the brain gets damaged, do you think the other structures can compensate enough for the person to function fairly normally? Explain your answer.

25. Examine the importance of the blood-brain barrier. Explain what you think would happen if this protective measure was no longer in place.

Lesson 6.4

Functional Anatomy of the Peripheral Nervous System

Learning Key Terms and Concepts

26. In a nerve, each axon fiber is covered by a fine sheath called the _____.

27. Groups of these sheathed fibers are bundled into fascicles surrounded by the _____.

28. Groups of fascicles and blood vessels are surrounded by the _____.

29. Mixed nerves carry both _____ impulses and _____ impulses.

30. The body has how many pairs of cranial nerves?

31. The body has how many pairs of spinal nerves?

32. Spinal nerves are divided into a(n) _____ ramus and a(n) _____ ramus.

33. The parasympathetic nervous system controls all of the automatic functions of the _____, _____, and _____ systems.

Thinking Critically

34. Explain what happens physiologically when the fight-or-flight response is activated in the body.

Lesson 6.5

Injuries and Disorders of the Nervous System

Learning Key Terms and Concepts

35. Name at least five symptoms of mild traumatic brain injury.

36. *True or False?* Cerebral palsy can be caused by several disorders or conditions.

37. Meningitis is inflammation of the _____ that surround the brain and spinal cord.

38. *True or False?* Multiple sclerosis (MS) is considered an autoimmune disease.

39. Alzheimer's disease is a progressive loss of brain function with consequences for _____, thinking, and _____.

Thinking Critically

40. Evaluate the cause and effect of cerebral palsy on the structure and function of cells, tissues, organs, and systems.

41. Explain the range of problems that can result from injuries to different parts of the spinal column.

42. Evaluate the cause and effect of TBI on the structure and function of cells, tissues, organs, and systems.

Building Skills and Connecting Concepts

Analyzing and Evaluating Data

The bar graph to the right shows approximate transmission speeds for several different types of nerve impulses. Use the graph to answer the following questions.

43. About how much faster do you *think* than *feel* pain?

44. Do nerve impulses signaling the sense of touch travel at approximately two, three, or four times the speed of thought impulses?

45. Assume that rising temperatures increase all the nerve impulse speeds by 5%. If the limb movement speed shown is 119 m/s (meters per second), what will it be at the higher temperature?

46. Give approximate fps (feet-per-second) speeds for each type of nerve transmission shown in the graph. (Use the conversion chart in the appendices if necessary).

Communicating about Anatomy and Physiology

47. **Speaking** Working in a group, brainstorm ideas for creating classroom tools (posters, flash cards, and/or games, for example) that will help your classmates learn and remember the different divisions and subdivisions of the nervous system. Choose the best idea(s), then delegate responsibilities to group members for constructing the tools and presenting the final products to the class.

48. **Reading** With a partner, make flash cards of the chapter terms for which phonetic spellings have been provided. On the front of the card, write the term. On the back, write the phonetic spelling as written in the text. (You may also choose to use a dictionary.) Practice reading aloud the terms, clarifying pronunciations where needed.

49. **Speaking** Pick 5–10 of the key terms that you practiced pronouncing. Write a brief scene in which those 5–10 terms are used as you imagine them being used by medical professionals in a real-life context. Then rewrite the dialogue using simpler sentences and transitions, as though an adult were describing the same scene to elementary or middle-school students. Read both scenes to the class and ask for feedback on whether the two scenes were appropriate for their different audiences.

Lab Investigations

50. Materials: large Styrofoam™ ball, scalpel or knife, markers, poster board, shower cap.
    A. Using the scalpel or knife, gently cut grooves in the Styrofoam™ ball and shape it to look like a brain.
    B. Using different colored markers, color each area of the brain: the four lobes (frontal, temporal, parietal, and occipital), the brain stem, cerebellum, and diencephalon.
    C. On a small piece of poster board, using the same colors to correspond to the different colored areas of the model brain, list the bodily functions that each lobe or area controls (some will overlap).
    D. Use the shower cap to illustrate meninges and how they protect and encase the delicate brain.

Expand your learning with additional online resources
- Supplemental Lab Activities
- Interactive Exercises
- Animations

www.g-wlearning.com/healthsciences

What do the eyes tell us?

The Sensory Systems

*W*ant to capture a picture or video? Use a camera, smartphone, or iPad™. Want to hear music from your portable music player? Use earphones.

The human eyes, ears, nose, and mouth far exceed the ability of current-day mechanical devices to capture and transmit special sensory information to the brain. The special senses, including vision, hearing, smell, and taste, involve extraordinarily well-designed sensory pathways in the nervous system. For each of these senses, highly specialized receptor cells communicate with neurons to begin the virtually instantaneous process of sending sensory messages to the brain. Once in the brain, the input from all the sensory systems is rapidly integrated and interpreted.

In this chapter, we will take a look at the anatomical structures and capabilities of the different components of the special sensory systems. In addition, we will discuss some of the common injuries and disorders of these systems, along with their symptoms and current treatments.

Chapter 7 Lessons

Lesson 7.1
The Eye

Lesson 7.2
The Ear

Lesson 7.3
Smell and Taste

While studying, look for the online icon **to:**

- **Practice** with e-flash cards and vocabulary games
- **Review** with interactive art labeling
- **Assess** with online exercises
- **Expand** with interactive activities and animated videos
- **Listen** to pronunciations of key terms in the audio glossary

www.g-wlearning.com/healthsciences

Study on the Go

Use a mobile device to practice vocabulary terms, listen to pronunciations, and review with self-assessment quizzes.

www.m.g-wlearning.com

Before You Read

Try to answer the following questions before you read this lesson.

What enables us to see colors?

What causes near- and farsightedness?

Lesson Objectives

1. Describe the external and internal anatomical structures of the human eye.

2. Explain how the sphincter pupillae and the dilator pupillae muscles work together to control the amount of light that is admitted to the eye.

3. Identify the anatomical structures associated with the retina and explain how they work together to produce vision.

4. Define *myopia*, *hyperopia*, and *presbyopia* and briefly explain what causes each of these common eye disorders.

5. Define *color blindness* and explain why it occurs more often in men than in women.

Key Terms

E-Flash Cards

aqueous and vitreous
  humors
choroid
ciliary body
ciliary glands
cones
conjunctiva
cornea
extrinsic muscles
iris
lacrimal glands

lens
optic chiasma
optic nerve
optic tracts
pupil
retina
rods
sclera
suspensory ligaments
tarsal glands

According to an old English proverb, "The eyes are the windows to the soul." Whether or not this is true, some people do indeed have expressive eyes that help to convey their emotional states. Eyes "twinkling with amusement" or "flashing with anger" are familiar descriptive phrases. A person can also be described as bright-eyed, dark-eyed, shifty-eyed, or eagle-eyed, all of which suggest distinctive images or characteristics.

The eyes obviously are important parts of our anatomy, with vision being an extremely useful sense. In this lesson we will describe the anatomical components of the eye and learn how they function together to produce the remarkable ability to see.

Anatomy of the Eye

The adult eye, sometimes referred to as the "eyeball," is about 2.5 cm (1 inch) in diameter and has a spherical shape. A variety of external structures serve to protect the eye, and specialized internal structures send sensory signals to the brain, enabling vision.

External Structures

The eye is a delicate structure and, fortunately, is well protected. The eye is encased in the bony, orbital socket of the skull and covered by an eyelid. The eyebrows also function as shields—for example, by protecting the eyes from dripping sweat on a hot day. The eyelashes provide considerable protection from circulating dust particles.

Several structures work together to lubricate the eyes (**Figure 7.1**). **Tarsal** (TAR-sal) **glands** in the eyelids produce an oily secretion, and modified sweat glands, called **ciliary** (SIL-ee-AIR-ee)

A.   Anterior view   **B.   Lateral view**

Figure 7.1 Lubricating structures of the eye. A—Anterior view. B—Lateral view. *Some of the structures identified in these drawings serve a function other than lubrication. What are these structures and what is their primary purpose?*

glands, are located between the eyelashes. The **conjunctiva** (KAHN-junk-TIGH-va), a delicate external membrane that covers the exposed eyeball and lines the eyelid, also secretes a lubricating mucus.

The **lacrimal** (LAK-ri-mal) **glands** above the lateral end of each eye continually release the familiar, salty solution known as tears through *excretory ducts*. Because tears contain antibodies and an enzyme called *lysozyme* that attacks bacteria, they not only lubricate the surface of the eye but also keep it clean.

Tears are flushed into tiny canals called *lacrimal canaliculi* in the medial corner of each eye. These canaliculi then drain into the *nasolacrimal* (NAY-zoh-LAK-ri-mal) *duct*, which empties into the nasal cavity.

Irritation to the eye produces extra tearing, which helps to wash away foreign substances. Under stressful conditions, tears may be produced at such a high rate that they cannot be drained away fast enough and spill over onto the cheeks.

Six **extrinsic muscles** attach to the outer surface of the eye and are responsible for moving the eye within the orbital socket (**Figure 7.2**). The specific functions of these muscles are listed in the table in **Figure 7.3** on the next page.

> **Check Your Understanding**
>
> 1. What do tarsal glands produce?
> 2. What are the two functions of tears?
> 3. Describe two different ways by which tears clean the eyes.

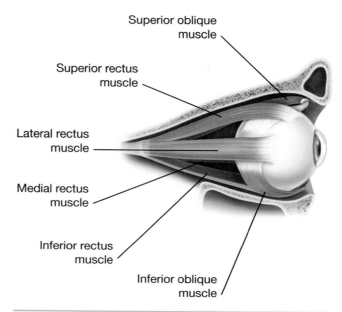

Figure 7.2 Lateral view of the extrinsic muscles of the eye.

Figure 7.3 The Extrinsic Eye Muscles

Muscle	Action
superior rectus	upward eye motion
inferior rectus	downward eye motion
lateral rectus	lateral eye motion
medial rectus	medial eye motion
superior oblique	downward and lateral eye motion
inferior oblique	upward and lateral eye motion

Internal Structures

The eyeball is a hollow chamber, somewhat oblong in shape, filled with fluids called **aqueous** (AY-kwee-us) and **vitreous** (VIT-ree-us) **humors**. These fluids help the eyeball to maintain its shape (**Figure 7.4**).

Three layers of tissue form the walls of the eyeball. The tough, fibrous **sclera** makes up the outer layer of the eye. The sclera includes the "white of the eye" as well as the transparent **cornea** over the anterior center of the eye. The cornea is called the "window of the eye" because light passes through it. The cornea has no blood supply and, therefore, is the one body tissue that can be transplanted from one person to another with no concern for rejection.

The middle layer of the eye, called the **choroid** (KOR-oyd), contains a rich supply of blood vessels that provide nourishment to the eye (**Figure 7.4**). These blood vessels

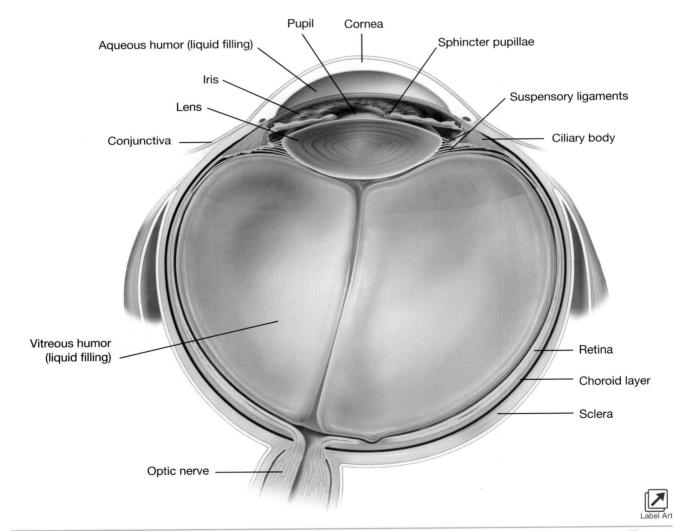

Figure 7.4 Internal structures of the eye. *How would our vision be affected if the iris lacked sphincter pupillae and dilator pupillae muscles to control the amount of light admitted to the eye?*

contribute to a crimson-purple pigmentation that darkens the interior of the eye, preventing light reflections. Anteriorly, the choroid also includes the **iris**, which gives the eye its color. The iris can widen or narrow to control the size of the **pupil**, the opening through which light passes into the interior of the eye.

Two sets of muscles within the iris work to control the amount of light admitted to the eye. The *sphincter pupillae* (pyoo-PIL-ay) contracts in the presence of bright light or when the eye focuses on an object within close range, causing the pupil to grow smaller. In the presence of dim light or when the eye focuses on a distant object, the *dilator pupillae* muscle contracts, causing dilation (enlargement) of the pupil.

The innermost layer of the eye, the **retina**, is located only around the posterior portion of the eye, anterior to the choroid (**Figure 7.4**). The retina is dense in specialized, light-sensitive nerve endings. These nerve endings send impulses through the optic nerve to the occipital lobe of the brain, where visual images are interpreted.

The sensory cells in the retina are called **rods** and **cones** (**Figure 7.5**). The rods are activated in dim light; the cones are sensitive to bright light and also provide color vision. As **Figure 7.5** shows, nerve ganglions (GAYNG-glee-ahnz) and bipolar neurons (discussed in chapter 6) provide connections between the retina and the rods and cones.

You may have heard of the "blind spot" on the retina. The physiological blind spot on each retina is called the *optic disc*. The optic disc is the junction between the optic nerve and the eye. Because there are no rods and cones in the optic disc, this tiny area is unable to transmit visual information—hence the term *blind spot*.

Under normal circumstances, we do not perceive the blind spot because the brain fills in the visual information from the other eye. Given the separation between the two eyes, the blind spots are missing different pieces of the combined visual field.

The **lens** of the eye is located behind the iris. It is a transparent, flexible, crystal-like structure curved outward on both sides (**Figure 7.4**). The lens is held in place by tiny **suspensory ligaments**

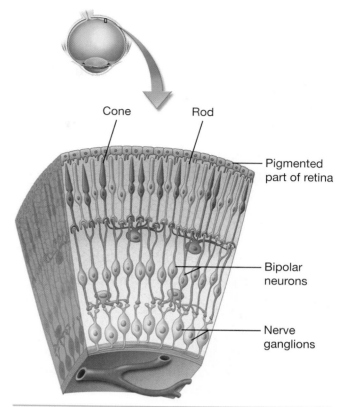

Figure 7.5 Rods and cones in the retina. *Which types of cells—cones or rods—are activated in dim light?*

that surround it. The ligaments attach to the **ciliary body**, which merges with the choroid layer.

When at rest, the eye is focused for distance vision. For the eye to clearly view objects closer than about 20 feet, the muscles of the ciliary body contract to change the shape of the lens. This process of contraction, known as *accommodation*, makes the lens thicker, enabling it to focus incoming light rays on the surface of the retina.

After about 40 years of age, the ability of the ciliary body muscles to appropriately contract diminishes. In the absence of other visual corrections, this causes people in the post-40 age group to need reading glasses for up-close vision.

 Check Your Understanding

1. Explain the purpose of aqueous and vitreous humors.
2. Name the three layers of the eye.
3. Which nerve is responsible for transmitting sensory signals to the brain?

Vision

You see an object when the light that is reflected from that object passes through your cornea, pupil, and lens to your retina. The rods and cones in the retina are stimulated and pass impulses to the **optic nerve**, which transmits sensory signals to the brain.

The optic nerves from the eyes cross at the **optic chiasma** (kigh-AZ-ma). The nerve fibers exiting the optic chiasma are called **optic tracts**. The optic tracts carry visual stimuli to the occipital lobe of the brain.

Injuries, Diseases, and Disorders of the Eye

Now that we understand the anatomy of the eye, we will take a look at some common injuries, disorders, and diseases that can affect the ways in which the eye functions.

Eye Injuries

The structure of the face and eyes helps protect the eyes from injury. The bony socket in which the eyeball is encased, the eyelid, the eyebrows, and the eyelashes all provide a barrier to foreign objects. In fact, these features are so effective in protecting the eye that many eye injuries do not affect the eyeball itself but, rather, the surrounding tissues and structures. Still, certain injuries can damage the eyeball, causing impairment or loss of vision.

Usually, minor irritants are flushed from the eye through tear production. Irritating chemicals, however, should be flushed with large quantities of water. Fragments of glass or other solid particles that become lodged in the eye should be removed only by a medical professional.

The cornea is well supplied with pain and touch receptors. Consequently, corneal injuries (abrasions or tears) are extremely painful. Fortunately, however, the cornea has an astonishing ability to self-repair; most injuries resolve themselves within 24 hours.

Trauma to the eye can cause a *detached retina*, in which the retina separates from the underlying support tissue. The detachment may be partial in the beginning, but without treatment it can rapidly progress to complete detachment. The associated vision loss can progress from minor to severe and even to blindness within a few hours or days.

Surgical techniques using lasers, air bubbles, or a freezing probe can be used to reattach the retina. In most cases, surgery can restore good vision. If unrepaired, a detached retina can cause loss of peripheral vision and, subsequently, loss of central vision.

Vision Disorders

A variety of relatively minor, common eye defects can impair vision. Many of these defects can be completely corrected with prescription lenses (**Figure 7.6**).

Myopia (Nearsightedness). Commonly known as nearsightedness, *myopia* (migh-OH-pee-a) results from an elongated eyeball shape, which causes the lens to focus objects in front of the retina rather than directly upon it (**Figure 7.7B**). Nearby objects can be seen clearly, but distant objects appear blurry.

The classic Snellen chart is used to diagnose myopia. This familiar chart includes rows of letters, with each successive row smaller than the one above. The Snellen chart and those similar

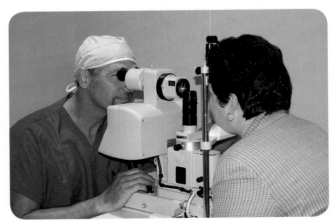

SandiMako/Shutterstock.com

Figure 7.6 Have your eyes examined on a regular basis and as soon as possible if you experience any of the problems discussed in this lesson. Note that several problems can be remedied if treated early but can be very damaging if left untreated.

A. **Normal vision:**
light rays focus on the retina

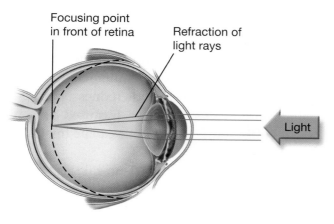

B. **Myopia (nearsightedness):**
light rays focus in front of the retina

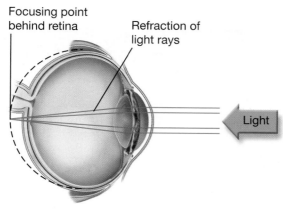

C. **Hyperopia (farsightedness):**
light rays focus beyond the retina

Animation

Figure 7.7 Common vision disorders. *If light rays focus on a point in front of your retina, do you have trouble seeing objects close to you or far away?*

Memory Tip

You may have heard middle-aged individuals joke that they are "getting old" because they need reading glasses. The word *presbyopia* comes from *presby-*, a combining form meaning "old," and *-opia*, a root word that means "the condition of having such a visual defect." The term was adopted in the late eighteenth century, when people in their forties were considered old!

The root *-opia* is used in conjunction with other combining forms to describe various eye disorders (*myopia, hyperopia,* and *amblyopia,* for example).

---

to it are used only as a first step in diagnosing myopia. Medical eye specialists perform a number of tests before they prescribe corrective lenses for visual defects. Laser surgery techniques also can be performed to correct myopia.

Hyperopia (Farsightedness). In the opposite condition, *hyperopia* (HIGH-per-OH-pee-a), also known as farsightedness, the distance from the lens to the retina is shortened because the shape of the eyeball is more flattened (**Figure 7.7C**). Light rays focus behind the retina instead of directly upon it. As a result, objects at a distance can be seen clearly, but objects close up appear blurry. Prescription lenses can correct this condition.

Presbyopia (Age-Related Farsightedness). Presbyopia (PREZ-bee-OH-pee-a) is an age-related version of farsightedness. Onset of presbyopia commonly occurs between 40 and 45 years of age because of changes that stiffen and discolor the lens of the eye. Presbyopia causes blurring of up-close vision that impedes the ability to read printed material or text on a computer screen.

Astigmatism. Irregular curvature of the cornea or lens causes *astigmatism* (a-STIG-ma-tizm), another common eye disorder. The result is blurred vision. Depending on the nature and extent of the curvature, vision may be proportionally affected. Corrective lenses can partially or completely correct astigmatism.

Amblyopia ("Lazy Eye"). *Amblyopia* (AM-blee-OH-pee-a), or "lazy eye," usually appears during childhood when one eye is extremely dominant and the other eye—the lazy eye—develops poor vision. If uncorrected, the lazy eye can become blind. Treatment generally consists of covering the "good" eye, requiring the extrinsic muscles of the lazy eye to function.

Diplopia (Double Vision). *Diplopia* (di-PLOH-pee-a), or double vision, results when one eye is misaligned, causing two images of the object to be perceived simultaneously. Treatment may involve wearing a temporary patch over the affected eye, corrective lenses, or surgery.

Strabismus ("Crossed Eyes"). A person with *strabismus* (strah-BIZ-mus) has an eye that drifts in different directions due to malfunctioning of the extrinsic muscles of that eye. The condition is treated with eye exercises, corrective lenses, or surgery.

Color Blindness. *Color blindness* affects the cone cells on the retina, impairing an individual's ability to distinguish colors. Red-green color blindness, the inability to distinguish red from green, is a common form of this disorder.

Color blindness is an inherited condition. For a son to be color blind, he needs to inherit the gene for color blindness only from his mother. By contrast, for a daughter to be color blind, she must inherit the gene from both parents. This explains why men have a higher incidence of colorblindness compared to women.

Night Blindness. With *night blindness*, the rods in the retina do not function optimally, making it difficult for a person to see well at night. Night blindness is associated with aging.

The table in **Figure 7.8** summarizes the characteristics of common eye disorders.

 Check Your Understanding

1. What is another name for nearsightedness?
2. What chart is used to check for myopia?
3. Presbyopia usually affects people in what age group? Explain.

Eye Diseases

Many diseases can affect the eye. We will briefly examine some of the more common eye diseases that require professional care.

Conjunctivitis. Commonly known as "pinkeye," *conjunctivitis* (kahn-JUNK-ti-VIGH-tis) is a highly contagious inflammation of the conjunctiva. Symptoms include redness, pain, swelling, and mucus discharge. If caused by a bacterial infection, conjunctivitis can be treated with antibiotics.

Cataracts. A cataract (KAT-uh-rakt) is the development of a progressive clouding of the transparent lens of the eye, causing obstruction of light. The result is blurred vision, poor night vision, yellowing of colors, and "halos" around lights. *Cataracts* are associated with aging and frequently occur in people older than 70 years of

Figure 7.8 Common Eye Disorders and Their Characteristics

Condition	Description	Cause
myopia	nearsightedness	elongated eyeball
hyperopia	farsightedness	shortened eyeball
presbyopia	age-related farsightedness	stiffness of the lens
astigmatism	blurred vision	irregular curvature of cornea or lens
amblyopia	lazy eye	abnormal dominance of one eye
diplopia	double vision	abnormal alignment of the eyes
strabismus	crossed eyes	muscles in one eye do not coordinate with those in the other eye
color blindness	inability to distinguish colors	disorder of the cone cells in the retina
night blindness	difficulty seeing at night	disorder of the rod cells in the retina

age. Exposure to bright sunlight can speed the development of cataracts. Cataracts are treated with laser surgery.

Glaucoma. *Glaucoma* (glaw-KOH-ma) is a condition of increased pressure within the eyeball caused either by overproduction of aqueous humor or blockage of normal aqueous humor drainage. The onset of symptoms is gradual and includes aching eyes, poor vision in dim light progressing to blurred vision, and the appearance of halos around lights.

As the condition progresses, tunnel vision—or loss of peripheral vision—occurs, and blindness eventually follows. Untreated glaucoma is a common cause of blindness. Glaucoma occurs in about 20 percent of adults older than 40 years of age. Early detection is a must! Glaucoma can be readily treated with medication or surgery.

Macular Degeneration. A progressive loss of central vision, the hallmark symptom of *macular* (MAK-yoo-lar) *degeneration,* occurs in about 10 percent of elderly people. Peripheral vision, however, remains unaffected. There are two types of macular degeneration: dry and wet.

Dry macular degeneration is caused by progressive thinning of the retina. Although no treatment currently exists, most individuals with this condition do not completely lose their eyesight and are able to function with vision aids. *Wet macular degeneration* involves leakage of small blood vessels within the eye. Some individuals with this condition respond favorably to medication or laser surgery (**Figure 7.9**).

Diabetic Retinopathy. Damage to the retina caused by long-term diabetes is called *diabetic retinopathy* (REHT-i-NAHP-a-thee). This condition is becoming increasingly prevalent and is currently the leading cause of blindness in American adults. Diabetic retinopathy involves swelling and leaking of the vessels that supply blood to the retina.

When diabetic retinopathy is sufficiently advanced, bleeding occurs, causing the individual to see red spots. Laser surgery typically is effective in treating the condition when it is caught early enough.

Monkey Business Images/Shutterstock.com

Figure 7.9 Eye disorders and diseases such as detached retinas, myopia, cataracts, and macular degeneration can be treated successfully with laser surgery.

Vitreous Floaters. *Vitreous floaters* are small, irregularly shaped specks that drift around within your field of vision. Floaters form when tiny chunks of the gel-like vitreous humor break off and float in the aqueous humor in the center of the eyeball.

Although sometimes distracting, ordinary eye floaters are common and normally not a cause for alarm. However, the sudden appearance of multiple floaters accompanied by what appear to be flashes of light on the lateral periphery of the eye can be symptoms of a retinal tear or retinal detachment. In such cases, immediate medical attention is required.

 Check Your Understanding

1. Which disease of the eye is highly contagious?
2. What are the signs and symptoms of cataracts?
3. Distinguish between dry macular degeneration and wet macular degeneration.

Lesson 7.1 Review and Assessment

Mini Glossary   Make sure that you know the meaning of each key term.

 Build vocabulary with e-flash cards and games

aqueous and vitreous humors   the watery fluid that fills the anterior and posterior chambers of the eye

choroid   the middle layer of the wall of the eye

ciliary body   the structure between the choroid and the iris that anchors the lens in place

ciliary glands   modified sweat glands located between the eyelashes

cones   sensory cells in the retina that are sensitive to bright light and provide color vision

conjunctiva   a delicate external membrane that covers the exposed eyeball and lines the eyelid

cornea   a transparent tissue over the anterior center of the eye

extrinsic muscles   muscles attached to the outer surface of the eye that are responsible for changing the direction of viewing

iris   the anterior portion of the choroid, which gives the eye its color

lacrimal glands   tear secretors; located above the lateral end of each eye

lens   a transparent, flexible structure that is curved outward on both sides

optic chiasma   the point at which the optic nerves cross

optic nerve   transmitter of visual sensory signals to the occipital lobe of the brain

optic tracts   the continuation of the optic nerve fibers beyond the optic chiasma

pupil   the opening through which light rays enter the eye

retina   the innermost layer of the eye, containing light-sensitive nerve endings that send impulses through the optic nerves to the brain

rods   sensory cells in the retina that are activated in dim light

sclera   the tough, fibrous outer layer of the eye

suspensory ligaments   tiny structures that attach the lens of the eye to the ciliary body

tarsal glands   secretors of an oily substance; located in the eyelids

Know and Understand

 Assess

1. What part of the eye is called the "window of the eye?"

2. Rods and cones are located in which layer of the eye?

3. Describe the pathway of vision.

4. Where are the extrinsic muscles and what is their purpose?

5. List the anatomical features that protect the eye from injury.

6. Which glands produce the salty solution known as *tears*?

7. What part of the eye has many pain receptors and is able to repair itself quickly?

Analyze and Apply

8. Compare and contrast myopia, hyperopia, and presbyopia.

9. Derrick has had to do a lot of reading in college. He never had a problem with his vision in the past, but lately he has had trouble reading the print in his textbook. When he noticed that he was holding his book farther and farther away from his eyes, he decided to see an ophthalmologist. What do you think the doctor told Derrick? Which injury, disorder, or disease that you read about in this chapter was the diagnosis? What treatment do you think the doctor prescribed?

In the Lab

10. Make a KWL chart like the one below. Fill in the chart, listing what you know about accommodation, what you want to know, and, after doing the demonstration below, what you learned.

Demonstration: Close one eye and stare at a point about 20 feet away. The point at which you are staring should be in focus. While concentrating on the point, raise one of your fingers into your line of sight just below the point. Your finger should be a bit blurred. Now, change focus—look at the tip of your finger instead of the point 20 feet away. Your finger will come into focus, but the distant point will be blurred.

K	W	L
What I **K**now	What I **W**ant to Know	What I **L**earned

The Ear

Before You Read

Try to answer the following questions before you read this lesson.

Why do we have earwax?

How does yawning wide while descending from a height help to equalize pressure in the ears?

Lesson Objectives

1. Describe the major anatomical structures of the outer ear, the middle ear, and the inner ear.

2. Explain the process by which hearing occurs, from the transmission of sound waves to the perception and interpretation of sound.

3. Explain the role of the inner ear in helping your body to maintain equilibrium, or balance.

4. Describe some common causes of deafness.

5. Describe some common ear infections.

Key Terms

E-Flash Cards

anvil	membranous labyrinth
auditory canal	organ of Corti
auricle	ossicles
bony labyrinth	oval window
ceruminous glands	perilymph
cochlea	semicircular canals
cochlear duct	stirrup
endolymph	tympanic membrane
Eustachian tube	vestibule
hammer	vestibulocochlear nerve

Just as vision is a highly useful sense, so is the sense of hearing. Our ears are remarkable in their ability to capture, amplify, and transmit sounds of varying loudness and pitch (high versus low tones) to the brain. Our ears also serve another important function, however. They play a central role in our ability to maintain physical balance or even to recognize which direction is up.

In this lesson, we will examine the anatomy and inner workings of the ear to learn how the functions of hearing and balance are carried out.

Anatomy of the Ear

The ear includes three anatomical regions—the external (outer) ear, the middle ear (tympanic cavity), and the internal (inner) ear. The external and middle ear contribute to our ability to hear. The internal ear plays roles in both hearing and equilibrium (balance).

External (Outer) Ear

The irregularly shaped, outer portion of the ear is called the **auricle** (AW-ri-kuhl), or *pinna*. In many animal species, the outer ear serves to channel sound waves into the ear, but in the human species this function is minimal. As **Figure 7.10** on the next page shows, the auricle connects with the **auditory canal,** also known as the *external acoustic meatus*.

The auditory canal is a short, tubelike structure about one inch long and one-quarter inch in diameter. The walls of this canal are lined with skin that contains **ceruminous** (seh-ROO-mi-nus) **glands**. The ceruminous glands secrete *cerumen*, also known as *earwax*. Earwax helps to clean, lubricate, and protect the ear.

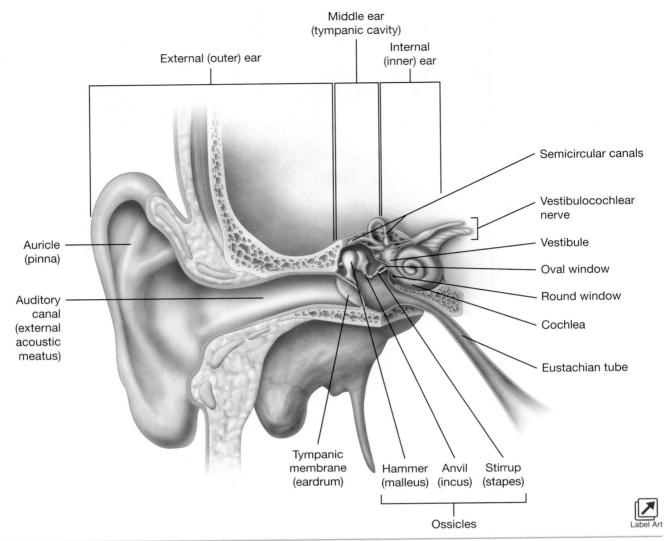

Middle ear
(tympanic cavity)

External (outer) ear

Internal
(inner) ear

Semicircular canals

Vestibulocochlear
nerve

Auricle
(pinna)

Vestibule

Oval window

Auditory
canal
(external
acoustic
meatus)

Round window

Cochlea

Eustachian tube

Tympanic
membrane
(eardrum)

Hammer   Anvil   Stirrup
(malleus) (incus) (stapes)

Ossicles

Label Art

Figure 7.10 Anatomy of the ear. *Which structure separates the outer ear from the middle ear?*

At the end of the auditory canal is the **tympanic** (tim-PAN-ik) **membrane**, commonly known as the *eardrum*. Sound waves entering the ear cause the tympanic membrane to vibrate. The eardrum also separates the outer ear from the middle ear.

Middle Ear (Tympanic Cavity)

The middle ear, or *tympanic cavity*, is a small, open chamber in the temporal lobe of the skull (**Figure 7.10**). The tympanic membrane is on the lateral side of the cavity. On the medial side is bone with a membrane-covered opening known as the **oval window**. Beneath the oval window is a *round window*.

Inside the tympanic cavity lie the three smallest bones in the body, known as **ossicles** (AHS-i-kuhls). The ossicles are named for their shapes—the **hammer**, or *malleus*; the **anvil**, or *incus*; and the **stirrup**, or *stapes*. Together, these bones connect the tympanic membrane to the membrane of the oval window. The hammer attaches to the tympanic membrane, the anvil attaches to the hammer, and the stirrup attaches to the anvil on one side and to the oval window on the other. Because of their mechanical arrangement, the ossicles not only transmit, but also amplify, sound waves.

The **Eustachian** (yoo-STAY-shuhn) **tube** connects the middle ear to the pharynx

(**Figure 7.10**). The pharynx is the part of the throat that connects the mouth and nasal cavity to the esophagus (the digestive tube between the throat and stomach). The Eustachian tube serves to equalize pressure on either side of the tympanic membrane. Yawning widely is a way to help bring pressure in the pharynx, Eustachian tube, and middle ear to the same level as pressure outside the ear. This is a good strategy to use when air (barometric) pressure changes rapidly, such as during an airplane descent or while driving down a mountain road.

Internal (Inner) Ear

The oval window connects the middle ear with the inner ear. The inner ear structures reside in a hollow tunnel that winds and twists like a bowl of interconnected spaghetti noodles. **Figure 7.11** shows a representation of these winding tunnels, known as the **bony labyrinth**. As this figure indicates, the three components of the inner ear are the **cochlea** (KAHK-lee-a), **vestibule** (VEHS-ti-byool), and **semicircular** (SEHM-ee-SIR-kyoo-lar) **canals**.

As **Figure 7.11** illustrates, the cochlear (KAHK-lee-ar) nerve and vestibular (vehs-TIB-yoo-lar) nerve transmit sensory information from the cochlea and vestibule, respectively. The cochlear nerve carries information about hearing,

and the vestibular nerve carries information about balance. These two nerves join to form a single cranial nerve, the **vestibulocochlear** (vehs-TIB-yoo-loh-KAHK-lee-ar) **nerve**.

The bony labyrinth is filled with a clear fluid called **perilymph** (PER-i-limf). Inside the bony labyrinth are membrane-covered tubes called the **membranous** (MEHM-bray-nus) **labyrinth**, which follow the course of the bony labyrinth. Inside the membranous labyrinth is a thicker fluid called **endolymph** (EHN-doh-limf).

Functions of the Ear

You know that the function of your ears is to detect sounds in your environment. But did you know that your ears also help your body to maintain its balance, or equilibrium? In this section, we will discuss these two important functions of the ear.

Hearing

When sound waves enter the ear, they are transmitted through the auditory canal, causing the tympanic membrane to vibrate. This motion stimulates the hammer, anvil, and stirrup to amplify and transmit these vibrations to the membrane of the oval window. This process of amplification and transmission sets in motion the fluids of the inner ear.

Our ability to hear resides within the snail-shaped cochlea of the inner ear. The portion of the membranous labyrinth inside the cochlea is called the **cochlear duct**. Within the cochlear duct is the spiral-shaped **organ of Corti**, which contains hearing receptors called *hair cells* (**Figure 7.12** on the next page). The short, stiff hair cells are stimulated by high-pitched sounds; the longer, more flexible hair cells are stimulated by low-pitched sounds.

Motion of the endolymph in the cochlear duct causes the *tectorial membrane* to move. As **Figure 7.12** shows, movement of the tectorial membrane stimulates the hair cells, which in turn stimulate the cochlear branch of the vestibulocochlear nerve. The cochlear nerve then transmits electrical impulses to the auditory region of the brain in the temporal lobe.

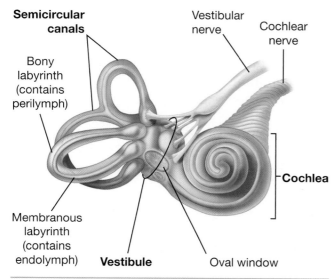

Semicircular canals

Vestibular nerve

Cochlear nerve

Bony labyrinth (contains perilymph)

Membranous labyrinth (contains endolymph)

Vestibule

Oval window

Cochlea

Figure 7.11 Structures of the inner ear. *What role, if any, do you think the inner ear plays in the development of a phobia such as a fear of heights?*

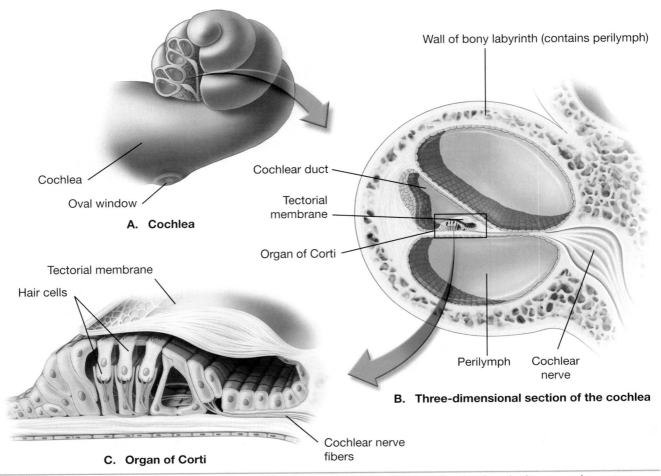

Wall of bony labyrinth (contains perilymph)

Cochlea

Oval window

A. Cochlea

Cochlear duct

Tectorial membrane

Organ of Corti

Tectorial membrane

Hair cells

Perilymph   Cochlear nerve

B.   Three-dimensional section of the cochlea

Cochlear nerve fibers

C.   Organ of Corti

Figure 7.12 Anatomy of the cochlea. *What role do different kinds of hair cells play in relaying sound messages to the brain?*

Equilibrium (Balance)

We tend to take our *equilibrium*, or ability to balance, for granted. Only when we are dizzy or disoriented do we typically even appreciate balance. The ability to balance comes from specialized structures in the inner ear.

The vestibule of the inner ear contains three semicircular canals (**Figure 7.11**). The hair cells in the semicircular canals are stimulated by movement of the endolymph in the canals, much like the hair cells in the organ of Corti are stimulated by motion of the endolymph to produce hearing. These hair cells, however, stimulate the vestibular nerve, which communicates with the cerebellum to provide information about the orientation and motion of the head. The semicircular canals play an important role in balance when a person is both stationary and moving.

Check Your Understanding

1. What are the two functions of the ear?
2. What is the function of cerumen?
3. List the ossicles and tell why they are important.
4. What is the significance of the Eustachian tube?
5. Which structure in the inner ear controls equilibrium?

Disorders and Infections of the Ear

A variety of conditions can affect hearing or balance. This section addresses some of the most common disorders and infections of the ear.

WHAT RESEARCH TELLS US

...*about* Tone-Deafness

You may have noticed that some people have difficulty singing in key with music. It is typically said of such people that they cannot "carry a tune."

A person who sings off-key has *amusia* (uh-MYOO-zee-uh). Amusia is characterized by the inability to distinguish differences in pitch (that is, how high or low a tone is) as well as the inability to remember melodies. Amusia is present in about 3% of people from birth, but it can also result from a brain injury.

Researchers studying this condition have tried to train amusic children to develop the ability to better hear and reproduce musical tones. One method used by the researchers consists of having the children repeatedly listen to popular music for one month. This training, however, has had no apparent effect. Studies of brain activity in amusic individuals indicate that this difficulty in processing musical tones is caused by poor neural connections between the auditory center in the brain and the other related areas of the brain.

Taking It Further

1. Can you carry a tune? Sing a favorite song to friends or relatives, then listen to them as they sing. Compare the results.

2. Do some research on the causes of and treatments for amusia. Share your findings with the class.

Deafness

Deafness is the term applied to any loss of hearing, ranging from a slight to a complete inability to hear. Injuries that affect the structures of the middle or inner ear can cause deafness. Regular exposure to extremely loud sounds such as construction noise or loud music can damage the hair receptor cells in the organ of Corti, leading to hearing loss. Other causes of deafness include excessive earwax, scarring of the tympanic membrane following inflammation, and damage to the auditory nerve or auditory region of the brain.

Presbycusis (PREHZ-bee-KYOO-sis) is the term for age-related hearing loss. Presbycusis usually can be improved through the use of hearing aids.

Hearing aids amplify and change sounds so that the wearer can better hear the sounds. Some hearing aids amplify all sounds; others specifically boost low- or high-frequency sounds.

Hearing aids are available in a variety of styles and sizes (**Figure 7.13**), and price ranges vary considerably. This is why you would want to carefully analyze all information (from healthcare workers and promotional materials) before making inferences about the best products and services for you or the person you are helping with the purchase.

"In-the-canal" hearing aids are custom-molded to fit inside the auditory canal. This type of hearing aid is recommended for mild to moderate hearing loss.

"Half-shell" hearing aids are custom-fit to sit inside the small, inner bowl-shaped area of the outer ear. These hearing aids are recommended for mild to moderately severe hearing loss. Somewhat larger hearing aids, called "in-the-ear" aids, are custom-designed to fill most of the bowl of the outer ear. This type of hearing aid is recommended for mild to severe hearing loss.

Finally, "behind-the-ear" hearing aids, designed to "ride" behind the ear, are capable of greater amplification than the other types of hearing aids. This model, which transmits amplified sound to a molded piece inside the auditory canal, is appropriate for most types of hearing loss.

Tinnitus

Tinnitus (TIN-i-tus) is a condition that causes a sound like ringing to be heard in the ear. Tinnitus occurs when the hair cells in the organ of Corti that stimulate the auditory nerve are damaged. Normal movement of the hair cells is triggered by sound waves. When the hair cells have been damaged, however, they sometimes move randomly, generating the ringing sound.

A.   **B.**

Figure 7.13 Hearing aid models. A—"Behind-the-ear" model. B—"In-the-canal" model.

What damages these hair cells? The most common culprit is repeated exposure to loud noise, such as loud music. Tinnitus is a common and growing problem. According to the American Tinnitus Association, some 50 million people in the US suffer from the disorder.

External Otitis (Swimmer's Ear)

Have you ever gone swimming in a lake and then later developed an earache? You might have had *swimmer's ear*, formally known as *external otitis* (oh-TIGH-tis). This bacterial or fungal infection of the auditory canal is caused by immersion in contaminated water. Symptoms may include pain, fever, and, in extreme cases, temporary hearing loss.

Swimmer's ear can be prevented by thoroughly cleaning and drying the ear canal with an alcohol-based solution after swimming, or by avoiding immersion of the ears.

Otitis Media (Middle Ear Infection)

Otitis media is an infection of the middle ear caused by bacteria or a virus. It is usually associated with an upper respiratory tract infection. Otitis media is relatively common in infants and toddlers because their Eustachian tubes are not yet fully developed. Symptoms of a middle ear infection may include pain, swelling, and production of pus.

A mild to moderate middle ear infection caused by bacteria is treated with antibiotics. More serious bacterial infections that do not respond well to antibiotics are frequently treated by a surgical procedure. During the surgery, tiny tubes are inserted into the tympanic membrane. These small tubes alleviate the elevated pressure in the inner ear.

Viral infections do not respond to antibiotics but often improve with time.

 Check Your Understanding

1. List the causes of deafness.
2. Define presbycusis.
3. The condition that causes ringing in the ears is called _____.
4. Why are infants and toddlers prone to otitis media?

Labyrinthitis (Inner Ear Infection)

Labyrinthitis (LAB-uh-rin-THIGH-tis) is an infection of the inner ear that produces inflammation (swelling). This condition affects the semicircular canals in particular and can disrupt their normal function, causing severe dizziness (*vertigo*) and even nausea and vomiting. Individuals with vertigo are unable to stand because their sense of orientation is severely compromised. Chronic inflammation of the semicircular canals of the inner ear is called *Ménière's disease*. This disease causes periodic but severe vertigo as well as progressive hearing loss.

An ear infection that causes vertigo is treated with antibiotics, if the infection is bacterial. If the ear infection is viral, certain medications may be prescribed to ease the discomfort caused by vertigo.

Lesson 7.2 Review and Assessment

Mini Glossary
Make sure that you know the meaning of each key term.

 Build vocabulary with e-flash cards and games

anvil tiny bone within the middle ear that transmits sound from the hammer to the stirrup

auditory canal a short, tubelike structure that connects the outer ear to the eardrum

auricle the irregularly shaped outer portion of the ear

bony labyrinth winding tunnels located in the inner ear

ceruminous glands secretors of cerumen, or earwax; located in the auditory canal

cochlea a snail-shaped structure in the inner ear that enables one to hear

cochlear duct the portion of the membranous labyrinth inside the cochlea

endolymph a thick fluid inside the membranous labyrinth

Eustachian tube a channel that connects the middle ear to the pharynx and serves to equalize pressure on either side of the tympanic membrane

hammer tiny bone in the middle ear that transmits sound from the tympanic membrane (eardrum) to the anvil

membranous labyrinth membrane-covered tubes inside the bony labyrinth

organ of Corti a spiral-shaped ridge of epithelium in the cochlear duct lined with hair cells that serve as hearing receptors

ossicles the body's three smallest bones—the hammer, anvil, and stirrup; found in the middle ear

oval window a membrane-covered opening that connects the middle ear to the inner ear

perilymph a clear fluid that fills the bony labyrinth

semicircular canals inner ear channels containing receptor hair cells that play an important role in balance

stirrup tiny bone in the middle ear that attaches to the anvil on one side and the oval window on the other

tympanic membrane a sheet of tissue at the end of the auditory canal; also known as the eardrum

vestibule a chamber in the inner ear that contains the three semicircular canals

vestibulocochlear nerve a cranial nerve comprising the cochlear nerve and the vestibular nerve

Know and Understand
 Assess

1. What are the three anatomical regions of the ear?
2. Name the two terms used to describe the outer portion of the ear.
3. Where are the ceruminous glands located?
4. The Eustachian tube connects _____ to the _____.
5. Define equilibrium.
6. Which part of the brain controls equilibrium?
7. Compare and contrast the function of the short, stiff hairs in the organ of Corti with that of its long, flexible hairs.
8. Describe the pathway of hearing.
9. What is the main function of the semicircular canals?

Analyze and Apply

10. Explain in detail the relationship between hearing and the brain.

11. Using a T-chart similar to the one here, list the differences between swimmer's ear, middle ear infection, and inner ear infection.

In the Lab

12. Research the products and services available for either deafness or otitis media. Collect promotional materials for a variety of products and services from product manufacturers and medical clinics. Analyze the data in these materials based on the knowledge gained from this lesson. Make inferences about the products and services and recommend the best ones to the class.

Lesson 7.3 Smell and Taste

Before You Read

Try to answer the following questions before you read this lesson.

How can a particular smell trigger an emotion?

How does the sense of smell influence taste?

Lesson Objectives

1. Describe the anatomy of the olfactory region and explain how it functions.
2. Explain why certain smells can trigger memories and emotions.
3. Describe the major anatomical structures of the gustatory sense and explain their functions.
4. Identify the five taste sensations.
5. Explain how we detect flavors in foods.

Key Terms

E-Flash Cards

antihistamines
gustatory cells
gustatory hairs
histamines
mucous layer
odor molecules
olfactory bulb
olfactory filaments
olfactory hairs

olfactory nerve
olfactory receptor cells
olfactory region
papillae
septum
tastants
taste buds
taste pores

Have you ever smelled your favorite food cooking and noticed that your mouth was watering? The sense of smell can stimulate your mouth to secrete saliva. Alternatively, imagine a perfectly cooked, scrumptious meal without the ability to smell or taste it.

Our senses of smell and taste enable us to enjoy what we eat and drink. These senses can also alert us to when food or drink has gone bad, as in the case of sour milk. In addition, our sense of smell can alert us to environmental dangers. For example, we will immediately leave an area in which we smell toxic fumes or another undesirable or potentially harmful scent.

How are we able to so rapidly interpret what we smell and taste? In this lesson we will explore the anatomy and physiology of the sensory pathways of smell and taste.

Olfactory Sense (Sense of Smell)

Have you ever noticed that when you have a cold, your ability to smell is considerably lessened? The sensors responsible for smell are located in a dime-sized area called the **olfactory** (ohl-FAK-toh-ree) **region**, on the top side of each nasal cavity (**Figure 7.14**). These sensors are called **olfactory receptor cells**. When your nasal cavity becomes congested with mucus from a cold, the olfactory receptors are covered and partially blocked. As a result, **odor molecules** from foods that normally would trigger your sense of smell do not reach the olfactory receptor cells.

The olfactory receptor cells are neurons. (For a definition of *neuron*, see chapter 6.) Tiny **olfactory hairs** extend from these neurons into

Nasal cavity

Olfactory bulb

Olfactory nerve

Bone

A. Olfactory region

Olfactory filaments of the olfactory nerve

Supporting cell

Olfactory receptor cell

Olfactory hairs

Mucous layer

Odor molecules

Label Art

B. Olfactory epithelium

Figure 7.14 The olfactory region. *Which labeled part of drawing B is covered with mucus when you have a cold? Why does this affect your sense of taste?*

the nasal cavity, where they are covered by a thin, protective layer of mucus. Whenever you inhale an odor, the chemicals that caused the odor dissolve in the **mucous layer** surrounding the olfactory hairs. This dissolving action stimulates the olfactory receptor cells, which send impulses through the **olfactory filaments** that make up the **olfactory nerve**. The olfactory filaments in turn feed impulses to the **olfactory bulb**, the thickened end of the olfactory nerve. The olfactory nerve sends impulses to the olfactory cortex of the brain.

The nerve pathway between the nose and the brain travels through the limbic system, the part of the brain responsible for emotions. A smell may trigger a positive or negative emotion because we have associated a particular experience with that scent. For instance, the scent of a Christmas tree or cookies baking in an oven may remind you of your family, bringing about a positive emotion. By contrast, the smell of an antiseptic ointment may remind you of an injury that you have experienced—one that you

would rather not remember because it triggers a negative emotion.

Although most animals have a much stronger sense of smell than humans, our olfactory receptors are actually quite sensitive. It takes only a few molecules of an inhaled odor to stimulate our olfactory receptors, which then fire a nerve impulse. Thus, the olfactory receptors can easily become used to an odor to which they are repeatedly exposed. This explains why people who habitually wear a certain perfume or cologne, for example, tend not to smell it on themselves.

Injuries and Disorders of the Nose

Your nose is important to your overall health. It acts as a filter to remove dust, irritants, and germs from the air that you breathe. A variety of problems, from the common cold to a deviated septum, can make breathing difficult.

WHAT RESEARCH TELLS US

...*about* Sense of Smell in Humans and Animals

How does the human olfactory sense compare to that of animals and fish? The human sense of smell is sufficiently powerful that it can detect the presence of a skunk with only 0.000,000,000,000,071 of an ounce of scent present. Because the sense of smell among many species of animals and fish may be related to survival, a larger portion of their brains is devoted to receiving and interpreting scents.

Dogs, for example, have about 125 to 220 million olfactory receptor cells. This is roughly 20 times the number of receptors that humans have. Dogs bred for hunting may have even more olfactory receptors; the bloodhound, for instance, has nearly 300 million (**Figure 7.15**). In fact, the percentage of a dog's brain that is responsible for smell is 40 times greater than the corresponding percentage of the human brain.

The dog's wet nose assists with scent detection by capturing odor particles. With all of these advantages, it has been estimated that a dog's sense of smell is 100 thousand to 1 million times more sensitive than that of a human. By comparison, the bloodhound's olfactory sense may be up to 100 million times more sensitive. This is why the bloodhound, referred to as "a nose with a dog attached," is often used in law enforcement to track down missing persons and criminals.

A horse's olfactory sense is not as sharp as that of a dog, but it is still stronger than our own sense of smell. Horses use their olfactory sense to identify other horses, people, predators, pastures, feeds, and water sources. A mare's sense

Degtyaryov Andrey Leonidovich/Shutterstock.com

Figure 7.15 The bloodhound has an extraordinarily well-developed sense of smell, making it ideal for law enforcement applications such as tracking missing persons and criminals. *How do you think "sniffer" dogs learn to track down a person they have never encountered?*

of smell is so discriminating that it enables her to pick out her own foal from a group of foals.

Fish such as salmon also have an extremely well-developed sense of smell. Salmon are born in small, freshwater streams. They then swim to the ocean, where they spend one to three years. After this period, they generally return to the same stream where they were born to lay eggs.

How does each salmon locate the exact same stream in which it was born? One hypothesis is

that the newborn salmon brain is imprinted with the distinctive odor of the water from the stream of its birth. Researchers tested this hypothesis by tagging a large number of young salmon and recording the location of their births. They then plugged the nostrils of 50 percent of these salmon to block their ability to smell. When the salmon returned to fresh water to lay their eggs, the researchers discovered that the salmon with plugged nostrils did not return to the same stream where they were born. By contrast, most of the salmon with unplugged nostrils returned to the site of their births. Although other factors may influence the salmon's remarkable ability to return to its birth stream, its sense of smell clearly plays a key role.

Taking It Further

1. Do some research to find out how "sniffer" dogs are trained to detect drugs or bombs with their noses. Share your findings with the class.

2. How strong is your own sense of smell? Open an alcohol swab packet near your belly button. Breathe in. Can you detect the odor from the swab? Begin moving it closer to your nose and continue trying to smell it. If you can detect the odor from a distance of 8 to 12 inches from your nose (around chest level), then your sense of smell is normal. If you find that you are having a hard time distinguishing the scent at 4 inches away from your nose, then you may have a loss of smell.

Rhinitis

Rhinitis (righ-NIGH-tis) is an inflammation of the mucous membranes that line the nasal passage. The most frequent cause of rhinitis is the common cold. However, the condition can be caused by anything that irritates these membranes. Possibilities include infections, allergies, strong chemical odors, and certain illegal drugs.

Irritation of the nasal membranes causes the release of **histamines** (HIS-ta-meenz), molecules that trigger a reaction that produces nasal congestion and drainage. Treatment of rhinitis requires removing or minimizing the original irritant and taking medications that contain **antihistamines** (AN-tee-HIS-ta-meenz), which work to curb the activity of histamines.

Septum Problems

The **septum** of the nose is the structure made of cartilage that divides the left and right air passages in the nose. It is normal for the septum not to be perfectly centered; a slight deviation to one side is common. However, a large shift in the position of the septum away from the center is called a *deviated septum*. Injury is usually, but not always, the cause of a deviated septum. When warranted, a deviated septum can be surgically repaired.

The septum may also develop one or more holes caused by injury, an ulcer, long-term exposure to toxic fumes, or illegal drug abuse. This condition is known as a *perforated septum*. A perforated septum can be surgically treated to close the open sores.

 Check Your Understanding

1. Where are sensors for smell located?
2. Explain the connection between smell and emotions.
3. What is the most common cause of rhinitis?
4. What are the two basic treatments for rhinitis?
5. What might cause a perforated septum?

Gustatory Sense (Sense of Taste)

The human mouth contains approximately 10,000 sensory receptors for the sense of taste. These **taste buds** are scattered throughout the interior of the mouth, including the lips and the sides, top, and back of the mouth. Most of the taste buds, however, reside on the familiar tiny bumps on the tongue known as **papillae** (pa-PIL-ee). Within each taste bud, **gustatory** (GUS-ta-TOH-ree) **cells** send tiny **gustatory hairs** up through the **taste pores**, very small openings in the top of the taste buds (**Figure 7.16**).

When you eat food, the food is mixed in your mouth with *saliva*, produced by the *salivary glands* in the mouth. Chemical molecules from food dissolve in the saliva to produce compounds called **tastants** (TAYS-tehnts). The tastants stimulate the gustatory hairs to send nerve impulses to the brain. Three of the cranial nerves—the *facial nerve*, the *glossopharyngeal* (GLAHS-oh-feh-RIN-jee-al) *nerve*, and the *vagus* (VAY-gus) *nerve*—are responsible for transmitting taste sensations to the brain.

Although we enjoy many foods and beverages because of the complexity of the taste sensations they generate, the gustatory sense comprises only five basic tastes. These are *sweet*, *salty*, *sour*, *bitter*, and *umami*. Umami is the taste of beef as well as the taste of monosodium glutamate, a seasoning commonly added to processed foods to enhance their taste. Although a single gustatory cell responds to only one of

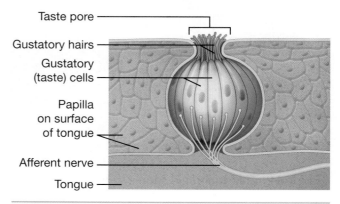

Figure 7.16 Anatomy of a taste bud. *Why do you think you like the tastes of certain foods and not those of other foods?*

the five taste sensations, individual taste buds contain 50 to 100 gustatory cells, which typically include all five taste sensations.

The flavors that we detect in food and beverages are influenced not only by sensations from our taste buds, but they are also strongly influenced by our sense of smell. An estimated 75% to 90% of what we attribute to taste is actually due to what we smell. In the absence of smell, we would be able to distinguish only the five basic tastes—sweet, salty, sour, bitter, and umami. But the average person is able to distinguish approximately 10,000 different flavors. The human mouth contains no taste receptors for the distinctly recognizable tastes of peach, tomato, lime, or chocolate, for example. Each of these flavors is produced by a combination of taste and smell. The brain receives sensory information from the receptors for both taste and smell, and then translates this information into the flavors that we recognize (**Figure 7.17**).

Flavor is actually a combination of taste, smell, texture or consistency, and temperature. Many people have aversions to food and beverages whose consistency they simply do not find

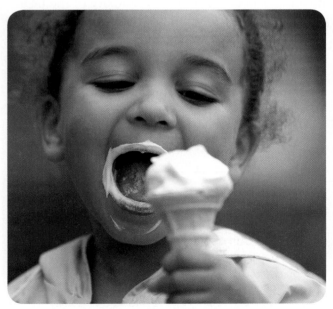

Darren Baker/Shutterstock.com

Figure 7.17 This young girl seems to be enjoying her vanilla ice cream cone, even though she is probably not aware of the many different factors affecting the taste. *What factors contribute to the tastes and flavors she is experiencing?*

appealing. A hot food or drink gives off odors that strongly activate the neural pathways for smell, whereas the same cold food or beverage gives off a much weaker odor, making it less appealing. Spicy foods stimulate not only gustatory cells but also pain receptors in the mouth. Because everyone perceives pain differently, some people enjoy the sensation of spicy foods and others do not.

Disorders of the Tongue

The powerful muscles of your tongue enable you to speak and to chew and swallow food. As discussed above, taste buds on the surface of your tongue allow you to experience different taste sensations. A variety of disorders, including infections, injuries, and abnormal tissue growth, can affect the appearance and function of the tongue. Some tongue disorders are short-lived and can be remedied with antibiotics. Other disorders require ongoing treatment for an underlying physical condition.

Infection of the tongue may follow severe biting of the tongue during a traumatic accident, or it may be associated with piercing of the tongue. Antibiotics are used to treat a tongue infection. Fortunately, the human tongue tends to heal quickly. In fact, it heals more quickly than any other part of the body.

Certain conditions can promote unnatural growth of the gustatory hairs of the tongue, causing the look and feel of a *hairy tongue*. The most common cause is inadequate oral hygiene, but other causes include use of certain medications, excessive drinking of coffee or tea, frequent tobacco use, or radiation treatments to the head or neck region. Good oral hygiene, including brushing the tongue, as well as the teeth, is both a prevention and cure for hairy tongue.

Burning mouth syndrome, as the name suggests, involves a sensation of moderate to severe burning in the mouth that may continue for months or even years. When the pain persists, anxiety and depression may develop. Related symptoms may include tingling, numbness, or dryness of the mouth and a bitter or metallic taste. The condition can arise from a variety of causes, including damage to the taste and pain receptors in the mouth, chronically dry mouth, nutritional deficiencies, hormonal changes, acid reflux, and infection in the mouth.

Treatment of burning mouth syndrome is based on the cause, so it may involve addressing an underlying disorder with nutritional supplements, hormone therapy, antibiotics, or other remedies. When no underlying cause is apparent, treatment is designed with the goal of reducing the pain associated with burning mouth syndrome.

 Check Your Understanding

1. What are papillae?
2. List three nerves responsible for sending taste sensory signals to the brain.

Lesson 7.3 Review and Assessment

Mini Glossary   Make sure that you know the meaning of each key term.

 Build vocabulary with e-flash cards and games

antihistamines medications that work to curb the activity of histamines

gustatory cells sensory receptors located within taste buds

gustatory hairs threads that emerge from the gustatory cells

histamines molecules that trigger a reaction to irritation of the nasal membranes, which produces nasal congestion and drainage

mucous layer a viscous coating that surrounds the olfactory hairs

odor molecules tiny airborne particles that trigger the sense of smell

olfactory bulb the thickened end of the olfactory nerve that sends sensory impulses to the olfactory region of the brain

olfactory filaments fibers in the olfactory nerve that receive impulses from olfactory receptor cells

olfactory hairs threads that extend from the olfactory receptor cells into the nasal cavity

olfactory nerve a cranial nerve that sends impulses to the olfactory cortex of the brain

olfactory receptor cells the sensors responsible for smell

olfactory region a dime-sized area at the top of each nasal cavity that houses sensors responsible for smell

papillae tiny bumps on the tongue that house taste buds

septum the structure made of cartilage that divides the left and right air passages in the nose

tastants compounds that stimulate the gustatory hairs to send nerve impulses to the brain

taste buds sensory receptors for taste

taste pores very small openings in the top of the taste buds through which gustatory hairs project

Know and Understand

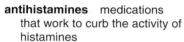
Assess

1. Define histamines and state the importance of antihistamines.

2. Which part of the brain is responsible for emotions related to scent?

3. What causes the blockage of the olfactory receptor cells when you have a cold?

4. What is the name of the structure that separates the right and left air passages of the nose?

5. The sense of taste is affected by the sense of _____.

6. Which disorder causes a bitter or metallic taste in the mouth?

Analyze and Apply

7. Describe in detail how you are able to taste food.

8. List the five basic tastes and give examples of each.

9. Natural gas has no smell. Explain why utility companies put an unpleasant smell in natural gas.

In the Lab

10. What is the difference between taste and flavor?

    While holding your nose, begin chewing a jelly bean. Can you identify the flavor of the jelly bean? Can you describe what you taste? You might say that you detect a sweet taste, which is due to the sugar in the jelly bean.

    Now, while continuing to chew, let go of your nose. What happens? Did you get a sudden rush of flavor? Can you better identify the flavor of the jelly bean?

    What did you learn from this experiment? Write a brief description of your findings.

Career Corner
Anatomy and Physiology at Work

A variety of career paths are available that involve working with and treating conditions of the sensory organs. A few of these options are discussed below.

Ophthalmologist

An ophthalmologist (AHF-thal-MAHL-oh-jist) is a medical doctor who specializes in treating injuries, disorders, and diseases of the eye through both medicine and surgery. Training for ophthalmologists in the United States includes a college degree, medical school, and a residency in ophthalmology.

Four years of residency training after medical school is required. The first year of residency training usually consists of a supervised internship in surgery, internal medicine, or pediatrics. During the following three years, residents receive specialized training in ophthalmology. Most residency programs are accredited by the Accreditation Council for Graduate Medical Education (ACGME) and are board-certified by the American Board of Ophthalmology.

Optometrist

Although optometrists (ahp-TAHM-eh-trists) are not doctors of medicine with the MD or OD credential, they are licensed medical professionals trained to prescribe and fit corrective lenses for improving vision (**Figure 7.18**). Optometrists can also diagnose and treat diseases of the eye and can prescribe needed medications. In some states in the US, optometrists can also perform certain types of laser surgery.

Training for optometrists begins with a four-year college degree that includes successful completion of required courses in math, chemistry, physics, physiology, anatomy, microbiology, and psychology. Students applying for admission to an optometry doctoral program must score well on the standardized Optometry Admission Test. Admission to optometry school is highly competitive, with

Figure 7.18 An optometrist tests a patient's vision.

many more candidates applying than can be accepted.

The four-year doctoral program in optometry involves specialized classroom and clinical training in all aspects of the anatomy and physiology of the eye, treatment of disorders and diseases of the eye, and procedures for screening and correcting vision deficits. In addition, students receive general training in anatomy, physiology, and systemic diseases of the entire human body. Upon completion of a four-year, accredited optometry program, the optometry degree (OD) is awarded.

To be certified to practice, optometrists must pass a national examination administered by the National Board of Examiners in Optometry (NBEO). This exam encompasses basic science, clinical science, and patient care. Some optometrists elect to complete one- to two-year residencies with training focused on pediatric or geriatric eye care, specialty contact lens prescription, or diseases of the eye.

Audiologist

An audiologist (AW-dee-AHL-oh-jist) is a healthcare professional who specializes in diagnosing and treating disorders of the ear, including problems with both hearing and balance. Audiologists perform screening programs for hearing and prescribe hearing aids. They can also provide custom-fitted earplugs and other hearing protection devices for individuals who work in noisy environments. Another job of the audiologist is counseling families to help them cope with the diagnosis of a hearing deficit in an infant, and counseling seniors to help them adapt to hearing loss, even after a hearing aid has been prescribed.

Training for audiologists currently requires a four-year college degree followed by a Doctor of Audiology (AuD) degree. Requirements for the AuD degree involve a minimum of 75 semester hours of postbaccalaureate study that includes anatomy and physiology (both general and specific to the ear) as well as diagnosis of hearing deficits and disorders of both hearing and balance. Training in counseling and sign language is required. In addition, the AuD degree requires completion of a 12-month, full-time, supervised practicum; 12 months of full-time, supervised experience with a professional practice; and successful completion of a national exam. To practice, audiologists must receive state licensure or registration.

Planning for a Health-Related Career

Do some research on the career of an ophthalmologist or audiologist. Alternatively, select a profession from the list of **Related Career Options**. Using the Internet or resources at your local library, find answers to the following questions:

1. What are the main tasks and responsibilities of this job?
2. What is the outlook for this career? Are workers in demand, or are jobs dwindling?

For complete information, consult the current edition of the *Occupational Outlook Handbook*, published by the US Department of Labor. This handbook is available online or at your local library.

3. What special skills or talents are required? For example, do you need to be good at biology or chemistry? Do you need to enjoy interacting with other people?
4. What personality traits do you think are needed to be successful in this job?
5. Does this career involve a great deal of routine, or are the day-to-day responsibilities varied?
6. Does the work require long hours, or is it a standard, "9-to-5" job?
7. What is the salary range for this job?
8. What do you think you would like about this career? Is there anything about it that you might dislike?

Related Career Options

- Biological Technician
- Health Educator
- Internist
- Laboratory Technologist
- Medical Assistant
- Nurse Practitioner
- Occupational Therapist
- Ophthalmic Assistant
- Ophthalmic Technician
- Optical Technician
- Optometrist
- Physician
- Physician Assistant
- Respiratory Therapist
- Surgeon

Chapter Summaries

Lesson 7.1   The Eye

Build vocabulary with e-flash cards and games

Key Points

- The eye is protected by the bony orbital socket, eyebrows, eyelashes, and eyelids.
- Tears produced by lacrimal glands act as a lubricant and have antibody properties that cleanse the eye.
- The sclera, choroid, and retina make up the three layers of the eye.
- Accommodation is a change in the shape of the lens to allow for near and distant vision.
- Myopia and hyperopia can be corrected with prescription lenses.
- Conjunctivitis is a highly contagious disease of the eye.
- Glaucoma is a disorder of the eye that will cause blindness if left untreated.

Key Terms

aqueous and vitreous humors
choroid
ciliary body
ciliary glands
cones
conjunctiva
cornea
extrinsic muscles
iris
lacrimal glands

lens
optic chiasma
optic nerve
optic tracts
pupil
retina
rods
sclera
suspensory ligaments
tarsal glands

Lesson 7.2   The Ear

Key Points

- The ear is divided into three parts—the external ear, middle ear, and internal ear.
- The middle ear contains the ossicles: anvil (incus), stirrup (stapes), and hammer (malleus).
- The external ear includes the auditory canal, which is lined with ceruminous glands.
- The inner ear is responsible for hearing and balance.
- Over time, loud music can cause hair receptor cells in the organ of Corti to no longer function, causing deafness.
- Ear infections are categorized according to their location: outer ear, middle ear, and inner ear.

Key Terms

anvil
auditory canal
auricle
bony labyrinth
ceruminous glands
cochlea
cochlear duct
endolymph
Eustachian tube
hammer

membranous labyrinth
organ of Corti
ossicles
oval window
perilymph
semicircular canals
stirrup
tympanic membrane
vestibule
vestibulocochlear nerve

Lesson 7.3 Smell and Taste

Key Points

- The olfactory receptor cells send impulses to the olfactory nerve, which then sends the stimuli to the olfactory cortex of the brain.
- The senses of smell and taste involve highly specialized, sensitive receptors.
- The nose filters dust, irritants, and germs from the air that we breathe.
- Taste buds are located on the papillae that cover the tongue.
- The five basic tastes are sweet, salty, sour, bitter, and umami.
- The facial nerve, the glossopharyngeal nerve, and the vagus nerve are responsible for sending sensory impulses from the taste receptors to the brain.
- The sense of smell contributes strongly to our sense of taste.

Key Terms

antihistamines
gustatory cells
gustatory hairs
histamines
mucous layer
odor molecules
olfactory bulb
olfactory filaments
olfactory hairs
olfactory nerve
olfactory receptor cells
olfactory region
papillae
septum
tastants
taste buds
taste pores

Chapter Assessments

Lesson 7.1

The Eye

Learning Key Terms and Concepts

1. The white of the eye is called the _____.
2. Of the following four words, which one doesn't belong? Why?
   - A. retina
   - B. rods
   - C. cones
   - D. choroid
3. Of the following four words, which one doesn't belong? Why?
   - A. cornea
   - B. sclera
   - C. retina
   - D. extrinsic muscles
4. The conjunctiva is a membrane that lines _____.
   - A. the eyelid
   - B. the innermost part of the eye
   - C. the iris
   - D. the rods and cones
5. The eyeball has three layers: the sclera, the choroid, and the _____.
   - A. iris
   - B. lens
   - C. orbit
   - D. retina

6. Maria wears contact lenses to see the whiteboard at school. She probably has an eye disorder called _____.
   - A. strabismus
   - B. hyperopia
   - C. myopia
   - D. presbyopia
7. Which part of the eye is removed during cataract surgery?
   - A. iris
   - B. lens
   - C. sclera
   - D. cornea
8. Which order below is the correct pathway of vision?
   - A. cornea, retina, optic nerve, pupil, lens
   - B. pupil, lens, retina, cornea, optic nerve
   - C. cornea, pupil, lens, retina, optic nerve
   - D. cornea, pupil, retina, lens, optic nerve

Thinking Critically

9. Compare the anatomy and functions of the iris and the pupil.
10. What would happen if a person had no lacrimal glands, or if the person's lacrimal glands were clogged?
11. What would be the result of the vitreous humor leaking out of the eyeball?

Lesson 7.2

The Ear

Learning Key Terms and Concepts

12. Another name for the eardrum is the _____.
13. The outer part of the ear is known as the _____.
14. The organ of Corti is located in which structure of the ear?
15. Where would you find cerumen?
    A. pinna   C. auditory canal
    B. Eustachian tube   D. middle ear
16. Which part of the ear carries sound impulses to the brain?
    A. pinna   C. cochlear nerve
    B. tympanic   D. auditory nerve
       membrane
17. In the pathway of hearing, sound waves travel from the tympanic membrane to the _____.
    A. ossicles   C. Eustachian tube
    B. cochlea   D. auditory nerve
18. What is the purpose of the Eustachian tube?
    A. to carry sound waves to the middle ear
    B. to carry sound waves to the inner ear
    C. to equalize pressure in the middle ear
    D. to protect the inner ear from microorganisms
19. An audiologist would examine someone with

    _____.

    A. hearing loss   C. blurred vision
    B. a sore throat   D. chest pain

Instructions: Write the **letter** of the name of the **part of the ear** on your answer sheet next to the corresponding number.

_____ 20. Auditory canal
_____ 21. Middle ear
_____ 22. Semicircular canals
_____ 23. Auricle
_____ 24. Vestibulocochlear nerve
_____ 25. Tympanic membrane

_____ 26. Cochlea
_____ 27. Eustachian tube

Thinking Critically

28. Mrs. Omar took her baby to the pediatrician because the baby had cried throughout the night and kept holding the left side of his head. Mrs. Omar told the doctor that her baby had suffered a cold for about a week. After examining the baby's ear, the doctor reported that the baby had a bulging, red eardrum. The doctor thought the cause was a middle ear infection and told the mother the baby was suffering from _____. What did the doctor say was the problem, and what treatment did she prescribe? Explain your reasoning.

Lesson 7.3

Smell and Taste

Learning Key Terms and Concepts

29. What percentage of taste is supplied by smell?
30. Describe at least three functions of your nose and sense of smell.
31. The gustatory sense comprises only five basic tastes. What are they?
32. A person has burned his tongue and has trouble tasting food. Which structures of his mouth were damaged?
    A. stapes   C. papillae
    B. pinna   D. palate
33. How would you prevent hairy tongue disorder?
34. What is the most common cause of rhinitis?
35. Which of the following would not cause a perforated septum?
    A. illegal drug use   C. histamines
    B. injury   D. an ulcer
36. Describe the taste of umami.
37. Where are taste buds not found?
    A. in the nose   C. on the lips
    B. on the tongue   D. on the roof of the
                               mouth

Thinking Critically

38. Explain why a particular smell might trigger a memory. Use the anatomy and physiology you learned in this lesson and previous lessons to support your hypothesis.

39. With a group of friends, taste various foods. Discuss and compare your sensitivity to the five basic tastes with your friends' sensitivity to these tastes. How would you describe your sense of taste compared with their sense of taste?

Building Skills and Connecting Concepts

Analyzing and Evaluating Data

The chart to the right shows the age ranges at which people begin to experience hearing loss. For each age range, percentages of the total population are given for both males and females. Use the chart to answer the following questions:

40. Which age range has the highest percentage of people (male and female combined) experiencing their first hearing loss?

41. Which group—men or women—tend to lose their ability to hear at an earlier age?

42. If you are a female, what are the approximate odds that you will retain your full hearing until you reach 65 years of age? if you are a male?
    A. 1 in 4
    B. 1 in 6
    C. 1 in 3
    D. 1 in 5

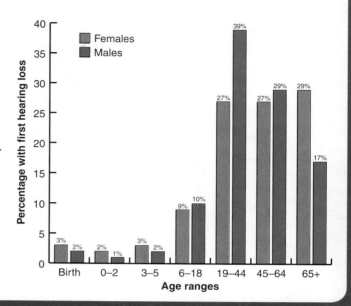

Communicating about Anatomy and Physiology

43. **Writing** Write a list of detailed instructions that you would give to a new mother regarding prevention and treatment of ear infections. After each instruction, explain why that particular instruction is important. In preparing your list, be sure to use the new vocabulary that you have learned in this chapter.

44. **Speaking and Listening** With two classmates, role-play a situation in which you are a physician's assistant counseling a young mother and father regarding ear infections. As a basic guide for your counseling, use the list that you developed for the writing activity in #43. Adjust your vocabulary as necessary while responding to their questions and clarifying information. Then switch roles.

Lab Investigations

45. Survey friends and family members to identify as many cases as possible of eye and ear diseases and disorders. For each case identified, document the person's disease or disorder, the person's gender, and the person's age at onset of the disease/disorder. Then, working with classmates who have conducted similar research and prepared similar documentation, compile and analyze the data. What conclusions can you draw from the data? For example, are there any correlations between age and a particular disease? gender and a disease? Working with your group, develop a graph or chart to summarize your findings and then present your results to the class.

46. Create a flyer highlighting strategies for preventing blindness. Target the flyer to senior citizens' groups. What key points would you include? How would you design the flyer to attract the attention of your intended audience? Share your flyer and the reasons for your content and design decisions with the class.

Expand your learning with additional online resources
- Supplemental Lab Activities
- Interactive Exercises
- Animations

Expand

www.g-wlearning.com/healthsciences

Would you want to become the tallest person on Earth?

266

The Endocrine System

8

*I*n 2010, the *Guinness Book of World Records* named Sultan Kosen, a 29-year-old man from Turkey, the world's tallest man, measuring 8 feet, 3 inches. Kosen also achieved the records for the largest hands (28.5 centimeters, or 11.22 inches) and largest feet (36.5 centimeters, or 14.4 inches). If you are a basketball player, you are probably thinking, *"Awesome!"*

A tumor caused Kosen's pituitary gland to secrete excessive amounts of growth hormone, resulting in gigantism, a condition in which a person grows to an exceptionally large size. The only way to treat this condition is to stop the excretion of growth hormone.

In 2010, doctors at the University of Virginia's Medical Center put Kosen on drugs to balance his hormone levels. Then they used a gamma knife, which emits focused beams of radiation, to target the tumor. Because the tumor was too deep for conventional surgery, the gamma knife was one of their only options. The surgery was a success, and Sultan stopped growing.

Sultan's story highlights the overwhelming effects that the small but powerful endocrine glands and organs can have on the body. In this chapter you will learn about these glands and organs and some diseases and disorders that can occur when the endocrine system does not function properly.

Chapter 8 Lessons

Lesson 8.1
Functions and Control of the Endocrine System

Lesson 8.2
Major Endocrine Organs

Lesson 8.3
Endocrine Disorders and Diseases

While studying, look for the online icon to:

- **Practice** with e-flash cards and vocabulary games
- **Review** with interactive art labeling
- **Assess** with online exercises
- **Expand** with interactive activities and animated videos
- **Listen** to pronunciations of key terms in the audio glossary

www.g-wlearning.com/healthsciences

Study on the Go

Use a mobile device to practice vocabulary terms, listen to pronunciations, and review with self-assessment quizzes.

www.m.g-wlearning.com

Functions and Control of the Endocrine System

Lesson Objectives

1. Explain how the endocrine and nervous systems work together to regulate bodily functions.
2. Describe the basic anatomy of the endocrine system.
3. Describe the functions of hormones, and explain how hormones move through the body.
4. Identify the two classifications of hormones.
5. Explain how hormones help maintain homeostasis.

Key Terms

E-Flash Cards

amino-acid hormones
downregulated
epinephrine
glucagon
hormonal control
hormones
humoral control

hypothalamic
  nonreleasing
  hormones
hypothalamic releasing
  hormones
insulin
neural control
steroid hormones
upregulated

Like the nervous system, the endocrine system controls and monitors organs, glands, and processes in the body. The endocrine system does this job by using hormones that first collect information and then stimulate organs, glands, and tissues.

The nervous and endocrine systems work together to regulate bodily functions, but they act in very different ways. The nervous system works quickly through electrical impulses, and its effects are short-lived. The endocrine system secretes hormones that are slower to react but whose effects are longer lasting.

It's likely that your body has initiated the fight-or-flight response at some point in your life. Perhaps you have encountered a dangerous situation, such as almost being hit by a car or being startled by something unexpected. Our bodies jump into action to move us out of the way from a speeding vehicle or other impending dangers—that's the nervous system at work. After the danger has passed, a racing heartbeat, an increased respiratory rate, and a thin layer of sweat on your skin may persist for a time. This slower, longer-lasting response is the work of the endocrine system.

Anatomy of the Endocrine System

The endocrine system is a collection of organs and small glands that directly or indirectly influence all the functions of the body. Some of the endocrine glands, such as the hypothalamus (HIGH-poh-THAL-a-mus), pituitary (pi-TOO-i-tair-ee), adrenal, and pineal (PI-nee-al) glands, are also part of the nervous system. This overlap allows the two systems to integrate their responses.

For instance, when the body temperature drops below normal, the sympathetic nervous system (SNS) springs into action. The SNS wants the thyroid gland to release heat-producing hormones, but the SNS cannot directly act on the thyroid. Instead, the hypothalamus receives sensory input from the SNS, which triggers the discharge of hypothalamic releasing hormones. These hormones cause the pituitary gland to secrete hormones that ultimately cause the thyroid to produce the heat desired by the SNS. We will learn more about this process later in this lesson.

Endocrine Glands

The endocrine system is made up of ductless glands called *endocrine glands*. Endocrine glands are glands of internal secretion; they secrete **hormones**, or chemical messengers, directly into the bloodstream. The endocrine glands include the hypothalamus, pancreas, pituitary gland, adrenal gland, thyroid gland, pineal gland, testes (male), and ovaries (female).

The organs and glands of the endocrine system are spread throughout the body and regulate many functions. **Figure 8.1** illustrates the location of the endocrine glands.

Exocrine Glands

Exocrine glands, which are glands of external secretion, are the counterpart to the endocrine glands. Unlike endocrine glands, which secrete hormones directly into the bloodstream, exocrine glands have a duct through which secretions are carried to the body's surface or to other organs. Examples of exocrine glands and their secretions include

- sweat glands (sweat);
- salivary glands (saliva);
- mammary glands (breast milk);
- lacrimal glands (tears); and
- pancreas glands (digestive enzymes).

The pancreas is unique because it functions as both an exocrine gland and an endocrine gland. The pancreas releases hormones that regulate blood glucose levels in the body. It also secretes digestive enzymes through a duct into the small intestine.

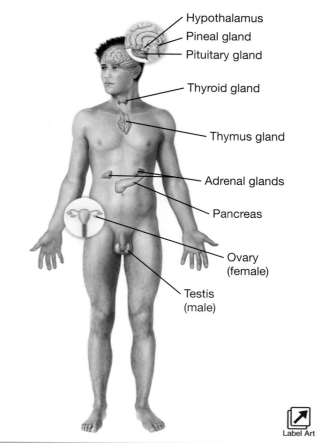

Label Art

Figure 8.1 The glands and organs of the endocrine system are located throughout the body. *What substances are produced by the glands of the endocrine system?*

Hormones

The glands of the endocrine system secrete many different hormones into the bloodstream. As stated earlier, hormones are chemical messengers that influence the activities of other tissues and organs.

Have you ever wondered what stimulates your thirst and hunger? It's the hypothalamus gland. Do you feel energized, refreshed, and happier after getting a good night's sleep? You can thank the pineal gland for secreting melatonin, a hormone that induces sleep. Some days, we are filled with energy; other days, we feel sluggish and tired. Your thyroid gland secretes several hormones that affect your energy level.

Generally, hormones regulate carbohydrate, fat, and protein metabolism; water and electrolyte balance; reproductive activity; growth and development; and energy balance. Hormones also aid in the body's response to infection and stress. These are just a few of the ways that the endocrine system affects everyday functions, emotions, and behaviors.

Hormones are usually classified in two ways—as lipid (fat-based) hormones called **steroid hormones**, or **amino-acid hormones** composed of protein or protein-related substances. Most hormones are amino-acid hormones, except those secreted by the adrenal cortex (the outer layer of the adrenal gland) and the reproductive glands.

Hormone Receptors

Hormones are transported throughout the body by the blood, which comes into contact with all the body's tissues and organs. However, hormones affect only the tissues and organs that have receptors specific to those particular hormones. As you learned in chapter 1, a receptor is a transmitter cell that senses and responds to certain stimuli. When the hormone binds with its receptor, the hormone is able to influence the activity of the cell. The hormone does so by changing the cell membrane's permeability, increasing or decreasing enzyme activity, increasing protein synthesis, or stimulating secretory activity.

The receptors for steroid hormones are found inside the cell nucleus. By contrast, the receptors for amino-acid hormones are found on the membrane, or surface, of the cell. When an amino-acid hormone binds with the cell surface receptor, it stimulates a second messenger. This second messenger works inside the cell to produce a cascade of responses. There are many secondary messengers, and they vary from cell to cell.

When a steroid hormone binds to the receptor inside a cell nucleus, the interaction between the hormone and receptor alters the cell's DNA and activates mRNA (messenger RNA). mRNA then travels to the cytoplasm and stimulates protein synthesis.

Some hormones, such as epinephrine (eh-pi-NEH-frin), have receptors at many different sites, making their effects widespread. Other hormones have fewer target sites, limiting their effects.

Upregulating and Downregulating Hormone Receptors. The activity of hormone receptors can be **upregulated** (increased) or **downregulated** (decreased), making them more or less sensitive to the hormone.

Exercise, for example, upregulates insulin receptors, making them more sensitive to **insulin** (a hormone that promotes the uptake of glucose in body tissues). Because exercise upregulates insulin receptors, less insulin is needed to promote glucose uptake in people who are physically active. However, obesity downregulates insulin receptors, so more insulin must be present to promote glucose uptake by cells. These two glucose-uptake scenarios have important implications for diabetics, particularly those who are overweight.

✓ Check Your Understanding

1. What is a hormone?
2. What is the difference between an endocrine gland and an exocrine gland?
3. Where are the receptors for steroid and amino-acid hormones located?
4. What serves as the transport system for hormones as they travel to their receptor sites?

Hormone Secretion Control

Now that we know what a hormone is and does, let's discuss what prompts a gland to secrete or inhibit a hormone. Endocrine glands are regulated in three different ways: **neural control**, **hormonal control**, and **humoral control**.

Neural Control

During instances of neural control, nerve fibers stimulate the endocrine organs to release hormones. Earlier in this lesson we talked about the fight-or-flight response, which helps us act quickly in potentially dangerous situations.

During the fight-or-flight response, the SNS stimulates the adrenal medulla to release **epinephrine** and norepinephrine (NOR-eh-pi-NEH-frin), hormones that prime the body to fight or flee from a stressful situation. The effects of these hormones include increased heart rate, blood pressure, respiration, and blood flow to muscles; decreased blood flow to organs; and dilation of the pupils.

The fight-or-flight response is just one example of neural control. There are other situations in which the nervous system acts on the hypothalamus, influencing hormone release in other organs and glands of the endocrine system.

Hormonal Control

Hormonal control of the endocrine glands and organs is achieved by a hierarchy, or chain of command, of the endocrine organs. During hormonal control, endocrine organs are stimulated by hormones from other endocrine organs, starting with the hypothalamus. This chain reaction seeks a response from the targeted tissue or organ.

Hormonal control can be likened to the hierarchy of a business. Think of the hypothalamus as the president of the company, the pituitary as the vice president, and the other endocrine glands as managers (**Figure 8.2**).

As "president" of the endocrine system, the hypothalamus directs the activities of the pituitary gland (the "vice president"). The hypothalamus does this through the secretion of hormones such as **hypothalamic releasing hormones** and **hypothalamic nonreleasing hormones**. The pituitary gland then releases its many hormones to direct the "managers"—the

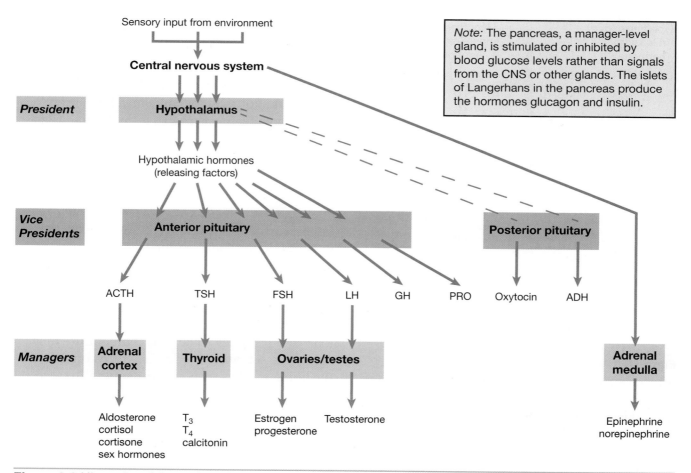

Figure 8.2 Hierarchy of the endocrine system. Each gland in the hierarchy controls the activities of the gland or glands below it. Each gland is controlled by the gland or glands above it. *Why is it appropriate to compare the relationship between endocrine glands to the hierarchy of a business?*

adrenal cortex, thyroid, reproductive organs, pancreas, and adrenal medulla.

When the hormones from the "managers" rise in the bloodstream, they have an end goal, such as stimulating target tissues. After the goal has been achieved, the pituitary and hypothalamus can receive signals from the "manager" hormones that inhibit, or turn off, the pituitary and hypothalamic hormones, thus ending the chain of hormonal control. Does this process sound familiar? If so, that's because it is a negative feedback loop, a concept discussed in chapter 1. An example of a negative feedback loop for the endocrine system is shown in **Figure 8.3**.

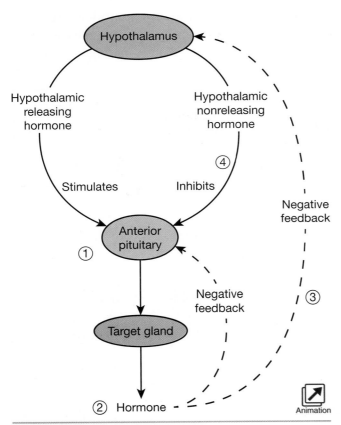

Figure 8.3 Negative feedback loop. 1—The hypothalamus and the pituitary gland direct the target gland to release hormones. 2—The target gland releases hormones to achieve a goal, such as the stimulation of target tissues. 3—After the goal is achieved, the target gland sends signals to the hypothalamus and the pituitary gland. 4—The hypothalamus inhibits the production of additional hypothalamic and anterior pituitary hormones. *What stimulates the hypothalamus to release its hormones?*

Humoral Control

Humoral control of the endocrine system is achieved by monitoring the levels of various substances in body fluids, such as the blood. If a homeostatic imbalance is detected, corrective actions are undertaken to help the body regain homeostasis.

For example, when blood glucose levels rise, the pancreas secretes insulin, stimulating the absorption of glucose in body tissues. Greater absorption of glucose in body tissues lowers blood glucose levels. By contrast, when blood glucose levels drop, the pancreas secretes the hormone **glucagon** (GLOO-kuh-gahn). Glucagon causes the breakdown of glycogen stored in the liver. The glycogen then enters the bloodstream and increases blood glucose levels.

Hormones and Homeostasis

Your body is constantly monitoring all of its systems to ensure that everything is working normally. This functional balance is called *homeostasis*. If the function of any one of the organ systems deviates from the normal range (triggering homeostatic imbalance), the body takes corrective measures to restore homeostasis. Neural, hormonal, or humoral controls trigger the release of hormones during homeostatic imbalance. Increased hormone levels affect the target sites, thereby restoring homeostasis. Homeostatic balance and rising hormone levels inhibit further hormone secretions via a negative feedback loop. The negative feedback loop causes the gland to stop secreting the hormone.

Hypothalamic Control of Body Temperature. In chapter 1 you learned that the thermostat in a home functions much like the negative feedback loop in our bodies. When the temperature falls below the set point, the furnace turns on. When the home reaches the desired temperature, the furnace turns off. As **Figure 8.4** shows, your hypothalamus—the "president" of the endocrine system—functions as a thermostat for your body. The hypothalamus works to maintain the homeostatic set point of the body by keeping its temperature at 37°C (98.6°F).

The hypothalamus monitors body temperature. If your body temperature drops

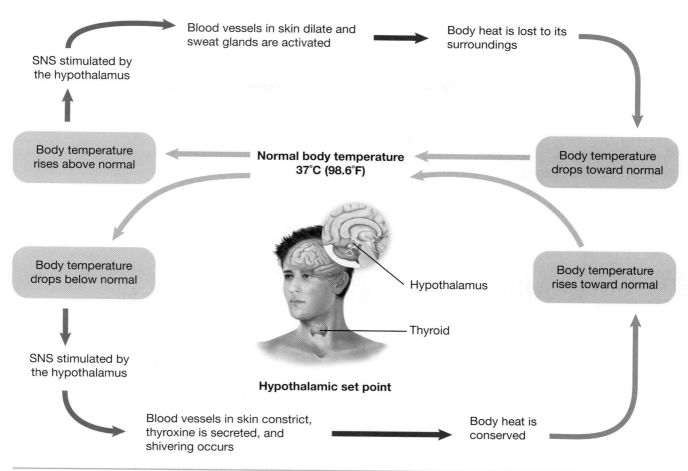

SNS stimulated by
the hypothalamus

Blood vessels in skin dilate and
sweat glands are activated

Body heat is lost to its
surroundings

Body temperature
rises above normal

**Normal body temperature
37°C (98.6°F)**

Body temperature
drops toward normal

Body temperature
drops below normal

Body temperature
rises toward normal

Hypothalamus

Thyroid

Hypothalamic set point

SNS stimulated by
the hypothalamus

Blood vessels in skin constrict,
thyroxine is secreted, and
shivering occurs

Body heat is
conserved

Figure 8.4 The hypothalamus serves as the body's thermostat. *The regulation of body temperature is an example of how the body maintains functional balance. What is this functional balance called?*

below 37°C (98.6°F), the hypothalamus sets in motion a series of responses.

The hypothalamus releases hormones that act on the thyroid gland. The thyroid gland produces thyroxine, a hormone that increases metabolic rate and heat production. The hypothalamus also stimulates the SNS, which initiates shivering and decreased blood flow to the skin. Shivering increases heat production and helps the body maintain core temperature. Once the body temperature has been restored to its hypothalamic set point (homeostasis), the hypothalamus signals the thyroid gland to stop releasing thyroxine. The hypothalamus also signals the SNS to send messages to the body that cause shivering to cease and blood flow to be restored to the skin.

When the body's thermal receptors sense an increase in body temperature above 37°C (98.6°F), the hypothalamus stimulates the SNS. The SNS increases sweat production by stimulating the sweat glands and widening the blood vessels of the skin, increasing blood flow to the area. In addition, the thyroid gland decreases thyroid hormone secretion.

Case Study: Jordan Romero. When Jordan Romero decided that he wanted to become the youngest person to climb Mount Everest at 13 years of age, he and his dad embarked on a training program to get Romero's body into shape. The 8,848-meter (29,029-foot) climb would challenge Romero's body, particularly because lower oxygen concentration in the air at high altitudes diminishes blood oxygen levels.

While at sea level, Romero spent many hours in an altitude tent, where he was exposed to a hypoxic environment (one with low oxygen content). The hypoxic environment of the altitude tent simulated the environment near the peak of Mount Everest. The low oxygen content of the air that Romero was breathing stimulated his kidneys to secrete the hormone erythropoietin. Erythropoietin stimulates bone marrow stem-cell production of red blood cells (RBCs).

The increased production of RBCs in Romero's blood increased the ability of his blood to carry oxygen. As a result, the effects of the hypoxic environment near the peak of Mount Everest were not as fatiguing and harmful to Romero. Thanks to this hormone response, Romero achieved his goal of becoming the youngest person to climb Mount Everest.

 Check Your Understanding

1. Which part of the brain maintains the homeostatic set point at 37°C (98.6°F)?
2. How does the secretion of thyroxine by the thyroid gland keep the internal body temperature from falling?
3. What are the three ways in which hormone secretions are controlled in the endocrine glands?
4. Which two endocrine glands exercise the most control over the others?

Lesson 8.1 Review and Assessment

Mini Glossary
Make sure that you know the meaning of each key term.

 Build vocabulary with e-flash cards and games

amino-acid hormones hormones composed of proteins, or protein-related substances

downregulated decreased

epinephrine the chief neurohormone of the adrenal medulla that is used as a heart stimulant, a vasoconstrictor (which narrows the blood vessels), and a bronchodilator (which relaxes the bronchial tubes in the lungs)

glucagon hormone secreted by the pancreas that causes the breakdown of glycogen stored in the liver

hormonal control type of endocrine control in which endocrine organs are stimulated by hormones from other endocrine organs, starting with the hypothalamus

hormones chemical messengers secreted by the endocrine glands

humoral control type of endocrine control in which levels of various substances in body fluids are monitored for homeostatic imbalance

hypothalamic nonreleasing hormones hormones produced in the hypothalamus and carried by a vein to the anterior pituitary, where they stop certain hormones from being released; hypothalamic inhibiting hormones

hypothalamic releasing hormones hormones produced in the hypothalamus and carried by a vein to the anterior pituitary, where they stimulate the release of anterior pituitary hormones

insulin a hormone that promotes glucose uptake in body tissues

neural control type of endocrine control in which nerve fibers stimulate the endocrine organs to release hormones

steroid hormones lipid (fat-based) hormones

upregulated increased

Know and Understand

 Assess

1. What is the endocrine system?
2. Which gland has both endocrine and exocrine functions?
3. Which endocrine glands are also parts of the nervous system?
4. Which gland is "president" of the endocrine system? Which is "vice president?"

Analyze and Apply

5. Identify similarities and differences between the nervous and endocrine systems.
6. Describe how the activity of a hormone receptor can be upregulated or downregulated.
7. Explain the role of neural control in a fight-or-flight response.

In the Lab

8. Following a December snowstorm in Wisconsin, Mark's parents ask him to help shovel the sidewalk in front of their home. After spending some time outside in the cold, Mark begins to shiver. In what other ways is Mark's body responding as his endocrine system works to raise his body temperature?

9. Working with a partner or in a small group, choose one of the following triggers: hunger, thirst, cold temperature, hot temperature, exhaustion, fear. Research how the endocrine system responds to the trigger. Prepare a PowerPoint® presentation and share your research with the rest of the class.

Before You Read

Try to answer the following questions before you read this lesson.

Which hormone makes you sleepy at night?

Which biological processes are associated with an "adrenaline rush"?

Lesson Objectives

1. Identify the organs and glands of the endocrine system.
2. Identify the six hormones of the anterior pituitary.
3. Describe the location and function of the thyroid, parathyroid, thymus, pineal, and adrenal glands. Identify the hormones produced by each of these glands.
4. Explain the endocrine and exocrine functions of the pancreas.
5. Identify the sex hormones produced by the gonads.

Key Terms

E-Flash Cards

adrenal cortex
adrenal glands
adrenal medulla
anterior pituitary
ovaries
pancreas
parathyroid glands
pineal gland

pituitary gland
posterior pituitary
scrotum
testes
thymus gland
thyroid gland
tropic hormones

As you learned in lesson 8.1, the endocrine system is run by the hypothalamus. The hormones of this tiny gland stimulate the pituitary gland, starting a chain reaction that affects organs and hormones throughout the endocrine system. Each organ plays an important role in ensuring that the endocrine system runs smoothly. In this lesson, we will learn about each of these organs, the hormones they produce, and the role they play in maintaining homeostasis.

The Hypothalamus

The hypothalamus is a very small gland (about 4 grams) buried deep in the brain below the thalamus. The job of the hypothalamus is to collect information from each body system and integrate the responses of the nervous and endocrine systems to maintain homeostatic balance. As you learned in chapter 6, the hypothalamus plays an important role in regulating everyday functions such as metabolism, heart rate, energy level, body temperature, thirst, nutrient intake, blood pressure, and blood composition. It even plays a role in our emotions and, to some degree, regulates our sleep.

Although the hypothalamus is part of the nervous system, it is also a key part of the endocrine system because it produces hypothalamic releasing hormones and hypothalamic nonreleasing hormones. These hormones stimulate or inhibit the release of hormones from the pituitary gland.

The Pituitary Gland

The **pituitary gland** is a pea-sized gland with two lobes—the **anterior pituitary** and the

posterior pituitary. It is located in the depression of the sphenoid bone and is suspended from the underside of the hypothalamus by a short stalk called the *infundibulum* (in-fun-DI-byuh-lum).

Hormones secreted by the pituitary gland function in two ways. They can act directly on target tissue to cause a specific metabolic response, or they can stimulate other endocrine glands (the "manager"-level glands discussed in lesson 8.1) to release their own hormones (**Figure 8.5**). Pituitary hormones that stimulate other endocrine glands are called **tropic hormones**, or *tropins*.

Hormones of the Anterior Pituitary

The anterior pituitary gland secretes six different hormones:

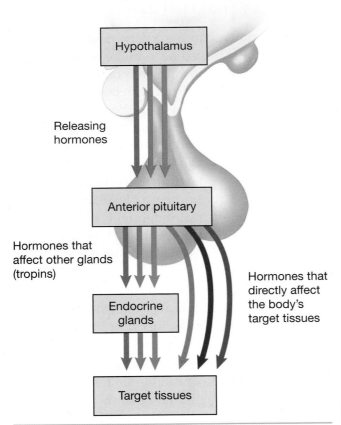

Figure 8.5 Some anterior pituitary hormones act on other glands, while other hormones act directly on the body's tissues. *Which hormones of the anterior pituitary act on other glands? Which hormones act directly on tissues?*

1. growth hormone (GH)
2. prolactin (PRO)
3. adrenocorticotropin (a-DREE-noh-KOR-ti-koh-TROH-pin) hormone (ACTH)
4. thyroid-stimulating hormone (also called *thyrotropin* or TSH)
5. follicle-stimulating hormone (FSH)
6. luteinizing (LOO-tee-in-ighz-ing) hormone (LH)

Follicle-stimulating hormone and luteinizing hormone are further categorized as gonadotropic (GOH-nad-ah-TROP-ik) hormones. **Figure 8.6** shows the hormones produced by the anterior pituitary and their target glands or tissues.

Of the six hormones secreted by the anterior pituitary, four of these are tropic hormones:

- *Adrenocorticotropin* (*ACTH*) acts on the adrenal cortex to stimulate release of steroid hormones.
- *Thyroid-stimulating hormone* (*TSH*) acts on the thyroid gland to stimulate release of two thyroid hormones, thyroxine (T_4) and triiodothyronine (T_3).
- *Follicle-stimulating hormone* (*FSH*) stimulates production of estrogen and eggs in women and production of sperm in men.
- *Luteinizing hormone* (*LH*) acts on the ovaries to produce progesterone and estrogen in women. It also signals the release of eggs. In men, LH stimulates the interstitial cells of the testes to produce testosterone.

Besides producing these four tropic hormones, the anterior pituitary also stores and releases hormones from the hypothalamus. These hormones are kept in the anterior pituitary until the hypothalamus stimulates their release.

Growth Hormone. Unlike the tropic hormones, *growth hormone (GH)* is an anterior pituitary hormone that acts directly on body tissues. In

Memory Tip
ACTH, TSH, FSH, and LH are called *tropic* hormones because they are produced by *gonadotropes*, cells in the anterior pituitary. Tropic hormones act on other endocrine glands, *not* body tissue.

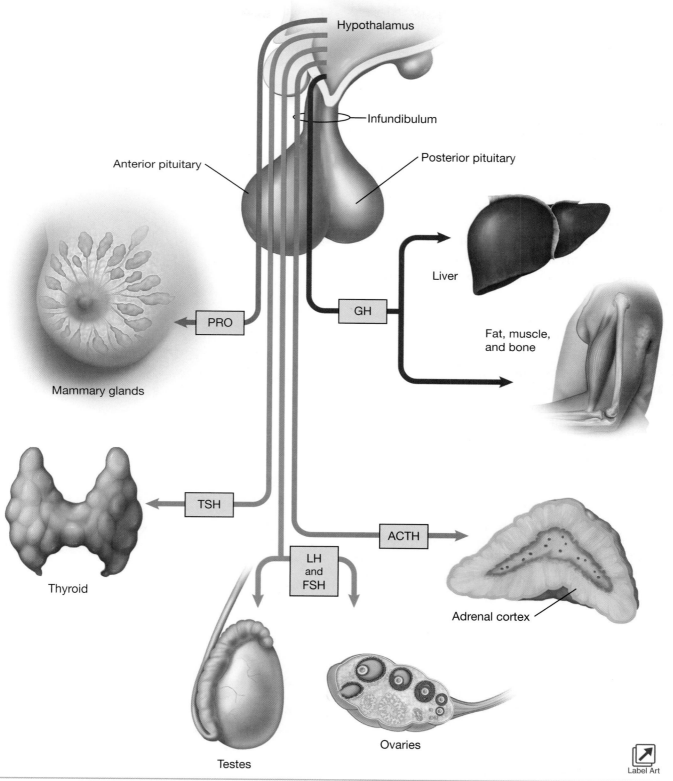

Figure 8.6 Hormones secreted by the anterior pituitary affect many parts of the body. *Of the six hormones shown, which two are not tropic?*

the chapter introduction, we talked about Sultan Kosen, the world's tallest man. Kosen's record-breaking height, hands, and feet are the result of excessive amounts of growth hormone (GH). GH is responsible for the growth and development of the muscles, cartilage, and long bones of the body.

GH also helps break down fats for use as a fuel source by the body. GH is released about 30 to 45 minutes after a person starts to exercise. By using fats as a fuel source, the body is able to spare the carbohydrates whose glucose is needed for energy by the brain. About 80 minutes into an exercise session, GH stimulates fats (in the form of glycerol) and proteins (in the form of amino acids) to be converted into glucose by the liver. This process is called *gluconeogenesis* (gloo-koh-nee-oh-JEH-neh-sis). By using fats and proteins as a fuel source, growth hormone plays an important role in our ability to maintain prolonged physical activity, such as running a marathon.

Prolactin. *Prolactin* stimulates the growth of mammary glands and milk production in a nursing mother. This hormone derives its name from its word parts: the prefix *pro-* means "for," and the combining form *-lact-* means "milk." Prolactin is also present in the male body, but its role in males is unclear.

Hormones of the Posterior Pituitary

The posterior pituitary is actually an extension of the hypothalamus. The posterior pituitary does not produce hormones. Rather, it *stores* two hormones—*antidiuretic* (an-tigh-digh-yoo-REH-tik) *hormone* (*ADH*) and *oxytocin* (AHK-see-TOH-sin)—produced by the hypothalamus.

> ### Memory Tip
> Gluconeogenesis, the process by which the liver converts fat and amino acids into glucose, can be easily remembered by examining the combining forms that make up this word. *Gluco-* refers to "glucose"; *-neo-* means "new"; and *-genesis* means "creation." Put the parts together, and you have the definition of *gluconeogenesis*!

Because it does not produce its own hormones, the posterior pituitary is not a true endocrine gland. Secretion of hormones from the posterior pituitary is the result of hypothalamic neuroendocrine input, or nervous system stimulation of the hypothalamus (**Figure 8.7**).

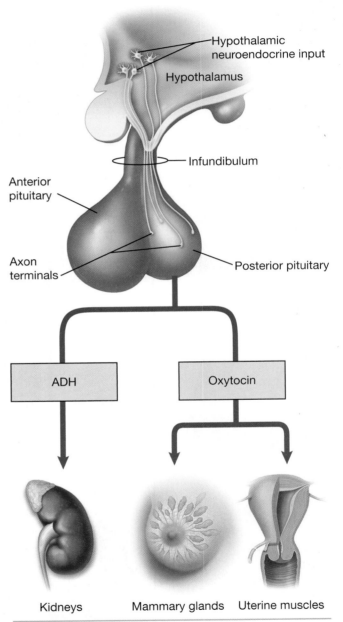

Figure 8.7 The posterior pituitary stores ADH and oxytocin secreted by the hypothalamus. These hormones help maintain the body's fluid balance. In addition, they stimulate uterine contractions in pregnant women and milk production in nursing women.

Antidiuretic Hormone. *Diuretics* are substances that stimulate urine production to decrease fluid retention in the body. Antidiuretic hormone (ADH) does the opposite—it decreases urine output, which increases body fluid volume.

ADH travels in the blood to its target organ, the kidneys. ADH stimulates the kidneys to increase water reabsorption and return the fluid to the blood. People who engage in regular physical activity have an increased sensitivity to ADH. As a result, they have a higher volume of blood plasma (the liquid portion of blood).

What stimulates the hypothalamus to trigger the release of ADH? ADH, which is subject to humoral control, is secreted when plasma volume decreases from dehydration or profuse sweating during exercise. ADH is also secreted when the solid particles in the blood become more concentrated.

ADH also plays an important role in blood pressure regulation. Blood pressure is the tension that blood places on the walls of arteries. ADH can raise blood pressure because it causes the arteries to narrow, thus increasing their resistance to blood flow. At the same time, ADH increases blood volume because of increased reabsorption of fluid and sodium by the kidney. The combination of increased blood volume and narrowed arteries leads to higher blood pressure because more blood is flowing through the smaller vessels.

Alcohol inhibits ADH, which leads to increased urination, dehydration, and a dry mouth the morning after a person drinks alcoholic beverages. Caffeine and foods such as asparagus have a similar effect on ADH and act as diuretics.

Oxytocin. Pregnant women produce oxytocin during labor, and the hormone stays in their bodies until they are finished nursing their child. Oxytocin facilitates childbirth by stimulating the muscles of the uterus to contract. Oxytocin release is also stimulated by the sucking mechanism of a nursing infant, causing the mammary glands to secrete breast milk from the mammary ducts.

Perhaps you have heard of a pitocin (pi-TOH-sin) drip. A pitocin drip is a synthetic, intravenous form of oxytocin that is administered to induce, or speed up, delivery of a baby.

Check Your Understanding

1. Describe the role of the hypothalamus in the endocrine system.
2. How are hormones secreted by the pituitary gland classified in relation to their targets?
3. What does *FSH* stand for, and what is its purpose?
4. Which parts of the body does growth hormone help to grow and develop? Name an additional function of GH.
5. Which two hormones does the posterior pituitary store?

Thyroid Gland

The **thyroid gland** is located inferior to the larynx, or *Adam's apple*, at the base of the throat. This butterfly-shaped gland is two inches long and lies at the front and sides of the trachea (**Figure 8.8A** on the next page). The two lobes of the thyroid gland are divided by a center band of tissue, called the *isthmus* (IS-mus).

The thyroid gland secretes two hormones: *thyroid hormone* and *calcitonin* (kal-si-TOH-nin). These hormones drive our metabolism. People often blame an underactive thyroid gland for their overweight condition, but the thyroid gland is rarely the reason that people become overweight or obese.

Thyroid Hormone

Thyroid hormone is actually two hormones—*thyroxine* (T_4) and *triiodothyronine* (T_3). Both of these hormones are responsible for controlling the rate of energy metabolism and heat production in the body. The follicular cells of the thyroid secrete T_4 and T_3. These hormones are formed from two linked tyrosine (TIGH-ruh-seen) amino acids with iodine atoms attached to the amino acids. T_4 has four iodine atoms, and T_3 has three iodine atoms. T_3 is the more powerful of the two hormones.

The iodine required to make T_4 and T_3 comes from your dietary intake, which is why salt is fortified with iodine in many countries. We will

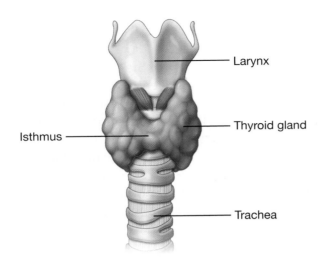

A. Location of the thyroid gland

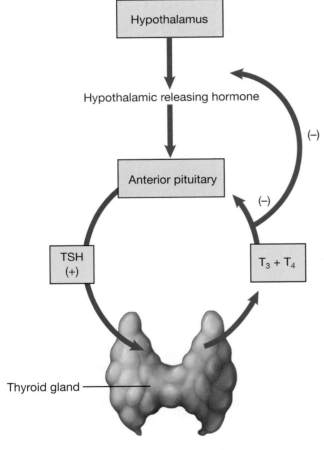

B. Regulation of thyroid hormone release

Figure 8.8 The thyroid gland. A—The thyroid gland is located below the larynx and above the trachea. B—The thyroid gland produces thyroid hormone when signaled by the hypothalamus and anterior pituitary. *Which hormones provide negative feedback to the anterior pituitary and hypothalamus?*

discuss the implications of an iodine deficiency in lesson 8.3.

Every cell in the body is affected by thyroid hormone because every living cell needs energy to survive. Thyroid hormone also plays a vital role in growth, development, and maturation.

Regulation of Thyroid Hormone Release. The release of thyroid hormone is controlled by the hypothalamus (**Figure 8.8B**). Hypothalamic releasing hormones signal the anterior pituitary to release thyroid-stimulating hormone (TSH). TSH triggers secretion of T_3 and T_4 by the thyroid gland. The increased levels of circulating T_3 and T_4 trigger a negative feedback loop, inhibiting further release of hormones from the hypothalamus (hypothalamic releasing hormone) and pituitary glands.

Calcitonin

Calcitonin is produced and released by the parafollicular cells of the thyroid gland. The parafollicular cells are located between the follicular cells in the connective tissue of the thyroid. Calcium homeostasis is maintained by calcitonin and *parathyroid hormone* (*PTH*), which is produced by the parathyroid glands.

When blood calcium levels rise, the thyroid gland releases calcitonin. Calcitonin causes calcium in the blood to be deposited and absorbed into the bone. As a result, blood calcium levels decrease. Calcitonin also reduces the absorption of calcium by the intestines and kidneys.

Once we reach adulthood and our bones are fully developed, very little (if any) calcitonin is released by the thyroid gland.

Parathyroid Glands

The **parathyroid glands** are two pairs of glands located on the posterior aspect of the thyroid gland. These four tiny glands (each is the size of a grain of rice) secrete parathyroid hormone (PTH) in response to low blood calcium levels. Parathyroid hormone increases blood calcium levels in three ways:

1. by stimulating breakdown of bone tissues by osteoclasts, thus moving calcium from the bone into the blood

2. by increasing calcium absorption in the intestines with the aid of vitamin D during digestion

3. by stimulating kidney resorption of calcium from urine and excreting phosphorus

Figure 8.9 illustrates the regulation of blood calcium levels by both PTH and calcitonin.

Thymus Gland

The **thymus gland** is both an endocrine gland and a lymphatic organ. It lies under the sternum, anterior to the heart. During childhood, the thymus gland is quite large, but it becomes smaller as we age. At the onset of puberty, the thymus begins to shrink; by adulthood, it is barely visible.

The thymus secretes *thymosin* (THIGH-muh-sin), a hormone essential for the development of white blood cells called *T lymphocytes*, or *T cells*. T cells play a key role in the body's immune system.

Pineal Gland

The **pineal** (PI-nee-al) **gland** is a pinecone-shaped gland in the brain. Its exact function remains unclear. However, we do know that when the body is exposed to darkness, the pineal gland releases the hormone *melatonin*, causing us to feel sleepy. Melatonin levels are highest at night.

Adrenal Glands

As **Figure 8.10** on the next page shows, the **adrenal glands** are a pair of glands that sit on top of the kidneys. The adrenal glands are actually two organs: the **adrenal cortex** functions as a gland, whereas the **adrenal medulla** is part of the nervous system.

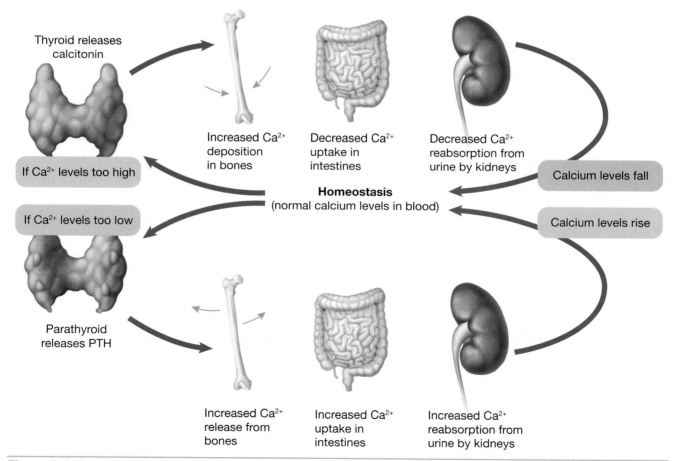

Thyroid releases calcitonin

Increased Ca²⁺ deposition in bones

Decreased Ca²⁺ uptake in intestines

Decreased Ca²⁺ reabsorption from urine by kidneys

Calcium levels fall

If Ca²⁺ levels too high

Homeostasis
(normal calcium levels in blood)

Calcium levels rise

If Ca²⁺ levels too low

Parathyroid releases PTH

Increased Ca²⁺ release from bones

Increased Ca²⁺ uptake in intestines

Increased Ca²⁺ reabsorption from urine by kidneys

Figure 8.9 The thyroid and parathyroid glands act together to maintain healthy blood calcium levels. *Which thyroid hormone is responsible for maintaining homeostatic blood calcium levels?*

Figure 8.10 The adrenal glands are located on top of both kidneys. The adrenal cortex (outer layer) is divided into three layers. The inner layer is the adrenal medulla. *Hormones released by the adrenal medulla are integral in initiating an "adrenaline rush". What is another name for this response?*

The adrenal cortex makes up the outer layer of each adrenal gland. The adrenal cortex itself comprises three layers that secrete three steroid hormones. The inner layer, the adrenal medulla, is stimulated by the sympathetic branch of the autonomic nervous system (ANS).

Hormones of the Adrenal Medulla

In lesson 8.1 we discussed the fight-or-flight response. This response occurs when the adrenal medulla secretes two hormones—epinephrine (commonly referred to as *adrenaline*) and norepinephrine (also known as *noradrenalin*). Epinephrine and norepinephrine are both *catecholamines* (kat-eh-KOH-la-meens), hormones released into the blood during times of physical or emotional stress.

The body's response to increased catecholamine levels is called an "adrenaline rush." The telltale signs of an adrenaline rush include increased heart rate, blood pressure, and breathing. In addition, changes that we cannot feel are occurring within the body. For example, blood flow is shunted to the heart, and our muscles prepare us to fight or take flight. Increases in metabolic rate and glucose production by the liver make more energy available for the potential brush with danger.

Hormones of the Adrenal Cortex

The adrenal cortex produces three groups of steroid hormones—*mineralocorticoids* (min-eh-ra-loh-KORT-i-koids), *glucocorticoids* (gloo-koh-KORT-i-koids), and *sex hormones*. Steroid

Memory Tip
The three substances regulated by the hormones of the adrenal cortex all start with an *S*—**S**odium, **S**ugar, and **S**ex hormones.

hormones are made from cholesterol and are lipid soluble (that is, they can dissolve in lipids).

The anterior pituitary controls the release of *corticoid hormones*—hormones of the adrenal cortex. Many of these hormones are vital to our survival, so a decrease in their production can be life threatening. These three types of hormones regulate sodium (mineralocorticoids), sugar (glucocorticoids), and sex hormone levels in the body.

Mineralocorticoids. The principal mineralocorticoid hormone is *aldosterone* (al-DAHS-ter-ohn). Aldosterone stimulates the kidneys to reabsorb sodium and water from urine and to eliminate potassium. It also plays a major role in blood pressure regulation and plasma levels. When sodium and water are reabsorbed by the kidneys, plasma volumes increase, raising blood pressure. Aldosterone also regulates concentration of blood electrolytes, such as sodium and potassium.

Glucocorticoids. The main glucocorticoid hormones, *cortisone* (KOR-ti-sohn) and *cortisol* (KORT-i-sahl), maintain blood glucose levels by converting fats and amino acids into glucose via gluconeogenesis. This ensures that the brain and nervous system have a constant supply of glucose, their only fuel source.

Sex Hormones. The adrenal cortex produces small amounts of female sex hormones (*estrogens*) and male sex hormones (*androgens*). However, most sex hormones secreted by the adrenal cortex are androgens, primarily *testosterone*.

The reproductive organs also produce sex hormones. The effects of sex hormones produced by the reproductive organs (discussed in Chapter 15: The Male and Female Reproductive Systems) usually mask the effects of sex hormones produced by the adrenal cortex. This is because the reproductive organs secrete higher volumes of hormones earlier in our lives. As we age, the reproductive organs secrete smaller quantities of sex hormones. The adrenal cortex, however, continues to produce the same amount of sex hormones; the effects of these hormones can become more noticeable with age. For example, because the adrenal cortex secretes

high quantities of androgen, some females develop facial hair and other masculine traits.

Check Your Understanding

1. Which two hormones are secreted by the thyroid gland?
2. Which chemical element found in certain foods is necessary for thyroid hormone production?
3. How does parathyroid hormone increase blood calcium levels?
4. Where is the thymus gland located?
5. Which component of the adrenal gland is actually part of the nervous system?

Pancreas

The **pancreas** is a long, thin gland located posterior to the stomach in the upper part of the abdominal cavity. It functions as an endocrine gland by secreting hormones that control blood glucose levels. The pancreas also functions as an exocrine gland that excretes digestive enzymes. You will learn more about the exocrine function of the pancreas in Chapter 13: The Digestive System and Nutrition.

The hormone-secreting cells of the pancreas are called the *islets* (IGH-lets) *of Langerhans* (LAHNG-er-hahnz). The islets of Langerhans are composed of *alpha cells* that secrete glucagon, which increases blood glucose levels, and *beta cells* that secrete insulin, which lowers blood glucose levels. Together, the alpha and beta cells work together to maintain blood glucose levels between the normal range of 70 and 105 mg/dL.

Regulation of blood glucose levels by the pancreas is shown in **Figure 8.11** on the next page. When blood glucose level is high (after a meal, for example), the pancreas secretes insulin to lower blood glucose level.

Insulin targets almost every cell in the body and promotes glucose uptake by cells. Once inside a cell, glucose is used for cellular energy. Insulin is essential for providing life-sustaining energy and health because it is the only hormone capable of getting glucose into the body cells.

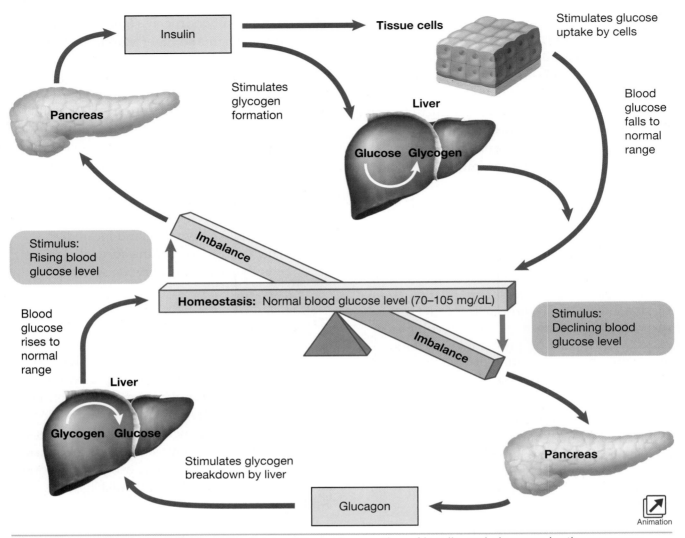

Figure 8.11 Blood glucose levels are maintained through secretion of insulin and glucagon by the pancreas. *What is the homeostatic set point for blood glucose levels?*

Insulin also stimulates the liver to convert excess glucose as glycogen, or fat.

Glucagon has the opposite effect of insulin. When blood glucose level is low, for example, the pancreas secretes glucagon, which increases blood glucose. Glucagon secretion is achieved primarily through gluconeogenesis. Other hormones can raise blood glucose level, but glucagon is the most effective.

Gonads

Gonads are sex glands. In men, gonads are called **testes**; in women, they are called **ovaries**.

The paired, oval testes are encased by the **scrotum**, a sac located outside the body. The testes produce sperm and androgen hormones such as testosterone. Testosterone is responsible for sperm production, development of the male reproductive system, and the emergence of male secondary sex characteristics during puberty. The testes release testosterone when they are stimulated by luteinizing hormone (LH) from the anterior pituitary gland.

The ovaries, which are located inside the female pelvic cavity, produce eggs and the hormones estrogen and *progesterone* (proh-JES-teh-rohn). Estrogen plays a key role in the development of the female reproductive glands and secondary sex characteristics. Along with progesterone, estrogen regulates the menstrual cycle and promotes breast development.

Other Hormones

Hormones are produced by other tissues in the body, such as adipose (fatty) tissue and tissues that line the heart, stomach, and intestines. For example, the kidneys secrete erythropoietin (eh-RITH-roh-POY-eh-tin), a hormone that stimulates red blood cell production. Fatty tissue secretes prostaglandins (prahs-tuh-GLAN-dins), which act at, or near, the site of production. Prostaglandins regulate the smooth muscle cells that line the blood vessels and respiratory passages, stimulate the muscles of the uterus, and activate the inflammatory response. In addition, adipose cells produce the hormone leptin, which suppresses appetite and increases energy production.

Lesson 8.2 Review and Assessment

Mini Glossary   Make sure that you know the meaning of each key term.

 Build vocabulary with e-flash cards and games

adrenal cortex   outer layer of the adrenal glands, which itself has three layers that secrete steroid hormones

adrenal glands   a pair of glands that sit on top of the kidneys; consist of the adrenal cortex and adrenal medulla

adrenal medulla   the part of the adrenal glands that functions as a part of the nervous system; it secretes the hormones epinephrine and norepinephrine (catecholamines) during the fight-or-flight response

anterior pituitary   one lobe of the pituitary gland that secretes six different hormones: growth hormone, prolactin, adrenocorticotropin hormone, thyroid-stimulating hormone, follicle-stimulating hormone, and luteinizing hormone

ovaries   the female sex glands

pancreas   a long, thin gland located posterior to the stomach. As an endocrine gland, the pancreas secretes insulin and glucagon, which control blood glucose levels; as an exocrine gland, the pancreas secretes digestive enzymes

parathyroid glands   two pairs of glands located on the posterior aspect of the thyroid gland that secrete parathyroid hormone in response to low blood calcium levels

pineal gland   a pinecone-shaped gland in the brain that releases the sleep-inducing hormone melatonin

pituitary gland   a pea-sized gland that activates a metabolic response in target tissues or stimulates other endocrine glands to release hormones

posterior pituitary   one lobe of the pituitary gland that stores two hormones produced by the hypothalamus: antidiuretic hormone and oxytocin

scrotum   a sac that encases the pair of oval testes

testes   the male sex glands

thymus gland   a gland that secretes thymosin, a hormone vital to the body's immune system; functions as both an endocrine gland and a lymphatic organ

thyroid gland   gland located below the larynx, or *Adam's apple*, that secretes thyroid hormones (T_3 and T_4) and calcitonin

tropic hormones   pituitary hormones that act on other endocrine glands; tropins

Know and Understand

Assess

1. Which tropic hormones are secreted by the anterior pituitary gland?
2. Which hormones are secreted when TSH acts on the thyroid gland?
3. What is the purpose of gluconeogenesis?
4. What two functions does prolactin play in a mother nursing an infant?
5. Which two hormones regulate the female menstrual cycle?

Analyze and Apply

6. Compare and contrast the adrenal cortex and the adrenal medulla.

7. Explain why the thyroid hormone affects all cells in the body.
8. Describe the regulation of calcium in the body.

In the Lab

9. Lena, a 70-year-old woman, visits her doctor because she is concerned about the slight appearance of facial hair. Explain why it is not unusual for older women to develop masculine traits.
10. Create a mock profile of an endocrine gland on your favorite social media site. Include the following: a brief summary of what it is, where it resides, what type of work it does, and who its friends are. Share your profile with the class.

Lesson 8.3 Endocrine Disorders and Diseases

Before You Read

Try to answer the following questions before you read this lesson.

What effect does an overactive thyroid gland have on the body?

What is the difference between diabetes mellitus and diabetes insipidus?

Lesson Objectives

1. Describe the following disorders of the pituitary gland: acromegaly, dwarfism, and diabetes insipidus.

2. Discuss the difference between hypothyroidism and hyperthyroidism. Name the disorders associated with each.

3. Identify disorders and diseases of the parathyroid and adrenal glands.

4. Identify the cause, symptoms, and treatment plan for someone with Cushing's syndrome.

5. Explain the difference between type I and type II diabetes mellitus.

Key Terms

E-Flash Cards

acromegaly	hypothyroidism
Addison's disease	insulin resistance
Cushing's syndrome	myxedema
diabetes insipidus	neonatal
diabetes mellitus	hypothyroidism
dwarfism	peripheral neuropathy
goiter	tetany
Graves disease	thyroiditis
hypercalcemia	type I diabetes mellitus
hyperglycemia	type II diabetes mellitus
hyperthyroidism	

Because the endocrine system is hierarchical in nature, many of its glands depend upon one another yet also act independently. Therefore, when an endocrine gland is not functioning properly, the effects of its malfunction can be felt throughout the body or at a specific site. In this lesson we will learn about some common disorders and diseases of the endocrine system.

Pituitary Disorders

The pituitary gland—divided into the anterior and posterior pituitary—releases many important hormones. Thus, a hypofunctioning (underactive) or hyperfunctioning (overactive) pituitary gland can have widespread effects.

Hyperfunction of the Pituitary Gland

Hyperfunction of the pituitary occurs when the gland secretes excessive amounts of a specific hormone. One of the most common disorders caused by hyperfunction of the pituitary is acromegaly (ak-roh-MEG-a-lee).

Acromegaly. When the anterior pituitary hypersecretes growth hormone, the result is a rare condition called **acromegaly**, or *gigantism*. Acromegaly causes an increase in overall body size, especially in the extremities.

Acromegaly is usually caused by a noncancerous tumor pressing on the pituitary gland. Pressure from the tumor can cause headaches, vision disturbances or loss of vision, seizures, and fatigue. This disorder most often affects middle-aged adults, but it may also affect children. In children, acromegaly causes unusually tall height, large hands, and large feet. In adults, acromegaly causes thickened bones and enlarged facial features, hands, and feet. Diagnosis of acromegaly in adults may take years because its effects appear gradually.

Treatment of acromegaly includes medications to shrink the tumor and decrease GH levels. Surgery may be performed to remove the tumor if it is operable. As you learned in the chapter introduction, surgeons may operate on a patient using a radiation beam, or gamma knife, when a tumor is located in a hard-to-reach place. Although medications and surgery will stop excessive growth, the effects of acromegaly cannot be reversed. Unfortunately, the strain that acromegaly places on the body often leads to a shortened life span.

Hypofunction of the Pituitary Gland

Hypofunction of the pituitary gland occurs when the pituitary gland secretes inadequate amounts of hormones. Hypofunction of the pituitary can cause several disorders, including dwarfism and diabetes insipidus.

Dwarfism. Hyposecretion of GH by the pituitary gland can cause **dwarfism**, a condition in which adult height reaches less than four feet (**Figure 8.12**). Dwarfism affects only a person's physical size; intellectual ability is normal.

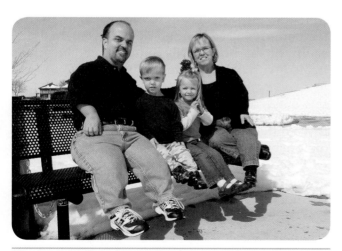

Figure 8.12 People who have a condition called dwarfism prefer to be referred to as "little people." *What is the impact of dwarfism on a person's intellectual abilities?*

Dwarfism may be congenital (acquired during development in the uterus). It can also be caused by brain injury or a medical condition, such as growth hormone deficiency. When diagnosed at an early age, dwarfism is usually treated with supplemental growth hormones.

Diabetes Insipidus. Hyposecretion of antidiuretic hormone from the posterior pituitary causes **diabetes insipidus**. ADH normally targets the kidneys, causing them to reabsorb water from urine. ADH deficiency can cause a large loss of water and electrolytes. People with diabetes insipidus experience excessive thirst, or *polydipsia* (pahl-i-DIP-see-a).

Diabetes insipidus is different from diabetes mellitus (MEL-it-uhs), a pancreatic disorder commonly referred to as *diabetes*, which we will learn about later in this lesson.

Thyroid Disorders

In lesson 8.2, we learned that the thyroid gland secretes thyroxine (T_4) and triiodothyronine (T_3), hormones that control the metabolism of every living cell in our bodies. When inadequate or excessive levels of these hormones are secreted, the result is a thyroid disorder.

Hyperthyroidism

Hyperthyroidism, or an *overactive thyroid*, is characterized by a visibly enlarged thyroid gland in the neck (**Figure 8.13**). An enlarged thyroid is called a **goiter** (GOY-ter). A goiter is caused by insufficient amounts of iodine, a chemical element necessary for the production of thyroid hormones, or by thyroid disorders.

Iodine is not produced by the body, so it is important that we eat foods containing iodine. This is one of the reasons that most countries, including the United States, add iodine to salt. An overactive thyroid works hard to secrete hormones, but without iodine from the diet, production of thyroid hormones is impaired.

Low levels of the hormones T_3 and T_4 cannot complete the negative feedback loop to "turn off" the hypothalamus and the pituitary glands. As a result, the hypothalamus and pituitary thyroid gland. A tumor on the thyroid gland causes oversecretion of the thyroid hormones.

Graves disease also causes the eyes to bulge outward, a condition called *exophthalmos* (EK-sahf-THAL-muhs). This may make it difficult or impossible to close the eyelid, which can lead to drying and scarring of the cornea. Loss of vision may result from this condition.

Hypothyroidism

Hypothyroidism, or *underactive thyroid*, is usually caused by **thyroiditis**, the result of inflammation that damages thyroid cells. Thyroiditis can be caused by the immune system attacking the thyroid, a cold, a respiratory infection, an inflammation that occurs after pregnancy (postpartum thyroiditis), or prescription drugs.

Hypothyroidism is most common in women and in people above 50 years of age. Symptoms of the disorder include fatigue, pale and dry skin, thin hair, brittle fingernails, increased sensitivity to cold temperatures, constipation, and weight gain. Treatment involves replacing the T_3 and T_4 hormones through supplemental hormone therapy. Most people with hypothyroidism will need lifelong supplemental hormone therapy to manage their disease.

Myxedema. Adults with hypothyroidism that goes undiagnosed or untreated will develop **myxedema** (MIKS-eh-DEE-ma). Myxedema is a severe form of hypothyroidism that causes weight gain; a swollen, puffy face; low body temperature; dry skin; and decreased mental acuity, or sharpness. This condition can be treated with an oral form of thyroxine.

Neonatal Hypothyroidism. Newborn children can develop **neonatal hypothyroidism**. This thyroid deficiency may develop congenitally (before birth) or soon after birth. Often, children with neonatal hypothyroidism have a poorly developed thyroid gland or ineffective thyroid hormones.

Untreated neonatal hypothyroidism can lead to mental and physical disability. Dull, dry skin and dry, brittle hair are also common. Early diagnosis is key because the effects of this disorder can be reversed. Like myxedema, neonatal hypothyroidism is treated with oral thyroxine.

Figure 8.13 This woman has a goiter, a result of insufficient iodine levels or thyroid disorders. A goiter may cause difficulty breathing and swallowing, as well as a cough. *How can large goiters be treated?*

gland continue to produce thyroid-releasing hormone and thyroid-stimulating hormone.

TSH causes the thyroid gland to enlarge. Increased heart rate, elevated body temperature, hyperactivity, weight loss, diarrhea, and difficulty concentrating are other side effects of hyperthyroidism.

Other causes of hyperthyroidism include noncancerous growths on the thyroid or inflammation of the thyroid gland. Treatments for hyperthyroidism include surgery to remove part, or all, of the thyroid gland or tumor, radioactive iodine to destroy thyroid cells, and thyroid drugs to reduce thyroid hormones.

Graves Disease. The most common cause of hyperthyroidism is **Graves disease**, an autoimmune disorder that leads to an overactive

Check Your Understanding

1. Which condition results from hypofunction of the pituitary gland?
2. Which endocrine disorder is caused by an ADH deficiency?
3. What is an enlarged thyroid gland called?
4. Which thyroid disorder causes exophthalmos?
5. How is myxedema treated?

Disorders of the Parathyroid Gland

In lesson 8.2, we learned that the parathyroid glands secrete parathyroid hormone and the thyroid gland secretes calcitonin. These hormones work together to regulate blood calcium levels.

Hypercalcemia. Hypersecretion of PTH causes too much calcium in the blood, a condition known as **hypercalcemia** (HIGH-per-kal-SEE-mee-a). Hypercalcemia leads to increased calcium absorption by the kidneys. The excess calcium in the kidneys, along with changes in the bones (which develop holes and become brittle), causes kidney stones to form. Hypercalcemia can also affect the nervous and cardiovascular systems, causing depression, decreased heart rate, and fatigue.

Hypocalcemia. Hypocalcemia (HIGH-poh-kal-SEE-mee-a), or low blood calcium, leads to unstable nerve and muscle membranes that continuously fire electrical signals. The result is a condition of sustained muscular contraction known as **tetany** (TET-a-nee). If left untreated, tetany can affect the respiratory muscles, leading to asphyxiation and death. Treatment for hypocalcemia includes PTH replacement therapy, vitamin D, and calcium. Blood tests to monitor calcium levels are also helpful in managing this disease.

Adrenal Medulla Disorders

In rare cases, individuals develop a tumor on the adrenal medulla called a *pheochromocytoma* (FEE-oh-KROH-moh-sigh-TOH-ma). A pheochromocytoma causes the adrenal medulla to hypersecrete the hormones epinephrine and norepinephrine.

High amounts of epinephrine and norepeinephrine in the bloodstream can produce life-threatening results: high blood pressure, rapid heart rate, weight loss, nervousness, and sleep disturbances. These symptoms are experienced intermittently (from time to time) and usually resolve within 15 to 20 minutes. Pheochromcytoma is diagnosed through an abdominal CT or MRI scan, catecholamine tests of blood or urine, or an adrenal biopsy. Treatment involves immediate lowering of blood pressure through prescription or IV medications and the removal of the tumor.

Disorders of the Adrenal Cortex

As with other disorders of the endocrine system, disorders of the adrenal cortex can result from any number of factors. Tumorous growths on the adrenal gland can cause an adrenal cortex disorder. Another cause of adrenal cortex disorders is irregular secretion of hormones from other glands that act on the adrenal cortex. Finally, the hyposecretion or hypersecretion of adrenal cortex hormones can cause a disorder in the body. Let's examine some common disorders of the adrenal cortex.

Cushing's Syndrome

Cushing's syndrome is a disorder of the adrenal cortex caused by hypersecretion of cortisol. This syndrome can be caused by

- oversecretion of adrenocorticotropin hormone (ACTH) by the pituitary gland, which stimulates hypersecretion of cortisol by the adrenal cortex;
- a tumor on the adrenal gland that stimulates hypersecretion of cortisol; or
- prolonged use of steroid drugs, such as those prescribed to treat arthritis and other autoimmune disorders. Steroid drugs can suppress the release of ACTH, thus preventing the production of cortisol.

Overproduction of cortisol causes many symptoms including a rounded, moon-shaped face; weight gain (especially in the upper body); high blood glucose levels; hypertension; osteoporosis; reddish-purple abdominal stretch marks; difficulty concentrating; and facial hair in women (**Figure 8.14**).

Cushing's syndrome is diagnosed by measuring cortisol levels in the saliva each morning or by obtaining a 24-hour urine collection sample. Treatment of Cushing's syndrome caused by a tumor includes surgical removal of the tumor.

It is important to exercise caution when taking steroid drugs. Prolonged use of a steroid drug, whether for illness or to enhance athletic performance, can inhibit the release of ACTH by the anterior pituitary, leading to a lack of cortisol. This puts a patient at risk for developing Cushing's syndrome. Therefore, it is very important that patients be slowly weaned from steroid drugs, giving the anterior pituitary time to begin producing ACTH again.

Athletes who use anabolic steroids often suffer numerous and long-lasting effects, including decreased heart function, elevated blood pressure, liver damage, premature bone plate closures, aggression, depression, impotence or decreased sperm count in males, and menstrual cycle abnormalities in females.

Addison's Disease

Hyposecretion of adrenal corticoid hormones can cause **Addison's disease**, which produces muscle atrophy, a bronze skin tone, low blood pressure, and kidney damage. Other symptoms include excessive levels of potassium in the blood; hypoglycemia (HIGH-poh-glih-SEE-mee-a); severe loss of fluids and electrolytes (especially sodium); and a general feeling of weakness. Addison's disease is life threatening because it can lead to low blood volume, electrolyte disturbances, or shock. Treatment for Addison's disease includes hormone replacement therapy.

Check Your Understanding

1. What causes the formation of kidney stones in people with hypercalcemia?
2. What is the cause of Cushing's syndrome?
3. What are the possible consequences of prolonged anabolic steroid use?

The Pancreas and Diabetes Mellitus

In lesson 8.1 we learned that the pancreas secretes two hormones that regulate blood glucose levels—insulin and glucagon. **Diabetes mellitus (DM)** is characterized by the body's inability to produce sufficient amounts of insulin to regulate blood glucose levels. There are two types of diabetes—**type I diabetes mellitus**, or *juvenile onset diabetes*, and **type II diabetes mellitus**, or *adult-onset diabetes*.

Figure 8.14 Cushing's syndrome is characterized by a rounded face and reddish complexion. *Which hormone is hypersecreted in a person who develops Cushing's syndrome?*

In the United States, 90% to 95% of diabetes cases are type II; the remaining 5% to 10% are type I. This disease is so common that almost everyone knows someone with diabetes. In 2010, the National Institutes of Health (NIH) reported that approximately 27% of adults 65 years of age and older were diabetic, and the numbers were rising. Diabetes is the seventh leading cause of death in the United States. It is also the leading cause of kidney failure, nontraumatic lower limb amputation, and new cases of blindness. Diabetes is also a major contributor to heart disease and stroke.

Symptoms and Diagnosis of Diabetes Mellitus

Diabetes mellitus is diagnosed through a fasting *blood glucose test*, a *glucose tolerance test*, and the *HbA1c test*, or *glycosylated* (gligh-koh-sih-LAY-tehd) *hemoglobin test*.

- Blood glucose test—a blood glucose level of 126 mg/dL or higher after an eight-hour fast is considered positive for diabetes.
- Glucose tolerance test—in this oral glucose tolerance test, a person's blood glucose level is measured two hours after drinking a liquid that contains 75 grams of glucose, or sugar. A blood glucose level of 200 mg/dL or greater is in the diabetic range.
- HbA1c test—this test measures average blood glucose levels over a three-month period. A glucose level of 5.6% or less is normal, 5.7%–6.4% is prediabetic, and 6.5% or greater indicates diabetes.

Generally, a family history of diabetes mellitus or symptom onset prompts people to be tested for this disorder. The primary symptoms of diabetes include

- *polyuria* (pahl-ee-YOOR-ee-a)—excessive urination to eliminate glucose;
- *polydipsia*—excessive thirst to replenish water lost through polyuria; and
- *polyphagia* (pahl-ee-FAY-jee-a)—increased hunger to replace fats and proteins used by the body as fuel sources.

Other symptoms of diabetes may include unexplained weight loss or gain, blurred vision, nausea, and slow-healing wounds.

Type I Diabetes Mellitus

Type I diabetes mellitus is an autoimmune disorder in which the immune system attacks and kills the insulin-secreting beta cells of the pancreas. Destruction of these cells causes insulin production to decrease or stop altogether. As a result, blood glucose levels rise from their normal circulating levels of 70–105 mg/dL to dangerously high levels exceeding 500 mg/dL.

Type I diabetics receive insulin through several injections over the course of a day. Insulin dosage levels are based on self-administered blood glucose checks. If blood glucose levels are high, a higher insulin dose is administered; if blood glucose levels are low, less insulin is taken (**Figure 8.15**). Type I diabetics may regulate their blood glucose levels through an externally worn insulin pump that continuously monitors glucose and delivers appropriate dosages of insulin.

It's unclear what causes the immune system to attack the insulin-secreting beta cells of the pancreas. However, we do know that type I diabetes mellitus is a hereditary condition. People with this disorder are usually diagnosed at a young age.

Type II Diabetes Mellitus

In people with type II diabetes, the pancreas secretes insulin, but the body's insulin receptors

Boscorelli/Shutterstock.com

Figure 8.15 Diabetics use a device called a glucometer to monitor fluctuations in their blood glucose levels. *If a glucometer shows a high blood glucose level, what action should a diabetic take?*

WHAT RESEARCH TELLS US

...*about* Managing Diabetes with Diet and Exercise

Diabetes mellitus has reached epidemic proportions in the United States, largely because of the increased rate of obesity and lack of physical activity. The NIH estimates that there are about 57 million prediabetic cases among people 20 years of age and older in the United States.

Recently, a study of 3,000 diabetic and prediabetic people investigated the effect of a low-fat diet and 30 minutes of moderately intense exercise five days a week (**Figure 8.16**). Most of the study participants chose walking as their exercise activity, and the results were dramatic. On average, participants lost 5% to 7% of their

Dotshock/Shutterstock.com

Figure 8.16 Regular exercise can decrease a person's risk of developing diabetes mellitus.

body weight. These two simple but effective lifestyle changes reduced

the incidence of type II diabetes in the sample group by nearly 60%.

Taking It Further

1. With a partner, discuss other health benefits of a diet low in fat and calories and a regular exercise routine. How might a healthful diet and regular exercise benefit people with diseases that you have learned about in other chapters of this book?

2. Why do you think obesity has reached epidemic proportions in the United States? Brainstorm ways in which our society can combat this problem.

---

are downregulated—a condition called **insulin resistance**. Insulin-resistant receptors won't take up glucose even when insulin is present, so blood glucose levels become elevated, a condition known as **hyperglycemia**. When glucose builds up in the blood, it is absorbed by the kidneys and excreted in urine.

It is unclear what causes the body's cells to become insulin resistant but we do know that insulin resistance is associated with obesity, physical inactivity, family history of diabetes, and old age. In fact, the NIH estimates that 80% of type II diabetics are overweight or obese.

Although large amounts of glucose are available in the body for energy production, diabetics are unable to use this glucose because insulin is unavailable or the body's cells are insulin resistant. When the body's cells are unable to use glucose as a fuel source, fats and proteins must be used instead.

Using fats for fuel produces ketone bodies that decrease the pH of the blood, making it

dangerously acidic. This condition is called *ketoacidosis* (keet-oh-as-i-DOH-sis). If left untreated, ketoacidosis can lead to diabetic coma and death. People with ketosis—high levels of ketones in the body—also have fruity-smelling breath because of the presence of acetone.

If adopting a healthful diet and getting adequate exercise are not sufficient for managing type II diabetes mellitus, oral hypoglycemic agents or injectable insulin are available.

Living with Diabetes Mellitus

Patient education is very important for diabetic care. People with diabetes who develop **peripheral neuropathy** (noo-RAHP-a-thee), which causes loss of feeling in the extremities, must take particularly good care of their feet. As a result, diabetics may be unaware when they get a cut or wound on their foot. Unnoticed cuts or wounds can become infected. Severely infected wounds often result in amputation of the affected limb.

There is no known cure for diabetes mellitus. Since there is no cure, the goal for patients is learning how to successfully manage this disorder. The cornerstones of managing diabetes mellitus are a healthful diet, physical activity to increase insulin sensitivity of the body's cells, weight loss, and taking medications as prescribed.

Lesson 8.3 Review and Assessment

Mini Glossary   Make sure that you know the meaning of each key term.

 Build vocabulary with e-flash cards and games

acromegaly   a rare condition in which the anterior pituitary hypersecretes growth hormone, causing an increase in overall body size; gigantism

Addison's disease   a condition caused by hyposecretion of adrenal corticoid hormones that causes muscle atrophy, a bronze skin tone, low blood pressure, kidney damage, hypoglycemia, severe loss of fluids and electrolytes, and a general feeling of weakness

Cushing's syndrome   a disorder of the adrenal cortex caused by hypersecretion of cortisol; symptoms include weight gain, high blood glucose levels, hypertension, and osteoporosis

diabetes insipidus   a disorder resulting from hyposecretion of antidiuretic hormone (ADH) by the posterior pituitary

diabetes mellitus   a disease that results from the body's inability to produce sufficient amounts of insulin to regulate blood glucose levels

dwarfism   a condition in which the pituitary gland hyposecretes growth hormone, resulting in an adult height of less than four feet

goiter   an enlarged thyroid gland caused by insufficient amounts of iodine or a thyroid disorder

Graves disease   an autoimmune disorder that causes an overactive thyroid gland and outward bulging of the eyes

hypercalcemia   a condition caused by the hypersecretion of parathyroid hormone (PTH), leading to increased blood calcium levels and increased calcium absorption by the kidneys

hyperglycemia   a condition in which blood glucose levels become elevated

hyperthyroidism   a condition characterized by a visibly enlarged thyroid gland in the neck; *overactive thyroid gland*

hypothyroidism   a condition caused by an underactive thyroid gland

insulin resistance   a condition common in type II diabetes in which the pancreas secretes insulin, but the body's insulin receptors are downregulated, causing elevated blood glucose levels

myxedema   a condition in adults with hyperthyroidism that causes weight gain; a swollen, puffy face; low body temperature; dry skin; and decreased mental acuity

neonatal hypothyroidism   hypothyroidism that occurs in infants and children; may develop congenitally or following birth

peripheral neuropathy   a disease or degenerative state of the peripheral nerves often associated with diabetes mellitus; marked by muscle weakness and atrophy, pain, and numbness

tetany   a condition of sustained muscular contraction

thyroiditis   inflammation of the thyroid gland

type I diabetes mellitus   juvenile-onset diabetes

type II diabetes mellitus   adult-onset diabetes

Know and Understand

 Assess

1. What causes diabetes insipidus?
2. Why are goiters uncommon in the United States today?
3. What are the symptoms of hypothyroidism?
4. Which disease is caused by the hyposecretion of adrenal corticoid hormones?
5. Which tests are used to diagnose diabetes mellitus?

Analyze and Apply

6. Compare and contrast type I and type II diabetes mellitus.
7. Why does hypercalcemia cause brittle bones?

In the Lab

8. Dominick, a 37-year-old male, has developed type II diabetes mellitus. Dominick is 5 feet, 8 inches tall and weighs 300 pounds. Make a list of questions that you would ask Dominick if you were counseling him about beneficial lifestyle changes. Also, make a list of guidelines that would help Dominick manage his disease.
9. Create a time line for a day in the life of a high school student with type I diabetes mellitus. Use text and images to describe the day's events. Pay special attention to how often the student checks her glucose levels, and determine how she receives insulin.

The organs and hormones of the endocrine system have wide-ranging effects on the body. Many careers require highly specific or general knowledge of this complex body system. We will explore two occupations involving work with patients who have endocrine system disorders and diseases: endocrinologist and physician assistant.

Endocrinologists use their advanced knowledge of the endocrine system to diagnose and treat hormonal imbalances and diseases. Physician assistants treat patients in a variety of settings and circumstances; thus, they need a broad understanding of the body.

Endocrinologist

Endocrinologists (EHN-doh-kri-NAHL-uh-jists) are medical doctors who specialize in the treatment of hormone imbalances with the goal of restoring hormonal activity to normal, homeostatic levels (**Figure 8.17**). Disorders commonly treated by endocrinologists include diabetes mellitus, obesity, osteoporosis, thyroid disorders, infertility, and other endocrine system disorders. Many of these disorders can affect other body systems, so a comprehensive understanding of human biology and anatomy and physiology is a must for endocrinologists.

Blaj Gabriel/Shutterstock.com

Figure 8.17 Endocrinologists work to diagnose and treat hormonal disorders.

Extensive education, beyond a four-year bachelor's degree in biology or a related field, is required to become an endocrinologist. After four years of medical school, future endocrinologists spend three to four years at an internship, or residency in internal medicine. The internship culminates with a two- to three-year fellowship spent focusing on hormone conditions and diseases.

Endocrinologists typically work in hospitals, private practices, or medical research facilities. They work closely with patients to diagnose and establish treatment plans for endocrine system diseases.

Physician Assistant

Physician assistants (PAs) practice medicine under the direction and observation of physicians and surgeons. Although they are formally trained to examine and treat patients, physician assistants do not attend medical school. Physician assistants diagnose and treat injuries and illnesses, take patients' medical histories, order and interpret test results, and give vaccinations. In some states they are allowed to write prescriptions. One example of the difference between a physician assistant and a doctor is that a physician assistant may perform the "prep" work on a patient right before surgery (making the opening incision) but a doctor performs the surgery.

To become a physician assistant, candidates must earn a bachelor's degree that includes coursework in biology, chemistry, anatomy and physiology, and other science-based courses. PAs must also complete an accredited two- to three-year physician assistant master's program and pass a national licensing exam.

PAs work in hospitals, clinics, emergency rooms, surgery centers, private physicians' offices, and schools. PAs may treat patients when a doctor is unavailable—for example, during house calls, nursing homes visits, or rural or inner-city clinics that a doctor might not visit daily (**Figure. 8.18**). In these circumstances, PAs communicate with the supervising physician on staff or other medical personnel as necessary, or as required by law.

Planning for a Health-Related Career

Do some research on the career of a physician assistant or an endocrinologist. Keep in mind that many practice specialties are available to endocrinologists. Some endocrinologists may focus on researching and treating one disease in particular—for example diabetes mellitus or thyroid disorders.

Otherwise, choose a profession from the list of **Related Career Options**. Using the Internet or resources at your local library, find answers to the following questions:

1. What are the main tasks and responsibilities of this job?
2. What is the outlook for this career? Are workers in demand, or are jobs dwindling?

For complete information, consult the current edition of the *Occupational Outlook Handbook*, published by the US Department of Labor. This handbook is available online or at your local library.

3. What special skills or talents are required? For example, do you need to be good at biology and chemistry? Do you need to enjoy interacting with other people?
4. What personality traits do you think are needed to be successful in this job? For example, a career as a physician assistant requires collaboration with other people, particularly a supervising doctor. Do you enjoy teamwork?
5. Does this career involve a great deal of routine, or are the day-to-day responsibilities varied?
6. Does the work require long hours, or is it a standard, "9-to-5" job?
7. What is the salary range for this job?
8. What do you think you would like about the career? Is there anything about it that you might dislike?

Related Career Options

- Gynecologist
- Nurse Practitioner
- Occupational Therapist
- Occupational Therapy Aide
- Paramedic
- Pediatrician
- Pharmacist
- Physician
- Registered Nurse
- Surgeon

Figure 8.18 When patients have difficulty leaving their homes, a physician assistant will sometimes make house calls.

Chapter Summaries

Lesson 8.1 Functions and Control of the Endocrine System

Build vocabulary with e-flash cards and games

Key Points

- The endocrine system is a collection of organs and small glands that directly or indirectly influence all the functions of the body.
- The endocrine system and the nervous system work together to regulate body functions.
- The glands of the endocrine system secrete many different hormones, or *chemical messengers*, into the bloodstream.
- When a hormone binds with a receptor in or on a cell, the hormone can influence the activity of the cell in various ways.
- Endocrine glands are stimulated or inhibited in three different ways: neural control, hormonal control, and humoral control.
- Hormones are used to maintain homeostasis.

Key Terms

amino-acid hormones
downregulated
epinephrine
glucagon
hormonal control
hormones
humoral control

hypothalamic nonreleasing hormones
hypothalamic releasing hormones
insulin
neural control
steroid hormones
upregulated

Lesson 8.2 Major Endocrine Organs

Key Points

- The major organs and glands of the endocrine system are the hypothalamus, pituitary gland, thyroid gland, parathyroid gland, thymus gland, pineal gland, adrenal glands, pancreas, and gonads.
- The anterior pituitary secretes six different types of hormones. The posterior pituitary gland stores ADH and oxytocin.
- The thyroid gland secretes two hormones: the thyroid hormone, which drives the metabolism, and calcitonin, which helps to maintain calcium homeostasis.
- The adrenal cortex secretes three steroid hormones, which regulate sodium, sugar, or sex hormone levels.
- The pancreas secretes hormones that regulate blood glucose levels.

Key Terms

adrenal cortex
adrenal glands
adrenal medulla
anterior pituitary
ovaries
pancreas
parathyroid glands
pineal gland

pituitary gland
posterior pituitary
scrotum
testes
thymus gland
thyroid gland
tropic hormones

Lesson 8.3 Endocrine Disorders and Diseases

Key Points

- Endocrine disorders and diseases are usually caused by hypersecretion or hyposecretion of hormones from a particular gland or organ.
- Major disorders of the pituitary gland include acromegaly, dwarfism, and diabetes insipidus.
- Major disorders of the thyroid gland are hyperthyroidism (goiter and Graves disease, for example) and hypothyroidism.
- Parathryoid gland disorders affect calcium levels in the blood.
- A tumor on the adrenal medulla can cause life-threatening hypersecretion of the hormones epinephrine and norepinephrine.
- Diabetes mellitus results from the inability of the pancreas to produce sufficient amounts of insulin to regulate blood glucose levels.

Key Terms

acromegaly	hyperthyroidism
Addison's disease	hypothyroidism
Cushing's syndrome	insulin resistance
diabetes insipidus	myxedema
diabetes mellitus	neonatal hypothyroidism
dwarfism	peripheral neuropathy
goiter	tetany
Graves disease	thyroiditis
hypercalcemia	type I diabetes mellitus
hyperglycemia	type II diabetes mellitus

Chapter Assessments

Lesson 8.1

Functions and Control of the Endocrine System

Learning Key Terms and Concepts

1. The chemical messengers secreted by the endocrine glands are _____.
   A. electrolytes
   B. enzymes
   C. hormones
   D. lacrimals

2. Which of the following is *not* an example of an exocrine gland?
   A. salivary glands
   B. sweat glands
   C. mammary glands
   D. adrenal glands

3. What are lipid-based hormones called?
   A. steroid hormones
   B. hypothalamic hormones
   C. amino-acid hormones
   D. glucagon

4. Receptors for _____ hormones are found on the surfaces of cells.

5. Which endocrine gland maintains the body's homeostatic set point at 37°C (98.6°F)?
   A. hypothalamus
   B. pituitary gland
   C. adrenal glands
   D. pancreas

6. Another name for the hormone epinephrine is _____.

7. _____ glands have ducts and are the counterpart to endocrine glands.

Thinking Critically

8. The body's fight-or-flight response can be triggered in situations that pose no real physical threat or danger. For example, think about the last time you were very anxious in a social situation. What physical sensations did you feel? Relate your sensations to the description of the fight-or-flight response in the chapter.

9. Contrast the three control systems (neural, hormonal, and humoral) of the endocrine system.

Lesson 8.2

Major Endocrine Organs

Learning Key Terms and Concepts

10. TSH is secreted by the pituitary gland and acts on the _____.
    A. pancreas
    B. testes
    C. thymus gland
    D. thyroid gland

11. The hormone prolactin, which stimulates milk production in a nursing mother, is produced by the _____.
    A. adrenal gland
    B. ovaries
    C. pituitary gland
    D. thyroid gland

12. Parathryoid hormone raises concentrations of _____ in the blood.
    A. calcium
    B. endorphins
    C. iron
    D. iodine

13. *True or False*? Antidiuretic hormone increases urine output and decreases body fluid volume.

14. The adrenal cortex produces three groups of steroid hormones—sex hormones, mineralocorticoids, and _____.

15. _____ is the hormone responsible for sperm production and the development of the male reproductive system.
    A. progesterone
    B. testosterone
    C. estrogen
    D. glycogen

16. Which endocrine gland is located in front of the trachea?
    A. adrenal gland
    B. thymus gland
    C. pituitary gland
    D. thyroid gland

17. Which two hormones are stored in the posterior pituitary?
    A. ADH and oxytocin
    B. ADH and LH
    C. TSH and oxytocin
    D. LH and oxytocin

18. *True or False*? The posterior pituitary gland is not a true endocrine gland.

19. The hormone-secreting cells of the pancreas are called the _____.

20. The hypothalamus is located _____.
    A. just below and to the right of the liver
    B. behind the sternum, above the diaphragm
    C. deep inside the brain
    D. inside the thyroid gland

21. Which of the following descriptions best describes the hormones secreted by the pituitary gland?
    A. They act directly on target tissues.
    B. They stimulate other endocrine glands.
    C. both A & B
    D. none of the above

22. Of the six hormones secreted by the anterior pituitary gland, which two are not tropic?

23. Which of the following glands does not secrete any hormones?
    A. parathyroid
    B. hypothalamus
    C. thyroid
    D. posterior pituitary

24. *True or False*? The adrenal cortex is part of the nervous system.

25. The hormone commonly referred to as adrenaline is secreted by which of the following?
    A. pineal gland
    B. adrenal cortex
    C. pancreas
    D. none of the above

26. Which of the following glands plays a key role in maintaining proper glucose levels in the blood?
    A. adrenal glands
    B. thymus gland
    C. pancreas
    D. pineal gland

Thinking Critically

27. Both antidiuretic hormone and aldosterone play major roles in blood pressure regulation. Explain the role of each hormone.

28. Explain the relationship between insulin and glucagon with regard to blood glucose levels.

Lesson 8.3

Endocrine Disorders and Diseases

Learning Key Terms and Concepts

29. Unusually tall height, along with enlargement of the hands, feet, and facial features, are common symptoms of _____.
    A. acromegaly
    B. Graves disease
    C. hypothyroidism
    D. goiter

30. Which of the following disorders is *not* associated with growth hormone imbalance?
    A. acromegaly
    B. diabetes
    C. dwarfism
    D. gigantism

31. When diagnosed at a young age, dwarfism is treated by _____.
    A. removal of the thyroid gland
    B. radiation therapy
    C. administering supplemental growth hormones
    D. administering iodine supplements

32. *True or False?* The pituitary gland controls the metabolism of every living cell in the human body.

33. A goiter is caused by a lack of _____ in the diet.
    A. sodium
    B. iodine
    C. iron
    D. potassium

34. *True or False?* A person suffering from hypothyroidism would most likely have a goiter.

35. Hypocalcemia, or low blood calcium levels, can cause _____.
    A. diabetes
    B. leukemia
    C. elevated blood sugar levels
    D. tetany

36. Which of the following is *not* a common symptom of Cushing's syndrome?
    A. weight gain
    B. moon-shaped face
    C. enlarged thyroid
    D. hypertension

37. Normal blood glucose levels fall in the range of 70 to _____ mg/dL.
    A. 500
    B. 105
    C. 80
    D. 135

Thinking Critically

38. A young woman is brought into a medical clinic by her husband. She complains of hyperactivity and weight loss. She also appears to be mentally sluggish and has difficulty concentrating when questioned by a nurse. There is a slight swelling in the anterior of her neck. Which condition do you suspect? What are some possible causes and treatment options?

Building Skills and Connecting Concepts

Analyzing and Evaluating Data

Use the bar graph from the Centers for Disease Control to answer the following questions.

39. How many new cases of type I diabetes mellitus occurred per 100,000 children under ten years of age? How many cases of type II occurred? What conclusion can you make from this data?

40. Which ethnic group experienced the highest number of new cases of type I diabetes? Which group experienced the fewest number of cases?

41. The number of new cases of type II diabetes increases dramatically in the 10 to 19 age group, as compared to the under 10 age group. Based on your reading of this chapter and any research you might need to do, develop reasons why new cases of type II diabetes mellitus are more prevalent in the older age group.

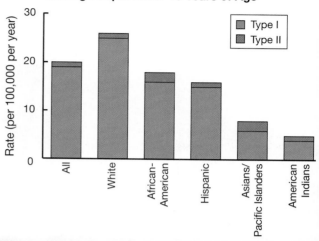

New Cases of Diabetes Mellitus among People under 10 Years of Age

Communicating about Anatomy and Physiology

42. **Writing** In the competitive world of professional sports, athletes are sometimes tempted to take performance-enhancing drugs. One such drug is human growth hormone, a manufactured version of growth hormone. Research the use of human growth hormone by professional athletes. Identify an athlete who has tested positive for human growth hormone. How did this revelation affect his or her career? Excessive amounts of growth hormone can lead to acromegaly. Does human growth hormone also cause this disease? What other negative side effects does this drug have on the body? Create a presentation and share your findings with the class.

43. **Listening and Speaking** Listen closely as your classmates present their findings on human growth hormone. Take notes on anything you find particularly interesting, or write down any questions you think of during their presentations. Once they are finished presenting, share with the class one thought or question you had regarding their research.

Lab Investigations

44. Visit the Centers for Disease Control (CDC) website and search for "age-adjusted prevalence of obesity and diagnosed diabetes among US adults." In the search results, locate and click on "Maps of Trends in Diabetes-Obesity." (Both PowerPoint® and PDF files are available.) Working with another student or in a small group, prepare a report on the steady rise in obesity and diabetes in the US. Start by making a list of states by region. Then study the CDC maps from years 2005–2010. What trends do you notice about the link between obesity and diabetes throughout the US? Share your findings with the class.

Expand your learning with additional online resources
- Supplemental Lab Activities
- Interactive Exercises
- Animations

Companion Website

www.g-wlearning.com/healthsciences

Can a larger lung volume contribute to athletic success?

The Respiratory System

*E*very breath that you take puts your respiratory system in direct contact with the environment. Have you ever stopped to think about what your lungs are exposed to on a daily basis? Do you walk to school along a busy street and breathe in exhaust fumes from cars? Does a friend or relative expose you to secondhand smoke? Through its anatomical structures and respiratory reflexes such as sneezing and coughing, your respiratory system filters everything that you breathe in from the environment.

The respiratory system has a big job to do; appropriately, it is one of the largest organ systems in the body. There are about 1,500 miles of airways and almost 1,000 miles of capillaries in the lungs. If we were to spread out the 300 million air sacs found in the lungs, they would cover the surface of nearly an entire tennis court. In fact, the surface area of your lungs is about 80 times greater than the surface area of your skin.

Because the body cannot go without oxygen for long, the respiratory system is vital to survival. Working with the cardiovascular system, the respiratory system ensures that a supply of fresh oxygen is always available, while removing harmful carbon dioxide from the body. Let's explore the anatomy of this body system to learn how it carries out the life-sustaining process of respiration.

Chapter 9 Lessons

Lesson 9.1
Functions and Anatomy of the Respiratory System

Lesson 9.2
Respiration: Mechanics and Control

Lesson 9.3
Respiratory Disorders and Diseases

While studying, look for the online icon **to:**

- **Practice** with e-flash cards and vocabulary games
- **Review** with interactive art labeling
- **Assess** with online exercises
- **Expand** with interactive activities and animated videos
- **Listen** to pronunciations of key terms in the audio glossary

www.g-wlearning.com/healthsciences

Companion Website

Study on the Go

Use a mobile device to practice vocabulary terms, listen to pronunciations, and review with self-assessment quizzes.

www.m.g-wlearning.com

G-W Mobile

Functions and Anatomy of the Respiratory System

Lesson Objectives

1. Explain how the respiratory and cardiovascular systems work together to conduct gas exchange.

2. Identify the main structures of the respiratory system.

3. Describe the functions and anatomy of the respiratory organs.

Key Terms
E-Flash Cards

alveolar capillary
  membrane
alveoli
bronchioles
cardiopulmonary
  system
conchae
epiglottis
larynx
mediastinum
nares

olfactory receptors
palate
pharynx
pleural sac
pores of Kohn
primary bronchi
sinuses
surfactant
thyroid cartilage
tonsils
trachea

Humans can survive for weeks without food and days without water, but only minutes without oxygen. In most cases the brain will cease to function, and death will occur, after the brain has been deprived of oxygen for five to six minutes. However, there have been incidents in which individuals have survived for longer durations with effective CPR and emergency medical treatments.

The main purpose of the respiratory system is to provide a constant supply of oxygen, while at the same time eliminating carbon dioxide, a waste product, from the body. This process is called *gas exchange*.

The respiratory system (sometimes called the *pulmonary system*) works cooperatively with the cardiovascular system to conduct gas exchange. These two systems are often collectively referred to as the **cardiopulmonary system**.

The blood, pumped through the body by the cardiovascular system, acts as the transport vehicle for oxygen and carbon dioxide. Fresh oxygen from the lungs is delivered to all cells of the body. The body's cells discharge carbon dioxide into the bloodstream, which then carries the carbon dioxide to the lungs for elimination.

Most people understand why we need sufficient amounts of oxygen, but they don't realize that removal of carbon dioxide from the body is equally important. Excessive levels of carbon dioxide can be toxic to the body, causing damage to cells and organs and even resulting in death.

Anatomy of the Respiratory System

The major organs of the respiratory system include the nose, pharynx, larynx, trachea, bronchi, bronchioles, and lungs (**Figure 9.1**). The respiratory system is divided into two parts: the upper respiratory tract and the lower respiratory tract. The upper respiratory tract includes the nose, mouth, nasal cavity, pharynx, and larynx. The lower respiratory tract consists of the trachea, bronchi, bronchioles, and lungs. The lungs contain alveoli (al-VEE-oh-ligh), air sacs in which the important gas-exchange function occurs.

The structures of the upper respiratory tract not only serve as a passageway for air moving in and out of the lungs, but they also perform other vital functions:

- filter and remove foreign particles from inspired (inhaled) air
- humidify and control the temperature of the inspired air
- produce sound (voice)
- provide a sense of smell (olfactory sense)
- aid in immune defense
- conduct air to the lower respiratory tract

As a result of these functions, the air that reaches the structures of the lower respiratory tract is warm, moist, and filtered—important qualities for the health of the lungs.

We will now examine the respiratory system organs that contribute to respiration, or *breathing*.

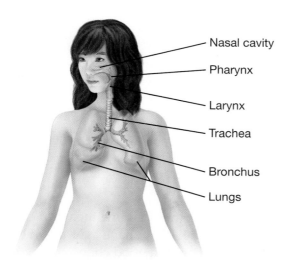

Figure 9.1 Simplified overview of the major respiratory structures. *What is another name for the respiratory system?*

The Nose

The nose is the only part of the respiratory system that is external to the body. During inspiration (inhalation, when breathing in), air enters the nose through two openings called **nares**, or *nostrils*. As we discuss the anatomy of the nose and its internal structures, refer to **Figure 9.2** on the next page.

The nose comes in many shapes and sizes. Some noses have bumps and others are small and turned up at the end. The nose's prominent location makes *rhinoplasty* (surgical modification of the nose) one of the most commonly performed plastic surgeries.

The Nasal Cavity

As you will recall from chapter 1, the nasal cavity occupies the space behind the nose. It is divided into a right and left chamber by the *nasal septum*.

The nasal cavity is lined with mucous membranes that filter and purify inspired air. At the front of the nasal cavity, just inside each naris (the singular form of *nares*), is the *vestibular* (vehs-TIB-yoo-lar) *region*. This region contains oily, coated nasal hairs called *cilia*, which trap and prevent particles from entering the nose.

Along the mucous membrane that lines the roof of the nasal cavity is an area called the *olfactory region*. **Olfactory receptors** located in this region provide our sense of smell. Our sense of smell is closely tied to our sense of taste. The next time you have a stuffy nose and your sense of taste seems "off," an accumulation of mucus on your olfactory receptors may be the culprit.

The rest of the nasal cavity is called the *respiratory cavity*, despite the fact that no respiration occurs there. The respiratory region is lined with a mucosal membrane occupied by a dense network of thinly walled veins. This mucosal membrane warms the air that we breathe, but the thin walls of these veins and their location can cause nosebleeds.

Conchae. Three uneven, scroll-like nasal **conchae** (KAHN-kee) bones extend down through the nasal cavity. The conchae are categorized into

The image labels read:
- Nasal cavity
- Pharynx
- Larynx
- Trachea
- Bronchus
- Lungs

A. Regions of the pharynx

B. The upper respiratory tract

Figure 9.2 Detailed overview of the major structures of the upper respiratory tract. A—Regions of the pharynx. B—The upper respiratory tract. *What normally passes through the pharynx? How might you describe the air that reaches the lower respiratory tract as a result of the work done by the upper respiratory tract?*

three types based on their location in the nasal cavity: superior, middle, and inferior conchae. These bones create three passageways that greatly increase the surface area available for filtering inspired air.

The conchae also increase the turbulence of the airflow in the nasal passage. This movement of air allows more particles to be trapped in the

mucous membranes that line the nasal cavity and the conchae. If you have ever flown on an airplane, there is a good chance that you have experienced turbulence. When a plane is subjected to turbulent airflow, the ride is bumpy. The erratic movement of the plane is similar to the turbulent movement of inspired air when it enters the conchae.

Check Your Understanding

1. List the structures that make up the respiratory system.
2. Besides serving as a passageway for air, what functions do the structures of the upper respiratory tract perform?
3. Which structures make up the lower respiratory tract?
4. What is the only external part of the respiratory system?

Figure 9.3 Front and side views of the sinuses. *Where do the names of the sinuses come from?*

The Palate. The **palate** (PAL-at) separates the nasal cavity from the mouth. It is commonly called the *roof of the mouth*. The anterior part of the palate is supported by bone; for this reason, it is called the *hard palate*. The posterior palate is called the *soft palate* because it is composed of soft muscle and tissue and is unsupported by bone.

Hanging from the end of the soft palate is the uvula, a small, conical mass of connective tissue and muscle fibers. The uvula is believed to play a small role in speech, but it also helps prevent food from entering the nasal cavity.

When the parts of the palate do not completely fuse together during fetal development, a *cleft palate* is the result. The upper lip can also be cleft, or separated. A cleft palate or lip leaves an opening in the roof of the mouth or a gap between the lip and nose. This condition occurs in 1 out of every 700 babies. Surgery to close and repair the cleft palate or lip typically fixes this problem.

The Sinuses. The **sinuses** are air-filled cavities that surround the nose. They are lined with mucous membranes and are connected to the nasal cavities by ducts that drain into the nose.

There are four sinuses. Each is named for the bone on which it lies: the *frontal sinus, ethmoidal sinus, sphenoidal sinus,* and *maxillary sinus* (**Figure 9.3**).

The sinuses lighten the weight of the head, warm and moisten inspired air, and amplify, or strengthen, the tone of the voice. Have you ever noticed how "nasal" a person's voice becomes during a sinus infection? That's because an infection causes the sinuses to become swollen and filled with fluid and germs. This prevents the voice from projecting in its normal tone.

The Pharynx

The **pharynx** (FAIR-ingks) is a muscular passageway that transports air, food, and liquids from the nasal and oral cavities to the trachea and esophagus. Thus, it is part of both the respiratory and digestive systems. The pharynx, commonly called the *throat*, is approximately 12.7 centimeters (5 inches) long. The pharynx is composed of an upper section called the *nasopharynx* (NAY-zoh-FAIR-ingks), a middle section called the *oropharynx* (OHR-oh-FAIR-ingks), and a lower region called the *laryngopharynx* (la-RING-goh-FAIR-ingks).

The nasopharynx is located behind the nasal cavity, superior and posterior to the soft palate. The *Eustachian tubes* of the middle ear drain into the nasopharynx. Because of this connection, an inner ear infection can cause an upper respiratory infection, or vice versa. Whereas air is the only thing that passes through the nasopharynx, the oropharynx and laryngopharynx are passageways for air, food, and liquid.

The Tonsils. The **tonsils** are clusters of lymphatic tissue in the pharynx (**Figure 9.2**). The pharyngeal tonsil is located in the upper part of the nasopharynx; the palatine and lingual tonsils lie in the upper portion of the oropharynx.

The tonsils are the first line of defense against infection. When bacteria and other pathogens enter the throat, they become trapped in the tonsils. This is why the tonsils themselves can become infected and inflamed, causing a condition called *tonsillitis*. We will learn about tonsillitis later in this chapter.

The Larynx

The **larynx** (LAIR-ingks), or *voice box*, routes air and food to the proper passageways and houses the structures that produce speech. It is a triangular-shaped space located inferior to the pharynx. The larynx is composed of eight cartilaginous plates. The largest plate, the **thyroid cartilage**, is commonly called the *Adam's apple*.

A flap of cartilaginous tissue called the **epiglottis** (EHP-i-GLAHT-is) lies between the root of the tongue and the larynx (**Figure 9.2**). The epiglottis acts as a "gatekeeper" by controlling the destination of ingested food and liquid and inspired air. As food or liquid is swallowed, the epiglottis covers the opening of the larynx, preventing the substance from entering the trachea. If food or liquid does enter the trachea, a cough is triggered to expel the substance so that it does not enter the lungs. When we are not swallowing food or liquid, the epiglottis allows air to flow freely into the lower respiratory tract.

The structures that produce the distinctive sound of your voice are located in the larynx. The larynx is lined with a mucous membrane that forms a pair of folds called the *vocal cords*. Between the vocal cords is a space called the *glottis*, which gives the vocal cords room to vibrate. When air enters the vocal cords, they vibrate, producing sound.

Check Your Understanding

1. Which two structures does the palate separate?
2. Where is the uvula located?
3. Which two body systems is the pharynx a part of?
4. What are the two major functions of the larynx?

The Trachea

The **trachea** (TRAY-kee-a), also called the *windpipe*, extends about 10 centimeters (4 inches)

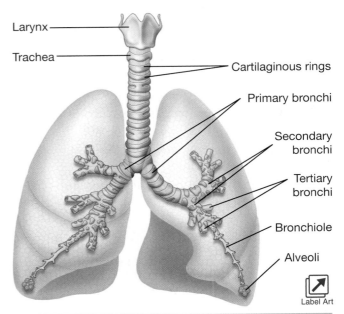

Figure 9.4 The larynx, trachea, and bronchial tree. The cartilaginous rings of the trachea continue throughout the passageways, ending at the bronchioles. *What is another name for cartilaginous rings? What purpose do they serve?*

from the end of the larynx to the fifth thoracic vertebra (mid-chest). The walls of the trachea are lined with a mucous membrane that contains ciliated epithelium, a covering with tiny, hair-like structures. The ciliated epithelium continuously sweeps foreign matter (such as dust) upward toward the larynx and pharynx, where it can be swallowed or coughed up.

The walls of the trachea are reinforced by a series of cartilaginous, C-shaped rings (**Figure 9.4** above). These C-shaped rings serve two functions. The C-shaped rings on the anterior side of the trachea contain rigid cartilage that provides support and prevents the airway from collapsing. The C-shaped rings on the posterior side of the trachea don't contain cartilage; they are flexible and allow the trachea to expand. This flexibility is helpful when large food particles pass through the esophagus, the structure that lies behind the trachea.

The Bronchi

At its bottom end, the trachea divides into right and left **primary bronchi** (BRAHNG-kigh). The primary bronchi lead to the right and left lungs (**Figure 9.4**). The wider, shorter bronchus (singular form of *bronchi*) on the right also hangs more vertically than the left bronchus. Because of these structural differences, inhaled substances are more likely to become lodged in the right bronchus. This understanding of the shape of the bronchi has helped doctors quickly locate and remove inhaled objects, preventing many choking deaths.

The bronchi subdivide into Y-shaped, smaller branches called the *secondary* and *tertiary bronchi*, until they end in the smallest conducting passageway—the **bronchioles** (BRAHNG-kee-ohls). The walls of the bronchial branches—but not the walls of the bronchioles—are reinforced by cartilaginous rings. The increasingly smaller branches of the bronchi are often compared to the branches of a tree. This is why the lungs are sometimes referred to as the *respiratory tree*.

The Alveoli. The bronchi and bronchioles are collectively known as the *conducting zone* because they are passageways that conduct air to and from the lungs. The terminal bronchioles lead into the *respiratory zone*. The respiratory zone contains the respiratory bronchioles, *alveolar ducts*, and grape-like clusters of **alveoli**. A limited amount of gas exchange occurs in the respiratory bronchioles, which are connected to the clusters of alveoli by the alveolar ducts.

The alveoli, or air-filled sacs, are the main sites of gas exchange in the lungs. Millions of alveoli clusters make up the bulk of the lung tissue. The alveoli walls are composed of very thin, squamous epithelial cells. The interior of these walls is coated with **surfactant**, a phospholipid. Surfactant reduces the surface tension in the alveoli and prevents them from collapsing.

The internal environment of the alveoli is kept clean and healthy by bacteria-ingesting cells called *macrophages*. Gases and macrophages travel between alveoli via the **pores of Kohn**, small openings in the alveolar wall.

The Alveolar Capillary Membrane. The alveoli and the capillaries that surround them make up the **alveolar** (al-VEE-oh-lar) **capillary membrane** (**Figure 9.5**). The alveolar capillary membrane is built for gas exchange. Oxygen easily diffuses across the membrane of the alveolar sacs into the capillaries, and carbon dioxide passes from the blood into the alveolar sac.

Gas exchange occurs rapidly for a few reasons. First, the surface area of the lungs is immense. If we were to lay the alveolar sacs side by side on the ground, they would cover almost the whole length of a tennis court. The millions of alveolar sacs provide an almost unlimited

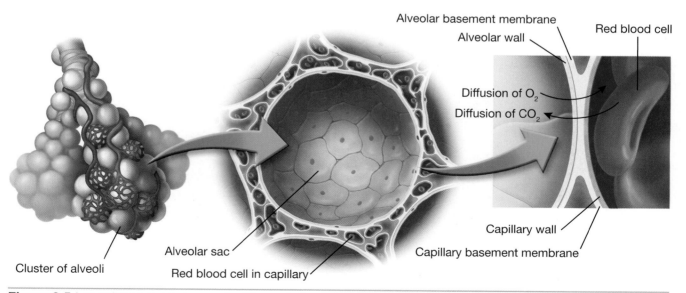

Alveolar basement membrane
Alveolar wall
Red blood cell
Diffusion of O_2
Diffusion of CO_2
Capillary wall
Capillary basement membrane
Cluster of alveoli
Alveolar sac
Red blood cell in capillary

Figure 9.5 Lung tissue is made up of millions of alveoli clusters. Pulmonary gas exchange occurs rapidly because the capillary walls of the alveolar sacs are much thinner than even a sheet of tissue paper. *What are other reasons that gas exchange occurs very rapidly?*

number of sites for gas exchange between the blood and alveolar sacs.

Second, the oxygen and carbon dioxide molecules only have to travel from the red blood cell, through the capillary wall and its membrane, and then through the alveolar wall and its membrane. These membranes are razor thin—thinner than even a sheet of tissue paper. This razor-thin quality makes it easy for oxygen and carbon dioxide to move freely between the alveoli and the bloodstream.

The third reason that gas exchange occurs rapidly is that gases always diffuse from areas of high concentration to areas of low concentration. Carbon dioxide has a high concentration in the capillary blood, but its concentration in the lungs is low. As a result, carbon dioxide diffuses rapidly from the blood into the alveolar sacs.

By contrast, there is a high concentration of oxygen in the alveoli sacs of the lungs, and a low concentration in the capillary blood. Thus, oxygen readily diffuses into the blood, where it binds with hemoglobin molecules in the red blood cells.

So just how fast does gas exchange occur in the lungs? Faster than you might think.

Our blood becomes 98% oxygenated in 0.75 seconds—in about the blink of an eye!

The Lungs

The lungs are large organs that occupy almost the entire thoracic (chest) cavity (**Figure 9.6**). The **mediastinum** (MEH-dee-as-TIGH-num), the central area of the thoracic cavity, lies between the lungs. It houses the heart, great blood vessels, trachea, esophagus, thoracic duct, thymus gland, and other structures. The mediastinum creates a deep, concave indentation (rounded inward) along the border of the left lung.

The upper part of the lung, called the *apex*, is located just below the clavicle, or collarbone. The broad base of the lung rests on the diaphragm. The lungs are divided into lobes by fissures. The right lung has three lobes: the superior, middle, and inferior lobes. The left lung has only two lobes: the superior left lobe and inferior left lobe.

Most of the tissue in our lungs is filled with air. In fact, the lungs weigh only 2.5 pounds and would float if placed in water.

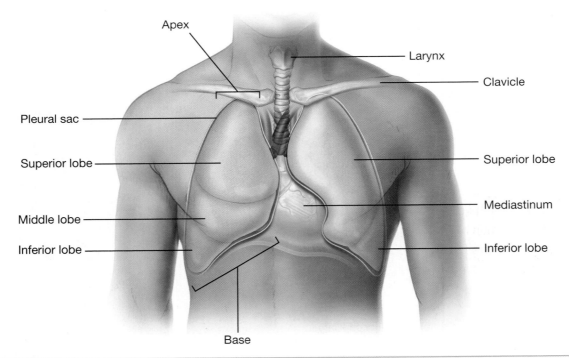

Figure 9.6 The lungs. The right lung has three lobes, but the left lung has only two lobes. *One lung is narrower than the other. Which lung do you think is narrower, based on the text description of the lungs?*

The Pleural Sac. The lungs are surrounded by a thin, double-walled **pleural sac**. The pleural sac is composed of two slippery, serous membranes. One membrane, the *parietal pleura*, lines the thoracic wall and diaphragm. The other membrane, the *visceral pleura*, covers the lungs and dips into the fissures. Both pleura membranes secrete a serous, or watery, fluid that allows the two linings to smoothly slide against each other as the lungs expand and contract during respiration. The serous fluid also acts like glue by keeping the two linings from pulling apart.

Lesson 9.1 Review and Assessment

Mini Glossary

Make sure that you know the meaning of each key term.

 Build vocabulary with e-flash cards and games

alveolar capillary membrane gas-exchange structure that contains the alveoli and the capillaries surrounding the alveoli

alveoli air sacs in the lungs from which gas is exchanged with the capillaries

bronchioles the thin-walled branches of the bronchi; the smallest air-conducting passageways of the bronchi. The terminal bronchioles conduct a small amount of gas exchange in the respiratory zone.

cardiopulmonary system the collective name for the respiratory and cardiovascular systems; these systems work together to conduct gas exchange

conchae three uneven, scroll-like nasal bones that extend down through the nasal cavity

epiglottis a flap of cartilaginous tissue that covers the opening to the trachea; diverts food and liquids to the esophagus during swallowing

larynx a triangular-shaped space inferior to the pharynx that is responsible for voice production; the *voice box*

mediastinum the area of the thoracic cavity between the lungs; houses the heart, great blood vessels, trachea, esophagus, thoracic duct, thymus gland, and other structures

nares the two openings in the nose through which air enters; nostrils

olfactory receptors sensory cells in the olfactory region that provide the sense of smell

palate the structure consisting of hard and soft components that separates the oral and nasal cavities; the *roof of the mouth*

pharynx the muscular passageway that extends from the nasal cavity to the mouth and connects to the esophagus; *the throat*

pleural sac the thin, double-walled serous membrane that surrounds the lungs

pores of Kohn small openings in the alveolar walls that allow gases and macrophages to travel between the alveoli

primary bronchi the two passageways that branch off the trachea and lead to the right and left lungs

sinuses the air-filled cavities that surround the nose

surfactant a phospholipid that reduces the surface tension in the alveoli and prevents them from collapsing

thyroid cartilage the largest cartilaginous plate in the larynx; the *Adam's apple*

tonsils clusters of lymphatic tissue in the pharynx that function as the first line of defense against infection

trachea the air tube that extends from the larynx into the thorax, where it splits into the right and left bronchi; the *windpipe*

Know and Understand

 Assess

1. What is the main purpose of the respiratory system?
2. Why are the bronchi and bronchioles together called the *conducting zone*?
3. How many lobes does each lung have?
4. What is the job of the cilia in the nasal cavity?
5. What is the common name for the palate?
6. Which structures are housed in the larynx?
7. Which structures provide rigid support for the trachea and prevent it from collapsing?

Analyze and Apply

8. Explain why a person's sense of taste is diminished when he or she has a stuffy nose.

9. Imagine that you are a doctor and one of your patients recently gave birth to an infant with a cleft palate and lip. How would you explain this condition and the treatment required?
10. Why is the epiglottis called the *gatekeeper*?
11. Explain the three reasons that the process of gas exchange occurs so rapidly.

In the Lab

12. Working in a group of three or four students, create a clay model of the respiratory system. Use different colored clay for each organ. Once you have created individual pieces for each major structure, connect all the clay organs to form the respiratory system. Then create a label for each organ. Share your model with your classmates.

Lesson Objectives

1. Understand the mechanics of respiration.
2. Explain how our breathing is affected by neural, chemical, and emotional factors as well as conscious control.
3. Explain the effects of central chemoreceptors, peripheral chemoreceptors, and mechanoreceptors on respiration.
4. Identify different methods of measuring lung volume and how each method works.

Key Terms
E-Flash Cards

central chemoreceptors
expiration
expiratory reserve
  volume (ERV)
external respiration
forced expiratory
  volume in one second
  (FEV$_1$)
forced expiratory
  volume in one
  second/forced vital
  capacity (FEV$_1$/FVC)
functional residual
  capacity (FRC)
Hering-Breuer reflex
inspiration

inspiratory reserve
  volume (IRV)
internal respiration
mechanoreceptors
peripheral
  chemoreceptors
pulmonary ventilation
residual volume (RV)
respiration
respiratory gas
  transport
tidal volume (TV)
total lung capacity
  (TLC)
vital capacity (VC)

Every minute of every day, our respiratory system works hard to deliver oxygen and dispose of carbon dioxide. Breathing may seem like a subconscious action—something you aren't even aware that you're doing—but there are actually many factors that control respiratory activity. In this lesson, we will explore the mechanics of breathing and the mechanisms by which it is controlled.

Respiration

As you learned in lesson 9.1, the main function of the respiratory system is gas exchange. Gas exchange is done through a process called **respiration**, or *breathing*.

The cardiovascular system and the respiratory system work together to accomplish respiration. There are four key tasks involved in this process:

1. **pulmonary ventilation**: air is continuously moved into and out of the lungs
2. **external respiration**: fresh oxygen from outside (*external* to) the body fills the lungs and alveoli, allowing gas exchange between the alveoli and pulmonary blood
3. **respiratory gas transport**: the oxygen and carbon dioxide gases in the blood are transported between the lungs and different body tissues
4. **internal respiration**: gas exchange occurs *inside* the body between the tissues and capillaries

In this chapter we will investigate the first two processes: pulmonary ventilation and external respiration. Respiratory gas transport and internal respiration are discussed in both Chapter 10: The Blood and Chapter 11: The Cardiovascular System.

Boyle's Law

The mechanics of breathing can be explained by Boyle's law. Boyle's law states that the volume of a gas is inversely proportional to its pressure. In simpler terms, as the volume of a gas increases, the pressure of the gas decreases.

Boyle's law affects breathing because of differences between atmospheric (outside) air pressure and intrapulmonary (lung) air pressure. At rest, both atmospheric and intrapulmonary air pressures are 760 millimeters of mercury (mmHg). When these pressures are the same, lung volume, or the amount of air in the lungs, does not change. At this point, there is no airflow (**Figure 9.7**).

For the lungs to be able to take in air, the intrapulmonary pressure must be *less than* the atmospheric pressure. When the direction of airflow is reversed to expel air from the lungs, the intrapulmonary pressure must be *greater than* atmospheric pressure.

Inspiration

Inspiration is the process by which air flows into the lungs; it is also called *inhalation*. Inspiration begins when the external intercostal muscles

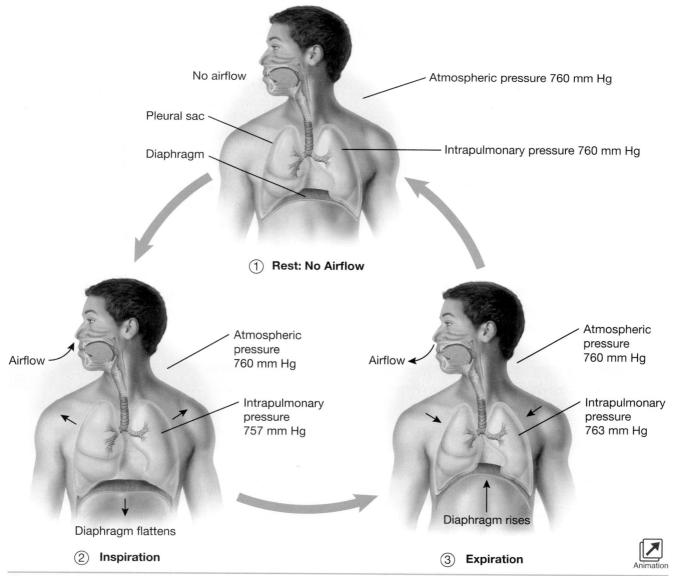

Figure 9.7 Changes in intrapulmonary and atmospheric pressure allow air to flow into and out of the lungs.
Explain the processes that cause intrapulmonary pressure to rise and fall.

contract, lifting the ribs upward and outward. At the same time, the dome-like diaphragm muscle contracts downward and flattens (**Figure 9.7**). Both of these maneuvers expand the thoracic cavity, decreasing its internal pressure. As the thoracic cavity expands, it pulls the lungs with it, and the lungs also expand.

As the lungs expand, the intrapulmonary pressure falls below the atmospheric pressure. When the intrapulmonary pressure is lower than the atmospheric pressure, a vacuum is created. The vacuum sucks air into the lungs until the pressure inside the lungs is equal to the atmospheric pressure.

Expiration

The process by which air is expelled from the lungs is called **expiration**, or *exhalation*. Expiration begins when the external intercostal muscles and the diaphragm relax, decreasing the space in the thoracic cavity and increasing the intrapulmonary pressure to 763 mmHg (**Figure 9.7**). When the intrapulmonary pressure exceeds the atmospheric pressure (760 mmHg), air is forced out of the lungs.

It is important to note that expiration does not require muscle contraction. This is because normal expiration is a *passive process*. When asthma or mucus accumulation narrows the respiratory passageways, or when your respiration rate increases during exercise, expiration becomes an *active process*. Active expiration requires the internal intercostal muscles to forcibly depress the rib cage to expel air from the lungs. At the same time, the abdominal muscles contract to push air out of the lungs.

Nonrespiratory Air Maneuvers

Did you know that a sneeze can travel up to 40 miles per hour? A sneeze is a nonrespiratory air maneuver. Besides breathing, there are other ways in which air moves into and out of the lungs.

You are familiar with coughing, sneezing, hiccupping, and yawning, but have you ever wondered why they happen? These nonrespiratory maneuvers often occur as a reaction, or reflexive response, to a stimulus (such as dust or debris) entering the respiratory passages. **Figure 9.8** explains how and why these nonrespiratory air maneuvers occur.

 Check Your Understanding

1. What is the main function of the respiratory system?
2. What does Boyle's law state?
3. For inspiration to occur, must the intrapulmonary pressure be higher or lower than atmospheric pressure?
4. Which process—inspiration or expiration— normally requires muscle contractions?

Figure 9.8 Nonrespiratory Air Maneuvers

Air Maneuver	Cause	Result
cough	a need to clear dust or other debris from the lower respiratory tract	a deep breath closes the epiglottis, and then a forceful exhalation is performed
sneeze	a need to clear the upper respiratory passageways of dust or other debris	the uvula closes off the oral cavity and routes air through the nose
hiccup	an irritation of the phrenic nerves that causes the diaphragm muscle to spasm	Sudden inspirations against the vocal cords of a closed glottis cause the hiccupping sound.
yawn	thought to be caused by a need for increased oxygen in the lungs	Prolonged, deep inspirations (taken with the jaws widely open) saturate the alveoli with fresh air.

Control of Breathing

Breathing is controlled mainly by neural and chemical factors, although our emotions and conscious control play a small role. The average respiratory rate for adults at rest is 12 to 15 breaths per minute. The average respiratory rate can vary based on biological and physical factors.

One biological factor that affects the way we breathe is gender. In general, women have higher respiratory rates because they have a smaller lung capacity than men. Age is another important biological factor. Infants take between 40 and 60 breaths each minute because they have a very small lung capacity.

A physical factor that influences respiratory rate is postural position (whether you are sitting or standing). When you move from a reclined position to a standing position, your breathing rate almost doubles. During maximal exercise, your respiratory rate can increase dramatically— by about 50 breaths per minute. However, respiration does not usually limit the exercise ability of people with healthy lungs.

Neural Factors

Rate and depth of breathing are controlled by inspiratory and expiratory breathing centers in the brain (**Figure 9.9** on the next page). These centers are located in the medulla oblongata and the pons, which are part of the brain stem.

The medulla oblongata and pons work as a team to make breathing a smooth, rhythmic process. The medulla is like the quarterback of the team, setting the normal breathing pace. By contrast, the pons is more of a utility player, fine-tuning respiratory rate and depth while also coordinating the transition between inspiration and expiration.

The medulla and pons work together to create a normal, rhythmic breathing pattern. The medullary inspiratory center stimulates the diaphragm and the external intercostals. This stimulation is achieved by afferent nerve impulses sent through the phrenic and intercostal nerves. As the lungs fill with air, *stretch receptors* in the bronchioles and alveoli

trigger the **Hering-Breuer reflex** to prevent overinflation of the alveolar sacs. Once activated, the stretch receptors send nerve impulses to the medulla via the vagus nerve. These impulses alert the medulla to stop inspiration and start exhalation (**Figure 9.9**). The pons works to achieve smooth transitions between inspiration and expiration.

Chemical Factors

Most people don't think of oxygen and carbon dioxide as chemicals, but when it comes to respiration, that is how they are classified. Oxygen (O_2) and carbon dioxide (CO_2) are chemicals that influence the inspiratory and expiratory centers of the brain. Because oxygen is essential for maintaining life, you might think it exerts greater control over the rate and depth of breathing than carbon dioxide. However, as **Figure 9.9** on the next page shows, several chemical factors regulate breathing.

Central Chemoreceptors. Within the respiratory centers of the brain are sensory cells called **central chemoreceptors** (KEE-moh-ree-SEHP-tors). Central chemoreceptors constantly monitor changes in cerebrospinal fluid pH (acidity or alkalinity). A decrease in cerebrospinal fluid pH indicates high amounts of carbon dioxide in the body.

When metabolism increases, oxygen consumption accelerates and the body produces more carbon dioxide. In excessive quantities, carbon dioxide can be dangerous because it is the only chemical that can cross the blood-brain barrier, a protective border between brain tissues and circulating blood.

High levels of carbon dioxide increase the number of hydrogen ions in the body. These hydrogen ions cause the pH of the cerebrospinal fluid to decrease. When the central chemoreceptors sense a decrease in cerebrospinal fluid pH, they stimulate the brain's inspiratory center. They do this by sending impulses to the inspiratory center via the vagus and glossopharyngeal nerves. When the inspiratory center receives this information, it stimulates an increase in the rate and depth of breathing.

① **Stimulus: Inspiration**

Peripheral chemoreceptors (O_2, CO_2, pH)

Mechanoreceptors in muscles

Central chemoreceptors in brain (CO_2, pH)

② **Response: Inspiration**
The external intercostal muscles and diaphragm contract.

Inspiratory center

Expiratory center

③ **Stimulus: Expiration**
Stretch receptors in the lungs stimulate the expiratory center.

④ **Response: Expiration**
The external intercostal muscles and diaphragm relax.

Figure 9.9 Regulation of breathing. The inspiratory and expiratory breathing centers, located in the medulla oblongata and pons, control the rate and depth of breathing. These centers are stimulated by sensory triggers (central chemoreceptors, peripheral chemoreceptors, and mechanoreceptors) and neural triggers (stretch receptors).

The result is a fresh supply of oxygen and lower carbon dioxide levels. As you can see, carbon dioxide is the chemical driving force behind respiration.

Peripheral Chemoreceptors. Located in the aorta and carotid arteries, **peripheral chemoreceptors** are sensitive to changes in blood oxygen level. Peripheral chemoreceptors are also mildly sensitive to carbon dioxide and pH, but less so than they are to oxygen. Like the central chemoreceptors, peripheral chemoreceptors stimulate respiration by sending sensory information via the vagus and glossopharyngeal nerves to the brain.

Memory Tip
Central chemoreceptors are sensitive to **C**arbon dioxide. Both of these terms start with C. **P**eripheral chemoreceptors are most sensitive to **O**xygen. P and O are close together in the alphabet.

Mechanoreceptors. Yet another type of sensory cells that play a role in regulating respiration are the **mechanoreceptors** (MEHK-a-noh-ree-SEHP-tors). Located in muscles and joints, mechano-receptors detect muscle contraction and force generation during exercise. Mechanoreceptors are responsible for the quick increase in ventilation that occurs when you first begin to exercise. As exercise continues and carbon dioxide builds up, the chemoreceptors help to regulate respiration.

 Check Your Understanding

1. By which two factors is breathing mainly controlled?
2. What is the average breathing rate for adults?
3. How many breaths per minute does an infant take?
4. Where are the inspiratory and expiratory control centers located?
5. What processes do the inspiratory and expiratory centers control?

Lung Volume

Now that you understand how breathing is regulated, let's turn our attention to lung volume measurement. Lung volume measurements are used to assess whether or not a person's lung capacity is normal. The total volume for a pair of healthy adult lungs is about six liters of air.

Do you think that lung volume plays a major role in an athlete's success? Does the swimmer with the largest lung volume have a better chance of winning an event than the one with a smaller lung capacity? Before answering these questions, it is important to understand how to measure and interpret lung volume.

Lung volume varies according to age, height, weight, gender, and race. Therefore, it is important that an appropriate set of normative values is used as a reference source. There are two types of lung volume: static and dynamic. *Static lung volume* measures only volume; *dynamic lung volume* measures volume based upon time. For instance, a dynamic lung volume measurement might assess the ability of the lungs to forcibly expire air in one second.

Static lung volume is measured by a *spirometer* (spigh-RAHM-eh-ter). Dynamic lung volume is measured using a *flow volume meter*.

Static Lung Volume

Measures of static lung volume are important because they can be used to determine whether or not a lung deficiency or disorder exists. In static lung volume measurement, a person performs a series of breathing maneuvers. First, the person is instructed to breathe normally for at least six breaths so that a measurement of **tidal volume (TV)** can be obtained. Tidal volume is the amount of air inhaled during a normal breath. Then, the person inspires maximally (breathes in as deeply as possible), followed by a maximal expiration. This last breathing maneuver helps identify the person's **vital capacity (VC)**, or the total amount of air that can be forcibly expired after a maximal inspiration.

The volume of air that never leaves the lungs, even after the most forceful expiration, is called the **residual volume (RV)**. Residual volume is important because it allows gas exchange to occur continuously between inspiration and expiration. Residual volume cannot be measured by a spirometer; it requires advanced measurement techniques.

Static lung volume can be measured in other ways:

- **functional residual capacity (FRC)**: the amount of air that remains in the lungs after a normal expiration; ERV + RV
- **inspiratory reserve volume (IRV)**: the amount of air that can be inhaled immediately after a normal inspiration
- **expiratory reserve volume (ERV)**: the amount of air that can be exhaled, or forced from the lungs, immediately after a normal expiration
- **total lung capacity (TLC)**: a combination of the vital capacity plus the residual volume; IRV + TV + ERV + RV (which usually measures about 6L of air)

Each of these forms of static lung volume measurement can be obtained with a spirometer except for the FRC, which requires more sophisticated equipment. See **Figure 9.10** for

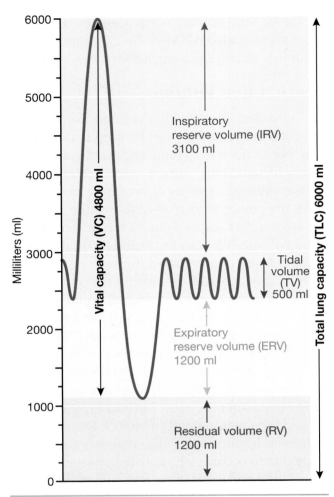

Figure 9.10 Lung volume chart. This lung volume tracing was obtained by a test using a spirometer. *How might a lung volume chart be used?*

measure dynamic lung volume. The pulmonary function test is very important because it can determine whether or not a person has asthma, obstructive lung disease, or restrictive lung disease. Like static lung volume measurements, dynamic lung volume measurements vary based on age, height, weight, gender, and race.

During a test of dynamic lung volume, a person is instructed to breathe normally into a mouthpiece connected to a flow volume machine. After several tidal (normal) respirations, the person is instructed to inspire maximally and then expire as long, hard, and fast as possible. The goal is for the person to breathe out for at least six seconds. This may not sound very hard, but most people cannot expire for six seconds on their first attempt. The most important measurements obtained from this test include the following:

- **forced expiratory volume in one second (FEV$_1$)**: the maximum amount of air that a person can expire in one second. This test measures the ability of the lungs to expel air
- **forced expiratory volume in one second/ forced vital capacity (FEV$_1$/FVC)**: measures the overall expiratory power of the lungs

People with chronic obstructive pulmonary disease (COPD) such as emphysema, asthma, or chronic bronchitis often have increased airway resistance because of an obstruction. As a result, their FEV$_1$ and FEV$_1$/FVC values are less than 80% of those for healthy individuals.

People with restrictive lung disease such as cystic fibrosis or pneumonia have an increased stiffness in the lungs, which prevents the lungs from expanding normally. Lung stiffness causes static and dynamic lung volume values to be much lower than normal. Lung volumes indicative of some pulmonary disorders will be discussed in greater length in lesson 9.3.

an example of spirometer test results of static lung volume. Test results are usually compared to normal values matched to the patient's age, height, weight, gender, and ethnicity.

Generally, lung volume does not predict the average athlete's performance. During maximal exercise, you use only about 65% of your lungs' vital capacity. Because high-intensity exercise does not require 100% of the lungs' vital capacity, lung volume is not a limiting factor for healthy individuals.

Dynamic Lung Volume

Dynamic lung volume is a measurement of flow rate during a forced vital capacity maneuver. Pulmonary function testing by a computerized flow-volume meter is used to

 Check Your Understanding

1. What does vital capacity (VC) measure?
2. Explain the difference between inspiratory reserve volume and expiratory reserve volume.
3. What can a pulmonary function test determine?

Lesson 9.2 Review and Assessment

Mini Glossary
Make sure that you know the meaning of each key term.

 Build vocabulary with e-flash cards and games

central chemoreceptor   a chemical receptor cell that monitors changes in the pH of the cerebrospinal fluid in an effort to regulate carbon dioxide levels and respiration

expiration   the process by which air is expelled from the lungs; exhalation

expiratory reserve volume (ERV)   the additional amount of air that can be exhaled, or forced from the lungs, immediately after a normal exhalation

external respiration   the process by which gas exchange occurs between the alveoli in the lungs and the pulmonary blood

forced expiratory volume in one second (FEV₁)   the amount of air that a person can expire in one second

forced expiratory volume in one second/forced vital capacity (FEV₁/FVC)   the overall expiratory power of the lungs

functional residual capacity (FRC)   the amount of air that remains in the lungs after a normal expiration; ERV + RV

Hering-Breuer reflex   an involuntary impulse triggered by stretch receptors in the bronchioles and alveoli that halts inspiration and initiates exhalation

inspiration   the process by which air flows into the lungs; inhalation

inspiratory reserve volume (IRV)   the amount of air that can be inhaled immediately after a normal inhalation

internal respiration   the process of gas exchange between the tissues and arterial blood

mechanoreceptors   chemical receptor cells that detect muscle contraction and force generation during exercise; they quickly increase respiration rates when exercise begins

peripheral chemoreceptors   sensory receptor cells located in the aortic arch and carotid arteries that are sensitive to changes in blood oxygen level

pulmonary ventilation   the process of continuously moving air in and out of the lungs

residual volume (RV)   the volume of air that never leaves the lungs, even after the most forceful expiration

respiration   the process by which the lungs provide oxygen to body tissues and dispose of carbon dioxide; breathing

respiratory gas transport   the process by which oxygen and carbon dioxide are transported to and from the lungs and tissues

tidal volume (TV)   the amount of air inhaled in a normal breath

total lung capacity (TLC)   a combination of the vital capacity plus the residual volume; IRV + TV + ERV + RV

vital capacity (VC)   the total amount of air that can be forcibly expired from the lungs after a maximum inspiration

Know and Understand
Assess

1. What are the four key tasks the cardiopulmonary system works to accomplish?
2. Describe the mechanics of a cough.
3. Why do women take more frequent breaths than men?
4. How does posture affect your breathing rate?
5. Where are the neural centers for breathing located?

Analyze and Apply

6. What are stretch receptors, and what role do they play in the Hering-Breuer reflex?
7. Explain Boyle's law and how it relates to breathing.
8. Imagine that you are a pediatrician. A frantic mother visits you in your office with her newborn son. The mother expresses concern that her baby's breathing rate is too high. She tells you that the baby takes many more breaths each minute than his older brother. After testing the baby's respiratory rate, you discover that it falls in the normal range for newborns. How do you explain this to the mother?

In the Lab

9. You can determine lung capacity with a balloon, ruler, pencil, and graph paper.

Take several deep breaths and then exhale as much air as possible into the balloon. Measure and record the diameter of the balloon, labeling it *vital capacity*. Repeat three times, and then calculate your average vital capacity.

Exhale normally. Before inhaling again, quickly put the balloon to your lips and exhale into the balloon. Measure the diameter of the balloon as before, and record this measurement as the *expiratory reserve*. Repeat three times and calculate your average expiratory reserve.

Take a normal breath, and as you exhale normally, put the balloon to your lips. Measure the diameter of the balloon as before, recording the measurement as *tidal volume*. Repeat three more times, then calculate your average tidal volume.

Make a bar graph that compares your three average lung volume measurements. Compare your results with those of your classmates.

Respiratory Disorders and Diseases

Lesson Objectives

1. Identify common illnesses of the upper respiratory tract.
2. Explain how proper respiratory etiquette and hand hygiene can help prevent transmission of the common cold.
3. Identify the most common form of chronic obstructive pulmonary disease and describe strategies for symptom management.
4. Understand the causes and symptoms of lung cancer and available treatment options for this disease.

Key Terms

E-Flash Cards

acute bronchitis
asthma
bronchospasms
chronic bronchitis
chronic obstructive
    pulmonary disease
    (COPD)
emphysema
hyperventilation

influenza
laryngitis
nasopharyngitis
pharyngitis
pneumonia
sinusitis
tonsillitis
tuberculosis (TB)

It's likely that you have had the common cold several times in your life—after all, it's called the *common* cold for a reason! In fact, you have probably had the flu, have a friend with asthma, or know someone whose tonsils have been removed. But do you know how to prevent the cold or flu? Do you know what causes your friend's asthma attacks?

In this lesson we'll discuss the causes and symptoms of several respiratory disorders, along with treatment options. You may be surprised to learn that some of these disorders cannot be cured, yet others can be prevented by behavior as simple as washing your hands.

Upper Respiratory Tract Illnesses

Upper respiratory tract illnesses, or URIs, are the most common acute illnesses. As you learned in lesson 9.1, the upper respiratory tract includes the nose, nasal cavity, sinuses, pharynx, and larynx. Infection and inflammation of the upper respiratory tract can lead to a variety of illnesses, such as

- **nasopharyngitis** (NAY-zoh-FAIR-in-JIGH-tis): the common cold;
- **pharyngitis** (FAIR-in-JIGH-tis): inflammation of the pharynx, or throat;
- **sinusitis** (SIGH-nus-IGH-tis): inflammation of the sinuses;
- **laryngitis** (LAIR-in-JIGH-tis): inflammation of the larynx, or *voice box*; and
- **tonsillitis** (TAHN-si-LIGH-tis): inflammation of the tonsils.

Figure 9.11 lists the causes and symptoms of upper respiratory tract illnesses. The chart also provides recommended treatments for these illnesses.

Figure 9.11 Common Upper Respiratory Tract Illnesses

Upper Respiratory Tract Illness	Cause	Symptoms	Treatment
Pharyngitis	infection from common cold or flu virus; bacterium such as group A strepto-coccus (strep throat)	sore, scratchy throat; fever; headache; swollen lymph nodes	gargle with saline solution; drink warm fluids; suck on freezer pops or throat loz-enges; take over-the-counter pain relievers and antibiotics if strep is diagnosed
Sinusitis	bacteria, viruses, and fungi	sinus pain; nasal stuffi-ness and discharge; head-ache; fever; sore throat; postnasal drip; fatigue	drink fluids; apply warm, moist cloth to face; use humidifier, nasal saline spray; see a doctor about severe symptoms
Laryngitis	viral infections such as common cold or flu, bacte-rial infections, allergies, or inhaled irritants	sore throat; hoarseness; loss of voice; fever	rest your voice; use humidi-fier, decongestants, or pain relievers
Tonsillitis	viral or bacterial infection; group A streptococcus is most common bacterial infection	red, swollen tonsils; white/yellow patches on tonsils; difficult, painful swallow-ing; bad breath; swollen neck glands	gargle with saline solution; drink warm fluids such as tea with honey; take over-the-counter pain medica-tions (no aspirin for those under 21 years of age), anti-biotic if strep is diagnosed; surgery

Avoiding URIs

Most people get between two and four colds each year. According to the Cleveland Clinic, there are 12 million medical visits for pharyngitis and 20 billion cases of bacterial sinusitis each year.

Transmission of upper respiratory illnesses such as nasopharyngitis occurs by direct hand-to-hand contact, handling a contaminated object, and airborne droplets produced by unprotected sneezing or coughing. Proper respiratory etiquette and hand hygiene are the most effective ways to prevent URIs (**Figure 9.12** and **Figure 9.13** on the next page):

- Cover your nose and mouth with a tissue when you cough or sneeze. If a tissue is unavailable, sneeze or cough into your sleeve to avoid contaminating your hands.
- Wash your hands often with soap and hot water. Use an alcohol-based hand sanitizer if soap and water are not available.
- Avoid touching your hands to your eyes, nose, or mouth to decrease the spread of germs.

Influenza

Influenza, or the *flu*, is a viral infection that affects the respiratory system. Unlike a cold, whose symptoms come on slowly, the flu strikes quickly. Symptoms include a fever above 38°C (100°F), headache, nasal congestion, alternating chills and sweats, dry cough, fatigue, and aching muscles, especially in the back, arms, and legs.

From November through March, the flu strikes the Northern Hemisphere in epidemic proportions. According to the Centers for Disease Control (CDC), 5% to 20% of the US population is infected with the flu each year, and more than 200,000 people are hospitalized because of flu-related complications. The CDC also reports that influenza-related deaths average about 25,000 annually in the United

Hannamariah/Shutterstock.com

Figure 9.12 Sneezing into your sleeve decreases the transmission of germs. *What other ways can you avoid spreading germs?*

icyimage/Shutterstock.com

Figure 9.13 Wash your hands with hot, soapy water for 20 seconds, about the length of time it takes to sing "Happy Birthday" twice.

States, although this number can vary greatly from year to year. The CDC also estimates that school-aged children (5 to 17 years of age) in the United States miss 38 million days of school each year because of the flu. The single best way to protect against seasonal flu is to get the seasonal influenza vaccine each year.

✓ **Check Your Understanding**

1. What is the scientific name for the common cold?
2. How many colds does the average person contract each year?
3. Which URI is characterized by red, swollen tonsils and swollen neck glands?

Lower Respiratory Tract Illnesses

Like the upper respiratory tract, parts of the lower respiratory tract are susceptible to certain ailments. Bronchitis, pneumonia, and tuberculosis are among the most common.

Acute Bronchitis

Generally, bronchitis is classified as either acute or chronic bronchitis. **Acute bronchitis** is an inflammation of the mucous membranes that line the trachea and bronchial passageways. You will learn about chronic bronchitis later in this lesson.

Acute bronchitis is characterized by a cough that may or may not produce mucus. This illness usually develops as a result of an ongoing viral infection such as influenza or a cold. Treatment for acute bronchitis varies based on the patient's symptoms. It often includes the use of nonsteroidal anti-inflammatory drugs (NSAIDs), decongestants, and expectorants (medications that expel mucus).

Pneumonia

Pneumonia (noo-MOH-nee-ah) is an infection of the lungs. It is usually caused by a virus or bacterium, but some pneumonia infections are caused by a fungus or parasites.

The immune response to the invading virus or bacterium damages and sometimes kills the cells of the lungs. Fluid also builds up in the lungs, making gas exchange difficult. Symptoms of pneumonia include cough, fever, chills, fatigue, shortness of breath, nausea, vomiting, and diarrhea. Diagnosis is made by examining chest X-rays and cell cultures.

Treatment of pneumonia includes antibiotics and supplemental oxygen, as necessary.

Tuberculosis

Tuberculosis (TB) is a highly contagious infection caused by *Mycobacterium tuberculosis*. It most commonly attacks the lungs, but it can spread to other organs such as those in the digestive, nervous, or lymphatic systems. TB is contracted by breathing in air droplets from the cough or sneeze of an infected person.

Symptoms of TB include fever, fatigue, unintentional weight loss, and excessive sweating, especially at night. People with TB also develop a cough that may produce mucus or blood.

Most forms of TB can be treated with antibiotics, but some new forms are drug resistant. Individuals with TB must be confined to their home or the hospital for two to four weeks to avoid spreading this contagious disease to others.

Chronic Obstructive Pulmonary Diseases

Chronic obstructive pulmonary disease (COPD) is any lung disorder characterized by a long-term airway obstruction, making it difficult to breathe. Two of the most common forms of COPD are **emphysema** (EHM-fi-SEE-ma) and **chronic bronchitis**. Bronchitis is classified as *chronic* when a person has a cough that has lasted from three months to two years.

The CDC reports that COPD is the third leading cause of death in the United States and a major cause of long-term disability. According to the World Health Organization, COPD accounts for 5% of all deaths worldwide.

Causes of COPD

The primary cause of COPD is cigarette, cigar, or pipe smoking. The longer that a person smokes, the more susceptible he or she becomes to COPD. The risk of developing COPD is also increased by long-term, regular exposure to secondhand smoke or occupational exposure to chemical fumes, dust, or pollution.

People with COPD are more likely to have frequent respiratory infections such as cold and flu viruses, pneumonia, or a cough that produces mucus. They also experience dyspnea (difficulty breathing), which progressively worsens. Breathing—something that many people take for granted—is an exhausting experience for COPD patients. Difficulty breathing leaves many COPD patients unable to participate in everyday activities. The challenges associated with managing COPD can also cause patients to develop depression.

Living with COPD

There is no cure for COPD. The main goals of treatment for COPD are to help the patient manage symptoms, improve the quality of life, slow the progression of the disease, and treat infections. The key factor in achieving these goals is *smoking cessation*. A person with COPD *must* stop smoking and avoid exposure to substances that may irritate the lungs.

Smoking causes 1 in 5 deaths annually, or 440,000 deaths each year. The CDC estimates that 25 million people alive today will die prematurely from the harmful effects of smoking. This includes 5 million people under 18 years of age.

The nicotine in tobacco is more addictive than cocaine, so a person may experience several failed attempts at quitting the smoking habit before success is achieved. The use of nicotine gum or patches increases the likelihood of smoking cessation; however, these can also be addictive.

COPD symptoms can be alleviated through a variety of methods. One technique, purse-lipped breathing, helps maximize breathing and ease shortness of breath. Patients using this technique are advised to inhale through their nose and then slowly release the air through pursed, or puckered, lips. Respiratory muscle training, pulmonary rehabilitation, and supplemental oxygen can also help reduce COPD symptoms. Pharmacological therapies such as bronchodilators, anti-inflammatory medications, and inhaled steroids can help expand airways and are often prescribed for COPD patients. However, none of these methods slows the progression of COPD more effectively than smoking cessation. Pulmonary function tests, X-rays, bronchoscopies (brahng-KAHS-koh-pees), and monitoring of gas levels in arterial blood are used in both the diagnosis and management of COPD.

Figure 9.14 illustrates the results of a pulmonary function test for normal individuals and those with emphysema, chronic bronchitis, and restrictive disease (any chest disease that reduces lung volumes). Note the concave-shaped expiration pattern for individuals with emphysema and chronic bronchitis. This is due to trapped air in the lungs. Additionally, when you examine the curve for restrictive disease, you will see how limited inspiration and expiration are as compared to the curve for normal individuals. This is because the lungs are unable to expand due to stiffness.

Emphysema

Commonly caused by tobacco smoke, emphysema is a form of COPD that leads

to chronic inflammation in the lungs. This inflammation damages the air passages distal to the terminal bronchioles, namely the alveolar ducts and the alveolar sacs (**Figure 9.15**). The pulmonary capillary bed is also damaged. This damage decreases the surface area of the lungs, limiting the number of sites available for gas exchange. As emphysema progresses, the alveolar sacs rupture, leading to poor gas exchange and buildup of carbon dioxide in the lungs.

To compensate for the poor gas exchange, the body triggers **hyperventilation**, which increases the respiratory rate. Hyperventilation brings in oxygen while allowing the lungs to dispose of accumulated carbon dioxide.

People with emphysema work so hard to breathe regularly that they often lose weight. This exertion also causes emphysema patients to develop a pink appearance to the face. The characteristic pink cheeks and labored breathing of the COPD patient have led to the descriptive term "pink puffers" among people in clinical circles.

Chronic Bronchitis

People with chronic bronchitis have an obstructed airway due to inflammation of the bronchi and excessive mucus production. The excessive mucus limits respiration and gas exchange. It also increases the risk of infection because bacteria can become trapped and breed in the warm, moist environment of the lungs. The body responds to the mucus accumulation by decreasing the respiratory rate and increasing

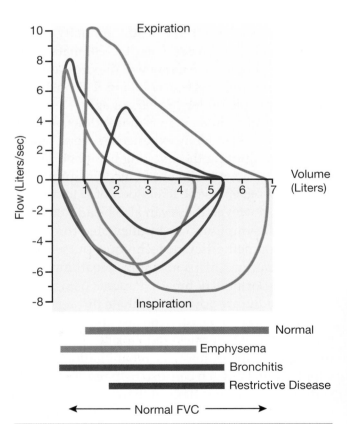

Figure 9.14 Results of a pulmonary function test for healthy individuals, and for people diagnosed with emphysema, chronic bronchitis, and restrictive disease. *Can you explain the concave-shaped expiration pattern for individuals with emphysema and chronic bronchitis?*

Figure 9.15 Lung of a smoker with emphysema. The accumulation of inhaled irritants from smoking blackened the lung. *What other diseases are associated with smoking?*

cardiac output. Unlike emphysema, chronic bronchitis does not damage the pulmonary capillary bed.

The face and lips of a person with chronic bronchitis develop a blue color due to *hypoxemia*, or lowered arterial blood oxygen content. Residual volume also increases, causing a bloated appearance. These two side effects have led to the description of chronic bronchitis patients as "blue bloaters."

 Check Your Understanding

1. What is the difference between acute and chronic bronchitis?
2. How is tuberculosis contracted?
3. What is the primary cause of COPD?
4. Which respiratory disease is associated with the term "pink puffer"?

Asthma

Asthma (AZ-ma) is a respiratory disease in which the airways of the lungs become narrow or inflamed during episodes called *asthma attacks*. During an asthma attack, the airways are temporarily constricted by **bronchospasms** (BRAHNG-koh-spazmz), contractions of the smooth bronchial muscles. Also, the lining of the inflamed airways produces mucus that causes further narrowing. Bronchospasms, inflammation, and mucus production result in symptoms such as wheezing, breathlessness, coughing, and tightness in the chest.

People with a family history of allergies are at an increased risk of developing asthma because many of the stimuli that trigger allergies also cause asthma attacks. A variety of substances can trigger an asthma attack. Asthma triggers include cigarette smoke, mold, air pollution, pet hair and dander, cold air, exercise, dust, pollen, and emotional stress.

If you lose your breath easily, feel very tired or weak when exercising, wheeze and cough after exercise, or experience a frequent cough (especially at night), these may be early symptoms of asthma. A school nurse or other healthcare professional can use a peak flow meter to measure the airflow from your lungs (**Figure 9.16**).

mayer kleinostheim/Shutterstock.com

Figure 9.16 A peak flow meter is used to measure airflow from the lungs. Blowing forcefully into the end of the device causes the marker to move up the numbered scale.

Your doctor may use a more detailed pulmonary function test to diagnose asthma. Proper diagnosis is important because it leads to treatment options that enable an asthmatic person to lead a healthy, productive life; participate in physical activity; and limit the frequency and severity of asthma attacks.

Treatments for asthma include limiting exposure to irritants that can trigger an asthma attack and using prescription medications such as bronchodilators, anti-inflammatory drugs, and inhaled steroids (**Figure 9.17**). These medications work by relaxing the muscles of the bronchi and expanding the airways.

The prevalence of asthma in the United States has risen dramatically in recent years, with a 50% increase in African-American children. About

xavier gallego morel/Shutterstock.com

Figure 9.17 A mother helps her child use an asthma inhaler with a spacer. The spacer allows more of the medicine to get into the child's lungs.

WHAT RESEARCH TELLS US

...*about* Exercise-Induced Asthma

Asthma attacks triggered by exercise are called exercise-induced bronchospasms (EIBs), or *exercise-induced asthma*. Exercise-induced asthma is not uncommon. Many people who exercise regularly have asthma, even professional athletes. For example, hundreds of athletes successfully compete at the Olympic Games despite having asthma.

Researchers investigated the incidence of EIBs among members of the US Olympic Winter Sports teams. The athletes tested for EIBs included members of seven different teams: biathlon, cross-country skiing, figure skating, ice hockey, Nordic combined events, long-track speed skating, and short-track speed skating (**Figure 9.18**).

steba/Shutterstock.com

Figure 9.18 United States speed skating team. Winter sport athletes often have higher rates of EIB.

All the athletes in the study were tested for EIBs during actual or simulated competition. The overall incidence of EIBs was 23%. This percentage included nearly half of the cross-country skiing

team as well as winners of gold, silver, and bronze medals. This study demonstrated that athletes can compete at the international level—even winning an Olympic gold medal—despite having exercise-induced asthma.

Taking It Further

1. Research the career of a famous athlete with asthma. Did the disease present challenges to the athlete? How did he or she cope with the disease? Present your findings in an oral report to the class.

2. If you were a coach and a member of your team showed symptoms of exercise-induced asthma, what advice would you give him or her for managing this disease?

8% of adults and 9% of children have asthma. This respiratory disease can be fatal; it kills more than 3,500 each year. In the United States, the costs associated with asthma treatments and lost productivity in the workplace amount to roughly $56 billion each year.

Lung Cancer

More people in the United States die from lung cancer than any other form of cancer. This statistic is particularly tragic because lung cancer is highly preventable. In about 90% of cases, smoking is the main cause of lung cancer. Exposure to secondhand smoke, radon, asbestos, and other toxins are other risk factors for lung cancer.

The majority of people with lung cancer die within a year because the cancer was not diagnosed at a treatable stage. Lung cancer

metastasizes (spreads) quickly to lymph nodes and other organs, such as the brain and the breasts.

Lung cancer is usually classified as non-small cell or small cell lung cancer. Non-small cell lung cancer is the more common of the two forms and is prevalent in smokers. Non-small cell lung cancer spreads more slowly than small cell lung cancer. Small cell lung cancer develops and spreads quickly in the early stage of the disease, often before a detectable tumor forms on one of the lungs. Because a tumor is usually the identifying element of lung cancer, small cell cancer has ample time to spread before it is detected.

Treatment options for both non-small cell and small cell lung cancer include radiation therapy and chemotherapy. In some cases, surgery is performed to remove the cancerous growth. However, surgery is usually not an option because the cancer typically is too advanced when it is diagnosed. Unfortunately, radiation therapy and chemotherapy are often not very effective because lung cancer tends to spread quickly throughout the body. Alternate treatment options have been developed, including an inhalable, dry chemotherapy drug. One promising treatment option involves tailoring chemotherapy drugs based on a patient's unique biological response to treatment methods.

 Check Your Understanding

1. What percentage of adults in the United States has asthma?
2. What are some treatments for asthma?
3. What causes nearly 90% of all lung cancers?
4. Why is lung cancer difficult to treat?

Lesson 9.3 Review and Assessment

Mini Glossary   Make sure that you know the meaning of each key term.

 Build vocabulary with e-flash cards and games

acute bronchitis   a temporary inflammation of the mucous membranes that line the trachea and bronchial passageways; causes a cough that may produce mucus

asthma   disease of the lungs characterized by recurring episodes of airway inflammation causing bronchospasms and increased mucus production

bronchospasms   spasmodic contractions of the bronchial muscles that constrict the airways in the lungs during an asthma attack

chronic bronchitis   a long-lasting respiratory condition in which the airways of the lungs become obstructed due to inflammation of the bronchi and excessive mucus production

chronic obstructive pulmonary disease (COPD)   any lung disorder characterized by a long-term airway obstruction, making it difficult to breathe

emphysema   chronic inflammation of the lungs characterized by an abnormal increase in the air spaces near the bronchioles; causes an accumulation of carbon dioxide in the lungs

hyperventilation   excessive ventilation that leads to abnormal expulsion of carbon dioxide

influenza   a viral infection that affects the respiratory system; the flu

laryngitis   inflammation of the larynx, or voice box

nasopharyngitis   inflammation of the nasal passages and pharynx; the common cold

pharyngitis   inflammation of the pharynx, or throat

pneumonia   an infection of the lungs that causes inflammation; caused by a virus, bacterium, fungus, or—in rare cases—parasites

sinusitis   inflammation of the sinuses

tonsillitis   inflammation of the tonsils

tuberculosis (TB)   a highly contagious bacterial infection caused by *Mycobacterium tuberculosis*

Know and Understand

 Assess

1. Which bacterium can cause both pharyngitis and tonsillitis?
2. Which upper respiratory tract illness can lead to voice loss?
3. Why is sneezing into your sleeve preferable to sneezing into your hands?
4. List some ways that upper respiratory tract illnesses can be prevented.
5. Which symptoms indicate influenza?
6. Name three lower respiratory tract illnesses.
7. How is pneumonia treated?
8. What is COPD?

Analyze & Apply

9. Montee has not been feeling well for a few weeks. He has been coughing frequently. His cough regularly produces mucus, but sometimes it also contains blood. Montee has been very tired and feverish, often waking in the middle of the night because he is warm and sweating profusely. After considering his symptoms, what disease do you think Montee has?

10. Explain how the results of a pulmonary function test differ between a person with healthy lungs and someone with emphysema or chronic bronchitis.

11. Why are people with a family history of allergies at a higher risk for having asthma?

12. Why is purse-lipped breathing recommended for people with COPD?

In the Lab

13. Create an informational pamphlet on the respiratory disorder of your choice. Research the causes of the disorder, symptoms, age groups affected, tests or scans used to diagnose the disorder, treatments, and prognosis. Include images in your pamphlet. Present your pamphlet to the class.

Career Corner
Anatomy and Physiology at Work

As we have learned in this chapter, the respiratory system is a vital system because it delivers life-sustaining oxygen to our body tissues and removes harmful carbon dioxide.

A number of careers are dedicated to the study of the respiratory system, the health and maintenance of its components, and the diagnosis and treatment of respiratory disorders and diseases. We will explore two of these careers.

Respiratory Therapist

A respiratory therapist (RT) is a healthcare professional who, under the supervision of doctors, cares for people with respiratory disorders. RTs also provide emergency care for people who have breathing problems resulting from heart attack, stroke, near-drowning, or other circumstances.

RTs perform diagnostic tests on patients. These tests include pulmonary function tests, static lung volume measurements, cardiopulmonary exercise testing, and arterial blood gas tests.

RTs also treat patients with poor pulmonary health. They control patients' supplemental oxygen levels and provide respiratory muscle training. In addition, RTs educate patients about effective ways to minimize symptoms and manage their pulmonary disease. RTs administer drug treatments to patients, including nebulizer therapy treatments. A nebulizer is a machine that turns liquid medication into a mist, which is breathed directly into the lungs.

To become a respiratory therapist, you need an associate's degree or a bachelor's degree in respiratory therapy from an accredited institution. RTs must also pass a national certification exam and meet the licensing requirements of their state. Most hospitals hire registered respiratory therapists (RRTs) who have passed the Registered Respiratory Therapist exam.

The demand for respiratory therapists is expected to increase by more than 25% in the next 10 years. Much of the growth in this field, and in other healthcare-related careers, is due to the aging of a large segment of the population called *baby boomers*. Baby boomers are people who were born in the decades after World War II, when the birth rate in the United States increased dramatically. The baby boomers are now moving into old age, a time when many people develop health problems, including respiratory system disorders.

Pharmacy Technician

A pharmacy technician assists licensed pharmacists in dispensing prescription medications. They work in hospitals and in retail pharmacies.

Because pharmacy technicians interact frequently with patients or customers, they must have excellent interpersonal, or "people," skills. After receiving a prescription from a customer, the pharmacy technician often must request additional information from the customer or a doctor. Prescriptions also come into the pharmacy electronically from doctors' offices, so pharmacy technicians must have a working knowledge of computers and fax machines.

Pharmacy technicians must be very attentive to detail. Dispensing the wrong medication or the wrong dosage (amount) to a customer or patient can cause illness or even death. After reading a prescription, the pharmacy technician retrieves the correct medication from the shelves. Under the supervision of a pharmacist, the pharmacy

Lisa F. Young/Shutterstock.com

Figure 9.19 A respiratory therapist assists her patient with a breathing exercise.

Dmitry Kalinovsky/Shutterstock.com

Figure 9.20 A pharmacy technician works under the direct supervision of a licensed pharmacist.

technician counts out the correct number of tablets or capsules, measures the prescribed amount of a liquid, or mixes substances to produce the drug. Pharmacy technicians who work in healthcare facilities may also dispense intravenous (IV) medications to patients.

After prescriptions have been packaged and labeled, a pharmacist checks them. The pharmacy technician then dispenses the medications to customers and takes payment. Pharmacy technicians may also create and maintain medical profiles of their customers or patients, prepare and submit health insurance forms, and manage the pharmacy inventory.

Pharmacy technicians must possess a high school diploma or its equivalent. Some pharmacy technicians receive on-the-job training; others attend a certificate program at a vocational school or community college. Certification for pharmacy technicians is offered by the National Pharmacy Technician Certification Board and the National Healthcare Association. To find out the certification requirements for your state, check the website of your state pharmacy board.

The job outlook for pharmacy technicians is promising. As we age, we often need more prescription medications. A shortage in the number of licensed pharmacists has also created a demand for pharmacy technicians.

Planning for a Health-Related Career

Do some research on the career of a respiratory therapist or a pharmacy technician. You may choose instead to research a profession from the list of **Related Career Options**. Using the Internet or resources at your local library, find answers to the following questions:

1. What are the main tasks and responsibilities of a person employed in the career that you chose to research?
2. What is the outlook for this career? Are workers in demand, or are jobs dwindling? For complete information, consult the current edition of the *Occupational Outlook Handbook,* published by the US Department of Labor. This handbook is available online or at your local library.
3. What special skills or talents are required? For example, do you enjoy research? Do you need to enjoy communicating with other people?
4. What personality traits do you think are necessary for success in the career that you have chosen to research? For example, are you meticulous and accurate? Pharmacy technicians must have these traits.
5. Does the work involve a great deal of routine, or are the day-to-day responsibilities varied?
6. Does the career require long hours, or is it a standard, "9-to-5" job?
7. What is the salary range for this job?
8. What do you think you would like about this career? Is there anything about it that you might dislike?

Related Career Options

- Athletic Trainer
- Medical Assistant
- Medical Records and Health Information Technician
- Occupational Therapist
- Pharmacist
- Physical Therapist
- Registered Nurse

Chapter Summaries

Lesson 9.1 Functions and Anatomy of the Respiratory System

> Build vocabulary with e-flash cards and games

Key Points

- Humans can survive only minutes without oxygen.
- Removal of carbon dioxide from the body is equally as important as maintaining sufficient amounts of oxygen.
- The respiratory system consists of several structures including the nose, pharynx, larynx, trachea, bronchi, bronchioles, and lungs.
- The larynx routes air, food, and liquids either to the trachea (air) or to the esophagus (food and liquids).
- The trachea is also called the *windpipe*. It serves as a passageway for air entering and leaving the lungs.
- The bronchioles, the smallest, terminating passageways of the bronchi, end in millions of air sacs called *alveoli*.
- Gas exchange takes place between capillary blood and the alveoli in the alveolar capillary membrane.

Key Terms

alveolar capillary membrane
alveoli
bronchioles
cardiopulmonary system
conchae
epiglottis
larynx
mediastinum
nares
olfactory receptors

palate
pharynx
pleural sac
pores of Kohn
primary bronchi
sinuses
surfactant
thyroid cartilage
tonsils
trachea

Lesson 9.2 Respiration: Mechanics and Control

Key Points

- The main function of the respiratory system is gas exchange. Gas exchange supplies the body with fresh oxygen while removing harmful carbon dioxide.
- The external intercostal muscles are involved in inspiration but not in expiration.
- Normal breathing is a passive process unless a person is exercising or has asthma. Under those circumstances, breathing becomes an active process.
- Neural and chemical factors play a key role in breathing control.
- The rate and depth of breathing are controlled by inspiratory and expiratory centers in the brain. These centers are located in the medulla and pons areas of the brain stem.
- Lung volume varies based on age, height, weight, gender, and race.

Key Terms

central chemoreceptors
expiration
expiratory reserve volume (ERV)
external respiration
forced expiratory volume in one second (FEV_1)
forced expiratory volume in one second/forced vital capacity (FEV_1/FVC)
functional residual capacity (FRC)
Hering-Breuer reflex

inspiration
inspiratory reserve volume (IRV)
internal respiration
mechanoreceptors
peripheral chemoreceptors
pulmonary ventilation
residual volume (RV)
respiration
respiratory gas transport
tidal volume (TV)
total lung capacity (TLC)
vital capacity (VC)

Lesson 9.3 Respiratory Disorders and Diseases

Key Points

- Upper respiratory tract illnesses are the most common acute illnesses.
- Upper respiratory tract illnesses are transmitted by hand-to hand contact, handling of a contaminated object, and airborne droplets from an infected person's cough or sneeze.
- Thorough hand washing is one of the most effective ways to prevent transmission of upper respiratory illnesses.
- Bronchitis, pneumonia, and tuberculosis are among the most common lower respiratory tract illnesses.
- Chronic obstructive pulmonary disease (COPD) is any lung disorder that causes long-term airway obstruction and difficulty breathing.
- The primary cause of COPD is smoking.
- The prevalence of asthma in the United States has risen dramatically in recent years.
- More people die from lung cancer in the United States than from any other form of cancer. Because it can quickly metastasize (spread) it is hard to diagnose lung cancer at an early, treatable stage.

Key Terms

acute bronchitis
asthma
bronchospasms
chronic bronchitis
chronic obstructive
   pulmonary disease
   (COPD)
emphysema
hyperventilation

influenza
laryngitis
nasopharyngitis
pharyngitis
pneumonia
sinusitis
tonsillitis
tuberculosis (TB)

Chapter Assessments

Assess

Lesson 9.1

Functions and Anatomy of the Respiratory System

Learning Key Terms and Concepts

1. The main purpose of the respiratory system is to provide a constant supply of oxygen while eliminating _____.

2. Which of the following is *not* part of the respiratory system?
   - A. nose
   - B. lungs
   - C. duodenum
   - D. trachea

3. The nasal cavity contains oily, coated hairs called _____ that trap and prevent particles from entering the nose.

4. *True or False?* The palate is commonly known as the *roof of the mouth*.

5. _____ are air-filled cavities that surround the nose.

6. *True or False?* The pharynx is part of both the respiratory and digestive systems.

7. The larynx is also called the _____.

8. The flap of cartilage that covers the opening of the larynx during swallowing to prevent food or liquids from entering the trachea is called the _____.
   - A. uvula
   - B. tonsils
   - C. epiglottis
   - D. pharynx

9. *True or False?* The trachea is commonly called the *windpipe*.

10. The trachea divides into right and left _____.

11. The air-filled sacs in the lungs are called _____.

12. *True or False?* The left lung is wider than the right lung.

Thinking Critically

13. Explain in your own words how the conchae filter inspired air. Why do you think this filtering method is so effective?

14. The anterior part of the trachea is supported by cartilaginous, C-shaped rings that prevent it from collapsing. On the posterior side, the C-shaped rings are open and contain no cartilage. Why is this beneficial?

Lesson 9.2

Respiration: Mechanics and Control

Learning Key Terms and Concepts

15. The main function of the respiratory system is to conduct _____.

16. Another name for breathing is _____.

17. _____ is the respiratory process by which air is continuously moved into and out of the lungs.
    A. pulmonary ventilation
    B. external respiration
    C. respiratory gas transport
    D. internal respiration

18. _____, also called *inhalation*, is the process by which air flows into the lungs.

19. *True or False?* Normal expiration is an active process.

20. Biological factors that influence breathing rate include _____.
    A. gender   C. both A and B
    B. age   D. none of the above

21. *True or False?* Your postural position affects your breathing rate.

22. _____ monitor cerebrospinal fluid pH to detect excess carbon dioxide levels in the body.
    A. Stretch receptors
    B. Central chemoreceptors
    C. Peripheral chemoreceptors
    D. Mechanoreceptors

23. Lung volume varies according to _____.
    A. weight   C. race
    B. height   D. all of the above

24. Explain in your own words the difference between each of the following pairs of lung capacity measurements.
    A. tidal volume and inspiratory reserve volume
    B. expiratory volume and vital capacity
    C. FEV1 and ERV

25. *True or False?* Lung volume generally does not predict the average athlete's performance.

26. During maximal exercise, we use only about _____ of our lungs' vital capacity.
    A. 30%   C. 65%
    B. 50%   D. 85%

Thinking Critically

27. Explain the following formula: IRV + TV + ERV + RV = TLC. What does each abbreviation mean? Why do these four elements equal TLC?

28. Recalling what you have learned about neural and chemical factors that control breathing rate, why is it not possible to hold your breath for long periods of time?

Lesson 9.3

Respiratory Disorders and Diseases

Learning Key Terms and Concepts

29. The most common respiratory tract illnesses occur in the _____.
    A. upper respiratory tract
    B. lower respiratory tract

30. Inflammation of the throat is called _____.

31. Laryngitis is an inflammation of the _____.

32. Sinusitis can be caused by _____.
    A. fungi   C. viruses
    B. bacteria   D. all of the above

33. *True or False?* Influenza causes white or yellow patches to form on the tonsils.

34. Acute bronchitis usually develops in response to an ongoing _____ infection.

35. *True or False?* People with tuberculosis must be confined to their home or the hospital for two to four years to avoid spreading this highly contagious disease.

36. The two most common forms of COPD are emphysema and _____.

37. Bronchitis is considered chronic when a person has a cough that has lasted _____.
    A. two to three   C. three months to
       weeks   two years
    B. five or six days   D. ten years or longer

38. The primary cause of COPD is _____.

39. About 8% of adults and _____ % of children in the United States have asthma.
    A. 3   C. 9
    B. 10   D. 14

40. *True or False?* Emotional stress can trigger an asthma attack.

41. *True or False?* Non-small cell lung cancer is prevalent among smokers.

42. Surgery, radiation therapy, and _____ are treatment options for lung cancer.

Thinking Critically

43. Imagine that you are a doctor, and a female patient visits your office with a complaint of headache, fatigue, sinus pain and stuffiness, body aches, and chills. You take her temperature and discover that she has a fever of 38.9°C (102°F). She tells you that she felt fine the night before but woke up that morning feeling terrible. Based on the patient's symptoms, what is your first diagnosis and why?

44. Identify the respiratory diseases associated with the terms "pink puffers" and "blue bloaters." Why are these terms appropriate for each disease?

Building Skills and Connecting Concepts

Analyzing and Evaluating Data

Imagine that you are a doctor and one of your patients is an active, 15-year-old boy named Toua. Toua complains of tightness in his chest, wheezing, and breathlessness. Using a spirometer, you test Toua's lung volume. His test results (shown below) confirm your suspicion—Toua has asthma. Review Toua's test results and then answer the questions that follow.

Tidal Volume (TV) = 200 ml (Normal = 500 ml)

Residual Volume (RV) = 600 ml (Normal = 1,200 ml)

Total Lung Capacity (TLC) = 4,400 ml (Normal = 4,400–6,400 ml)

Vital Capacity (VC) = 3,000 ml (Normal = 4,500–5,500 ml)

Inspiratory Reserve Volume (IRV) = 1,500 ml (Normal = 3,000 ml)

45. Why do Toua's symptoms indicate asthma?

46. Look at Toua's tidal volume. What explains this low level?

47. What does his vital capacity indicate? Why does a below-average VC suggest asthma?

48. Why is Toua's TLC in the normal range even though he has asthma?

Communicating about Anatomy and Physiology

49. **Speaking and Writing** Working in a group of three or four students, recall the last time that you had a cold or the flu. Discuss common symptoms. Write down the five most common symptoms. Do research to find out why these symptoms occurred. For example, a sore throat is caused by mucus dripping into your pharynx (throat), producing irritation and inflammation. Share your findings with the class.

50. **Reading and Writing** In this chapter, you learned that the respiratory and cardiovascular systems work together to conduct gas exchange. Think about the body systems that you have studied so far and skim ahead looking for similar relationships between the structures and functions of systems. Write a detailed report that describes and analyzes one or more of these relationships.

Lab Investigations

Work with a partner to determine breathing recovery rates after exercise.

Take turns measuring your resting breathing rate. Count the number of breaths in one minute. Do this three times, find the average, and then record your resting breathing rate.

Next, do 25 jumping jacks. Immediately afterward, have your partner count the number of breaths that you take in one minute. Record this number. Continue to record the number of breaths that you take each minute after that. Then count the number of minutes that it takes you to return to your resting breathing rate. Record this number.

Finally, run in place for two minutes. Immediately afterward, have your partner count the number of breaths that you take during the first minute. Record this number. Then record the number of breaths that you take each minute until you have returned to your resting breathing rate. Record these numbers.

51. Compare your average resting rate, your respiratory rate one minute after doing the jumping jacks, and your respiratory rate after running in place. Is there a great difference between these numbers? Explain your results.

52. Examine the number of minutes that it took to return to your resting rate after doing 25 jumping jacks and after running in place. Are these numbers higher or lower than you expected?

53. The faster that your respiratory rate returns to its resting value, the more physically fit you are. Based on your results, what do you think your level of physical fitness is? If your physical fitness is lower than you'd like, what are some strategies that you can undertake to improve it?

Expand your learning with additional online resources
- Supplemental Lab Activities
- Interactive Exercises
- Animations

Companion Website

www.g-wlearning.com/healthsciences

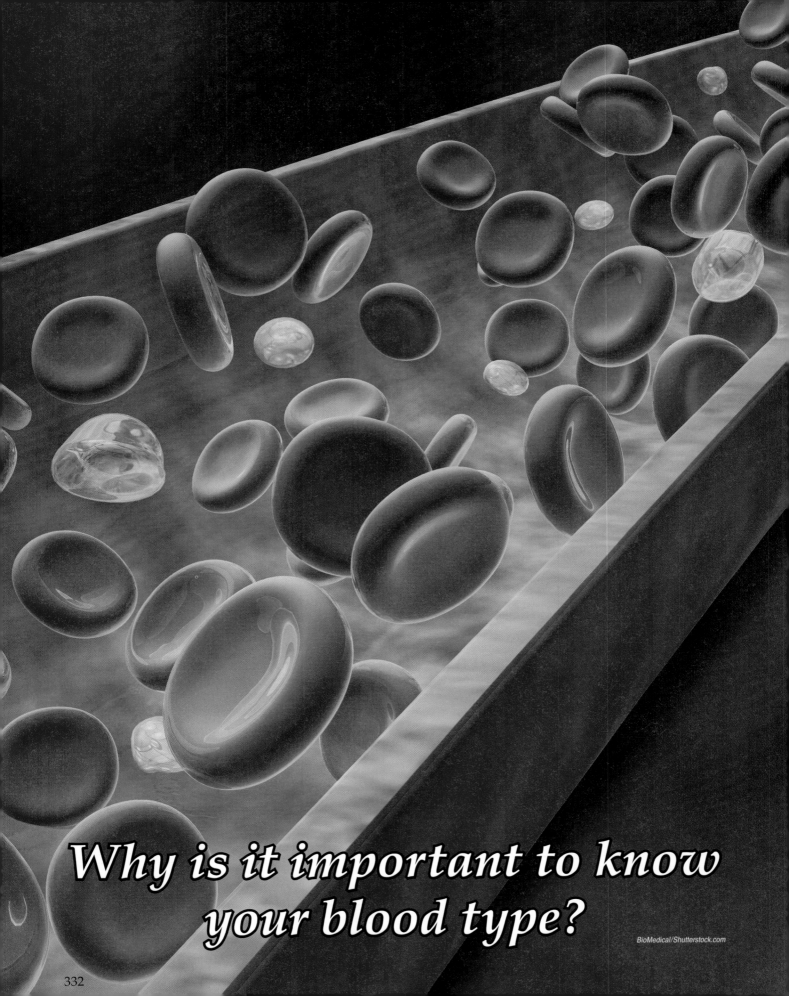

Why is it important to know your blood type?

The Blood

*O*ur understanding of the life-giving functions of blood has not always been clear. As early as Greek times, physicians thought that draining blood from the body, a procedure known as *bloodletting*, would cure the sick and restore health to the body. This practice continued into the late 1800s.

As you might suspect, some individuals did not fare well from bloodletting. Bloodletting contributed to the death of President George Washington. During a brief illness that began with a sore throat and fever, Washington's physicians bled him. Over the course of 16 hours, physicians drained 5 to 7 pints of Washington's blood. That's equivalent to 40% to 60% of the body's supply of blood! Not surprisingly, President Washington died shortly thereafter.

Today we understand the important role that blood plays in maintaining a person's health and sustaining life. For this reason, many people donate their blood to organizations such as the American Red Cross, which maintains blood banks. When you donate blood, you really are giving the gift of life: one pint can feed, protect, clean, and heal up to three people.

In this chapter you will learn about the functions and composition of blood, blood types, and common blood disorders and diseases.

Chapter 10 Lessons

Lesson 10.1
The Function and Composition of Blood

Lesson 10.2
Blood Types

Lesson 10.3
Blood Disorders and Diseases

While studying, look for the online icon **to:**

- **Practice** with e-flash cards and vocabulary games
- **Review** with interactive art labeling
- **Assess** with online exercises
- **Expand** with interactive activities and animated videos
- **Listen** to pronunciations of key terms in the audio glossary

www.g-wlearning.com/healthsciences

Study on the Go

Use a mobile device to practice vocabulary terms, listen to pronunciations, and review with self-assessment quizzes.

www.m.g-wlearning.com

The Function and Composition of Blood

Lesson Objectives

1. Explain how blood transports nutrients and waste products, regulates body temperature, and fights infection.
2. Identify the solid and liquid components of blood.
3. Describe how the body manufactures blood cells.
4. Explain the physical properties and function of red blood cells, white blood cells, and platelets.
5. Describe the process of coagulation.

Key Terms

E-Flash Cards

buffy coat
coagulation
diapedesis
erythropoiesis
erythropoietin (EPO)
fibrin
formed elements
hematocrit

hemoglobin
hemolysis
hemostasis
plasma
platelet plug
platelets
red blood cells
white blood cells

Every day, our body undergoes so many changes that it would be hard to quantify them. Even with all of these changes, however, the body maintains homeostasis through many dynamic regulatory systems. Blood is one of our body's regulatory and transport systems. Our blood plays a vital role in gas exchange; body temperature maintenance; and acid-base, fluid, and electrolyte balance.

The Function of Blood

The blood is responsible for providing transportation, regulation, and protection throughout the body. It plays a key role in gas exchange, which, as you will recall from chapter 9, involves supplying oxygen and other nutrients to cells, while also removing carbon dioxide and other waste products. The blood carries waste to the kidneys and carbon dioxide to the lungs, where both the waste and carbon dioxide are eliminated from the body.

Blood also protects the body against infection and regulates body temperature by directing heat toward the skin and lungs. In addition, buffers and amino acids transported in the blood help maintain the body's pH at healthy levels between 7.35 and 7.45.

Figure 10.1 summarizes the different roles that blood plays in maintaining homeostasis.

The Formed Elements

There are two basic components of blood: the liquid component, called **plasma**, and the solid components, collectively referred to as the **formed elements** (**Figure 10.2**). The formed elements consist of **red blood cells** (*erythrocytes*), **white blood cells** (*leukocytes*), and **platelets**. Red

Figure 10.1 Functions of the Blood

Transports	oxygen and carbon dioxide
	waste products of metabolism (urea and lactic acid)
	hormones
	enzymes
	nutrients (glucose, fats, amino acids, vitamins, and minerals)
	blood cells (white and red)
	plasma proteins (fibrinogen, albumin, globulin)
Regulates	body temperature
	acid-base balance (pH)
	fluid and electrolyte balance
Protects	white blood cells protect against infection
	antibodies detect foreign material
	clotting factors prevent excessive bleeding

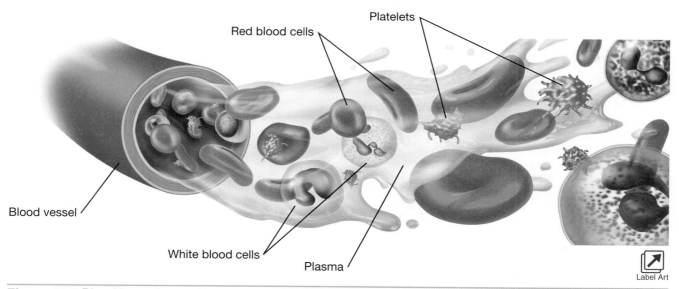

Label Art

Figure 10.2 Blood is made up of both liquid (plasma) and solid components (the formed elements). *What three substances comprise the formed elements?*

blood cells carry oxygen to tissue, white blood cells protect the body, and platelets play a vital role in blood clotting. The formed elements make up about 45% of the blood's content, and plasma comprises the remaining 55%.

Components of blood are readily identified when a blood sample is taken and spun down in a centrifuge. A centrifuge is a machine that spins rapidly, generating centrifugal force and separating elements in the blood. The centrifugal force separates the blood into three layers: liquid plasma rises to the top of the tube, red blood cells settle at the bottom of the tube, and a thin layer called the **buffy coat** settles between the red blood cells and plasma. The buffy coat contains white blood cells and platelets (**Figure 10.3**).

Alexander Raths/Shutterstock.com

Blood draw

Suthep/Shutterstock.com

Centrifuge

Plasma (55%)

Buffy coat — White blood cells and platelets (<1%)

Red blood cells (45%) (hematocrit)

Formed elements

Functions of the formed elements

Cell type	Number per µL (mm³) of blood	Functions
Red blood cells (erythrocytes)	4–6 million	Carry oxygen and carbon dioxide
White blood cells (leukocytes) — Basophil, Neutrophil, Eosinophil, Lymphocyte, Monocyte	4,000–11,000	Immune response–fight infection, produce antibodies, and intensify inflammatory response
Platelets	150,000–440,000	Form and dissolve blood clots

Figure 10.3 Drawn blood is spun through a centrifuge to separate the plasma and formed elements. *What property of blood does hematocrit measure?*

Separating these blood elements allows us to take a common blood measurement called **hematocrit** (hee-MAT-oh-krit). Hematocrit is the proportion of the total blood volume that is composed of red blood cells. This proportion of red blood cells is expressed as a percentage of total blood volume.

Hematocrit averages 45% of total blood volume in men and 40% of total blood volume in women. Hematocrit is fairly constant, but dehydration can cause hematocrit to increase due to loss of blood plasma, or decreased blood volume. However, if you live at a high altitude, your hematocrit may increase to 60% or 65% of your total blood volume because altitude exposure increases red blood cell production.

Physical Properties of Blood

Blood is a sticky, thick fluid that makes up roughly 8% of our total body weight. Both men and women have, on average, between 4 and 5 liters of blood in their bodies. However, blood volume depends on body size, muscle mass, and physical fitness. Athletes, for example, have higher blood volumes.

Blood is slightly salty, with a sodium chloride concentration of 0.9%. It has a pH between 7.35 and 7.45 and an average temperature of 38°C (100.4°F). The color of blood varies based on the oxygen level in the bloodstream. Oxygen-rich blood in the arteries is a brighter red than the oxygen-poor blood in the veins.

The old saying that "blood is thicker than water" is literally true. At 38°C (100.4°F), the viscosity (thickness) of blood is about five times thicker than that of water. This is because blood contains solid components such as the formed elements, plasma proteins, and electrolytes. Blood viscosity contributes to blood flow resistance. In general, the thicker the blood, the harder the heart has to work to maintain blood flow. Factors that increase blood viscosity are decreased blood temperature, prolonged exposure to a high altitude, and an elevated hematocrit level.

 Check Your Understanding

1. The functions of blood can be divided into what three major categories? Give two specific examples for each category.
2. What are the two basic components of blood?
3. Typically, what percentage of the blood is made up of plasma?
4. Which physical property of blood is affected by differences in the blood oxygen level?

Plasma

The formed elements are transported in the plasma, or liquid part of the blood. Plasma is a pale yellow fluid composed of 90% water and 8% plasma proteins; the remaining 2% is a mixture of electrolytes, nutrients, ions, respiratory gases, hormones, and waste products.

Blood plasma contains three types of proteins: fibrinogen, albumin, and globulin (**Figure 10.4** on the next page). These proteins perform a variety of functions, including transporting lipids (fats) and fat-soluble vitamins, regulating blood pressure and volume, and assisting in blood clot formation.

Besides water and plasma proteins, blood plasma contains a mixture of electrolytes and buffers. The electrolytes include sodium, potassium, chloride, magnesium, and calcium, all of which help maintain fluid and electrolyte balance. Buffers such as bicarbonate, phosphate, and sulfate regulate blood pH.

As blood travels through the body, it collects and removes carbon dioxide, a waste product. Plasma contains a bicarbonate that provides the primary means for carbon dioxide transport. Because of gas exchange and different substances being added to or removed from plasma, its composition can vary from minute to minute. However, homeostatic mechanisms monitor and maintain relatively constant plasma composition. In short, blood plasma transports elements throughout the body in an effort to maintain homeostasis.

Figure 10.4 Plasma Proteins

Protein	Percent of Plasma Composition	Origin	Function
albumin	58%	liver	regulates osmotic pressure of blood and blood volume; transports lipids, hormones, and other solutes
globulin alpha	38%	liver	aids in blood clot formation; transports lipids and fat-soluble vitamins
beta		liver	transports lipids and fat-soluble vitamins
gamma		plasma cells	helps fight infection
fibrinogen	4%	liver	aids in blood clot formation

Maintaining homeostasis requires constant effort. Think about all the changes that take place in the body during a 30-minute run, for example. Blood glucose levels decline, blood pH becomes more acidic, and blood temperature increases. The body's feedback systems sense these changes and respond accordingly. To maintain homeostasis in this situation, gluconeogenesis begins, respiration increases to buffer (balance) the acidic pH of the blood, the sweat glands are activated, and blood flow is shifted to the skin to cool the body. Plasma plays an important role in each of these responses. It would be impossible to maintain homeostasis without it.

Manufacturing Blood Cells

Each blood cell has a limited life span, so it is important that the body has the ability to create new blood cells. New blood cells are created in a process called *hematopoiesis* (HEE-ma-toh-poy-EE-sis). You first learned about hematopoiesis in chapter 4.

Blood cells are manufactured in bone marrow, a soft, spongy substance inside the bones. Bone marrow contains fat, blood, and stem cells—cells that create other cells. There are two types of bone marrow: yellow and red. Only red bone marrow (found in the vertebrae, ribs, hips, sternum, and skull) can produce stem cells and blood cells. Lymphatic tissue in the lymph nodes, tonsils, spleen, and thymus gland also produces blood cells, but the majority of blood cells are manufactured by stem cells in the bone marrow.

Each of the formed elements in the blood starts as a hematopoietic stem cell, which morphs into another type of stem cell before it develops into a blast cell. Depending on which growth or stimulating factors and hormones influence the blast cell, it matures into a red blood cell, white blood cell, or platelet (**Figure 10.5**). As blood cells develop from the stem cell, they enter the bloodstream by seeping into the blood as it flows through the bone.

Check Your Understanding

1. Which three proteins are found in plasma?
2. Where are blood cells manufactured?
3. How do new blood cells enter the bloodstream?

Red Blood Cells (Erythrocytes)

Red blood cells (RBCs) are also called *erythrocytes*. RBCs perform one of the most important functions in the body—gas exchange. They carry oxygen to every living cell in the body and carry carbon dioxide away. RBCs are the most abundant cells in the blood, numbering between four and six million per cubic millimeter.

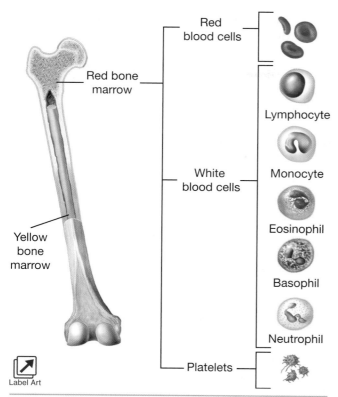

Label Art

Figure 10.5 Red blood cells, white blood cells, and platelets develop from stem cells in bone marrow. *In which color bone marrow are stem cells manufactured?*

To put this number into perspective, a cubic millimeter is so small that it is almost invisible to the naked eye. Imagine four to six million cells in a tiny, nearly invisible speck!

Shape and Size

Mature red blood cells are disk-shaped cells that look like a doughnut without the hole in the center. They are small, measuring only 7 or 8 micrometers in diameter. To put this measurement into perspective, 1 millimeter is equal to 1,000 micrometers.

As RBCs develop, the nucleus is forced out of the cell, causing the center of the cell to collapse. This mechanism of development serves three important functions:

1. It increases the surface area of the cell, providing a larger binding area for oxygen and carbon dioxide.
2. It increases the flexibility of the cell, allowing it to change shape so it can fit into capillary openings that are half the size of the cell.

3. It limits the cell's life span to 120 days; without a nucleus, the cell is unable to replicate.

Hemoglobin

The **hemoglobin** (HEE-moh-GLOH-bin) molecule is the "workhorse" of the red blood cell because it carries out the important job of gas exchange. Oxygen and carbon dioxide attach to the hemoglobin molecules of the RBC; thus, hemoglobin is known as the *binding site.*

Hemoglobin is actually composed of two molecules: a large protein called *globin* (GLOH-bin) and an iron molecule called *heme* (heem). Each hemoglobin molecule has four heme binding sites for oxygen (**Figure 10.6**).

One RBC contains approximately 250 million hemoglobin molecules. This means that one RBC carries almost one billion oxygen molecules. Before you donate blood, your hemoglobin level is measured. Hemoglobin levels differ between men and women. In men, they range from 12 to 16 grams per deciliter (g/dL); in women, hemoglobin levels range from 13 to 18 grams per deciliter.

Oxygen binds to hemoglobin, forming an *oxyhemoglobin* (AHK-see-HEE-moh-GLOH-bin) *molecule* in the capillaries of the lung. The oxygen-rich RBCs then travel to tissue capillaries. The oxygen is unloaded from the

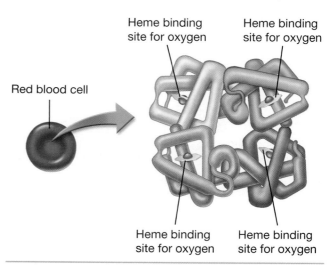

Figure 10.6 During gas exchange, oxygen binds to hemoglobin at each of the four heme binding sites.

hemoglobin, diffusing from the blood into the oxygen-deprived tissues.

The globin protein serves as the binding site for carbon dioxide. Once carbon dioxide has attached to the hemoglobin molecule, a *carbaminohemoglobin* (kar-BAM-i-noh-HEE-moh-GLOH-bin) *molecule* is formed. The carbaminohemoglobin molecule transports carbon dioxide back to the lungs. Keep in mind, however, that the bicarbonate ion in plasma is the chief means by which carbon dioxide is transported.

Erythropoiesis

The kidneys regulate red blood cell production through a process called **erythropoiesis** (eh-RITH-roh-poy-EE-sis). When blood oxygen content decreases—as it does where the altitude is above 5,000 feet—the kidneys secrete a hormone called **erythropoietin** (eh-RITH-roh-POY-eh-tin), or **EPO**.

Erythropoietin stimulates stem cell production of RBCs in the red bone marrow (**Figure 10.7**).

When additional RBCs are produced and blood oxygen levels rise, erythropoietin levels diminish, slowing RBC production. Thus, any condition or factor that lowers blood oxygen levels (such as emphysema or high altitude exposure) will cause the kidneys to release erythropoietin and stimulate RBC production. If an excess of RBCs is produced, polycythemia (PAHL-ee-sigh-THEE-mee-ah) can develop. We will discuss polycythemia, a condition marked by an increased level of RBCs circulating in the bloodstream, in more depth in lesson 10.3.

Iron, folic acid, vitamin B_{12}, and protein are needed for RBC production, as well as for red bone marrow. People who are anemic, and potentially those with an iron-deficient diet, lack enough iron to properly form the heme component of hemoglobin. The result is iron-deficient anemia, a blood disorder that you'll learn more about later in this chapter.

Figure 10.7 The endocrine system works with the blood to release the hormone erythropoietin, which stimulates red blood cell production.

WHAT RESEARCH TELLS US

...*about* Bioengineering Red Blood Cells to Create an Unlimited Supply

Since Roman times, scientists have been looking for viable (usable) substitutes for blood. Doctors and scientists have experimented with animal blood and animal milk. Even wine has been suggested as a possible alternative to blood.

Researchers at the Université Pierre et Marie Curie in Paris, France, have been studying the possibility of manufacturing red blood cells from stem cells. The researchers at this university were able to generate billions of RBCs from a single stem cell. The RBCs were then injected into the stem cell donor. The stem cells were treated with several different growth factors to stimulate them to develop into mature RBCs.

After 5 days, the survival rate of the human-engineered RBCs was 94% to 100%. Of this number, 41% to 63% were still alive after 26 days. This is similar to the survival rate of a normal RBC. This research is critical, especially when you consider how these engineered RBCs might be used.

vladm/Shutterstock.com

Figure 10.8 Every day, many units of blood are needed for transfusions and surgeries around the world.

Each year, the American Red Cross alone distributes about six million units of RBCs (**Figure 10.8**). According to the World Health Organization (WHO), each year more than 90 million blood donations are made at hospitals, clinics, blood banks, and donation centers around the world. However, some of these donations come from paid donors. In addition, the majority of blood donations are made in high-income countries.

Successful engineering of RBCs would limit dependence on paid donors, especially in low-income nations where voluntary donation is less common. Research continues, but this first successful attempt holds promise for a new way to achieve an unlimited blood supply.

Taking It Further

1. According to WHO, most blood transfusions in low-income countries are given to children with severe anemia and to women during childbirth. By contrast, the main reasons for blood transfusion in high-income countries are physical trauma (such as from a car accident), blood loss during organ-transplant surgeries, and blood disorders that require transfusion therapy. With your classmates, brainstorm possible reasons that donated blood is used for different purposes in low-income and high-income countries.

Your Body Goes Green: Recycling Red Blood Cells

Red blood cell molecules have the remarkable ability to bend, twist, and turn, allowing them to fit into capillaries half their size. All these contortions take their toll on the RBC, causing its membrane to quickly become ragged. The ragged membrane, coupled with the lack of a nucleus, seals the fate of the RBC—death by phagocytosis.

Phagocytosis (FAG-oh-sigh-TOH-sis) is the process by which macrophages (MAK-roh-fayj-ez) in the liver and spleen eat and recycle old RBCs, as well as other types of cells. Macrophages are cells that play a major role in immune system function. You will learn more about macrophages, phagocytes, and phagocytosis in Chapter 12: The Lymphatic and Immune Systems.

Hemolysis (hee-MAHL-i-sis) is the rupture of RBCs. It occurs when RBCs approach the end of their 120-day life span. Hemolysis can also result from diseases of the RBCs caused by antibodies, infections, or blood transfusion complications.

With the exception of the hemoglobin molecules, the RBC membrane breaks down quite easily. For a hemoglobin molecule to be recycled, it must first be separated into its two parts—globin and heme. The globin protein is further broken down into amino acids that are later used to make new proteins. The heme is broken down into iron and bilirubin (BIL-i-ROO-bin), a waste product.

The iron is stored in the liver until the bone marrow needs it to manufacture new RBCs. The bilirubin is excreted into bile. The bile is transported to the gallbladder and then travels through the intestines, before finally being excreted in the feces.

 Check Your Understanding

1. Which blood cells are most abundant in the blood?
2. Which two substances make up hemoglobin?
3. Which organ regulates red blood cell production through the process of erythropoiesis?
4. What is the name of the process in which red blood cells rupture when they reach the end of their life span?

White Blood Cells (Leukocytes)

White blood cells, or *leukocytes*, serve as the body's infection fighters and, therefore, play an important role in immune response. At any given time, blood contains about 4,300 to 10,800 white blood cells (WBCs) per cubic millimeter. For every 1 white blood cell in your blood, there are approximately 700 red blood cells.

Although RBCs far outnumber WBCs, the ratio of 1 WBC for every 700 RBCs is a bit misleading. That's because WBCs can leave the blood, but RBCs cannot. Through a process called **diapedesis** (DIGH-a-peh-DEE-sis), WBCs slip through spaces in the capillary walls as they move from the blood to infection sites in body tissues. Therefore, the ratio stated above doesn't really tell the complete story of the prevalence of WBCs in the body.

As stated earlier, WBCs play an important role in the body's defense systems and immune response. When a foreign microorganism, such as a virus or bacterium, is detected, the body dramatically increases WBC production. Within a matter of hours, the number of WBCs doubles. The WBCs then race to battle the infection.

WBCs have an arsenal of weapons that they use to fight infection. Some WBCs engulf and digest bacteria and other antigens in a process called *phagocytosis* (**Figure 10.9**). Other WBCs produce antibodies, intensify the inflammatory response (which increases swelling and draws more white blood cells to the site of an injury or infection), play a role in allergic reactions, or destroy parasitic worms.

Classifying White Blood Cells

There are five different types of white blood cells. Each type varies by size, appearance, and function.

1. neutrophils (NOO-troh-fils)
2. eosinophils (EE-oh-SIN-oh-fils)
3. basophils (BAY-soh-fils)
4. lymphocytes (LIM-foh-sights)
5. monocytes (MAHN-oh-sights)

① White blood cell engulfs enemy cell (bacteria, dead cells)

② Enzymes start to destroy enemy cell

③ Enemy cell breaks down into small fragments

④ Indigestible fragments are discharged

Figure 10.9 White blood cells engulf foreign antigens, such as bacteria, in an effort to fight infection and keep the body healthy.

Neutrophils, eosinophils, and basophils are classified as *granulocytes* (GRAN-yoo-loh-SIGHTS). Granulocytes have granules in their cytoplasm. Lymphocytes and monocytes are classified as *agranulocytes* (ay-GRAN-yoo-loh-SIGHTS) because their cytoplasm lacks granules.

Unlike RBCs, WBCs have a nucleus. The nucleus of a WBC is visible under a microscope when exposed to Wright's stain, a staining solution that scientists use to differentiate blood types. The size of a WBC, the shape and color of its nucleus, and the color of any granules after staining help scientists classify the WBC (**Figure 10.10** on the next page).

Neutrophils. Neutrophils are the most abundant type of white blood cells and are the most important component of the body's immune system because they are the "first responders." Neutrophils are active phagocytes, cells that engulf and kill foreign invaders such as bacteria, viruses, and fungi. Neutrophils are vital to fighting infection; therefore, a neutrophil deficiency is a life-threatening condition.

Eosinophils. Eosinophils make up only a small portion of our white blood cell count—about 1% to 3%. Eosinophils participate in many inflammatory processes, especially allergic reactions, and are capable of phagocytosis. They are particularly active in the presence of parasites and worms.

Basophils. Basophils are the least abundant white blood cells in the body. They produce histamine, which induces an inflammatory response and summons more infection-fighting WBCs to a site of injury or infection. Basophils also produce heparin, an anticoagulant that prevents blood clotting. Basophils are often associated with allergic reactions and asthma. They also play an important role in T cell adaptive immune responses.

Lymphocytes. Lymphocytes are the second most abundant white blood cells in the body. There are two types of lymphocytes: T cells and B cells. More than 80% of lymphocytes are T cells. Lymphocytes play an important role in the immune response by forming antibodies to fight antigens. Lymphocytes are also essential in fighting cancer cells.

Monocytes. Monocytes, the largest white blood cells in the body, are produced in red bone marrow and then move to the blood, where they remain for one to three days before migrating into body tissues. Once they have arrived in the tissues, monocytes develop into hungry macrophages that devour microorganisms.

Check Your Understanding

1. List the five different types of white blood cells.
2. What is the difference between a granulocyte and an agranulocyte?

Platelets (Thrombocytes)

Platelets (or *thrombocytes*) are part of the formed elements of the blood. They are small, irregularly shaped cell fragments. As cell fragments, platelets do not have a nucleus. Old platelets are removed from the body by phagocytosis in the spleen and liver.

Platelets are derived from multinucleated megakaryocytes (MEHG-a-KAIR-ee-oh-sights), which are specialized bone marrow cells. Like red and white blood cells, megakaryocytes develop from a hematopoietic stem cell. The hormone *thrombopoietin* (THRAHM-boh-POY-eh-tin) regulates platelet production from megakaryocytes. Thrombopoietin is produced by the liver and kidneys.

Platelets play an important role in **hemostasis** (HEE-moh-STAY-sis), the sequence of events that causes blood clots to form and bleeding to stop (**Figure 10.11** on page 345). Hemostasis involves four key steps.

1. **Vessel wall injury and constriction.** When the endothelium, or inner lining of a blood vessel, is injured, it releases endothelin (EHN-doh-THEE-lin). Endothelin is a hormone that causes the blood vessel to constrict and spasm for several minutes. This constriction helps reduce blood loss at the site of the vessel wall injury. Under normal circumstances, platelets don't adhere to the blood vessel wall because the wall is coated with a platelet repellent

Figure 10.10 Characteristics of White Blood Cells

Type	Microscopic appearance	Percentage of WBCs	Diameter	Function
Granulocytes				
neutrophil	pale pink stain with fine granules in the cytoplasm; multi-lobed, deep purple nucleus	55%–77%	10–12 micrometers	performs phagocytosis; kills bacteria and fungi
eosinophil	rose-colored stain with coarse granules in the cytoplasm; two blue-red, irregularly shaped nuclei	1%–3%	10–12 micrometers	destroys parasitic worms; controls allergic responses
basophil	dark blue stain with large purple granules in the cytoplasm; nucleus with 2–3 lobes	<1%	8–10 micrometers	releases histamine, intensifying the inflammatory process; liberates the anticoagulant heparin; active in allergic reactions
Agranulocytes				
lymphocyte	light blue-stained cytoplasm and dark blue, disk-shaped nucleus	25%–33%	7–8 micrometers	B cells produce antibodies; T cells and natural killer cells fight cancerous tumors and viruses
monocyte	grayish-blue cytoplasm; blue-purple stained, kidney-shaped nucleus	2%–10%	7.5–10 micrometers	performs phagocytosis; lives longer than neutrophil; morphs into macrophage that removes dead cell debris and attacks microorganisms

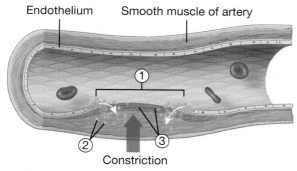

Endothelium   Smooth muscle of artery

① Constriction

1. Vessel wall injury and constriction
① Site of injury
② Endothelin release causes constriction
③ Collagen fibers exposed

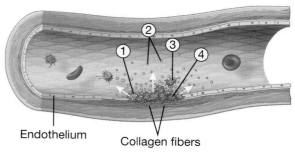

Endothelium   Collagen fibers

2. Platelet aggregation
① Platelet adhesion
② Chemicals released by platelets
③ Platelets gather
④ Platelets cluster to repair wall

Fibrin mesh secures platelet plug

3. Platelet plug formation and coagulation
① Tissue factor released
② Clotting factors released

4. Blood clot formation
① Red and white blood cells are trapped in mesh
② Release of coagulation inhibitors and other chemicals

Figure 10.11 Injured vessel walls are repaired during a process called *hemostasis. When a blood vessel wall is injured, what hormone is released to initiate constriction of the vessel wall?*

called *prostacyclin* (PRAHS-ta-SIGH-klin). When the blood vessel wall is injured, collagen fibers along the wall are exposed.

2. **Platelet aggregation.** Platelets stick to these collagen fibers as well as to the rough edges of the blood vessel wall (platelet adhesion). The platelets act like a spackling compound to repair the hole or tear. In addition, the platelets release chemicals that maintain constriction of the blood vessel and attract more platelets to the damaged wall.

3. **Platelet plug formation and coagulation.** This gathering of platelets forms a small, loose mass at the site of the injury called a **platelet plug**. To initiate **coagulation** (KOH-ag-yoo-LAY-shun),

the injured blood vessel releases a chemical called *tissue factor*. Tissue factor activates eleven different clotting factors, or proteins, in the blood. These clotting factors combine an enzyme called *thrombin* (THRAHM-bin) with the protein *fibrinogen* (figh-BRIN-oh-jehn). The combination of thrombin and fibrinogen produces **fibrin**, a long, thread-like fiber.

The fibrin strands weave in and around the platelet plug, forming a strong, tightly woven fibrin mesh. The process can be compared to throwing a fishing net around the platelet plug.

4. **Blood clot formation and retraction.** Red and white blood cells get trapped in the fibrin mesh, giving the blood clot a red color.

When coagulation is complete—usually somewhere between 2 and 15 minutes—the blood clot has formed. Shortly after the fibrin mesh is in place, the blood clot begins to retract, or shrink in size. This process normally takes 30 to 60 minutes.

As the blood clot retracts, platelets pull the fibrin threads together. This, in turn, draws the edges of the ruptured vessel together. Meanwhile, the factors that started the hemostasis sequence are rapidly inactivated to prevent excessive clotting. In addition, coagulation inhibitors are released to prevent further clot formation. Eventually, other chemicals serve to cut the fibrin strains and dissolve the blood clot completely.

Lesson 10.1 Review and Assessment

Mini Glossary   Make sure that you know the meaning of each key term.

 Build vocabulary with e-flash cards and games

buffy coat   a thin layer of white blood cells and platelets that lies between the red blood cells and plasma in a blood sample that has gone through a centrifuge

coagulation   the process by which the enzyme thrombin and the protein fibrinogen combine to form fibrin, a fiber that weaves around the platelet plug to form a blood clot; takes between 2 and 15 minutes to complete

diapedesis   the passage of blood, or any of its formed elements, through the blood vessel walls into body tissues

erythropoiesis   the process by which red blood cells are produced

erythropoietin (EPO)   a hormone secreted by the kidneys that stimulates the production of red blood cells

fibrin   a long, thread-like fiber created by the combination of thrombin and fibrinogen; weaves around the platelet plug to form a blood clot

formed elements   the solid components of blood; red blood cells, white blood cells, and platelets

hematocrit   the percentage of total blood volume that is composed of red blood cells

hemoglobin   an essential molecule of the red blood cell that serves as the binding site for oxygen and carbon dioxide; composed of two molecules: globin and heme

hemolysis   the rupture of red blood cells as a result of disease or old age

hemostasis   the sequence of events that causes a blood clot to form and bleeding to stop

plasma   the liquid component of blood

platelet plug   gathering of platelets that forms a small mass at the site of an injury

platelets   part of the formed elements of the blood; play a vital role in blood clotting

red blood cells   part of the formed elements of the blood; contain hemoglobin, a protein responsible for oxygen and carbon dioxide exchange; erythrocytes

white blood cells   part of the formed elements of the blood; fight infection and protect the body through various mechanisms; leukocytes

Know and Understand

Assess

1. List at least six functions of blood, two in each of the three major categories described in this lesson.

2. A centrifuge is used to separate the elements of blood into three layers. Describe the components of each layer.

3. Name at least four physical properties of blood.

4. Where are blood cells manufactured?

5. What does hematocrit measure? List the normal ranges for males and females.

Analyze and Apply

6. Compare and contrast the different functions of red blood cells, white blood cells, and platelets.

7. Explain in your own words the blood clotting process.

In the Lab

8. Draw and color an example of each type of white blood cell listed below. Identify the function of each next to its image: neutrophil; eosinophil; basophil; lymphocyte; monocyte.

Lesson 10.2

Blood Types

Before You Read

Try to answer the following questions before you read this lesson.

Why can't someone with type A blood receive blood from a person with type B blood?

What role does the Rh factor play in pregnant women?

Lesson Objectives

1. Identify the four blood types.
2. Describe the role of antigens and antibodies in the blood.
3. Explain the Rh classification system and why it is important.
4. Identify the purpose of a complete blood count.

Key Terms

E-Flash Cards

agglutination
antibody
antigen
erythroblastosis fetalis

Rh factor
RhoGAM
universal donor
universal recipient

Blood Types

You learned in lesson 10.1 that everyone's blood contains some similar elements—red blood cells, white blood cells, and platelets. But when blood from different people is viewed under a microscope, there are distinct differences. This is because there are four blood types: A, B, AB, and O.

Do you know your blood type? Have you ever wondered what determines your blood type? Like your eye or hair color, your blood type is inherited. **Figure 10.12** provides a list of possible blood types that a person may have based on the blood types of his or her parents.

Blood typing was made possible by the groundbreaking work of Karl Landsteiner, an Austrian scientist who won the Nobel Prize for his discovery. In 1901, Landsteiner classified blood according to the microscopic differences he found on the surface of the red blood cell.

The presence of molecule A on the red blood cell indicates type A blood, molecule B indicates type B blood, and the presence of both A and B molecules indicates type AB blood. Some people have neither A nor B molecules on their red blood cells. These people have type O blood.

Of the four blood types, type O is the most common in the United States, and type AB is the rarest. Blood types tend to vary among ethnic groups and regions of the world (**Figure 10.13**).

Antigens and Antibodies

The molecules on the surface of the red blood cells are called **antigens**. Antigens are large, complex molecules, such as proteins and glycolipids, that identify cells as "self" or "nonself." In this way, antigens make it possible for the body to tell the difference between its own cells and any nonself, or foreign, cells. The

Figure 10.12 Inherited Blood Type

	Parent 1	AB	AB	AB	AB	B	A	A	O	O	O
	Parent 2	AB	B	A	O	B	B	A	B	A	O
Possible blood type of child	**O**					X	X	X	X	X	X
	A	X	X	X	X		X	X		X	
	B	X	X	X	X	X	X		X		
	AB	X	X	X			X				

Figure 10.13 Blood Type Prevalence by Ethnicity

Blood Group	Prevalence (% of US Population)				
	Caucasian	African-American	Hispanic	Asian	Native American
AB	3	4	2	5	1
B	9	20	10	27	4
A	41	27	31	28	16
O	47	49	57	40	79

presence of foreign antigens causes the immune system to produce **antibodies** that mark the foreign cells for destruction. The antibodies circulate in plasma and mark any cells with antigens different from those found in the host's blood (or blood recipient during a transfusion). You will learn more about antigens and antibodies in the immune system in chapter 12.

Figure 10.14 on the next page shows the antigens and antibodies associated with each blood type. People with AB blood have antigens A and B on their red blood cells, but neither A nor B antibodies in their plasma, making them a **universal recipient**. A universal recipient can safely receive blood of any type due to the lack of attacking antibodies. People with type O blood have neither antigen A nor antigen B on their red blood cells, but both A and B antibodies in their plasma. Because type O blood has no antigens that can be attacked by the host's blood, anyone can receive type O blood. Thus, people with type O blood are **universal donors**.

Blood Transfusions

Understanding blood types is critical for blood transfusions and surgery. If we look at the history of blood transfusions, we see that the earliest outcomes of this technology were grim. In the fledgling days of medicine, physicians didn't know about the different blood types. Some transfusions were successful due in large part to luck, but others resulted in serious complications or death.

When a person with type A blood is transfused with blood from a type B blood donor, the recipient's anti-B antibodies attack the donor's red blood cells. This causes the donated red blood cells to clump together in a process called **agglutination** (ah-GLOO-ti-NAY-shun). Agglutination creates blockages in smaller blood vessels and is potentially fatal.

Agglutination also causes hemolysis, or destruction, of the donated red blood cells. Hemolysis releases hemoglobin into the bloodstream. Hemoglobin can accumulate in the kidneys, causing kidney damage and failure, or even death. Usually, however, blood transfusion

Figure 10.14 The ABO Blood Group System

Blood Type	Erythrocyte (Red Blood Cell) Antigens	RBC Antigens	Antibodies	Blood That Can Be Received
AB	A and B	A ——— B ———	Neither anti-A nor anti-B antibodies	A, B, AB, O (Universal recipient)
B	B		Anti-A	B, O
A	A		Anti-B	A, O
O	Neither A nor B	No antigens	Anti-A and Anti-B	O (Universal donor)

reactions are milder, with symptoms ranging from fever and chills to vomiting. Regardless, it is *extremely important* that blood types are classified and matched *before* transfusion.

The Rh Classification System

Besides the antigen that determines your blood type, there is another antigen on the surface of the red blood cells. This second antigen is called the **Rh factor**. The Rh factor is named after the rhesus monkey in which it was first discovered.

Not everyone possesses the Rh factor. Those who have the Rh factor on the surface of their red blood cells are classified as *Rh-positive*; those who lack it are classified as *Rh-negative*. The majority of people (approximately 85%) are Rh-positive.

When writing out a blood type, you drop the "Rh" and simply add a plus or minus superscript to the blood type's letter. For example, a person who has the Rh factor and type AB blood would say that she or he is AB+.

Rh Factor Complications

Plasma does not naturally contain an antibody for the Rh factor. However, antibodies to the Rh factor can develop if a person with Rh− blood is transfused with Rh+ blood. After exposure to the Rh+ blood, antibodies begin to form against the positive Rh factor. If the person is exposed to Rh+ blood again, the antibodies will cause agglutination and hemolysis.

Females can become sensitized to the Rh factor during pregnancy. If a mother who is Rh− has a baby who is Rh+, her first pregnancy will not cause a problem because the mother's blood has not yet developed antibodies, or a sensitivity to the Rh+ blood. However, some of the baby's Rh+ blood may come in contact with the mother's Rh− blood through the placenta, the organ that transports nutrients from the mother to her child. Once the mother's blood has been exposed to the Rh+ blood, she will develop anti-Rh+ antibodies.

If the mother becomes pregnant with another child who is Rh+, the mother's anti-Rh+ antibodies will attack the red blood cells of the fetus, causing agglutination and hemolysis. This action by the antibodies depletes the number of mature RBCs in the fetus. As a result, erythroblasts (immature RBCs) leave the bone marrow of the fetus before they are mature. If left untreated, the baby will develop **erythroblastosis fetalis** (eh-RITH-roh-blas-TOH-sis fee-TAL-is), or *hemolytic disease of the newborn (HDN)*. Erythroblastosis fetalis can be fatal.

Fortunately, erythroblastosis fetalis is becoming increasingly less common due to the development of the immune serum **RhoGAM**. RhoGAM is administered to the Rh⁻ mother shortly after she has given birth to her first child. The addition of RhoGAM prevents the mother's blood from becoming sensitized to the child's antibodies.

Any woman considering pregnancy should know her blood type and get early prenatal healthcare. It is essential for the health of the mother and her baby.

Check Your Understanding

1. What determines a person's blood type?
2. What molecules are found on the surface of red blood cells?
3. Which blood type classifies someone as a universal recipient? a universal donor?
4. Besides blood transfusions, what other condition can sensitize the body to the Rh factor?
5. What might a low platelet count indicate?

Complete Blood Count

A complete blood count (CBC) helps detect blood disorders or diseases such as anemia, abnormal blood cell counts, clotting problems, immune system disorders, and cancers of the blood (**Figure 10.15**). The test measures the number of RBCs, WBCs, and platelets.

Complete Blood Count Example Test Results

Test	Results	Low/High	Units	Normal Ranges
CBC with Differential				
Red Blood Count		3.5 (L)	× 10-6/µl	4.1–5.1 (F) / 4.70–6.10 (M)
Hemoglobin		10.8 (L)	g/dl	12.0–16.0 (F) / 14.0–18.0 (M)
Hematocrit		31.1 (L)	%	37.0–48.0 (F) / 42.0–52.0 (M)
Platelets	302		× 10-3/µl	140–415
White Blood Count	7.2		× 10-3/µl	4.5–11
Lymphocytes		48 (H)	%	17–44
Monocytes	7.0		%	3–10
Neutrophils		43 (L)	%	45–76
Eosinophils	2.0		%	0–4
Basophils	0		%	0–2

M = Male   F = Female

Low red blood count, hemoglobin, and hematocrit signal anemia.

Elevated white blood count may signal disease or infection.

Figure 10.15 The results of a complete blood count can be used to determine the presence of a disease or disorder. The Low/High column shows counts lower (L) or higher (H) than normal. *What are some diseases that can be identified by examining the results of a complete blood count?*

A low RBC count may indicate anemia, bleeding, or dehydration. In addition the number of each of the five different types of WBCs is measured for signs of infection, blood cancer, or immune disorder. A reduced platelet count may indicate a bleeding or a thrombotic (clotting) disorder. Hemoglobin and hematocrit levels are also measured for signs of anemia, sickle cell anemia, or Cooley's anemia. In the next lesson, we will discuss some of the disorders and diseases identified through a CBC.

Figure 10.15 illustrates the results of a complete blood count test. Values that are higher or lower than the normal range appear in red.

Lesson 10.2 Review and Assessment

Mini Glossary   Make sure that you know the meaning of each key term.

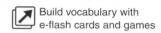 Build vocabulary with e-flash cards and games

agglutination the process by which red blood cells clump together, usually in response to an antibody; can block small blood vessels and cause hemolysis

antibody a cell that circulates in plasma and attacks red blood cells with foreign antigens, or antigens that are different from those of the host

antigen a protein on the surface of RBCs that is used to identify blood type; a molecule on the surface of cells that identifies cells as either "self" or "nonself" (foreign) cells

erythroblastosis fetalis a severe hemolytic disease of a fetus or newborn caused by the production of maternal antibodies against the fetal red blood cell antigens, usually involving Rh incompatibility between the mother and fetus

Rh factor the antigen of the Rh blood group that is found on the surface of red blood cells; people with the Rh factor are Rh$^+$ and those lacking it are Rh$^-$

RhoGAM an immune serum that prevents a mother's blood from becoming sensitized to foreign antibodies from her fetus

universal donor a person with type O blood; type O blood has no antigens that can be attacked by the host's blood, so it can be donated to anyone

universal recipient a person with type AB blood; type AB blood has neither A nor B antibodies, so a universal recipient can safely receive a transfusion of any blood type

Know and Understand

 Assess

1. What is an antigen?
2. Explain the process of agglutination.
3. What are the four blood types?
4. Besides the antigen that determines blood type, what other antigen is sometimes found on the surface of red blood cells?
5. Define *RhoGAM* and explain its use.
6. What does a complete blood count detect?
7. If a person's parents both have type B blood, what blood types might that person have?
8. If you have type B blood, what kind of an antibody do you have?
9. *True or False?* If you are Rh-positive, you have a higher than normal amount of Rh factor.

Analyze and Apply

10. What is the difference between an antigen and an antibody?
11. Explain why a person with type AB blood is a universal recipient.
12. Explain why a person with type O blood is a universal donor.

In the Lab

13. Using the information that you learned in this lesson, complete the chart shown here. Identify whether or not the recipient (column A) can safely receive a blood donation from each potential donor (column B).

Blood Donation		
Recipient Blood Type	**Potential Donor Blood Type**	**Safe to Receive Blood from Donor?**
B-	A	
AB	O	
AB	B	
O	AB	
O	O	
A-	B+	
B-	O-	

Lesson 10.3 Blood Disorders and Diseases

Before You Read

Try to answer the following questions before you read this lesson.

What does it mean to be anemic?

Which blood disorder causes yellowing of the whites of the eyes and skin?

Lesson Objectives

1. Describe the differences between chronic and inherited anemias.

2. Identify common blood disorders and diseases.

3. Explain the difference between leukemia and multiple myeloma, two forms of blood cancer.

Key Terms

E-Flash Cards

acute lymphocytic leukemia (ALL)
acute myeloid leukemia (AML)
anemia
aplastic anemia
chelation therapy
chronic lymphocytic leukemia (CLL)
chronic myeloid leukemia (CML)

Cooley's anemia
hemophilia
iron-deficient anemia
jaundice
leukemia
multiple myeloma
pernicious anemia
phlebotomy
polycythemia
sickle cell anemia

Blood disorders and diseases can be diagnosed in a variety of ways, including a complete blood count test, as we learned in the last lesson. But what causes a disorder or disease of the blood? Many health problems affecting the blood are inherited, but some are caused by environmental factors, poor diet, or even old age. In this lesson we will explore some of the most common disorders and diseases of the blood and their causes, symptoms, and treatments or management strategies.

Anemia

Anemia is a condition characterized by a decrease in the number of RBCs or an insufficient amount of hemoglobin in the RBCs. In both cases, the oxygen-carrying capacity of the RBCs is reduced.

Anemia can be acquired or inherited. There are three main causes of anemia: excessive blood loss, decreased RBC production, or a high rate of RBC destruction. Symptoms of anemia include headache, dizziness, weakness, fatigue, and difficulty breathing or shortness of breath.

There are several types of anemia. Some forms are mild and easily treated by adopting a healthful diet; others can be severe, debilitating, and even life-threatening if they remain undiagnosed or untreated. A healthful diet provides the building blocks for RBC production: iron, folic acid, and vitamin B.

Acquired Anemias

Anemia can be caused by a dietary deficiency or exposure to parasitic worms. It can also be a symptom of another disease.

Iron-Deficient Anemia. The most common type of anemia, **iron-deficient anemia**, accounts for nearly 50% of all anemias worldwide. Iron-deficient anemia results from an insufficient dietary intake of iron or loss of iron from intestinal bleeding.

Parasitic worms that result in intestinal bleeding are the main cause of iron-deficient anemia worldwide. Parasitic worms are most commonly found in developing, or low-income, countries.

Pregnant women may also suffer from iron-deficient anemia. This happens because their bodies supply the fetus with hemoglobin, which depletes the mother's iron levels. (Recall from lesson 10.1 that the heme molecule in hemoglobin is composed of iron.)

If iron-deficient anemia is caused by a poor diet, an iron supplement can be prescribed. Foods rich in iron (such as leafy, green vegetables) are also recommended (**Figure 10.16**).

Aplastic Anemia. A rare but serious condition, **aplastic anemia** is caused by damage to the stem cells in the bone marrow. When bone marrow stem cells are damaged, they cannot produce a sufficient number of RBCs, WBCs, and platelets. The blood cells manufactured in the bone marrow have problems developing into mature blood cells, resulting in aplastic anemia. Causes of aplastic anemia include

- toxins (such as those found in pesticides);
- radiation therapy or chemotherapy;

Nikola Bilic/Shutterstock.com

Figure 10.16 Spinach is an iron-rich food. Adopting a diet rich in leafy, green vegetables such as spinach is one way to help fight iron-deficient anemia. *What other foods are high in iron?*

- infectious diseases (for example, hepatitis; Epstein-Barr virus; human immunodeficiency virus, or HIV; and autoimmune disorders such as rheumatoid arthritis and lupus); and
- heredity.

Treatments for aplastic anemia include toxin removal, discontinuing radiation or chemotherapy, and blood transfusions. In severe cases, bone marrow stem-cell transplants can be performed.

Pernicious Anemia. When the intestines are unable to absorb B_{12}, a vitamin essential for RBC production, the result is **pernicious anemia**. This condition develops when the stomach stops producing intrinsic factor, a key protein in vitamin B_{12} absorption. A weakened stomach lining or an autoimmune disorder may cause the body to attack intrinsic factor.

Pernicious anemia usually develops later in life; on average, diagnosis occurs in patients around 60 years of age. Certain diseases, such as type I diabetes mellitus, Addison's disease, and chronic thyroiditis, can increase the risk of developing pernicious anemia.

Signs and symptoms common among people with pernicious anemia include a red, swollen tongue; pale skin; fatigue; and shortness of breath. Diarrhea or constipation are other symptoms. Treatment usually consists of vitamin B_{12} supplements.

Anemias Caused by Chronic Disease. Chronic illnesses such as rheumatoid arthritis or kidney disease can cause anemia. For example, kidney disease may lower production of the hormone erythropoietin, which regulates RBC production. Inflammatory conditions associated with diseases such as rheumatoid arthritis can affect the bone marrow's response to erythropoietin. As a result, RBC production can decrease. Diseases characterized by chronic infections, such as HIV, tuberculosis, cirrhosis of the liver, and certain cancers, also can cause anemia.

Treatment of anemia caused by chronic disease involves diagnosing and resolving the underlying disease. In the short term, blood transfusions may be used as part of the treatment plan for managing anemia.

Check Your Understanding

1. What are the three main causes of anemia?
2. Which type of anemia is the most common worldwide?
3. Which anemia is caused by the inability of the intestines to absorb vitamin B$_{12}$?
4. Why might a person with rheumatoid arthritis be more likely to develop anemia than someone without rheumatoid arthritis?

Inherited Anemias

Inherited anemias are determined by genetic makeup. A child must receive an anemia gene from both parents to experience symptoms of an inherited anemia. If an anemia gene is received from only one parent, the child will be a carrier but will not experience symptoms. Two commonly inherited anemias are sickle cell anemia and Cooley's anemia.

Sickle Cell Anemia. As you will recall from lesson 10.1, normal RBCs are disk shaped. However, the RBCs of a person with **sickle cell anemia** are shaped like a crescent or sickle, a large cutting instrument with a curved metal blade (**Figure 10.17**). This is because the hemoglobin molecules in the RBCs of a patient with sickle cell anemia are misshaped, causing the RBCs to take on the abnormal shape.

Sickle-shaped hemoglobin molecules carry less oxygen than normal hemoglobin molecules. Because of their shape and sticky texture, sickle-shaped RBCs easily get stuck in small blood vessels, disrupting normal blood flow. **Figure 10.17** illustrates how the sickle-shaped RBCs become lodged in blood vessels.

Symptoms of sickle cell anemia include excruciatingly painful episodes called *crises*.

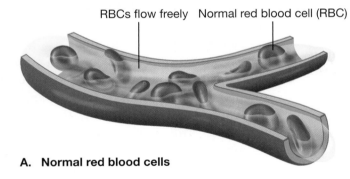

RBCs flow freely   Normal red blood cell (RBC)

A. Normal red blood cells

Cross section of RBC

Normal hemoglobin

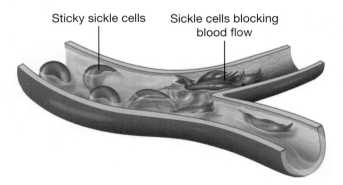

Sticky sickle cells   Sickle cells blocking blood flow

B. Abnormal red blood cells (sickle cells)

Cross section of sickle cell

Abnormal hemoglobin forms strands, causing the sickle, or crescent shape

Animation

Figure 10.17 Sickle-shaped red blood cells get stuck more easily in smaller blood vessels, causing painful episodes called *crises. Why does sickle cell anemia increase the risk of stroke?*

WHAT RESEARCH TELLS US

...*about* Extending Life Expectancy of Patients with Sickle Cell Anemia

People with sickle cell anemia are prone to life-threatening infections, fatigue, and painful episodes called *crises*. Historically, this has meant that people with sickle cell anemia have a shortened life span.

In the 1960s, 15% of children born with sickle cell anemia died before two years of age; many more died as teenagers. Since that time, research funded by the National Heart, Lung, and Blood Institute (NHLBI) has shown that infants given daily doses of penicillin have an 84% reduction in infections, thus greatly improving their life expectancy.

Because sickle-shaped RBCs can become lodged in the blood vessels of the brain, people with sickle cell anemia are prone to stroke. NHLBI-funded research led to the development of the Transcranial Doppler (TCD) screening test, which can identify whether or not a patient with sickle cell anemia is at risk for stroke. Frequent blood transfusions have proven to lower the risk of stroke and increase life expectancy.

In another effort to increase the life expectancy of patients with sickle cell anemia, NHLBI researchers performed a partial stem-cell transplant on ten individuals with severe sickle cell disease; nine of them were cured.

Research continues with the goal of finding a permanent cure for sickle cell anemia. Meanwhile, a disease that was once associated with an early death is now a manageable condition, with life expectancies ranging from 40 to 50 years of age and beyond.

Taking It Further

1. Research treatment options for sickle cell anemia that are not discussed in this chapter. Are any advanced technologies available? Write a report on your findings and present it to the class.

2. Denzel and Maya are considering having a baby. Denzel has the sickle cell trait. Do you think the couple should seek genetic counseling? Why or why not? Do research to support your case. Share your argument with the class.

Crises can last anywhere from a few hours to several days, and require hospitalization. The pain usually occurs in the back and around long bones, such as the femur, where tissues can be damaged from oxygen deprivation. Other symptoms include bacterial infection, fatigue, shortness of breath, rapid heart rate, and jaundice, a yellowing of the skin and eyes. Strokes may also occur if RBCs become lodged in the small vessels of the brain.

Treatment of sickle cell anemia may require daily doses of antibiotics to prevent bacterial infection, especially in small children with the disease. Folic acid supplements are also recommended. In the event of a crisis, the patient is given blood transfusions, pain medications, and fluids. In addition, blood transfusions are given frequently to increase the patient's RBC count.

Individuals who inherit the sickle cell gene from only one parent have the sickle cell trait,

which means they are a carrier but won't develop any of the symptoms of the disease. Sickle cell anemia is most common in African-Americans and individuals of Mediterranean descent.

In the past, sickle cell anemia resulted in death at an early age, but medical advances are helping people with this disease live into their fifties and beyond.

Cooley's Anemia. This condition, also called *thalassemia* (THAL-a-SEE-mee-a) *major*, is a type of anemia that affects hemoglobin proteins. **Cooley's anemia** limits the body's ability to produce fully developed hemoglobin and the proper number of RBCs. As a result, the blood's oxygen-carrying capability is reduced.

People with Cooley's anemia require frequent blood transfusions to increase their RBC counts. However, these transfusions can be dangerous because they can increase the iron in the blood to toxic levels. Excessive amounts of iron are especially harmful to the heart, liver, and endocrine organs. Iron accumulation leads to heart attack and death in 50% of people with Cooley's anemia before they reach 35 years of age.

Chelation therapy is a special procedure that removes excess metals, such as iron, from the blood. Chelation therapy is essential for preventing organ damage and failure. During this therapy, the chelating drug is pumped into the body either intravenously (through an IV) or subcutaneously (by injection). It then binds with whatever metal is present in excess amounts.

In the case of iron poisoning, the chelating drug binds with the iron and prepares it for elimination from the body via the urine. The drug is usually administered at night and is infused slowly over an eight-hour period, four to six nights a week.

Jaundice

Jaundice is a blood disorder characterized by yellow-colored skin and whites of the eyes. It can be caused by an excess of bilirubin—a byproduct of RBC breakdown—in the bloodstream. Bilirubin is typically excreted through bile in the liver, so jaundice can result from liver damage or disease.

Jaundice is common in newborns and is usually the result of an immature liver. A newborn is more likely to be jaundiced when his or her Rh factor is different from that of the mother's. If the mother is Rh-negative and the baby is Rh-positive, the mother's antibodies may attack the baby's red blood cells.

Infant jaundice is treated with phototherapy using ultraviolet light, which lowers the bilirubin levels in the baby's blood (**Figure 10.18**). Infant jaundice is usually resolved within two to four weeks of birth.

Hemophilia

Hemophilia (HEE-moh-FIL-ee-a) is a disorder in which the blood does not clot properly because one of the clotting factors responsible for coagulation is missing. There are 13 clotting factors involved in the coagulation process. As

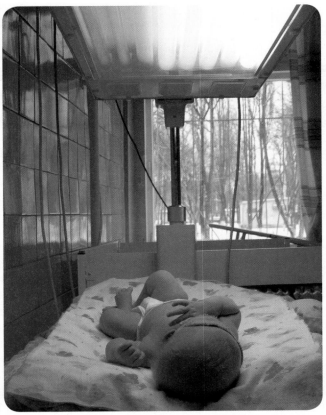

photobank.kiev.ua/Shutterstock.com

Figure 10.18 Phototherapy helps break down excess bilirubin so that it can be excreted in the urine and feces.

we learned in lesson 10.1, platelets and clotting factors form a blood clot to stop an injured blood vessel from bleeding. People with hemophilia typically lack either clotting factor VII or IX.

Hemophilia is usually inherited, but in very rare cases may be acquired if the body forms antibodies that fight one of the clotting factors. This disease is more common in males, and occurs in one out of every 5,000 births each year.

Polycythemia

Polycythemia (PAHL-ee-sigh-THEE-mee-a), also known as *polycythemia primary* or *polycythemia vera*, is a condition in which the bone marrow manufactures too many red blood cells.

Living at a high altitude contributes to polycythemia because long-term exposure to high altitude causes the kidneys to produce more erythropoietin. Erythropoietin stimulates stem cell production in the bone marrow, leading to increased RBC production. However, people who live at a high altitude will not develop polycythemia unless they also have a rare genetic mutation that increases bone marrow sensitivity to erythropoietin, causing even more RBCs to be produced. High RBC counts cause blood to thicken and increases the likelihood of blood clot formation.

Polycythemia is diagnosed by testing hemoglobin or hematocrit levels. Unusually high levels of hemoglobin or hematocrit indicate excessive RBC production.

Phlebotomy (fleh-BAHT-oh-mee), the *drawing of blood*, is the standard treatment for polycythemia. Phlebotomy reduces the number of RBCs circulating in the body. This helps achieve the goal of correcting hematocrit levels. Aspirin has also been used to thin the blood, but aspirin therapy is not advised for anyone with a history of spontaneous bleeding or stroke.

Check Your Understanding

1. Why does a sickle-shaped red blood cell take on its abnormal structure?
2. What type of drug therapy is used to remove excess metals, such as iron, from the blood?
3. What distinct changes in a person's physical appearance indicate jaundice?
4. Which disease do people suffer from if their blood does not clot properly?

Leukemia

Leukemia is a cancer of the blood. It is caused by the production of an extremely high number of immature white blood cells in the bone marrow. These immature, cancerous WBCs grow larger and faster than normal WBCs, but they lack the infection-fighting ability of normal WBCs. The cancerous WBCs live longer than healthy WBCs, crowding the healthy blood cells and making it hard for them to do their job. Cancerous WBCs can spread to lymph nodes (resulting in lymphocytic leukemia) and to other organs and tissues, causing swelling and pain.

Leukemia is classified as either *acute* or *chronic*. Acute leukemia worsens quickly, while chronic leukemia progresses more slowly. Children with leukemia usually have acute leukemia. Adults may contract either acute or chronic leukemia. There are four types of leukemia. Two are acute and two are chronic.

- **Acute lymphocytic leukemia (ALL)**: Most common in adults over 70 years of age, ALL is characterized by an overproduction of lymphocytes.
- **Acute myeloid leukemia (AML)**: AML is the most common form of leukemia in adults. It develops when the bone marrow produces too many myeloblasts, cells that fight bacterial infections. Myeloblasts are blast cells that later develop into RBCs, platelets, and some WBCs.
- **Chronic lymphocytic leukemia (CLL)**: Like acute lymphocytic leukemia, CLL is characterized by extremely high levels of lymphocytes. CLL is rare in children and most often affects middle-aged adults (**Figure 10.19** on the next page).
- **Chronic myeloid leukemia (CML)**: CML is a type of leukemia in which the bone marrow manufactures too many granulocytes (neutrophils, eosinophils, and basophils).

People with chronic leukemia may not experience any symptoms, sometimes even for years after they develop the disease. By comparison, people with acute leukemia often seek medical care because they feel sick. Symptoms of both chronic and acute leukemia include weakness, fever, bone and joint pain, and stomach swelling and pain from an enlarged spleen or liver. People with leukemia also have frequent infections because cancerous WBCs are unable to aid in the immune response.

A complete blood count is often used to help diagnose leukemia. This disease increases the number of WBCs and decreases platelet and hemoglobin counts. A physical examination is done to check for swelling in the lymph nodes, spleen, or liver. In addition, doctors may perform a biopsy (removal and examination of body tissues) and other tests to look for cancerous cells.

Figure 10.19 This micrograph shows a blood sample from a person with chronic lymphocytic leukemia (CLL). Notice the disproportionate number of WBCs (lymphocytes, which are purple in this micrograph) to RBCs. In a healthy person, RBCs far outnumber WBCs. CLL results from the creation of a high number of lymphocytes, which causes a reduction in the number of RBCs.

Treatment options for leukemia vary, but often include chemotherapy, radiation therapy, and stem cell transplants. The five-year survival rate for acute myeloid leukemia varies with age. Those *under* 50 years of age at the time of diagnosis have a survival rate of 25% over a five-year period, while those *over* 50 years have a survival rate of 50% over a five-year period. New drug treatments for chronic myeloid leukemia have led to a promising 90% survival rate over the course of five years.

Multiple Myeloma

Multiple myeloma (MIGH-eh-LOH-ma) is a cancer of the plasma cells in bone marrow. The plasma cells of a person with this disease divide many times, creating even more cancerous plasma cells, called *myelomas*.

Myeloma cells deposit in the bone marrow, forming tumors that can damage the bone. As a result, people with multiple myeloma are prone to bone fractures and bone pain, particularly in the back and ribs. Other symptoms of this

disease include excess blood calcium levels, kidney damage, and frequent infections.

Multiple myeloma is a treatable but incurable condition. It is treated with steroid drugs, chemotherapy, and stem cell transplants (**Figure 10.20**).

Multiple myeloma is the second most common blood cancer in the United States, accounting for 15% of all blood cancer cases. Each year, this disease affects between 1 and 4 out of every 100,000 people. African-Americans are twice as likely as Caucasians to develop multiple myeloma. Survival rates continue to improve as a result of new drug therapies and stem-cell transplant techniques.

 Check Your Understanding

1. What is the difference between acute and chronic leukemia?
2. Which cancer affects the plasma cells in bone marrow?

Li Wa/Shutterstock.com

Figure 10.20 Bone marrow is harvested (removed) from a healthy individual in preparation for a stem cell transplant. Transplanted bone marrow replaces the diseased bone marrow of a person with leukemia or multiple myeloma and produces healthy WBCs, RBCs, and platelets.

Lesson 10.3 Review and Assessment

Mini Glossary Make sure that you know the meaning of each key term.

 Build vocabulary with e-flash cards and games

acute lymphocytic leukemia (ALL) the most common form of leukemia in adults over 70 years of age; characterized by overproduction of lymphocytes

acute myeloid leukemia (AML) the most common form of leukemia in adults; develops when the bone marrow produces too many myeloblasts

anemia a condition characterized by a decrease in the number of red blood cells or an insufficient amount of hemoglobin in the red blood cells

aplastic anemia a rare but serious condition in which the bone marrow is incapable of making new red blood cells

chelation therapy a procedure in which excess metals, such as iron, are removed from the blood

chronic lymphocytic leukemia (CLL) a form of leukemia characterized by extremely high

levels of lymphocytes; most often found in middle-age adults

chronic myeloid leukemia (CML) a form of leukemia characterized by overproduction of granulocytes

Cooley's anemia a condition that affects the body's ability to produce fully developed hemoglobin and red blood cells; thalassemia major

hemophilia a condition in which blood does not clot properly due to the absence of a clotting factor

iron-deficient anemia the most common anemia; caused by an insufficient dietary intake of iron, loss of iron from intestinal bleeding, or iron-level depletion during pregnancy

jaundice a blood disorder characterized by yellow-colored skin and whites of the eyes

leukemia a cancer caused by the production of an extremely high

number of immature white blood cells in the bone marrow

multiple myeloma a cancer of the plasma cells in bone marrow

pernicious anemia a severe anemia caused by the inability of the intestines to absorb vitamin B_{12}, which is essential for the formation of red blood cells; usually develops in older adults

phlebotomy the drawing of blood; a standard treatment for polycythemia

polycythemia a condition in which the bone marrow manufactures too many red blood cells; caused by prolonged altitude exposure and a genetic mutation

sickle cell anemia a disease in which the red blood cells are shaped like a sickle, or crescent, rather than a disk; caused by irregularly shaped hemoglobin molecules in the red blood cells

Know and Understand

 Assess

1. What condition is characterized by a decreased number of red blood cells, fatigue, shortness of breath, and dizziness?

2. What type of food and what mineral supplement are recommended for a person with iron-deficient anemia?

3. What is another name for Cooley's anemia?

4. What condition results from damage to bone marrow stem cells, making them unable to produce mature blood cells?

5. Diseases such as type I diabetes mellitus, Addison's disease, or chronic thyroiditis increase the risk of developing which type of anemia?

6. What factor might increase the likelihood that a newborn will develop jaundice?

7. A crisis is a symptom of what disease? How would you describe a crisis?

8. What are the major treatments for sickle cell anemia?

9. What disease would cause people with that disease to be more concerned than normal about skin punctures and cuts?

10. Who is more likely to seek medical care—the person with acute leukemia or the one with chronic leukemia? Why?

Analyze and Apply

11. How does long-term exposure to high altitude contribute to polycythemia?

12. Explain the cause of leukemia.

13. Using what you have learned about stem cells, explain why a stem cell transplant would help a person with multiple myeloma.

In the Lab

14. Using your textbook, library resources, or the Internet, research multiple myeloma. Focus on any developing therapies and stem-cell transplant techniques. What do these new treatment options involve? How do they work? Create a poster to illustrate your findings and present it to the class.

Career Corner
Anatomy and Physiology at Work

As you know, the blood touches every cell and tissue in the body. Therefore, blood samples can be used to diagnose many disorders and diseases.

Phlebotomists are people who collect blood samples. These samples are then analyzed frequently and evaluated by medical technologists. Let's learn more about what people in these professions do each day.

Phlebotomist

Phlebotomists are trained in blood collection techniques and in the handling and storage of blood. Phlebotomists collect blood for diagnostic tests, blood banks, transfusions, and clinical research. Phlebotomists must also verify patient records.

Phlebotomists can collect blood in different ways. For example, they might simply stick a finger to draw a small amount of blood. To take more blood they would draw it from a vein, usually in the arm (**Figure 10.21**).

It is critical that phlebotomists follow proper procedures and safety precautions for collecting blood. They must also ensure that their equipment is sterile and safe for use.

Phlebotomists work in a variety of settings, including hospitals, medical clinics, and private practices. Some doctors do not have phlebotomists on staff, so they send their patients to laboratory companies, which employ phlebotomists. These laboratories specialize in collecting and analyzing blood samples for doctors' offices and blood banks.

Students interested in a career as a phlebotomist must possess a high school diploma or its equivalent. They must also complete a brief certification program.

Each state has different program and licensure requirements. States that do require a license to be a phlebotomist may require successful completion of an exam administered by an accrediting agency such as the American Society for Clinical Pathology.

Most licensing exams have questions about specimen collection, clinical laboratory procedures, proper handling of blood samples, and safety protocols. Some employers prefer to hire phlebotomists who are not only state licensed but also nationally certified.

Medical Technologist

Medical technologists analyze human blood and tissue specimens. They perform a full range of laboratory tests on these specimens. For example, they match blood types before transfusions or surgery. They also check blood samples for signs of disease, parasites, drugs, chemicals, and other elements. Medical technologists must also confirm the accuracy of their test results and report laboratory findings to doctors and pathologists.

The medical technology laboratory has a wide array of instruments, including microscopes and complex, computerized equipment. Therefore, medical technologists must be comfortable operating such machines.

Medical technologists must be precise, thorough, and able to handle high levels of stress. Doctors often need lab results quickly, so medical technologists must be comfortable working in a fast-paced, sometimes stressful

Orchidflower/Shutterstock.com

Figure 10.21 Phlebotomists collect and store patients' blood samples.

environment. Medical technologists are employed in hospitals, clinics, independent laboratories, and public health facilities (**Figure 10.22**).

Students interested in pursuing a career as a medical technologist should establish a strong science foundation in high school by taking courses such as biology, chemistry, math, and computer science. A Bachelor of Science degree in medical technology from a program recognized by the national accrediting agency for clinical laboratory sciences is also required. Aspiring medical technologists must also pass a national certification exam administered by the American Society for Clinical Pathology.

Planning for a Health-Related Career

Do some research on the career of a phlebotomist or a medical technologist. You may choose instead to research a profession from the list of **Related Career Options**. Using

michaeljung/Shutterstock.com

Figure 10.22 Medical technologists analyze samples of blood, urine, saliva, and tissue.

the Internet or resources at your local library, find answers to the following questions:

1. What are the main tasks and responsibilities of a person employed in the career that you chose to research?
2. What is the outlook for this career? Are workers in demand, or are jobs dwindling? For complete information, consult the current edition of the *Occupational Outlook Handbook*, published by the US Department of Labor. This handbook is available online or at your local library. More specific information for your state or local area may also be available.
3. What special skills or talents are required? Does the idea of working with blood make you feel queasy?
4. What personality traits do you think are necessary for success in the career that you have chosen to research? Some people are afraid of sharp instruments such as needles. Would you be able to calm a person's fear of needles and make them feel comfortable as you take a blood sample?
5. Does the work involve a great deal of routine, or are the day-to-day responsibilities varied?
6. Does the career require long hours, or is it a standard, "9-to-5" job?
7. What is the salary range for this job? Is this salary range in line with your expectations?
8. What do you think you would like about this career? Is there anything about it that you might dislike?

Related Career Options

- Biological Technician
- Chemical Technician
- Emergency Medical Technician (EMT)
- Epidemiologist
- Medical Assistant
- Medical Transcriptionist
- Occupational Health and Safety Technician

Chapter Summaries

Lesson 10.1 The Function and Composition of Blood

Build vocabulary with e-flash cards and games

Key Points

- The average adult has 10 to 12 pints of blood in the body, which makes up approximately 8% of total body weight.
- Red blood cells (erythrocytes) carry oxygen and other essential nutrients to every cell of the body. White blood cells (leukocytes) protect against infection. Platelets promote blood clotting.
- Blood cells are manufactured by stem cells in the bone marrow. This process is called *hematopoiesis*.
- Red bone marrow in the vertebrae, ribs, hips, sternum, and skull produce stem cells that, in turn, create red blood cells, white blood cells, and platelets.
- Besides red bone marrow, elements such as iron, folic acid, vitamin B_{12}, and protein are needed for red blood cell production.
- Red blood cells are the most abundant cells in the blood. They are disk-shaped and have a life span of approximately 120 days.
- White blood cells produce antibodies, intensify the inflammatory response, play a role in allergic reactions, and destroy parasitic worms.
- There are five different types of white blood cells, each of which is characterized by size, appearance, and function.

Key Terms

buffy coat	hemoglobin
coagulation	hemolysis
diapedesis	hemostasis
erythropoiesis	plasma
erythropoietin (EPO)	platelet plug
fibrin	platelets
formed elements	red blood cells
hematocrit	white blood cells

Lesson 10.2 Blood Types

Key Points

- There are four blood types: A, B, AB, and O.
- Antigens are molecules on the surface of the red blood cells; they determine a person's blood type.
- Antibodies are produced by the immune system in response to the presence of foreign antigens, such as viruses, bacteria, and fungi. Antibodies attack foreign antigens.
- When a person is transfused with blood from a donor with a different blood type, agglutination—the clumping of red blood cells—can occur.

Key Terms

agglutination	Rh factor
antibody	RhoGAM
antigen	universal donor
erythroblastosis fetalis	universal recipient

- Hemolysis—the rupture of red blood cells—occurs when the red blood cell has reached the end of its life span or is exposed to infection or disease. Hemolysis can also result from blood transfusion complications.
- The Rh factor is an antigen on the surface of red blood cells. People with the Rh factor are Rh-positive (Rh⁺). People without it are Rh-negative (Rh⁻).
- A complete blood count is a test that measures the number of red blood cells, white blood cells, and platelets. It is often used to diagnose blood disorders and diseases.

Lesson 10.3 Blood Disorders and Diseases

Key Points

- Anemia is characterized by a decreased number of red blood cells or an insufficient amount of hemoglobin in red blood cells. There are many different types of anemia.
- The three main causes of anemia are decreased production of red blood cells, excessive blood loss, or a high rate of red blood cell destruction.
- Iron-deficient anemia results from an insufficient dietary intake of iron or loss of iron from intestinal bleeding.
- Sickle cell anemia is an inherited condition that causes the red blood cells to be shaped like a sickle, or crescent, rather than shaped like a disk. The disease is most common in African-Americans and people of Mediterranean descent.
- Hemophilia is a genetic disease characterized by impaired blood clot formation due to a lack of one of the clotting factors responsible for coagulation. It is more common in males and occurs in one out of every 5,000 births each year.
- Leukemia is a cancer caused by increased production of immature white blood cells in the bone marrow. It is classified as either *acute* or *chronic*.

Key Terms

acute lymphocytic leukemia (ALL)
acute myeloid leukemia (AML)
anemia
aplastic anemia
chelation therapy
chronic lymphocytic leukemia (CLL)
chronic myeloid leukemia (CML)
Cooley's anemia
hemophilia
iron-deficient anemia
jaundice
leukemia
multiple myeloma
pernicious anemia
phlebotomy
polycythemia
sickle cell anemia

Chapter Assessments

Assess

Lesson 10.1

The Function and Composition of Blood

Learning Key Terms and Concepts

1. *True or False*? Blood is considered a regulatory system.
2. Which of the following is a basic component of blood?
   A. plasma
   B. formed elements
   C. both A and B
   D. none of the above

3. What percentage of blood is composed of plasma?
4. Blood makes up approximately what percentage of total body weight?
   A. 15%
   B. 12%
   C. 3%
   D. 8%
5. Which of the following is *not* a protein in blood plasma?
   A. fibrinogen
   B. sodium
   C. albumin
   D. globulin
6. *True or False*? Red blood cells have an unlimited life span.

7. Only _____ bone marrow is capable of producing blood cells and new stem cells.

8. The kidneys regulate red blood cell production through a process called _____.

9. _____ are the most abundant type of white blood cells in the body.

10. Basophils are white blood cells that _____.
    A. attack invading microorganisms
    B. produce histamine
    C. give red blood cells their disk shape
    D. give blood its color

Thinking Critically

11. A healthy blood vessel normally repels platelets to prevent unnecessary clotting. Explain hemostasis when a blood vessel wall has been injured.

Lesson 10.2

Blood Types

Learning Key Terms and Concepts

12. *True or False*? There are three major blood types.

13. _____ are molecules on the surface of cells that help the body distinguish between "self" and "nonself" cells.

14. A universal blood donor has which of the following blood types?
    A. type A   C. type AB
    B. type B   D. type O

15. *True or False*? The term *Rh factor* was inspired by the rhesus monkey.

16. The potentially fatal process that causes blood to clump and create blockages is called _____.
    A. coagulation   C. erythroblastosis
    B. agglutination   fetalis
                       D. hemolysis

17. *True or False*? Blood type was first classified according to type by an Austrian scientist named Karl Landsteiner in 1901.

18. Which of the following is *not* measured in a complete blood test?
    A. red blood cells   C. anemia
    B. platelets   D. white blood cells

19. Agglutination can cause _____ of donated red blood cells.

20. A universal recipient has which of the following blood types?
    A. type A   C. type AB
    B. type B   D. type O

Thinking Critically

21. Explain the characteristic that is used to identify the different blood types. Why is it dangerous to mix certain blood types for blood transfusions?

22. Identify the characteristic that makes blood types either positive (+) or negative (−). Explain the significance of these classifications.

Lesson 10.3

Blood Disorders and Diseases

Learning Key Terms and Concepts

23. Which of the following is one of the three main causes of anemia?
    A. increased production of white blood cells
    B. platelet destruction
    C. decreased production of red blood cells
    D. blood vessel injury

24. *True or False*? Iron-deficient anemia accounts for 50% of all anemias.

25. Aplastic anemia is caused by the inability of the bone marrow to make new _____.
    A. white blood cells   C. hemoglobin
    B. plasma   D. proteins

26. Pernicious anemia is caused by the inability of the intestines to absorb _____.

27. *True or False*? It is possible to inherit an anemic condition.

28. To develop sickle cell anemia, you must inherit the sickle cell gene from _____.
    A. your mother   C. both parents
    B. your father   D. grandfather

29. _____ is a disease that affects proteins in hemoglobin and prevents the body from producing fully developed hemoglobin.

30. Which type of therapy is used to remove excess iron from the blood?
    A. chemotherapy   C. chelation therapy
    B. radiation therapy D. vitamin B_{12} injection therapy

Thinking Critically

31. Kelsey is a fifteen-year-old girl whose parents moved to Chicago from their native Sicily five years before she was born. When Kelsey was a baby, she was diagnosed with a blood disorder. As a result of this disorder, Kelsey experiences back and leg pain. She is often short of breath and tired. Which blood disorder is Kelsey living with? What can she do to manage her disease?

32. Rachael is a young mother with Rh-negative blood. Her first child, Hazel, was born two years ago and has Rh-positive blood. Rachael is now pregnant with her second child. What complications might arise if her second baby also has Rh-positive blood? What can Rachael's doctor can do to avoid these complications?

Building Skills and Connecting Concepts

Analyzing and Evaluating Data

The chart on the right shows survival rates for leukemia and multiple myeloma patients from 1960–2007. Use this chart to answer the following questions.

33. By what percentage did survival rates for multiple myeloma cases improve between the 1960s and 2007?

34. If a person was diagnosed with leukemia in 1976, what survival rate could they expect?

35. If a person was diagnosed with multiple myeloma in 2003, what survival rate could they expect?

36. Survival rates for both multiple myeloma and leukemia have consistently risen since the 1960s. Why do you think this is?

37. What are the current five-year survival rates for multiple myeloma and leukemia? Research the statistics online and determine the survival-rate percentage for both diseases. Then, recreate the chart shown here on a sheet of paper. Add a new bar to represent the current survival rates.

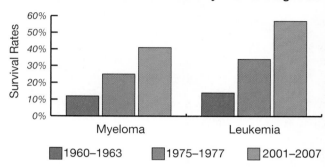

Five-Year Relative Survival Rates by Year of Diagnosis

Source: *SEER (Surveillance, Epidemiology and End Results) Cancer Statistics Review, 1975–2008.* National Cancer Institute; 2011.

Communicating about Anatomy and Physiology

38. **Reading and Writing** In 1985, the United States established mandatory screenings of donated blood for blood-borne diseases, such as HIV. Research the blood donation process. For what other diseases must donated blood be screened to prevent transmission of diseases? Besides screening for blood-borne diseases, what steps must be taken to ensure that donors are healthy candidates for donation? Can people with tattoos donate blood? What about someone with a cold virus? Write a report highlighting the precautions that are taken to ensure that donated blood is healthy and free of disease.

39. **Writing** Hemophilia is a genetic blood disorder that is usually inherited. One of the most well-known carriers for hemophilia was Queen Victoria of England. Research the history of hemophilia in Queen Victoria's family. Did this disease affect royal families in other nations? If so, why? Also, look into which members of her family were carriers and which suffered from the disease. Create a family tree that incorporates your findings and present it to the class.

Lab Investigations

40. Working in a small group, research the history of blood transfusions from the 1600s to the present. Why did some transfusion efforts fail? What technological developments improved transfusion success rates? Create a time line highlighting the major successes and failures. Present your time line to the class.

41. Working with a partner, create clay models of red blood cells, platelets, and each type of white blood cell. Pay special attention to the presence of granules in the white blood cells, as well as their stain color. Use the illustrations in this chapter to help you create your models.

Once you have finished constructing the models, label each model with its name and a brief description of the purpose that it serves in the body. Share your models with the class. Do your models resemble those of other groups? If not, what is different and why?

Expand your learning with additional online resources
- Supplemental Lab Activities
- Interactive Exercises
- Animations

www.g-wlearning.com/healthsciences

Could your heart be as powerful a pump as these oil wells?

The Cardiovascular System

"You gotta have *heart!*"

"Follow your *heart.*"

"Know it by *heart.*"

"Let's get to the *heart* of the matter!"

Is there an organ in the human body that is referenced in everyday language more often than the heart? What does this say about the function and importance of the heart?

The beating heart is just one part of the complex cardiovascular system. The system—comprising the heart, blood, and blood vessels—has a major impact on every living cell in the body.

Your heart beats 24 hours a day, 7 days a week. It pumps approximately 1.3 gallons (5 liters) of blood per minute, or approximately 2,000 gallons (7,571 liters) of blood each day. By comparison, a typical oil well pumps about 94 gallons of oil a day. The amount of blood pumped through your heart can fill 45 oil barrels a day and 2 oil super tankers in your lifetime. Isn't that an extraordinary feat for a muscle that is the size of a fist and weighs less than one pound? The heart is an amazing pump!

In the previous chapter, you learned about blood and how it feeds, protects, and heals your body. In this chapter, you will learn how blood is pumped through thousands of miles of passageways in the body to nourish every cell.

Chapter Lessons

Lesson 11.1
Heart Anatomy and the Function of the Cardiovascular System

Lesson 11.2
Regulation of the Heart

Lesson 11.3
Blood Vessels and Circulation

Lesson 11.4
Heart Disease

While studying, look for the online icon ![icon] **to:**

- **Practice** with e-flash cards and vocabulary games
- **Review** with interactive art labeling
- **Assess** with online exercises
- **Expand** with interactive activities and animated videos
- **Listen** to pronunciations of key terms in the audio glossary

www.g-wlearning.com/healthsciences

Companion Website

Study on the Go

Use a mobile device to practice vocabulary terms, listen to pronunciations, and review with self-assessment quizzes.

www.m.g-wlearning.com

G-W Mobile

Heart Anatomy and the Function of the Cardiovascular System

Before You Read

Try to answer the following questions before you read this lesson.

Besides serving as the transportation system of the body, what are the functions of the cardiovascular system?

Why does blood flow in only one direction in the heart?

What activities can make your heart stronger?

Lesson Objectives

1. Describe the function of the cardiovascular system.
2. Describe the location, size, and structures of the heart.
3. Outline the flow of blood through the cardiopulmonary system.
4. Describe how blood flows from the arteries to the veins.

Key Terms

E-Flash Cards

aorta
aortic valve
atrioventricular (AV) valves
cardiac output
diastole
endocardium
epicardium
inferior vena cava
interatrial septum
interventricular septum

mitral valve
myocardium
papillary muscle
semilunar valves
stroke volume
superior vena cava
systole
tricuspid valve
vasoconstriction
vasodilation

The cardiovascular system, also called the *circulatory system*, consists of a strong, muscular pump (the heart), an extensive network of pipes (blood vessels), and fluid (blood). The system transports oxygen, hormones, and other nutrients to cells and rids the body of carbon dioxide and other metabolic waste products. Additionally, the cardiovascular system helps to regulate body temperature by **vasodilation** (VA-soh-digh-LAY-shun) and **vasoconstriction** (VA-soh-kun-STRIK-shun) of blood vessels. Vasodilation is the expansion in the diameter of blood vessels, which increases blood flow. Vasoconstriction is the decrease in the diameter of blood vessels, which decreases blood flow.

The cardiovascular system has many functions including

- transportation of oxygen and other nutrients;
- removal of carbon dioxide and other waste products;
- regulation of body temperature;
- maintenance of the body's acid-base balance;
- transportation of hormones; and
- assistance with immune function.

The Heart: Location and Size

The heart is the hardest-working organ in the human body. A normal adult heart beats 72 to 82 times per minute (bpm), or approximately 3 billion times in a person's lifetime. This fatigue-resistant organ is about the size of a clenched fist. It weighs a little less than the combined weight of two baseballs, or about 8 to 10 ounces in women and 10 to 12 ounces in men.

The heart is located in the thoracic cavity under the *sternum*, or breastbone. It is centered in the chest and tilted slightly to the left. The heart is flanked on either side by the lungs and sits on top of the diaphragm. The broad *base* of the heart is positioned closer to the neck, at the second rib. The pointed *apex*, or bottom of the heart, lies at approximately the fifth rib and points down toward the left hip (**Figure 11.1**).

The Four Chambers of the Heart

The heart has an atrium and a ventricle on its right side and an atrium and a ventricle on its left side. The two atria (plural for *atrium*) act as low-pressure collecting chambers, while the two ventricles act as powerful pumps.

An **interatrial** (IN-ter-AY-tree-al) **septum** separates the right and left atria, and the two ventricles are divided by a much thicker **interventricular septum** (IN-ter-ven-TRIK-yoo-lar SEP-tum). The septal walls prevent oxygen-rich blood from mixing with oxygen-poor blood.

The right atrium receives deoxygenated blood from the venous system (system of veins)

via the **inferior vena cava** and the **superior vena cava** after the blood has made its trip around the body. The right ventricle then pumps the blood to the lungs. The left atrium receives the oxygenated blood from the lungs, and the left ventricle then pumps the blood through the **aorta** (ay-OR-ta) to the body. The two ventricles contract almost simultaneously—as the right ventricle pumps blood to the lungs, the left ventricle pumps blood to the body.

The Heart Valves

The heart is outfitted with four valves, which permit blood to flow in only one direction. **Figure 11.2** on the next page shows the heart valves in open and closed states.

The AV Valves

The **atrioventricular** (AY-tree-oh-vehn-TRIK-yoo-lar) **valves**, or AV valves, are the two valves located between the atria and the ventricles. When these valves are open, they allow blood to

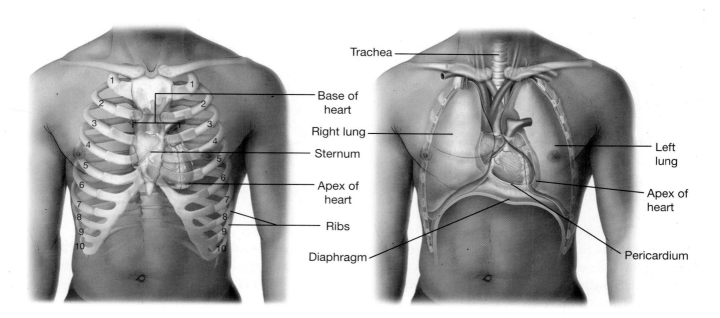

A. Position of the heart in the thoracic cavity

B. Position of the heart in relation to the lungs and diaphragm

Figure 11.1 Position of the heart. A—Position of the heart in the thoracic cavity. B—Position of the heart in relation to the lungs and diaphragm. *Write one sentence describing the position of the heart in relation to a structure(s) in the thoracic cage (see chapter 4 if necessary) and one sentence describing the location of the apex of the heart in relation to the lungs.*

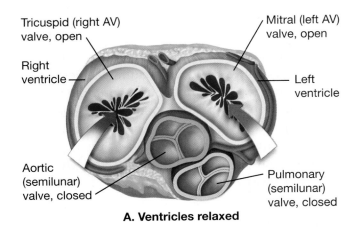

Tricuspid (right AV) valve, open

Mitral (left AV) valve, open

Right ventricle

Left ventricle

Aortic (semilunar) valve, closed

Pulmonary (semilunar) valve, closed

A. Ventricles relaxed

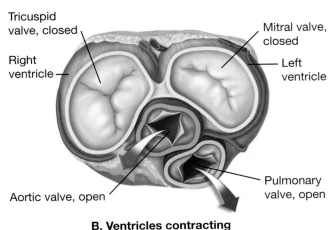

Tricuspid valve, closed

Mitral valve, closed

Right ventricle

Left ventricle

Aortic valve, open

Pulmonary valve, open

B. Ventricles contracting

Figure 11.2 Anterior superior view of the heart valves. The red arrows indicate the flow of oxygenated blood. The blue arrows indicate the flow of deoxygenated blood. *When the ventricles are relaxed, are the AV valves open or closed? When the ventricles contract, are the semilunar valves open or closed?*

flow from the atria into the ventricles. When they are closed, the AV valves prevent blood from flowing from the ventricles backward into the atria, as the ventricles contract.

On the right side of the heart the AV valve is called the **tricuspid** (trigh-KUS-pid) **valve** because it has three cusps, or flaps. The AV valve on the left side of the heart is called the *bicuspid* (bigh-KUS-pid) *valve*, or the **mitral** (migh-tral) **valve**, because it has two cusps.

Attached to these cusps are *chordae tendineae* (KOR-dee TEHN-di-nee), which are thin, fibrous cords, connected to the **papillary** (PAP-i-LAIR-ee) **muscles**. When the ventricles contract, the papillary muscles contract. These contractions pull on the chordae tendineae, which prevents

the valve cusps from swinging into the atria. If the valves were not secured by the chordae tendineae and the papillary muscles, the AV valve cusps would be pushed upward into the atria, allowing blood to flow backward into the atria. This backward blood flow is what happens when you have a heart murmur.

The Semilunar Valves

The next set of valves, the **semilunar** (SEHM-ee-LOO-nar) **valves**, allows blood to flow from the ventricles to the lungs and the rest of the body. The *pulmonary* (PUL-muh-NAIR-ee) *valve* and **aortic** (ay-OR-tik) **valve** each have three semilunar (half-moon) cusps that don't need to be anchored. When they close, the cusps are strong enough to brace each other, similar to the three legs of a stool.

The pulmonary valve is located at the opening of the pulmonary artery on the right side of the heart. The aortic valve is located at the opening of the aorta on the left side of the heart.

Memory Tip

These tips should help you remember the locations of the different heart valves. You can remember that the **T**ricuspid valve is on the **R**ight side of heart by noting that the letters **R** and **T** are close together in the alphabet. The **M**itral valve is on the **L**eft side of heart, so remember that **L** and **M** are side by side in the alphabet.

Blood Flow through the Heart

Now let's follow the flow of blood, step by step, through the heart. The steps are numbered and shown in **Figure 11.3** on the next page.

1. Deoxygenated blood enters the right atrium from both the inferior vena cava and the superior vena cava. The blood collects in the right atrium.
2. The collecting blood increases the pressure against the tricuspid (AV) valve, causing the valve to open. At this stage, with the tricuspid

valve open, the right ventricle fills passively. Then, the right atrium contracts, forcing the remaining blood into the ventricle.

3. Now the right ventricle contracts, and pressure increases in the chamber. This causes the tricuspid valve to close and the pulmonary valve to open, forcing blood into the pulmonary artery.

4. The pulmonary artery carries the blood to the lungs, where it becomes oxygenated in the capillary network of the lungs.

5. Oxygenated blood returns to the left atrium via the pulmonary veins.

6. Blood collects in the left atrium, causing pressure to increase in the chamber, thereby forcing the mitral (AV) valve to open.

7. At this stage, the left ventricle is filling passively. Atrial contraction forces the remaining blood into the left ventricle.

8. The ventricle contracts, and the pressure increases in the chamber. The increased pressure in the chamber causes the mitral

Figure 11.3 Heart chambers, great vessels, and blood flow through the heart. The arrows indicate the direction of blood flow through the heart. The blue arrows indicate deoxygenated blood. The red arrows indicate oxygenated blood. *Has the blood that is shown in the left ventricle already been through the lungs, or is it on its way to the lungs?*

valve to close and the aortic valve to open. The blood is forced into the aorta.

9. Oxygenated blood begins its journey of supplying oxygen to all parts of the body.

Walls of the Heart

The heart is a hollow organ enclosed in a fluid-filled, double-walled sac called the pericardium (PER-i-KAHR-dee-um). The fibrous outer wall of the sac anchors the heart to surrounding structures such as the sternum, diaphragm, and lungs. The inner wall of the sac is divided into two layers, which are separated by a fluid-filled cavity that allows the heart to beat in a frictionless environment.

The heart has three layers, or walls, of tissue. The **epicardium** (EHP-i-KAHR-dee-um) is the outermost layer of the heart, and it is also the innermost layer of the pericardial sac (**Figure 11.4**). The coronary arteries lie on the epicardial surface.

The **myocardium** (MIGH-oh-KAHR-dee-um), the middle layer of the heart, makes up about two-thirds of the heart muscle. It is the workhorse of the heart, contracting with enough force to pump blood through the 60,000 miles of vessels and back to the heart.

The innermost layer, the **endocardium** (EHN-doh-KAHR-dee-um), lines the interior of the heart chambers and covers the valves of the heart. The endocardium helps the blood to flow smoothly through the heart.

 Check Your Understanding

1. When a pulmonary valve opens, blood is forced into which artery and which main respiratory organ?
2. Is the blood leaving the left ventricle oxygenated or deoxygenated?
3. Which valve does blood move through as it goes from the right atrium to the right ventricle?
4. What is the name of the sac that encases the heart?
5. Name the three layers of the heart.

Figure 11.4 Layers of the walls of the heart. *Which layer of the heart can be described as the "workhorse"?*

Cardiac Cycle

The cardiac cycle consists of two phases: contraction and relaxation. During one complete cardiac cycle, the four chambers of the heart undergo a period of relaxation called **diastole** (digh-AS-toh-lee) when the chambers are filling with blood. Each cycle also includes a period of contraction called **systole** (SIS-toh-lee), when the chambers are pumping blood out of the heart.

The terms *systole* and *diastole* usually refer to what is happening in the ventricles because they are the major pumps of the heart. In a healthy heart, when the atria contract, the ventricles are relaxed. When the ventricles contract, the atria are relaxed.

One cardiac cycle is approximately 0.81 seconds in duration. In general, for an individual who has a resting heart rate of 72 to 82 bpm, approximately two-thirds of the cardiac cycle is spent in diastole, and one-third is spent in systole. This ratio is the basis for the formula for *mean arterial pressure*:

$$\text{Mean Arterial Pressure (MAP)} = \frac{2/3 \text{ Diastolic Blood Pressure}}{} + \frac{1/3 \text{ Systolic Blood Pressure}}{}$$

The mean arterial pressure measures the overall pressure within the cardiovascular system,

WHAT RESEARCH TELLS US

...*about* How the Hearts of Athletes Adapt to Exercise

An *echocardiogram* (EHK-oh-KAHR-dee-oh-GRAM) is an ultrasound test that looks at the structures of the heart to determine whether or not the heart valves are opening and closing properly. This test can also measure the pumping capacity of the heart.

Echocardiogram studies have shown that athletes who train aerobically (by running, cycling, or swimming, for example) have increases in both the size of their left ventricular chamber and in the thickness of the left ventricular wall. However, athletes who train using resistive exercise (weight lifting) have an increase in the left ventricular wall thickness but not in the size of the ventricular chamber.

Figure 11.5 A cardiovascular technologist performs an echocardiogram. *What can an echocardiogram reveal about a person's heart?*

Athletes also have an increase in their parasympathetic tone, causing their resting heart rate to decrease to 30 to 40 beats per minute. These adaptations are one

of the reasons why stroke volume among athletes is almost twice that of untrained individuals.

Taking It Further

1. Working with a partner, research the impact of regular exercise on the hearts of individuals who ordinarily do not exercise. What types of exercise bestow the greatest benefit? Develop a report for the class on the benefits of exercise and on exercise recommendations for different age groups.

2. Investigate the different types of echocardiogram tests and what each test reveals. Report your findings to the class.

---

which determines blood flow to various organs. If this pressure falls below 60 mmHG (millimeters of mercury), the organs of the body will become damaged from lack of oxygen. A lower blood pressure also means that the body will not receive the nutrient-rich blood flow that it needs.

At your next physical examination, your doctor may use a stethoscope to listen to your heart. During the cardiac cycle, the AV valves and the semilunar valves make sounds when they close. The sounds are referred to as "lub-dub" sounds. The "lub" sound is produced when the AV valves (tricuspid and mitral) close, and the "dub" sound is produced when the semilunar valves (pulmonary and aortic) close. If the valves don't close properly, there may be an additional sound, called a *heart murmur*. Many children are told by their doctors that they have a heart murmur. Most of these murmurs are harmless and are not caused by a heart abnormality, but, rather, a rapid growth spurt.

Cardiac Output

The amount of blood pumped from the heart per minute is called **cardiac output** (Q). Cardiac output is an important measurement because it can have an effect on blood pressure, cardiovascular fitness level, and body temperature.

The unit of measurement for cardiac output is liters per minute (L/min). The number of units is determined by multiplying the heart rate (HR) and the stroke volume (SV). **Stroke volume** is the amount of blood pumped from the heart per *beat*, and the units are milliliters per beat (mL/beat).

The average heart rate and stroke volume for a typical 154-pound male are approximately 72 beats/min and 70 mL/beat, which means that the cardiac output is 5,040 liters per minute (L/min). Women, because of their generally shorter stature and smaller size, have lower cardiac outputs than men do. Cardiac output is influenced by many factors, such as body size, exercise training, emotions, diet, and physical activity.

You would calculate the cardiac volume in the following way:

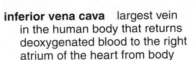

$$\begin{array}{ccc} \text{SV} & & \text{HR} & & \text{Q (cardiac} \\ \text{(mL/beat)} & \times & \text{(beats/min)} & = & \text{output)} \end{array}$$

$$\begin{array}{ccc} 70 & & 72 & & 5,040 \\ \text{mL/beat} & \times & \text{beats/min} & = & \text{mL/min} \end{array}$$

Check Your Understanding

1. Why do *systole* and *diastole* typically refer to what is happening in the ventricles?
2. What produces the "dub" sound heard through a stethoscope?
3. What is the formula for cardiac output?

Lesson 11.1 Review and Assessment

Mini Glossary   Make sure that you know the meaning of each key term.

 Build vocabulary with e-flash cards and games

aorta   a large arterial trunk that arises from the base of the left ventricle and channels blood from the heart into other arteries throughout the body

aortic valve   the semilunar valve between the left ventricle and the aorta that prevents blood from flowing back into the left ventricle

atrioventricular (AV) valves   the two valves (tricuspid and mitral) situated between the atria and the ventricles

cardiac output   the amount of blood pumped from the heart per minute

diastole   the period of relaxation in the heart when the chambers are filling with blood

endocardium   the innermost layer of the heart, which lines the interior of the heart chambers and covers the valves of the heart

epicardium   the outermost layer of the heart and the innermost layer of the pericardial sac

inferior vena cava   largest vein in the human body that returns deoxygenated blood to the right atrium of the heart from body regions below the diaphragm

interatrial septum   the wall that separates the right and left atria in the heart

interventricular septum   thick wall that divides the two ventricles in the heart

mitral valve   the valve that closes the orifice between the left atrium and left ventricle of the heart; bicuspid valve

myocardium   the middle layer of the heart, which makes up about 2/3 of the heart muscle

papillary muscle   one of the small muscular bundles attached at one end to the chordae tendineae and at the other to the innermost or endocardial wall of the ventricles; maintains tension on the chordae tendineae as the ventricle contracts

semilunar valves   valves situated at the opening between the heart and the aorta and at the opening between the heart and the pulmonary artery; they prevent backflow of blood into the ventricles

stroke volume   the volume of blood pumped from the heart per beat

superior vena cava   second largest vein in the body that returns deoxygenated blood to the right atrium of the heart from the upper half of the body

systole   a period of contraction when the chambers are pumping blood out of the heart

tricuspid valve   the valve that closes the orifice between the right atrium and right ventricle of the heart; composed of three cusps

vasoconstriction   narrowing of the blood vessels, which decreases blood flow

vasodilation   widening of the blood vessels, which increases blood flow

Know and Understand

 Assess

1. What are the names of the large blood vessels that bring blood back to the heart and empty it into the right atrium?
2. Which muscles control the AV valves?
3. What kind of vessels carry blood to the lungs?

Analyze and Apply

4. What are the main differences between the AV valves and the semilunar valves?
5. What does the name *chordae tendineae* tell you about the characteristics of these structures?
6. What have echocardiogram studies revealed about the different effects of exercise on the

hearts of aerobic athletes (runners, for example) and anaerobic athletes (weight lifters)?

7. Calculate cardiac output for a person with 40 beats/min and 93 mL/beat.

In the Lab

8. Create a hemisectional diagram of the heart (imagine cutting from top of right atrium to bottom of left ventricle). Label the three layers and the following structures: chambers, valves, septums, major blood vessels, and pericardium.
9. Starting with the inferior and superior venae cavae, trace the pathway of the blood through the heart diagram.

Lesson 11.2 — Regulation of the Heart

Before You Read

Try to answer the following questions before you read this lesson.

What is the internal (intrinsic) mechanism that allows the heart to beat on its own?

What are the two external (extrinsic) systems that regulate the heart?

Lesson Objectives

1. Describe the mechanisms that regulate the heart.
2. Describe different types of arrhythmia, or abnormal contractility conditions that can be detected via electrocardiogram.
3. Identify the components of the conduction system of the heart.

Key Terms

E-Flash Cards

arrhythmia
atrial fibrillation
atrioventricular node (AV node)
baroreceptors
bradycardia
bundle of His
depolarize
heart block
left bundle branches
premature atrial contractions (PACs)

premature ventricular contractions (PVCs)
Purkinje fibers
repolarize
right bundle branches
sinoatrial node (SA node)
tachycardia
ventricular fibrillation
ventricular tachycardia

The heart is regulated by three different mechanisms. One is inside the heart; the other two are outside of the heart.

Internal Control of the Heart

When the heart is transplanted from one individual to another, it will still beat on its own. How is this possible? The heart will continue to beat on its own because of a very important internal control mechanism called the *pacemaker*, alternately known as the **sinoatrial** (SIGH-noh-AY-tree-al) **node**, or SA node. The SA node is located at the top of the right atrium, slightly lateral and inferior to the opening of the superior vena cava (**Figures 11.6** and **11.7**). The SA node sends out an electrical impulse that tells the heart to beat at a rate between 60 and 100 bpm. You will learn more about the SA node and the internal control system a little later in this chapter.

External Control

The heart is also regulated by two external mechanisms: the cardiac center located in the medulla oblongata, and by the endocrine system.

The Cardiac Center

The cardiac center has sympathetic and parasympathetic branches, which are collectively referred to as the *autonomic nervous system* (**Figure 11.6**). (For a discussion of the autonomic nervous system, see chapter 6.) The cardiac center is always making adjustments in heart rate, contraction strength, and stroke volume. It gives the heart a "green light" (sympathetic

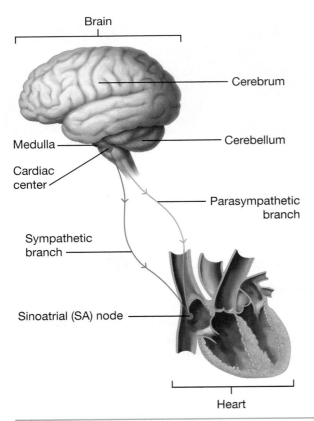

Figure 11.6 Location of the cardiac center in the medulla of the brain. *What type of stimulation—sympathetic or parasympathetic—causes the heart rate to increase?*

stimulation) when it wants the heart rate to increase, or a "red light" (parasympathetic stimulation) when the heart rate needs to slow down.

Baroreceptors (BAIR-oh-ree-SEP-ters) that are sensitive to pressure are located in the atrium of the heart, aortic arch, and carotid arteries. The baroreceptors constantly monitor blood pressure and send sensory information back to the cardiac center stimulating either the parasympathetic or sympathetic branches.

The parasympathetic branch is the dominant branch while you are at rest, which is why your heart rate is low at rest. As necessary, the parasympathetic branch releases acetylcholine, which decreases heart rate.

The cardiac center is also affected by emotions and physical activity. The sympathetic branch takes over during exercise or if you are emotionally stressed.

Memory Tip

Barometers measure the atmospheric pressure. Baroreceptors measure blood pressure.

In chapters 6 and 8, we discussed the characteristics of the fight-or-flight response. When faced with a dangerous situation, the body has to prepare itself to fight or run from the danger at hand. In such a situation, a set of brain structures called the *limbic system* stimulates the sympathetic branch in the cardiac center. The sympathetic nerve fibers stimulate the SA node, which causes the heart rate to increase.

The Endocrine System

The endocrine system is composed of many glands that secrete hormones, which can cause many changes within the body. The adrenal medulla and the thyroid glands, for example, can affect the cardiovascular system. When the adrenal medulla secretes epinephrine (ehp-i-NEHF-rin) and norepinephrine (NOR-ehp-i-NEHF-rin), heart rate increases. Similarly, when the thyroid gland releases thyroxine (thigh-RAHK-seen), heart rate increases.

✓ Check Your Understanding

1. What three different mechanisms regulate the heart?
2. Which structure is known as the "pacemaker" of the heart?
3. Which part of the nervous system signals the heart to increase the number of beats per minute?
4. Name three hormones released by the endocrine system that affect heart rate.

The Conduction System

Conduction is the process of conveying or transmitting types of energy, such as electrical impulses. The conduction system in the heart transmits signals that control both heart rate and contraction strength of the muscle tissues.

The conduction system of the heart includes two areas of nodal tissue and a network of conduction fibers. These structures allow the electrical impulses formed by the SA node to travel to the ventricles, telling the ventricles to contract. Let's trace the pathway of an electrical impulse generated by the SA node (**Figure 11.7**).

Once the SA node fires, the electrical impulse is carried to the left atrium via Bachmann's bundle. The impulse also goes to the **atrioventricular** (AY-tree-oh-vehn-TRIK-yoo-lar) **node**, or AV node, via three internodal pathways. The AV node is a very dense network of fibers, which causes the electrical impulse to get "tied up," or delayed there, for approximately a tenth of a second.

Once the electrical impulse leaves the AV node, it is carried through conducting fibers called the **bundle of His**, or the common bundle, in the ventricular septum. (The bundle of His is alternately known in scientific circles as the atrioventricular bundle.) The common bundle then divides, and the electrical impulse travels down the **left bundle branches** and the **right bundle branch** to millions of **Purkinje fibers** in both

ventricles. When the Purkinje fibers receive the impulse, they stimulate the ventricles to contract.

The Electrocardiogram

The *electrocardiogram* (ee-LEHK-troh-KAHR-dee-oh-gram), known as an ECG or EKG, is a recording of the electrical activity of the heart (**Figures 11.8** and **11.9** on the next page). In a sense, an ECG speaks the language of the heart. It illustrates what is happening electrically in the conduction system and mechanically in the atria and ventricles when they **depolarize** (contract) and **repolarize** (relax).

 Check Your Understanding

1. What role does the AV node play in the conduction system of the heart?
2. Which structures carry electrical impulses from the common bundle to the individual Purkinje fibers, causing the ventricles to contract?
3. What does *ECG* stand for and what is it used for?

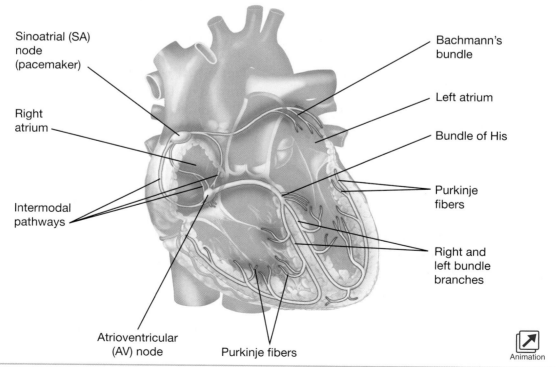

Sinoatrial (SA) node (pacemaker)

Right atrium

Intermodal pathways

Atrioventricular (AV) node

Purkinje fibers

Bachmann's bundle

Left atrium

Bundle of His

Purkinje fibers

Right and left bundle branches

Animation   Label Art

Figure 11.7 Conduction system of the heart. *Describe the pathway of an electrical impulse generated by the SA node.*

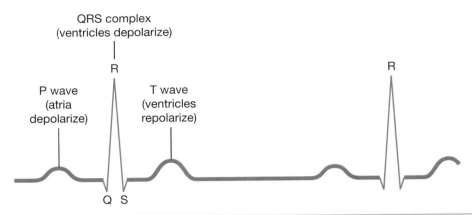

Figure 11.8 An ECG is a piece of graph paper containing a record of the electrical events in the heart. The placement of the electrodes on the body surface affects the size and shape of the waves recorded. This example shows a normal ECG.

Figure 11.9 Summary of Electrical and Mechanical Events and the ECG		
Electrical Event	**Mechanical Event**	**ECG Recording**
SA node fires	atria contract	P wave
impulse travels to Purkinje fibers	ventricles contract	QRS complex
ventricles relax	atria and ventricles fill	T wave

Cardiac Arrhythmias

Usually the heart follows a sequence of events at regular intervals. In a normal, healthy heart the rhythm is regular, and the rate is between 60 and 100 beats per minute. **Figure 11.10A** shows an ECG of a normal sinus rhythm, or *normal contractility condition.*

Sometimes, however, a beat comes too soon, or the conduction system may not work properly, and an abnormal heartbeat occurs. This irregularity is called an **arrhythmia** (ay-RITH-mee-a), or *abnormal contractility condition.* Generally, arrhythmias that originate in the atria or AV node aren't a problem, but those that originate in the ventricle are more dangerous and can be life threatening. Ventricular arrhythmias can affect blood flow to the heart and to the rest of the body, whereas atrial arrhythmias do not.

Arrhythmias have many causes, including damage to the heart muscle (such as from a heart attack); coronary artery disease; hypertension; smoking; excessive alcohol consumption; excessive caffeine ingestion from coffee or soft

drinks; electrolyte imbalances; illicit drug use; dietary supplements that contain stimulants; stress; and medications.

The ECG is the best tool for detecting abnormal rhythms. Listed below, and shown in **Figure 11.10**, are several types of arrhythmias. A normal rhythm is shown in **Figure 11.10A**.

B. **Bradycardia** (BRAD-ee-KAHR-dee-a)—a normal heart rhythm but with a rate below 60 bpm. This condition is common in athletes.

C. **Tachycardia** (TAK-i-KAHR-dee-a)—a normal rhythm but the rate is above 100 bpm.

D. **Premature atrial contractions (PACs)**—a condition in which an irritable piece of atrial heart tissue fires before the SA node. This causes the contraction to occur too early in the rhythm. Usually PACs are harmless. Caffeine ingestion, other types of stimulants, and stress can increase their likelihood.

E. **Atrial fibrillation**—a condition in which the atrial tissue is very irritated, causing the atria to beat at a rate greater than 350 bpm. The atria don't beat in a coordinated manner; they simply quiver. On an electrocardiogram, the baseline is a wavy line, and the rhythm is irregular. Atrial fibrillation is the most common type of arrhythmia worldwide. In fact, many people with atrial fibrillation go about their daily routine without any symptoms. But if the ventricular rate is too low or too high, pharmacological intervention or a pacemaker may be needed.

F. **Premature ventricular contractions (PVCs)**—a condition in which Purkinje fibers fire before the SA node, causing the ventricles to contract prematurely. Single PVCs are not dangerous. However, frequent PVCs (more than six per minute) or multifocal PVCs (those that occur at multiple sites in the ventricle) may be dangerous and therefore require treatment.

G. **Ventricular tachycardia (VT)**—a life-threatening arrhythmia in which the ventricles, rather than the SA node, initiate the beat. The heart rate is between 150 and 250 bpm, requiring immediate medical intervention such as intravenous lidocaine (LIGH-doh-kayn) or *cardioversion* (KAHR-dee-oh-VER-zhun).

H. **Ventricular fibrillation (VF)**—a life-threatening condition in which the ventricles quiver at a rate greater than 350 bpm. Essentially, there is no cardiac output in this condition. Immediate steps to *defibrillate* (stop) the heart must be undertaken, with the hope that the system will regain a normal, healthy rhythm.

I. **Heart block**—a condition in which the impulses traveling from the SA node to the ventricles are delayed, blocked intermittently, or completely blocked by the AV node. These are commonly called *first-* (impulse-delayed), *second-* (intermittently blocked) and *third-degree* (completely blocked) *heart blocks*. Third-degree heart block is a dangerous arrhythmia because there is no electrical communication between the atria and the ventricles. The atria fire at the rate of the SA node between 60 and 100 bpm, and the

A.   Normal sinus rhythm

B.   Sinus bradycardia

C.   Sinus tachycardia

D.   Sinus rhythm with PACs

E.   Atrial fibrillation

F.   Every other beat is a PVC

G.   Ventricular tachycardia

H.   Ventricular fibrillation

I.   Third-degree heart block

Figure 11.10 A shows a normal ECG. B through I—Different types of arrhythmias.

WHAT RESEARCH TELLS US

...*about* How Transplanted Hearts Function

Research on heart-transplant patients found that their resting heart rates are higher than normal at approximately 90 bpm. According to exercise stress-test studies, increases in heart rates occur more slowly in transplant patients, and recovery heart rates remain elevated for longer periods of time.

Why are the hearts of transplant patients different in this way? The parasympathetic and sympathetic systems do not

regulate heart rate in a transplanted heart. This means that heart rate is higher at rest, and it only begins to rise during exercise from an increase in hormones such as epinephrine and norepinephrine.

Taking It Further

1. Research the development of the total artificial heart (TAH). How do these hearts function in patients awaiting heart transplantation? Present your findings to the class.

Figure 11.11 A heart patient undergoes an exercise stress test.

ventricles beat at their own rate, between 15 and 40 bpm. Because the ventricles fire at such a slow rate, cardiac output is too low to adequately supply blood to the rest of the body. A pacemaker is usually inserted into the heart to remedy this condition.

 ### Check Your Understanding

1. What are PACs?
2. Which type of heart block is life-threatening and why?

Defibrillators and Life-Threatening Arrhythmias

A *defibrillator* is a device that can deliver a therapeutic dose of electrical current that momentarily stops the heart, allowing its built-in pacemaker, the SA node, to assume control and produce a normal rhythm. Automatic external defibrillators (AEDs) are available in many public gathering places, such as airports, shopping malls, and schools. These devices automatically detect the type of arrhythmia present and deliver an electrical shock if

appropriate, thus allowing people with little to no training to use them (**Figure 11.12**).

The American Heart Association offers a basic cardiopulmonary resuscitation (CPR) course that can train you to perform CPR and use an automatic external defibrillator. This course is recommended for everyone. If, however, you are involved in a rescue and have not taken such a course, you can still use the AED. With its foolproof, two- to three-step process, it is simple to use.

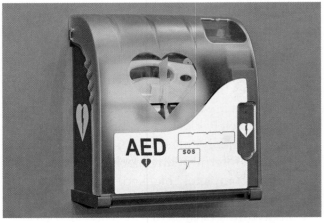

Baloncici/Shutterstock.com

Figure 11.12 An automated, external defibrillator, or AED. *In what types of public places are defibrillators often available?*

Lesson 11.2 Review and Assessment

Mini Glossary
Make sure that you know the meaning of each key term.

arrhythmia an irregular heartbeat or rhythm

atrial fibrillation condition in which the atria contract in an uncoordinated, rapid manner (rate above 350 bpm), causing the ventricles to contract irregularly

atrioventricular node (AV node) a small mass of tissue that transmits impulses received from the sinoatrial node to the ventricles via the bundle of His

baroreceptors pressure-sensitive nerve endings in the atrium, aortic arch, and carotid arteries

bradycardia a normal heart rhythm but with a rate below 60 bpm; a condition common among athletes

bundle of His a slender bundle of modified cardiac muscle that conducts electrical impulses from the AV node to the left and right bundle branches to Purkinje fibers in the ventricle

depolarize to contract; the atria and ventricles depolarize as the heart beats

heart block a condition in which the impulses traveling from the SA node to the ventricles are delayed, intermittently blocked, or completely blocked by the AV node

left bundle branches the left limbs or branches through which electrical impulses are transmitted from the bundle of His through the left ventricle

premature atrial contractions (PACs) condition in which an irritable piece of atrial heart tissue fires before the SA node, causing the atria to contract too soon

premature ventricular contractions (PVCs) condition in which Purkinje fibers fire before the SA node, causing the ventricles to contract prematurely

Purkinje fibers part of the impulse-conducting network of the heart that rapidly transmits impulses throughout the ventricles, causing ventricular contraction

repolarize to relax; the atria and ventricles repolarize as the heart beats

right bundle branches the right leg or branch through which electrical impulses are transmitted from the bundle of His through the right ventricle

sinoatrial node (SA node) a small mass of specialized tissue located in the right atrium that normally acts as the pacemaker of the heart, causing it to beat at a rate between 60 and 100 bpm

tachycardia a normal heart rhythm but with a rate above 100 bpm

ventricular fibrillation a life-threatening condition in which the heart ventricles quiver at a rate greater than 350 bpm

ventricular tachycardia a life-threatening arrhythmia in which the ventricles, rather than the SA node, initiate the heartbeat; the heart rate is between 150 and 250 bpm, requiring swift medical attention

Know and Understand

1. What do baroreceptors monitor and where do they send messages?
2. Which two endocrine system glands release hormones that affect heart rate?
3. List in order the structures through which an electrical impulse travels on its way to the muscle fibers of the ventricles.
4. What are the differences between atrial and ventricular fibrillation?
5. Further investigate AEDs. What are their therapeutic uses and effects?

Analyze and Apply

6. How does the nervous system help to regulate heart rate?
7. Using figures 11.8, 11.9, and 11.10, explain how you would interpret normal and abnormal contractility conditions.
8. What happens to an electrical impulse when it reaches the AV node in the conduction system of a normally functioning heart?

In the Lab

9. While sitting at your desk, take your heart rate at your carotid artery/pulse and record it. (You may want to refer to the information on taking a pulse later in this chapter.) Now run in place for 45 to 60 seconds. Take and record your heart rate again. Sit down and wait two minutes before taking and recording your heart rate again. Did your resting heart rate qualify as bradycardia? Did your exercising heart rate qualify as tachycardia? What happened to your heart rate after you sat down for two minutes? Explain the role of the sympathetic and parasympathetic nervous systems during this experiment. Share your answers with your lab group.

Using the data that you and your lab partners collected, your own experimental testing, your observations, and logical reasoning, analyze and evaluate the explanations given by your partners. Provide each partner with a critique of his or her explanation.

Before You Read

Try to answer the following questions before you read this lesson.

What are the three types of blood vessels and the most important function of each?

Why are capillaries well suited for gas exchange?

Can you trace the journey of a red blood cell through your heart?

Which artery can be used to measure both pulse and blood pressure?

Lesson Objectives

1. Identify the differences among the three types of vessels.
2. Outline the flow of blood through the cardiopulmonary system.
3. Describe how blood flows from the arteries to the veins.
4. Describe how the veins return blood to the heart.
5. Describe the distribution of blood at rest and during exercise.

Key Terms

E-Flash Cards

aortic arch	precapillary sphincter
arteries	pulmonary circulation
arterioles	radial artery
brachial artery	systemic circulation
capillaries	tunica externa
capillary beds	tunica intima
carotid artery	tunica media
coronary sinus	veins
ductus arteriosus	venules
foramen ovale	vital signs

Blood Vessels: The Transport Network

Three types of blood vessels form a closed loop of tubes that carry blood from the heart to the rest of the body and back to the heart. These vessels are the **arteries**, **capillaries**, and **veins**. Two other important subdivisions of vessels are the **arterioles** (ar-TAIR-ee-ohls), or microscopic arteries, and **venules** (VEN-yools), or smallest veins. **Figure 11.13** summarizes the structure and function of each of these types of blood vessels.

The Three Layers of Blood Vessels

All blood vessels, with the exception of capillaries, are composed of three layers that surround the blood-filled opening called the *lumen* (LOO-mehn). **Tunica intima** (TOO-ni-ka IN-ti-ma), the innermost layer, is composed of a single layer of squamous (flattened) epithelial cells over a sheet of connective tissue. The tunica intima provides a smooth, frictionless surface that allows blood to flow smoothly through the vessel (**Figure 11.14**).

Tunica media, the middle layer of blood vessels, is a thicker layer containing smooth muscle cells, elastic fibers, and collagen. The smooth muscle cells in this layer are directed by the sympathetic nervous system to *vasodilate* (increase the opening of the lumen) and *vasoconstrict* (decrease its opening). This process allows blood flow to be increased to certain tissues and decreased to other tissues as needed.

Vasodilation and vasoconstriction of the vessels also play a major role in regulating and determining blood pressure. When a vessel vasodilates, blood pressure is lowered; when the vessel vasoconstricts, blood pressure is increased.

Figure 11.13 Structure and Function of Vessels

Vessel Type	Structure	Function
*Artery**	three-layered vessel (intima, media, adventitia); thick, elastic, muscular walls	transports oxygen-rich blood away from heart to arterioles; influenced by the sympathetic nervous system (contraction/dilation)
Arteriole	thinner, three-walled vessel, mostly smooth muscle cells	transports blood from arteries to capillaries; greater impact by the sympathetic nervous system; acts to direct blood flow in the body
Capillary	single layer of epithelial cells	gas/nutrient and waste-product exchange between blood and tissues
Venule	thin-walled vessels bundled together to form a vein	transports blood from capillary to vein
Vein	three-layered (intima, media, externa), thin-walled vessel with one-way valves	transports oxygen-poor blood back to the heart

*Exception: Pulmonary arteries carry deoxygenated blood.

Figure 11.14 Sizes and layers of different types of blood vessels. *What size differences do you notice between the red and the blue vessels?*

The **tunica externa**, the outermost layer of blood vessels, is composed mostly of fibrous connective tissue, which serves to support and protect the vessels.

Differences between Arteries and Veins

Although arteries and veins both have three layers, the relative thickness and composition of the layers differ, as does the size of the lumen. These differences exist because the two vessels have very different functions in the cardiovascular system.

Figure 11.15 details the structural difference between arteries and veins. The arterial vessels carry blood away from the heart, so they must withstand large increases in pressure when the heart contracts. The aorta, the largest artery, leaves the heart and branches into progressively smaller arteries that eventually become arterioles (**Figure 11.16**). Arteries have the thickest, strongest, most elastic walls.

The venous system (system of veins) carries blood back to the heart. Unlike arteries, veins do not have to deal with large increases in pressure. Thus, the walls of the veins are thinner and less elastic than those of the arteries. The venous system acts as a reservoir, housing 65% of the blood in the body.

The blood enters the venules from the capillaries. The venules merge together to form progressively larger veins until they reach the largest veins, the inferior and superior venae cavae. These two veins empty into the right atrium of the heart.

The venous system is able to pump blood back to the heart because it has one-way valves that allow blood to flow only toward the heart. In addition, when the muscles that surround the veins contract, they *milk* the blood toward the heart (**Figure 11.17**).

Venous return of blood is also assisted by the pump-like action of the respiratory system. Changes in abdominal and thoracic pressure that occur with breathing help to pump blood back to the heart.

✓ Check Your Understanding

1. All blood vessels, with the exception of capillaries, consist of what three layers?
2. What is the name of the smallest type of artery?
3. What type of vessel carries blood back to the heart?
4. What is the largest type of artery?

Figure 11.15 Differences between Arteries and Veins

Structures	Arteries	Veins
walls	strong, thick, elastic	thin, less elastic
pressure	high	low
lumen	small	large
valves	no	yes

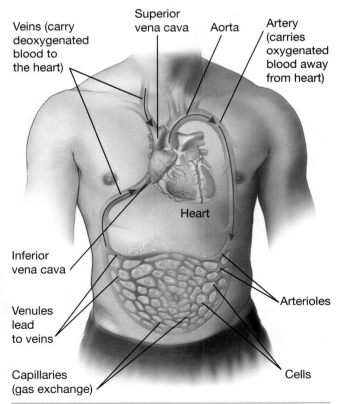

Figure 11.16 Network of blood vessels in the cardiovascular system. *Which group of vessels—the red or the blue—acts as a reservoir, holding over 60% of the body's blood?*

Muscle milking action on vein promotes venous return to heart

Muscle surrrounding the vein contracts, forcing blood to flow towards the heart

Figure 11.17 Muscle milking action. *Where is the muscle in relation to the vein on which it performs its milking action?*

Capillaries

Arterioles connect with the smallest and most numerous vessels in the body—the capillaries. Capillaries range in size from 0.0025 to 0.25 cm. Capillaries are so narrow that red blood cells must pass through them in a single line, one at a time.

Capillaries are called *exchange vessels* because oxygen and carbon dioxide gas exchange occurs between the capillaries and the tissues. Capillaries in the kidneys, liver, small intestines, and endocrine glands also have microscopic pores that allow the passage of small molecules. For instance, these pores allow hormones to pass into the bloodstream when the pores come in contact with endocrine glands, and they allow white blood cells to pass into tissue to kill harmful bacteria.

Blood flow through the capillaries is controlled by a **precapillary sphincter** (pree-KAP-i-LAIR-ee SFINGK-ter), a band of smooth muscle fibers that encircles the capillaries at

the arteriole-capillary junctions. Contraction of the precapillary sphincter stops blood flow to the capillary; relaxation increases blood flow. Contraction or relaxation of the precapillary sphincter is based on the local chemical conditions (pH, oxygen, carbon dioxide, temperature) in the tissue. For instance, approximately 15% of blood flow goes to your muscles at rest. During exercise, however, when the metabolic needs of the muscles dramatically increase, approximately 85% of the blood flow goes to the working muscles.

Capillaries don't operate separately; they form an expansive network of intertwined vessels called **capillary beds**. Blood begins its journey back to the heart when the capillaries merge with venules. The venules then merge with larger, thicker-walled veins that eventually lead back to the heart.

Circulation: Moving Blood around the Body

As you read earlier, the circulatory system is an extensive network of blood vessels that stretches 60,000 miles within the body. In this section you will learn

- how blood flows to various organs, including the heart;
- the unique characteristics of the hepatic portal circulatory system; and
- how a fetus receives blood from the mother's placenta.

To gain a better understanding of this vast network, we will break it down into manageable parts.

Cardiopulmonary Circulation

As you learned earlier in the chapter, the right side of the heart pumps oxygen-poor blood to the lungs (**pulmonary circulation**), and the left side of the heart pumps oxygen-rich blood to the rest of the body (**systemic circulation**). We will first explore the pulmonary system, part of which will be a review of what you learned earlier (**Figure 11.18** on the next page).

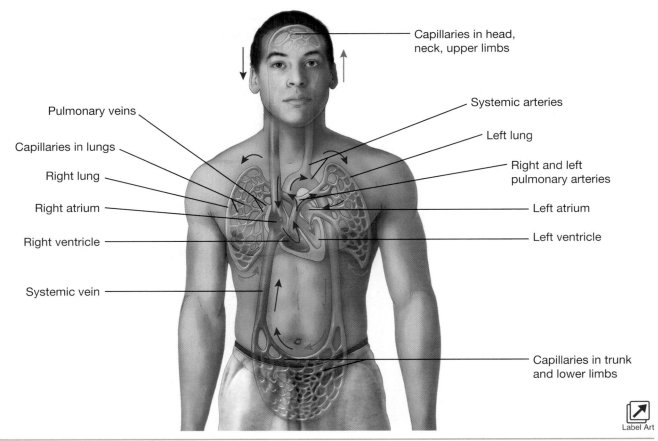

Pulmonary veins

Capillaries in lungs

Right lung

Right atrium

Right ventricle

Systemic vein

Capillaries in head, neck, upper limbs

Systemic arteries

Left lung

Right and left pulmonary arteries

Left atrium

Left ventricle

Capillaries in trunk and lower limbs

Label Art

Figure 11.18 The heart pumps blood through two major circuits: the pulmonary circuit and the systemic circuit. The right side of the heart pumps blood to the lungs (pulmonary circulation), and the left side of the heart pumps blood throughout the body (systemic circulation). *Is the blood entering the lungs in the pulmonary circuit oxygen rich or oxygen poor? Is the blood pumped from the left side of the heart to the rest of the body in the systemic circuit oxygen rich or oxygen poor?*

1. Deoxygenated blood enters the right atrium from the inferior and superior venae cavae.
2. Deoxygenated blood flows through the tricuspid valve into the right ventricle.
3. The right ventricle contracts, and deoxygenated blood is ejected through the pulmonary valve into the pulmonary artery.
4. The pulmonary artery splits into smaller arteries, which carry the deoxygenated blood to the lungs.
5. The two smaller pulmonary arteries branch into arterioles that merge with the capillary network in the lungs.
6. The blood becomes oxygenated in the lungs and then flows through the venules, which merge with the four pulmonary veins that carry the oxygenated blood back to the heart.

7. The pulmonary veins empty oxygenated blood into the left atrium.
8. Oxygenated blood flows through the mitral (AV) valve into the left ventricle.
9. The left ventricle contracts and ejects oxygenated blood through the aorta to the rest of the body.

Systemic Circulation

The systemic circulatory system refers to the closed-loop network of arteries, arterioles, capillaries, venules, and veins that circulate oxygen, hormones, water, and other nutrients to tissues and then carries carbon dioxide and waste products back to the heart. We will now trace the journey of a red blood cell. Keep in mind that we've got 60,000 miles to go!

WHAT RESEARCH TELLS US

...*about* Why Records Aren't Broken on Hot, Humid Days

Marathoners will not soon forget the environmental conditions at the 2012 Boston Marathon: direct sunlight, temperatures in the mid-80s, and high humidity. This was a recipe for slow race times and heat-related mishaps! Geoffrey Mutai, the 2011 winner, dropped out with heat-related cramps at mile 18, and the 2012 winner was 10 minutes slower than Mutai's 2011 time. Why do you think this occurred?

Research indicates that exercise in a heated environment causes internal competition in the body for blood supply. As body temperature increases, a greater percentage of blood goes to the skin to cool the body. In addition, increased sweat rates cause blood volume to decrease. The result of these conditions is that less blood goes back to the heart. Less blood to the heart means that the stroke volume must decrease.

How does the heart react to a decrease in stroke volume? For sufficient cardiac output to be maintained, heart rate must

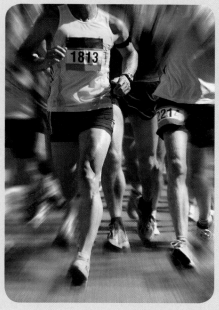

Mikael Damkier/Shutterstock.com

Figure 11.19 These runners are attempting to complete a marathon, which is just over 26 miles.

increase. This means that the heart has to work harder, causing the body to use fuel more quickly. Over time performance declines.

What can we learn from this research? To minimize performance declines during severe heat conditions, keep hydrated by drinking plenty of plain water or water that contains a mixture of salt and carbohydrates (electrolytes).

Taking It Further

1. Research how the cardiovascular system reroutes blood through the body as body temperature increases. Describe your findings in a report.

2. Besides excessively warm temperatures, what other environmental factors can affect heart rate?

3. Use a heart-rate monitor to measure your heart rate at various times over several days. Note any patterns. For example, is your heart rate higher or lower in the morning than later in the day? Do you notice a relationship between your body temperature and heart rate?

Our journey begins when the left ventricle pumps blood through the aorta, the largest artery in the body. The ascending branch of the aorta rises up from the heart, arches to the left (thus the term **aortic arch**), and then proceeds downward through the descending aorta into the thorax along the spine, through the diaphragm, and into the abdomen. Once this vessel reaches the abdomen, it is called the *abdominal aorta*.

There are many other arteries that arise from the aorta:

- The right and left coronary arteries branch from the ascending aorta and supply the

heart with blood, as you will learn in the next section.

- The brachiocephalic (BRAY-kee-oh-seh-FAL-ik), left common carotid, and left subclavian (sub-KLAY-vee-an) arteries branch from the aortic arch and supply the head, neck, and arms with blood. These arteries subdivide into many more arteries. **Figure 11.20** illustrates the arteries that arise from the aorta.

- Many arteries branch from the descending aorta, supplying blood to various organs including the liver, spleen, kidneys, stomach, and the rest of the lower body.

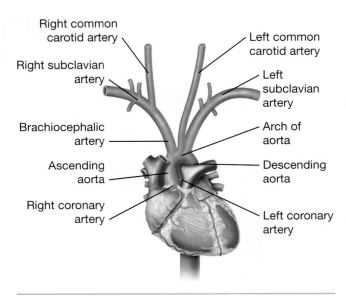

Figure 11.20 Arteries arising from the aorta. *To which areas of the body will these arteries supply blood? Which of the arteries labeled in this drawing is the major artery supplying blood to the lower limbs?*

The major arteries of the body are shown in **Figure 11.23** on page 390. As you can see, these arteries branch into smaller and smaller vessels, eventually becoming arterioles. The arterioles will merge with capillaries, where tissue and blood exchange nutrients and waste materials. The journey back to the heart begins with blood draining into the venules, which merge to form veins.

Figure 11.24 on page 391 illustrates the major veins that drain from the head and the trunk, as well as the upper and lower limbs. Generally, the names of the veins are the same as their arterial counterparts (for example, *renal* artery and *renal* vein). The systemic circulatory journey ends when the blood from the lower veins enters the inferior vena cava and blood from the upper veins empties into the superior vena cava. Both the inferior and superior venae cavae drain into the right atrium.

Cardiac Circulation

You now know that oxygen is supplied to the body by the arteries, which carry blood away from the heart. But how does the heart receive its oxygen supply?

Perhaps you thought that the blood that circulates through the chambers of the heart

provides the oxygen for the heart, but it does not. The oxygen-rich blood that nourishes the heart is supplied by the right and left coronary arteries that lie on the epicardial (outermost) surface of the heart (**Figure 11.21**).

The right coronary artery has two main branches, which supply blood to the inferior and posterior walls of the heart. The left main coronary artery divides into two arteries (the left anterior descending artery and the circumflex artery) that supply oxygen-rich blood to the anterior, lateral, and posterior walls of the heart.

The coronary arteries arise from the base of the aorta and fill when the ventricles are relaxed. The coronary arteries are closed when the ventricles contract, so they are protected from the high pressure that is generated during contraction. Blood from the coronary arteries

Memory Tip

Keep in mind that the names of the arteries and veins often refer to the organ or location that they supply with blood. For example, the *femoral* artery supplies blood to the femoral region of the leg, and the *lumbar* artery supplies blood to the lumbar area of the back.

Figure 11.21 Anterior view of the coronary arteries. *How would you respond if someone told you that this drawing represents both pulmonary and systemic circulation because it shows both arteries and veins?*

empties into several cardiac veins, which drain into a large vessel called the **coronary sinus**, which is located on the posterior wall of the right atrium.

Check Your Understanding

1. Why are the capillaries called *exchange vessels*?
2. Which structure controls blood flow between arterioles and capillaries?
3. Is the blood in the pulmonary veins oxygenated or deoxygenated? Explain your answer.
4. Which arteries arise from the ascending aorta?
5. Where are the coronary arteries located in the heart?

Hepatic Portal Circulation

So far, you have learned how oxygen is supplied to the tissues of the body. Now let's look at the way in which other nutrients, such as carbohydrates, fats, and proteins, are stored in or released into the bloodstream. Storage and circulation of these valuable nutrients is critical if you are to have the energy you need to perform your daily activities.

Hepatic portal circulation plays a vital role in maintaining proper carbohydrate, fat, and protein levels in the blood. The hepatic portal circulation system does something unusual. Whereas the arteries of the cardiovascular system deliver blood to different parts of the body, the veins of the hepatic portal circulation system supply the blood to the liver. Let's take a look at how this system works.

The veins that drain the stomach, spleen, pancreas, small intestine, and colon deliver blood to the liver through the hepatic portal vein (**Figure 11.22**). This blood is rich with nutrient sources from carbohydrates and fats. As the blood percolates through the liver, some of the nutrients are removed, stored, or repackaged for another use.

The best example is the fate of glucose. After a meal, the blood that drains into the liver may be high in glucose. The liver, which plays a role in regulating blood glucose levels, stores glucose as glycogen until a later date, when the body needs the glucose for energy. Let's suppose that a person is exercising and her blood glucose level starts to drop. As this happens, the liver breaks down its stored glycogen and releases it into the bloodstream as glucose, thereby maintaining blood glucose levels.

Once blood has been filtered by the liver, it returns to the inferior vena cava through the hepatic veins. You will learn more about this process in chapter 13.

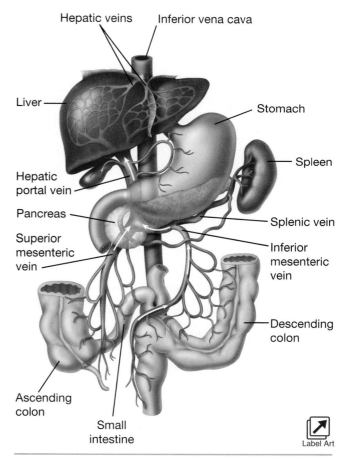

Figure 11.22 Hepatic portal circulation. Veins from the stomach, spleen, pancreas, small intestine, and colon drain into the hepatic portal vein. The liver filters the blood before the blood empties into the inferior vena cava. *What is the vital role of hepatic portal circulation?*

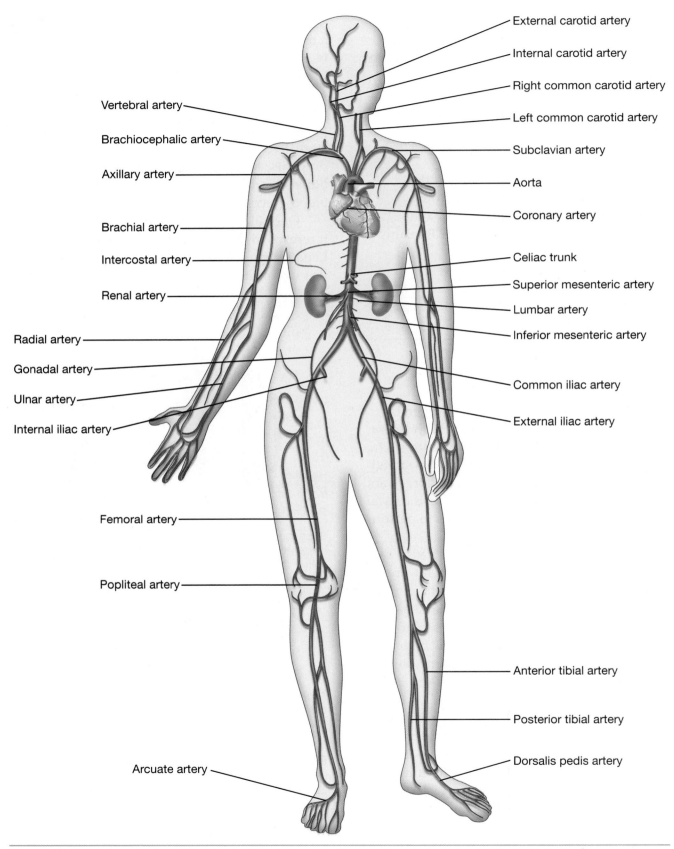

External carotid artery

Internal carotid artery

Right common carotid artery

Left common carotid artery

Subclavian artery

Aorta

Coronary artery

Celiac trunk

Superior mesenteric artery

Lumbar artery

Inferior mesenteric artery

Common iliac artery

External iliac artery

Anterior tibial artery

Posterior tibial artery

Dorsalis pedis artery

Vertebral artery

Brachiocephalic artery

Axillary artery

Brachial artery

Intercostal artery

Renal artery

Radial artery

Gonadal artery

Ulnar artery

Internal iliac artery

Femoral artery

Popliteal artery

Arcuate artery

Figure 11.23 Major arteries of the body. *What do we call arteries as they get smaller and smaller?*

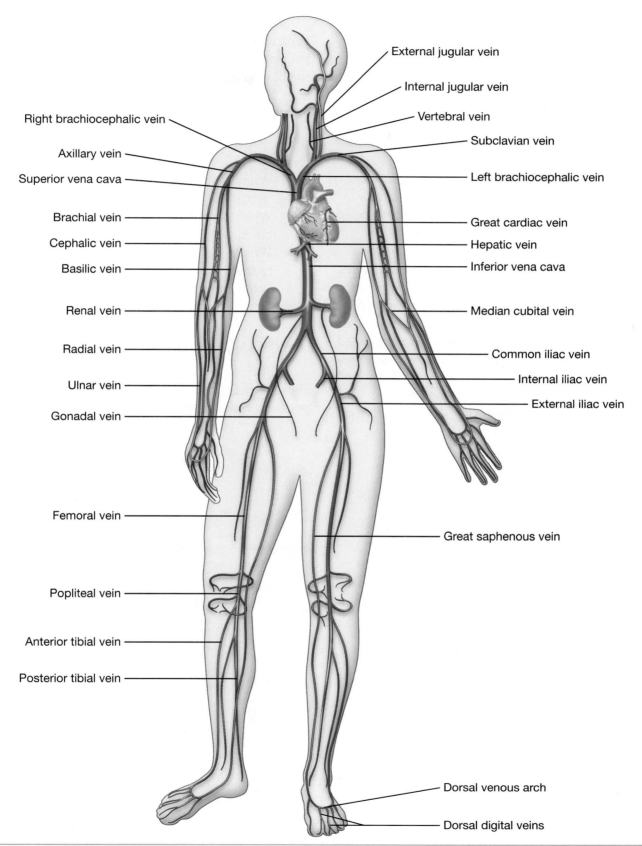

Figure 11.24 Major veins of the body. *Which two veins represent the end of the blood's journey through the body?*

Fetal Circulation

Fetal circulation is the process by which an unborn infant receives oxygen and nutrients and disposes of waste products. The infant receives oxygen and nutrients from the mother's blood through one large umbilical vein. The waste products are cleared through the two umbilical arteries in the placenta that pass through the umbilical cord to the fetus (**Figure 11.25**). This process is necessary because the lungs and digestive system of the fetus are underdeveloped and not yet functioning.

Most blood enters the fetus through the ductus venosus vein, bypassing the liver and going directly to the right atrium by way of the inferior vena cava. Blood bypasses the right ventricle and is shunted (diverted) to the left atrium because of an opening in the septal wall, between the atria, called the **foramen ovale**. A small amount of blood does go to the right ventricle, but it is drained through the **ductus arteriosus**, a vessel that connects the pulmonary artery to the aorta.

Once the blood is pumped from the left ventricle, the oxygenated blood flows through the infant's body. Deoxygenated blood returns to the placenta via the umbilical arteries. Shortly after birth, the ductus arteriosus and ductus venosus close, as does the foramen ovale.

 Check Your Understanding

1. What is the role of hepatic portal circulation?
2. What is unusual about hepatic circulation?
3. What type of blood vessel delivers blood to the liver?
4. What is the purpose of fetal circulation?

Taking Vital Signs

For those who are interested in—and proactive about—their health, pulse monitoring and blood pressure measurement are important skills to

Figure 11.25 Fetal circulation. Here you see the circulation of blood in a full-term fetus (before birth). *Describe how blood flows into and through the fetal heart during the development of the fetus. How does this process change after the baby is born?*

acquire. These skills are even more important for many of those who are interested in pursuing a healthcare career.

Have you ever taken your pulse? Pulse monitoring is essential if you want to ensure that you are exercising at an intensity level that will improve your cardiovascular fitness. Blood pressure measurement is a simple procedure that can provide lifesaving information about one's physical condition.

So, let's learn how to monitor your pulse and measure your blood pressure. Pulse and blood pressure measurements are commonly referred to as **vital signs**.

Taking Your Pulse

Pulse is a rhythmic, throbbing sensation that can be felt when the heart contracts and blood is forced through the arteries. To measure your pulse, use your index and third fingertips to apply light pressure to any point where an artery comes close to your skin. Count the number of beats for 15 seconds and multiply that number by 4. The most common anatomic locations for measuring your pulse are as follows:

- **Radial artery**: With your palm facing upward, feel for your pulse on the thumb side of your wrist (**Figure 11.26A**).
- **Carotid artery**: On the side of your neck, feel for your pulse to the right of your trachea, or windpipe (**Figure 11.26B**).

Memory Tip

What makes your body healthy?

Your body **MENDS** itself with the right lifestyle!

Make sure that your weight, blood pressure, cholesterol, and glucose are normal.

Exercise most days for 30 minutes at a moderate intensity level.

No smoking or use of tobacco products.

Diet should be rich in fruits and vegetables and low in saturated fat and sodium.

Stress less, laugh more. Recent research shows that laughter may lower disease risk!

- **Brachial artery**: At the fold of your elbow, feel for your pulse along the inner portion of your arm.

Measuring Blood Pressure

Blood pressure is measured at the brachial artery using a stethoscope (STETH-oh-skohp) and a sphygmomanometer (SFIG-moh-ma-NAHM-eh-ter), or *blood pressure cuff*. Inflating the cuff causes the brachial artery to collapse. As the cuff is deflated, the brachial artery gradually reopens, and you can hear the pulse, which creates a tapping sound. When the artery is completely open, the tapping sound disappears. Following are the steps for measuring blood pressure (**Figure 11.27** on the next page):

A.

B.

Figure 11.26 Measuring pulse. A—Radial artery. B—Carotid artery. *What are other sites on the body where pulse can be taken?*

Pump cuff to 150 mmHg

Lower cuff pressure

Cuff pressure continues to lower

Inflatable cuff

Brachial artery

Air valve

Squeezable bulb inflates cuff with air

Brachial artery closed; no "tapping" sound.

Blood is pushed into constricted artery when heart contracts. The 1st tapping sound heard is systolic blood pressure (120 mmHg).

Artery completely open; blood flows freely; no tapping sound is heard. This is diastolic blood pressure (80 mmHg).

Sounds are heard with stethoscope

Figure 11.27 Blood pressure measurement. *Explain the difference between systolic and diastolic blood pressure measurements.*

- Place the blood pressure cuff around the arm, with the arrow on the cuff pointed toward the brachial artery. Place two fingertips above the fold in the elbow.
- Make sure that your stethoscope is in the "on" position by gently tapping the diaphragm of the chest piece.
- Place the head of the stethoscope over the brachial artery.
- Squeeze the bulb of the sphygmanometer repeatedly while listening for a "tapping" sound.
- Continue to pump up the cuff 30 millimeters of mercury (mmHg) more after the "tapping" sound stops. This would be approximately 150 mmHg for someone with a normal blood pressure of 120/80 mmHg (**Figure 11.28**).
- Open the release valve so that the cuff deflates at a rate of about 2 mmHg/second.
- The first "tap" that you hear is the systolic blood pressure (120 mmHg). The last muffled sound that you hear is the diastolic blood pressure (80 mmHg).

Figure 11.28 Blood Pressure Classification		
Normal	**Pre-Hypertension**	**Hypertension**
<120/80 mmHg	120—130/ 80—89 mmHg	>140/90 mmHg

The systolic blood pressure is the pressure in the brachial artery when the left ventricle contracts. The diastolic blood pressure is the pressure in the brachial artery when the left ventricle is relaxed and filling with blood.

Know Your Numbers

In addition to knowing how to measure vital signs, you should know and monitor some other key numbers. These numbers will give you an indication of how healthy you are compared to the general population. Let's look at numbers for weight, blood pressure, cholesterol, and glucose.

Weight

An adult's body mass index (BMI) should range from 18.0 to 24.9, which represents a healthy weight. BMIs less than 18 are classified as thin. BMIs equal to or greater than 25 are considered overweight. BMIs greater than 30 are classified as obese.

To calculate your body mass index, divide your weight in kilograms by your height in meters squared.

$$\text{BMI} = \frac{\text{wt (kg)}}{\text{ht (m}^2)}$$

If you are an athlete or you have a lot of muscle mass, this BMI calculation method may incorrectly classify you as overweight or obese. This could happen because the formula does not take into account your body composition. The same incorrect result could occur if you used height and weight tables whether or not you were in the normal range for your age and size.

Body composition is a way of identifying your body's proportion of lean tissue to fat tissue. If you want to know your body composition, you can measure it using a weight scale that has bioelectric impedance technology. These special scales are available in many pharmacies and schools. Another way to measure body composition is to use a caliper to do a skinfold test.

Blood Pressure

Optimal blood pressure for an adult is 110/70 mmHg. Generally, lower blood pressure is not a problem, but it could cause you to become dizzy if you get up too quickly. Adults with blood pressure in excess of 140/90 mmHg should consult their physician. You will learn more about the risk factors for developing high blood pressure in the next lesson.

Cholesterol

As you learned in chapter 2, cholesterol is a steroid found in blood. Cholesterol is essential for cell function and for absorption of fat-soluble vitamins. It is also a precursor to the development of steroid hormones. Cholesterol is carried in the blood by lipids.

Memory Tip

To remember the differences between HDL (the good type of cholesterol) and LDL (the bad type), keep in mind the following hint: HDL is healthy, and LDL is lousy.

You can learn the cholesterol level in your blood by having your blood drawn and tested. The amount of cholesterol in the blood is represented by a number. Knowing your total cholesterol number is helpful.

It is more helpful, however, to know how much of your total cholesterol consists of high-density lipoprotein (HDL) and how much of it consists of low-density lipoprotein (LDL). HDL is the "good type" of cholesterol, and LDL is the "bad type."

LDL carries fat to the arterial walls and deposits it. Over time, these fatty deposits can cause buildup of plaque leading to blockages in the arteries. HDL removes fat from the arterial walls and brings it back to the liver, where it is broken down. Triglycerides are another form of fat that can increase your risk of cardiovascular disease.

The figures that follow represent desirable levels for each of these substances.

Cholesterol: less than 200 mg/dL
LDL: less than 100 mg/dL
HDL: more than 40 mg/dL
Triglycerides: less than 50 mg/dL

✓ Check Your Understanding

1. What two measurements are often referred to as *vital signs*?
2. A person's pulse is taken by placing the fingertips over the skin near which type of blood vessel?
3. What is the medical term for a blood pressure cuff?
4. What does systolic blood pressure measure?
5. What is the good type of cholesterol and what does it do?

Lesson 11.3 Review and Assessment

Mini Glossary
Make sure that you know the meaning of each key term.

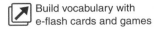 Build vocabulary with e-flash cards and games

aortic arch   the curved portion of the aorta between the ascending and descending parts of the aorta

arteries   vessels that carry blood away from the heart

arterioles   microscopic arteries that connect with capillaries

brachial artery   the artery located at the fold of the elbow where the brachial pulse is detected

capillaries   small, thin-walled vessels where oxygen and carbon dioxide gas exchange occurs

capillary beds   network of intertwined vessels formed by multiple capillaries

carotid artery   the artery located on the side of the neck, where the carotid pulse is felt

coronary sinus   large venous channel between the left atrium and left ventricle on the posterior side of the heart that empties into the right atrium at the junction of the four chambers

ductus arteriosus   a short, broad vessel in the fetus that connects

the left pulmonary artery with the descending aorta, allowing most of the blood to bypass the infant's lungs

foramen ovale   opening in the septal wall between the atria; normally present only in the fetus

precapillary sphincter   a band of smooth muscle fibers that encircles the capillaries at the arteriole-capillary junctions and controls blood flow to the tissues

pulmonary circulation   circulation of oxygen-poor blood from the right ventricle, through the lungs, and returning to the left atrium with oxygen-rich blood

radial artery   the artery located on the thumb side of the wrist, where the radial pulse is detected

systemic circulation   circulation of oxygenated blood through the arteries, capillaries, and veins of the circulatory system, from the left ventricle to the right atrium

tunica externa   the outermost layer of a blood vessel, composed mostly of fibrous connective tissue that supports and protects the vessel

tunica intima   the innermost layer of a blood vessel, composed of a single layer of squamous epithelial cells over a sheet of connective tissue; its smooth, frictionless surface allows blood to flow smoothly through the vessel

tunica media   the thicker middle layer of a blood vessel that contains smooth muscle cells, elastic fibers, and collagen; its muscle cells are directed by the sympathetic nervous system to increase or decrease blood flow to tissues as needed

veins   vessels that carry blood to the heart

venules   the smallest veins; connect the capillaries with the larger systemic veins

vital signs   measurements of pulse and blood pressure

Know and Understand

Assess

1. Which layer of the blood vessel is responsible for vasodilation and vasoconstriction?

2. Starting at the heart, list the vessels through which blood travels and returns to the heart during systemic circulation.

3. Which structures in the venous system prevent blood from flowing away from the heart? How is this accomplished?

4. How many pulmonary veins take blood back to the heart? Is the blood oxygenated or deoxygenated? Explain your answer.

Analyze and Apply

5. Explain why capillaries are called *exchange vessels*.

6. Calculate your BMI. Do you think it is accurate? What fact, which may skew the results, is not taken into account when calculating a person's BMI?

7. Suppose that you are at baseball practice and it is extremely hot and humid. What can you do to ensure that you perform at the top of your game?

8. The carotid pulse is stronger than the radial pulse. Why do you think that is the case?

In the Lab

9. **Taking Blood Pressure.** Following the steps described in this lesson, take your lab partner's blood pressure at rest. Next, ask your partner to run in place for one minute and repeat the same steps. Analyze the results. Did your partner's blood pressure change? If so, why?

Before You Read

Try to answer the following questions before you read this lesson.

Do heart murmurs typically cause serious health problems?

Why does your body create plaque?

What is the window of time, after cardiac symptoms begin, for preventing irreversible tissue damage?

Lesson Objectives

1. Identify several common types of heart diseases and disorders and their symptoms.
2. Explain the causes of and remedies for different heart conditions.
3. List and discuss strategies for preventing heart disease.
4. Describe the buildup of plaque in the arteries and the problems that can occur as a result.

Key Terms

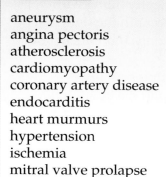
E-Flash Cards

aneurysm	myocardial infarction
angina pectoris	myocarditis
atherosclerosis	palpitations
cardiomyopathy	pericarditis
coronary artery disease	peripheral vascular
endocarditis	disease (PVD)
heart murmurs	stroke
hypertension	transient ischemic
ischemia	attack (TIA)
mitral valve prolapse	valvular stenosis

Cardiovascular diseases account for one in six deaths in the United States, or approximately 2,200 deaths per day, according to the American Heart Association. To put this statistic into perspective, someone will have a coronary event—a heart attack or chest pain, for example—approximately every 25 seconds. Also, every minute someone will die from a coronary event. Heart disease is not only epidemic but is also costly: the direct and indirect costs of heart disease in the United States are estimated at $300 billion annually.

Let's briefly look at some of the more common types of heart disease.

Valve Abnormalities

In lesson 11.1, you read about the valves that regulate the flow of blood through the heart. Improper functioning of these valves can cause a variety of problems. We will discuss three common abnormalities of the heart valves.

Heart murmurs—whooshing or swishing sounds heard upon *auscultation* (AWS-kul-TAY-shun)—the act of listening to internal sounds of the body using a stethoscope—that are caused by one of the heart valves not closing properly. Heart murmurs are common in young children and usually do not require any special treatment. They can also be caused by congenital heart defects, which are present at birth, and valvular disease as a result of aging, infection, rheumatic fever, or other disease.

Valvular stenosis—a narrowing of the heart valve due to stiff or fused valve cusps (**Figure 11.29** on the next page). Valvular stenosis can occur in one or more of the valves, making the heart work very hard to pump blood through the smaller-than-normal valve opening. People

A.

B.

Figure 11.29 Valve abnormalities. A—Normal aortic valve, closed. B—Aortic valve with stenosis. The white areas show calcification of the valve leaflets (flaps), which makes them stiff and unable to open properly. *What physical symptoms might be experienced by a person with stenosis of the aortic valve?*

with a mild case of stenosis may be symptom free. Those with a moderate form, however, may have to restrict their physical activity, and those with a severe case may need surgery to replace the valve.

Mitral valve prolapse—an incomplete closing of the mitral valve. Mitral valve prolapse is fairly common, occurring in up to 10% of the population. It is usually benign and does not require any restrictions. In a small number of cases, mitral regurgitation occurs. This is a disorder in which blood flows backward through the valve into the left atrium when the ventricle contracts. Symptoms may include shortness of breath, **palpitations** (sensation of rapid heartbeat), fatigue, and chest pain. In some instances the valve has to be repaired or replaced.

Diseases Ending in *-itis*

The suffix *-itis* means "inflammation". So if you have **pericarditis** (PER-i-kahr-DIGH-tis), you have an inflammation of the pericardial sac that surrounds your heart. This condition causes the heart to rub against the pericardial sac as the heart contracts, producing a stabbing pain in the chest. Shortness of breath, fatigue, and rapid pulse may also occur. Drugs are usually prescribed to fight the infection and to decrease inflammation and pain.

Myocarditis (MIGH-oh-kahr-DIGH-tis) is an inflammation of the myocardium, the middle layer of the heart. Myocarditis can cause symptoms similar to those of pericarditis.

Endocarditis (EHN-doh-kahr-DIGH-tis) is an inflammation of the innermost lining of the heart, including the inner surface of the chambers and the valves. It can destroy the heart valves and cause life-threatening complications if left untreated.

Heart Failure

Heart failure is a condition in which the heart cannot adequately pump blood to meet the oxygen needs of the body, or the heart muscle becomes stiff and has difficulty filling with blood. Heart failure can occur in the right or left ventricle. More commonly, it occurs in both ventricles.

When the heart's pumping ability diminishes, fluid backs up in the lungs, liver, arms, legs, and gastrointestinal tract. Other symptoms include shortness of breath, cough, edema (excessive fluid) in the ankles, weight gain, and frequent waking at night to urinate.

Several different drugs are used to treat heart failure with very good outcomes. These include diuretics to prevent water retention, vasodilators, and cardiostimulatory and cardioinhibitory drugs. Cardiostimulatory drugs enhance heart function by increasing heart rate; cardioinhibitory drugs reduce heart rate.

The most common cause of heart failure is coronary artery disease, but heart failure can also be caused by infection that weakens the heart muscle. This condition is called **cardiomyopathy** (KAHR-dee-oh-migh-AHP-a-thee). Heart failure usually happens gradually, but it can develop quickly after a heart attack has damaged the heart muscle.

Heart transplants are usually performed on individuals with end-stage heart failure and, in some rare cases, on children with congenital heart defects. Open-heart surgery is performed, and the patient's diseased heart is replaced with the donor's heart while the patient is hooked up to a heart-lung machine. The first-year survival rate among heart-transplant patients (81%) has greatly improved with the advent of immunosuppressant drugs. Five-year survival rates are 75%, and most individuals are able to return to their normal activities of daily living. However, they need to stay on a lifelong regimen of multiple medications to prevent rejection of the donated heart.

✓ Check Your Understanding

1. According to the American Heart Association, how many people in the United States die each day due to cardiovascular disease?
2. Name three common types of valve abnormalities.
3. What is the name of the condition in which the sac covering the heart is inflamed?
4. Of the three *-itis* diseases you read about, which is potentially the most dangerous?
5. What is the most common cause of heart failure?

Diseases of the Arteries

As you know, the arteries transport blood throughout the body. Here are some of the most common problems and diseases that can inhibit or prevent this vital function.

Weakened, bulging artery wall

Fatty deposit

Figure 11.30 Aneurysm. *Describe in your own words how this drawing would look if the aneurysm did not exist.*

Aneurysms

An **aneurysm** (AN-yoo-rizm) is an abnormal ballooning of a blood vessel—usually an artery—due to a weakness in the wall of the vessel (**Figure 11.30**). Although the causes of an aneurysm are unclear, hypertension, high cholesterol, and cigarette smoking increase the risk of developing an aneurysm.

Pain and swelling are common symptoms of an aneurysm, but some individuals have no symptoms. Common locations for aneurysms include the aorta, the brain, the artery behind the knee, and the intestine. Imaging techniques such as computed tomography (CT), ultrasound, and magnetic resonance angiography (MRA) are used to diagnose an aneurysm.

Aneurysms can rupture, causing sudden death or life-threatening side effects. This condition requires immediate surgical attention to repair the ruptured wall of the artery.

Coronary Artery Disease

Coronary artery disease (also called *coronary heart disease*) is caused by a narrowing of one or more of the coronary arteries from a buildup of plaque (obstruction). This buildup hardens over the course of many years, becoming the disease known as **atherosclerosis** (ATH-er-oh-skler-OH-sis), or *hardening of the arteries*.

The buildup of arterial plaque usually starts with an injury to the tunica intima, the innermost lining of the artery. The injury can be caused by high blood pressure, smoking, high blood glucose levels from insulin resistance or diabetes, or high levels of fats and cholesterol in the blood.

Once an injury to an artery occurs, the body tries to repair it by applying its version of a spackling compound, which consists of certain fats and cholesterol, calcium, and other substances in the blood. LDL cholesterol is one of the main culprits in the formation of plaque because it enters the intimal wall and starts to accumulate (**Figure 11.31**). White blood cells digest the LDL particles, become engorged with fat, and create a foamy substance, which is why they are called

foam cells. In addition, smooth muscle cells migrate from the tunica media of the vessel wall into the intimal lining where they ingest fats, multiply, and deposit collagen and elastin fibers.

The arterial plaque grows gradually, narrowing the channel through which the blood flows. When the vessel opening is decreased by 50% or more, the heart may not receive a sufficient amount of blood at certain times, such as during exercise or stressful situations. This insufficient blood supply may cause **angina** (AN-ji-na) **pectoris**, commonly referred to as *chest pain*. The drug nitroglycerine can be given to dilate (open) the coronary arteries, which helps to alleviate the pain.

Chest pain is the most common symptom arising from lack of oxygen and **ischemia** (is-KEE-mee-a), lack of blood flow to the heart. Other symptoms include throat dryness, jaw

Normal coronary artery

Atherosclerosis — Plaque buildup narrows the lumen of the artery

Atherosclerosis increasing — Plaque increasing

Artery occluded

Myocardial tissue dies due to ischemia (lack of blood flow)

Atherosclerosis with blood clot — Artery occluded. Myocardial infarction occurs

Figure 11.31 Progression of atherosclerosis and development of myocardial infarction. *How does LDL cholesterol cause the formation of plaque in blood vessels?*

pain, pain going down the left arm, nausea, increased perspiration, shortness of breath, and fainting. These are all "classic" symptoms because they are the symptoms that men typically experience. It was long thought, mistakenly, that heart disease was primarily a problem for men. By contrast, women often do not have any of the classic symptoms. Instead, they may feel unusually fatigued, have flu-like symptoms, or experience no pain at all.

 ### Check Your Understanding

1. Name three factors that can increase the risk of someone developing an aneurysm.
2. What is another name for *atherosclerosis*?
3. What materials contribute to the buildup of plaque?
4. What is the undesirable result of plaque buildup?

Heart Attack

If an artery becomes completely blocked, a **myocardial infarction**, or heart attack, occurs. This can happen suddenly when a piece of arterial plaque ruptures and occludes (closes) the artery. Many people who have had a heart attack remark that they "felt like an elephant was sitting

on [their] chest" or that "the pain was crushing." Morphine and/or other pain medications are administered to diminish the pain.

You may not think that people who have symptoms such as chest pain or shortness of breath before a heart attack are lucky, but in a way they are. These symptoms are early warnings, giving the person a chance at survival. Others are not so lucky: in approximately one-third of all heart attacks, the first symptom is death.

People with cardiac symptoms should take an aspirin and call 911 within five minutes of onset of the symptoms. Time is of the essence. The first two phases of a heart attack—ischemia and injury to the heart tissue—are reversible with proper intervention. But there is only a 20- to 60-minute window before death of cardiac tissue occurs, which is irreversible.

A goal of the American College of Cardiology (ACC) is to ensure that heart attack patients receive treatment within 90 minutes of their arrival at a hospital. Within 30 minutes of their arrival in the emergency room, patients should receive fibrinolytic (FIGH-brin-oh-LIT-ik) therapy, the use of special drugs to dissolve the clot. This therapy minimizes the threat of permanent damage to the heart. The ACC also recommends that heart attack patients receive *balloon angioplasty* to open the blocked vessel and that a *stent* (a circular, hollow, wire mesh tube) be inserted within 90 minutes of arrival in the ER (**Figure 11.32**).

A.

B.

C.

Pathompong Chaionnom/Shutterstock.com, Bryant Jayme/Shutterstock.com, Stephen Mahar/Shutterstock.com

Figure 11.32 Surviving a heart attack. A—Within 5 minutes of symptom onset, take aspirin and call 911. B—Within 30 minutes of symptom onset, get to a hospital; start fibrinolytic therapy, if appropriate. C—Within 90 minutes of arrival at the hospital, receive balloon angioplasty. *Why is time of the essence in providing treatment to someone who has just had a heart attack?*

Hypertension

Hypertension is another word for high blood pressure. It occurs when the force of blood against the arterial wall remains elevated for an extended period of time. In many cases, doctors are unable to determine what causes hypertension. Individuals with a blood pressure reading greater than 140/90 mmHg on three separate occasions are considered to have high blood pressure.

Many people don't know that they have high blood pressure because there are often no symptoms. This is why hypertension is called the *silent killer*. In fact, the Centers for Disease Control (CDC) estimates that one in five US adults has high blood pressure and doesn't know it. Approximately one-third of the people in the United States have high blood pressure, and the risk of developing it increases substantially with age. Risk factors for developing hypertension include a family history of hypertension, obesity, smoking, physical inactivity, and sensitivity to salt.

When energy intake exceeds the body's energy needs, the excess energy is stored for future use, in the form of triglycerides or glycogen. Because the body's glycogen storage capacity is limited, chronic energy excess leads to fat formation and obesity. In turn, obesity increases the risk of hypertension, stroke, and coronary artery disease.

Peripheral Vascular Disease (PVD)

Peripheral vascular disease (PVD) is a condition caused by a narrowing of the arteries in the legs. PVD usually results in a lack of blood flow to the thighs, calf muscles, and feet. Symptoms generally include pain, fatigue in the lower extremities, and a burning sensation in the calf muscle. Initially, these symptoms may be apparent only while walking, but they may also occur at rest as the condition worsens.

The disease strikes both men and women, but African-Americans are at greater risk. Smoking greatly increases a person's risk of developing PVD. Exercise lowers the risk and lessens the symptoms. Medications to dilate the arteries and prevent blood-clots help control the disorder. In severe cases, surgery or the placement of a stent to open the narrowed artery may be required.

Stroke

A **stroke**, or cerebral vascular accident, is a medical emergency that occurs when blood flow to the brain stops. There are two different types of strokes. An *ischemic stroke* occurs when one of the arteries of the brain becomes blocked. A *hemorrhagic stroke* occurs when one of the arteries ruptures, causing bleeding in the brain. Within minutes, the brain is deprived of oxygen, causing many complications and possibly death.

According to the CDC, stroke is the fourth leading cause of death in the United States and the leading cause of long-term, severe disability. The CDC estimates that the cost of care for stroke survivors in the United States is approximately $20 billion annually.

Paralysis, loss of speech, problems walking, uncontrolled emotional outbursts, depression, and coma are some of the potential side effects of stroke. These side effects may be temporary if a person experiences a **transient ischemic attack (TIA)**, a temporary lack of blood flow to the brain. In this case, symptoms usually will disappear within one to two hours. TIAs are a warning sign that stroke could occur in the future, so steps should be taken to correct the underlying condition and risk factors.

Memory Tip

Signs of a stroke are easy to remember if you use the F.A.S.T. tip developed by Methodist Health Systems.

F—Face   Is one side drooping?

A—Arms   Is one arm weak or numb?

S—Speech   Is speech slurred?

T—Time   Time is critical. Call 911 or get to the hospital quickly.

Risk factors for stroke include family history of stroke, high blood pressure, diabetes, high cholesterol, use of birth control pills, and race (specifically, African-American ancestry). Smoking, excessive alcohol consumption, illicit drug use, overweight or obese conditions, and physical inactivity also increase the risk of stroke.

Lesson 11.4 Review and Assessment

Mini Glossary   Make sure that you know the meaning of each key term.

 Build vocabulary with e-flash cards and games

aneurysm   abnormal ballooning of a blood vessel, usually an artery, due to a weakness in the wall of the vessel

angina pectoris   condition characterized by severe, constricting pain or sensation of pressure in the chest, often radiating to the left arm; caused by an insufficient supply of blood to the heart

atherosclerosis   hardening of the arteries

cardiomyopathy   heart failure caused by infection and weakening of the myocardium, or heart muscle

coronary artery disease   a narrowing of one or more of the coronary arteries due to a buildup of plaque; coronary heart disease

endocarditis   inflammation of the innermost lining of the heart, including the inner surface of the chambers and the valves

heart murmurs   extra or unusual sounds heard by a stethoscope during a heartbeat; may be harmless or indicative of a problem with one of the heart valves

hypertension   condition that occurs when the force of blood against the arterial wall remains elevated for an extended period of time; high blood pressure

ischemia   a lack of blood flow, usually due to the narrowing of a blood vessel

mitral valve prolapse   an incomplete closing of the mitral valve, causing blood to flow backward into the left atrium when the left ventricle contracts

myocardial infarction   tissue death that occurs in a segment of heart muscle from blockage of a coronary artery; heart attack

myocarditis   inflammation of the myocardium, the middle layer of the heart (also known as the heart muscle)

palpitations   sensation of rapid heartbeat

pericarditis   inflammation of the pericardial sac that surrounds the heart

peripheral vascular disease (PVD)   condition caused by a narrowing of the arteries in the legs

stroke   a sudden blockage of blood flow, or rupture of an artery in the brain, that causes brain cells to die from lack of oxygen

transient ischemic attack (TIA)   a temporary lack of blood flow to the brain

valvular stenosis   a narrowing of the heart valve due to stiff or fused valve cusps

Know and Understand

Assess

1. What percentage of deaths in the United States are caused by cardiovascular disease?

2. What surgical method can be used to remedy some valve abnormalities?

3. What fluid-related problem results from the heart's inability to pump sufficient blood to meet the body's oxygen needs?

4. What happens to an artery to cause a heart attack?

5. What is the five-year survival rate for heart transplant patients?

6. What is the maximum amount of time that should elapse before a heart attack patient arriving at the hospital receives a stent?

7. What disease is known as the "silent killer"?

Analyze and Apply

8. Explain why the body's attempt at repairing an injury to an artery can become a problem.

9. Compare and contrast a stroke and an aneurysm.

10. Explain how the cholesterol level in a person's blood makes the person susceptible to coronary artery disease.

In the Lab

11. Working with a partner, create a new-patient questionnaire for a medical center, focusing on questions to detect high blood pressure. Share and compare your questionnaire with the questionnaires created by other teams. Compile the best questions into one final questionnaire.

12. Working with a small group of students, pick one of the conditions discussed in this lesson that is of particular interest to you and the members of your group. Create a collage that represents the causes, symptoms, anatomy, physiology, and remedies for that condition. Share your collage with the class.

Career Corner
Anatomy and Physiology at Work

The cardiovascular system, which consists of the heart, blood, and blood vessels, influences every living cell in the body. Many people have found challenging and fulfilling careers in the promotion of cardiovascular health and the diagnosis and treatment of cardiovascular diseases. In this section we will explore three of these careers.

Clinical Exercise Physiologist

A clinical exercise physiologist performs many tasks, including exercise screening, clinical exercise testing, exercise prescription, and health education. The clinical physiologist does this for individuals with cardiovascular, pulmonary, metabolic, orthopedic, musculoskeletal, and hematologic diseases. These physiologists work in hospitals, physical therapy clinics, rehabilitation programs, corporate health programs, and colleges and universities.

Clinical exercise physiologists monitor heart rate and blood pressure responses to exercise, perform electrocardiogram monitoring, and supervise exercise participation for at-risk and diseased populations.

Clinical exercise physiology is a relatively new medical career that requires a master's degree in exercise science, exercise physiology, or kinesiology from an accredited institution. The Registered Clinical Exercise Physiology Certification from the American College of Sports Medicine is recommended. Job prospects are considered to be very good in the near future. This is largely due to the emphasis placed on exercise as a rehabilitative tool.

Exercise Specialist

An exercise specialist works with patients with cardiovascular, pulmonary, and metabolic diseases and disorders. These specialists also work with people who are concerned about maximizing their health (**Figure 11.33**).

The exercise specialist performs evaluations such as health screenings and graded exercise tests and assesses strength, flexibility, and

Tyler Olson/Shutterstock.com

Figure 11.33 Exercise specialist

body composition. These specialists educate people about exercise training and lifestyle modifications designed to promote health.

Exercise specialists must possess a bachelor's degree in exercise science, exercise physiology, or kinesiology from an accredited college or university. The Exercise Specialist Certification through the American College of Sports Medicine is recommended.

Cardiovascular Technologist and Technician

Professionals who perform—or assist in performing—diagnostic tests on patients with cardiovascular diseases are referred to as *cardiovascular technologists* and *technicians* (**Figure 11.34**). These tests may include electrocardiograms, cardiac catheterizations, pulmonary function tests, echocardiograms, and graded exercise testing.

Figure 11.34 Cardiovascular technologist/technician.

Most cardiovascular technologists have a two-year associate's degree from an accredited community college. Some institutions offer a four-year degree in cardiovascular technology. Cardiovascular technicians, also known as EKG technicians, may have a one-year certificate or receive on-the-job training. Certification can be obtained from the American Board of Cardiovascular Perfusion, American Society of Phlebotomy Technicians, or the American Certification Agency for Healthcare Professionals.

Planning for a Health-Related Career

Do some research on the career of a clinical exercise physiologist, an exercise specialist, or a cardiovascular technologist/technician.

Alternatively, select a profession from the list of **Related Career Options**. Using the Internet or resources at your local library, find answers to the following questions:

1. What are the main tasks and responsibilities of a person employed in the career that you chose to research?
2. What is the outlook for this career? Are workers in demand, or are jobs dwindling?

For complete information, consult the current edition of the *Occupational Outlook Handbook*, published by the US Department of Labor. This handbook is available online or at your local library.

3. What special skills or talents are required? For example, do you need to be good at biology and anatomy and physiology? Do you need to enjoy interacting with other people?
4. What personality traits do you think are necessary for success in the career you have chosen to research? For example, a career as an exercise specialist involves educating people about exercise training and lifestyle modifications designed to promote health. Do you enjoy teaching or coaching others?
5. Does the work involve a great deal of routine, or are the day-to-day responsibilities varied?
6. Does the career require long hours, or is it a standard, "9-to-5" job?
7. What is the salary range for this job?
8. What do you think you would like about this career? Is there anything about it that you might dislike?

Related Career Options

- Athletic Trainer
- Cardiovascular Nurse
- Diagnostic Medical Sonographer
- Electrocardiographic (ECG) Technician
- Fitness Trainer
- Kinesiotherapist
- Physical Therapist
- Radiologist
- Recreational Therapist
- Vascular Technologist

Chapter Summaries

Lesson 11.1 **Heart Anatomy and the Function of the Cardiovascular System**

 Build vocabulary with e-flash cards and games

Key Points
- The heart is located in the center of the thoracic cavity and is encased in the pericardium.
- The heart is made up of three layers: the epicardium, myocardium, and endocardium.
- The heart has four chambers: two atria and two ventricles.
- The "lub-dub" sounds of the heart are the closing of one-way valves between the atria and ventricles and the ventricles and blood vessels.
- Cardiac output is calculated by multiplying stroke volume and heart rate.

Key Terms
aorta
aortic valve
atrioventricular (AV) valves
cardiac output
diastole
endocardium
epicardium
inferior vena cava
interatrial septum
interventricular septum

mitral valve
myocardium
papillary muscle
semilunar valves
stroke volume
superior vena cava
systole
tricuspid valve
vasoconstriction
vasodilation

Lesson 11.2 **Regulation of the Heart**

Key Points
- The heart is regulated internally by the sinoatrial node (SA node), which sends an impulse through the atrioventricular node (AV node) to the bundle of His and down the left and right bundle branches to the Purkinje fibers.
- Externally, the heart is controlled by the nervous and endocrine systems.
- An electrocardiogram (ECG) records the electrical activity of the heart.
- There are many different types of arrhythmias, which can be detected with an ECG.

Key Terms
arrhythmia
atrial fibrillation
atrioventricular node (AV node)
baroreceptors
bradycardia
bundle of His
depolarize
heart block
left bundle branches
premature atrial contractions (PACs)

premature ventricular contractions (PVCs)
Purkinje fibers
repolarize
right bundle branches
sinoatrial node (SA node)
tachycardia
ventricular fibrillation
ventricular tachycardia

Lesson 11.3 **Blood Vessels and Circulation**

Key Points
- Arteries carry blood away from the heart and have thick, strong, elastic walls.
- Veins carry blood back toward the heart and have thin, less elastic walls and one-way valves.

Key Terms
aortic arch
arteries
arterioles
brachial artery
capillaries

capillary beds
carotid artery
coronary sinus
ductus arteriosus
foramen ovale

- Cardiopulmonary circulation is the process of transporting deoxygenated blood from the right side of the heart to the lungs and then transporting oxygenated blood back to the left side of the heart.
- Systemic circulation is the process of transporting oxygenated blood from the left side of the heart out to the rest of the body. Systemic circulation includes cardiac and hepatic portal circulation.
- Vital signs are assessed by taking both blood pressure and pulse.

precapillary sphincter
pulmonary circulation
radial artery
systemic circulation
tunica externa

tunica intima
tunica media
veins
venules
vital signs

Lesson 11.4 Heart Disease

Key Points

- Heart disease is associated with obesity and with behaviors such as smoking and eating a high-fat diet.
- Valve conditions are often not life threatening, but in some cases they require surgical repair or replacement.
- Inflammatory conditions in the heart can be treated with drugs that decrease inflammation.
- Heart failure can result from any variety of causes, such as inflammation, cardiomyopathy, or arterial disease.

Key Terms

aneurysm
angina pectoris
atherosclerosis
cardiomyopathy
coronary artery disease
endocarditis
heart murmurs
hypertension
ischemia
mitral valve prolapse

myocardial infarction
myocarditis
palpitations
pericarditis
peripheral vascular
    disease (PVD)
stroke
transient ischemic attack
    (TIA)
valvular stenosis

Chapter Assessments

Lesson 11.1

Heart Anatomy and the Function of the Cardiovascular System

Learning Key Terms and Concepts

1. The myocardium is the _____.
   A. sac surrounding the heart
   B. thick, muscular wall of the heart
   C. inner lining of the heart
   D. septum between the chambers of the heart

2. The bicuspid (mitral) valve is located between the _____.
   A. right and left ventricles
   B. left atrium and left ventricle
   C. left and right atria
   D. left ventricle and the aorta

3. The fluid-filled, double-walled sac that surrounds the heart is called the _____.
   A. pericardium   C. myocardium
   B. endocardium   D. epicardium

4. The heart is flanked on either side by the _____.
   A. diaphragm   C. hips
   B. lungs   D. sternum

5. The "lub" of the heart's "lub-dub" sound is caused by the closing of the _____ valves.

6. The wall that separates the atria from each other is called the _____.

7. Attached to the cusps of heart valves are thin, fibrous cords called _____, which are connected to _____ muscles.

Thinking Critically

8. What do you think would happen if the interventricular septum had a hole in it?

9. It is widely believed that arteries carry only oxygenated blood and veins carry only deoxygenated blood. Is this a correct statement? Explain and defend your answer.

Lesson 11.2

Regulation of the Heart

Learning Key Terms and Concepts

10. The "pacemaker" of the heart is the _____.
    A. mitral valve   C. sinoatrial node
    B. atrioventricular   D. bundle of His
       node

11. The SA node is _____.
    A. located at the top of the right atrium
    B. the pacemaker
    C. located near the bundle of His
    D. the origin of Purkinje fibers

12. Sympathetic nerve fibers stimulate the SA node, which _____.
    A. increases the heart rate
    B. decreases the heart rate
    C. causes the ventricles to contract
    D. makes the heart rate irregular

13. Which of the following is not considered a component of the heart conduction system?
    A. sinoatrial (SA) node
    B. epicardium
    C. Purkinje fibers
    D. atrioventricular (AV) node

14. The cardiac center of the brain is made up of the _____ and _____ branches of the nervous system.

15. The _____, which are sensitive to pressure, are located in the aortic arch and carotid arteries.

Thinking Critically

16. What would happen if a person's parasympathetic nervous system did not function?

17. How do the endocrine and limbic systems work together to help a person escape from a dangerous situation?

Lesson 11.3

Blood Vessels and Circulation

Learning Key Terms and Concepts

18. Which layer provides a smooth, frictionless surface for the flow of blood in a vessel?
    A. tunica media
    B. tunica intima
    C. tunica externa
    D. medulla oblongata

19. Which vessel has the thickest, strongest, and most elastic walls?
    A. artery
    B. capillary
    C. exchange vessel
    D. vein

20. Blood is carried to the lungs by the _____.
    A. pulmonary vein
    B. pulmonary artery
    C. aorta
    D. inferior vena cava

21. The arteries carry blood _____.
    A. away from the heart
    B. to the lungs
    C. to the lungs only
    D. to the heart

22. The smallest, most numerous vessels in the body are the _____.
    A. venules
    B. arterioles
    C. capillaries
    D. veins

23. Blood returning to the heart via the inferior vena cava and the superior vena cava collects in the _____.
    A. left ventricle
    B. right ventricle
    C. right atrium
    D. left atrium

24. Blood pressure measured when the left ventricle contracts is called _____ pressure.
    A. diastolic
    B. stroke
    C. systolic
    D. mean

25. The artery located on the side of your neck, where you can clearly feel your pulse, is called the _____.

Thinking Critically

26. Why is blood considered a connective tissue?

27. Drawing on the information you studied in the first three lessons, explain why low blood pressure is considered a potentially dangerous condition.

Lesson 11.4

Heart Disease

Learning Key Terms and Concepts

28. Inflammation of the middle layer of the heart is called _____.

29. The most common cause of heart failure is _____.

30. Infection that weakens the heart muscle is called _____.

31. Listening to heart sounds using a stethoscope is called _____.

32. One common location for an aneurysm is the _____.
    A. carotid artery
    B. aorta
    C. jugular vein
    D. brachial artery

33. Atherosclerosis is also known as hardening of the _____.
    A. veins
    B. blood vessels
    C. arteries
    D. athero

34. What is the term for a narrowing of the heart valve due to stiff or fused valve cusps?
    A. valve prolapse
    B. valvular stenosis
    C. palpitations
    D. heart murmurs

Thinking Critically

35. How is the function of the heart affected by a myocardial infarction?

36. Compare and contrast a TIA and a hemorrhagic stroke.

37. How would having too much LDL cholesterol in your blood vessels increase your risk of having a myocardial infarction?

Building Skills and Connecting Concepts

Analyzing and Evaluating Data

This bar graph shows the number of deaths from heart disease for selected years. Use the graph to answer the following questions.

38. How many people died from heart disease in 1980?

39. Between which years do we see the greatest reduction in the number of heart disease-related fatalities?

40. Between which 10-year periods do we see the smallest reduction in the number of heart disease-related fatalities? How might this be interpreted in a positive way?

41. What is the difference in the number of heart disease-related fatalities between 1950 and 2008?

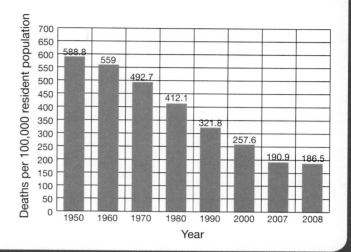

Communicating about Anatomy and Physiology

42. **Writing**. Create a children's story describing the adventures of a red blood cell as it travels through the human cardiovascular (circulatory) system. Include as many of the following terms as possible in your story: *aorta, atria, ventricles, tricuspid valve, bicuspid valve, semilunar valves, pulmonary circulation, systemic circulation, hepatic portal circulation, arteries, veins, venules, arterioles, capillaries, superior vena cava,* and *inferior vena cava*. Include other terms as desired. Devise a creative way to tell your story. For example, you may want to include color illustrations or make a pop-up book. Include brief descriptions of the roles of one or two body systems in addition to the cardiovascular system. Share your story with the class.

Lab Investigations

43. The graph above shows the number of deaths from heart disease between 1950 and 2008. With a small group of classmates, discuss the data in the graph. Then create a list of possible explanations for the dramatic decrease in the number of heart disease-related fatalities. Expand your list into a poster for your classroom.

44. Draw a human form on a large sheet of paper. Then draw and label the following structures of the cardiovascular system. Make the veins blue and the arteries red. Add arrows to show the direction of blood flow. Use your textbook as a guide and do Internet research if necessary.

structures of/circulation through the heart: *right atrium, left atrium, right ventricle, left ventricle, inferior vena cava, superior vena cava, aorta, tricuspid valve, bicuspid valve, pulmonary veins, pulmonary artery, aortic valve, pulmonary circulation, pulmonary valve, myocardium, endocardium, pericardium, apex, interventricular septum*

structures/circulation throughout the body: *brachial artery, femoral artery, radial artery, popliteal artery, dorsalis pedis artery, temporal artery, carotid artery, renal artery, hepatic vein, renal vein, jugular vein, portal vein, cerebral circulation, coronary circulation*

In your drawing, write the name of each of the following conditions on the part of the cardiovascular system in which the condition originates or occurs: *aneurysm, atherosclerosis, hypertension, pericarditis, ischemic stroke, hemorrhagic stroke, myocardial infarction*.

Expand your learning with additional online resources
- Supplemental Lab Activities
- Interactive Exercises
- Animations

Expand

www.g-wlearning.com/healthsciences

How does the lymphatic system work with the immune system to help keep your body healthy?

Dmitry Naumov/Shutterstock.com

The Lymphatic and Immune Systems

12

*T*he world can be a dangerous place—full of bacteria, viruses, fungi, and toxins. Because the human body is an attractive host for these and other infectious agents, your body must defend itself against constant assault by disease-producing microbes. You are usually unaware of this battle, which takes place on a microscopic level. Like a medieval town protected by walls, pots of burning oil, and soldiers, your body is protected by physical and chemical barriers and a cellular defense system.

In this chapter we will explore the lymphatic system and the body's defense systems against infection and disease. First, we will discuss the anatomy and basic physiology of the lymphatic system and related lymphatic tissues. Next, we will discuss the nonspecific defense system, whose mechanisms work without regard for the specific identity of an infectious agent. Finally, we will examine the body's specific defense system, which generates cells and antibodies that are custom-made for targeting an invading organism.

Chapter 12 Lessons

Lesson 12.1
The Lymphatic System

Lesson 12.2
Nonspecific Defenses

Lesson 12.3
Specific Defenses

Lesson 12.4
Disorders and Diseases of the Immune System

While studying, look for the online icon to:

- **Practice** with e-flash cards and vocabulary games
- **Review** with interactive art labeling
- **Assess** with online exercises
- **Expand** with interactive activities and animated videos
- **Listen** to pronunciations of key terms in the audio glossary

www.g-wlearning.com/healthsciences

Companion Website

Study on the Go

Use a mobile device to practice vocabulary terms, listen to pronunciations, and review with self-assessment quizzes.

www.m.g-wlearning.com

G-W Mobile

The Lymphatic System

The lymphatic system performs two vital functions in the human body: it solves a "plumbing" problem, and it constantly remains on the lookout for foreign invaders that can cause infection and disease.

The plumbing problem is caused by capillaries that naturally leak. As blood travels through the blood capillaries, a small amount of blood plasma leaks out of the capillaries and into the surrounding tissue. The normal leakage rate, across the entire body, is 2 to 3 mL per minute, a tiny amount compared to the 5,000 mL of blood that pass through capillaries each minute. But even this tiny amount would, in less than one day, cause a potentially fatal drop in blood pressure if the excess fluid were not returned to the cardiovascular system.

The lymphatic system also manages the challenge of quickly recognizing and mounting a counterattack against infectious agents. As the lymphatic system reabsorbs fluid from the leaking capillaries, it removes bacteria and virus-infected cells from body tissues. It also "sounds the alarm" that activates specific immune defenses. As we will see, the lymphatic system plays a vital role in the body's immune system, which provides protection against disease.

Organization of the Lymphatic System

The lymphatic system includes lymphatic vessels, lymphatic fluid (called *lymph*), and lymphatic organs such as lymph nodes and the spleen (**Figure 12.1**). The cells that fight infection develop within, and travel through, the organs and vessels of the lymphatic system.

The lymphatic system resembles the cardiovascular system in that both

Figure 12.1 The lymphatic system includes lymph, lymphatic vessels, lymphatic cells and tissues, and lymphatic organs. *Is a lymph node an organ?*

extend throughout almost all parts of the body. Both systems also have a network of vessels that vary in size from microscopic capillaries to large vessels. Unlike the circulatory system, however, the lymphatic system is not a closed loop.

Lymph Formation and Flow

Lymph formation begins with fluid that leaks out of *blood vessel capillaries*, the tiniest blood vessels in the body that connect the smallest arteries to the smallest veins

Memory Tip

The word *lymph* comes from the Latin word *lympha*, which means "water." Most of the time, lymph is a clear fluid that resembles water. However, its composition, produced by a combination of chemical substances, differs throughout the body. When lymph drains from the small intestine, for example, it takes on a milky appearance from the lipids (fats) that it collects as it travels through the small intestine.

(**Figure 12.2**). When this fluid is inside the blood vessels, it is called *blood plasma*. When it leaks out and enters the spaces between cells, it is called **interstitial** (IN-ter-STISH-al) **fluid**.

The slow but steady trickle of fluid out of the blood vessel capillaries amounts to about four liters per day. Because the average adult has only about three liters of blood plasma, all of a person's blood plasma would be lost in less than a day, if there were not a way for the fluid to return to the circulatory system.

As the fluid builds up in the interstitial space, some of it enters the *lymphatic capillaries* through small gaps between the **endothelial** (EHN-doh-THEE-lee-al) **cells**, which form the walls of the lymphatic capillaries (**Figure 12.2**). These endothelial cells overlap and are tethered to one another in a way that makes it easy for

fluid to enter the lymphatic capillaries but hard for it to leave. Once the fluid is in the lymphatic capillaries or the larger **lymphatic vessels**, it is called *lymph*. The lymphatic capillaries join together to form *collecting vessels*, which in turn link together to form even larger vessels called **lymphatic trunks**. The lymphatic trunks drain lymph from different parts of the body.

The human body does not have a pump similar to the heart to help propel lymph through this network of vessels. However, muscular contractions and movement of organs compress the lymphatic vessels, advancing the lymph along its route. This process is aided by **lymphatic valves**, tissue flaps that act as one-way valves inside the lymphatic vessels (**Figure 12.2**). When a lymphatic vessel is compressed by surrounding tissue, the valves

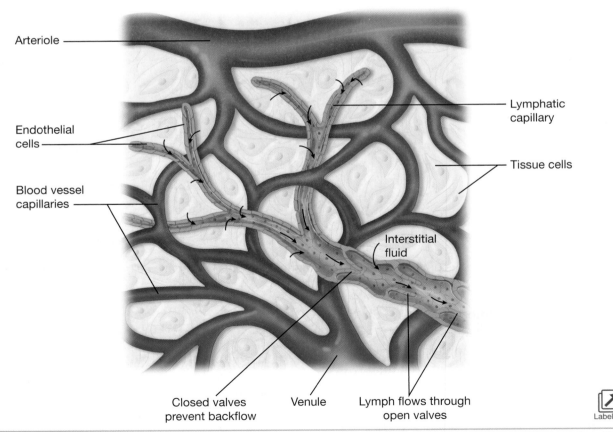

Figure 12.2 Lymph formation and flow. Blood plasma leaks out of blood capillaries and mixes with the interstitial fluid. It then enters lymphatic capillaries. The overlapping endothelial cells of the lymphatic capillaries make it easy for fluid to enter the capillaries but hard to leave. Lymph flows from lymphatic capillaries to progressively larger lymphatic vessels. Lymphatic vessels have internal flaps that act as one-way valves, which prevent lymph from flowing backward to the capillaries.

allow the lymph to go only in one direction—away from the lymphatic capillaries.

Lymph Drainage

The lymphatic trunks are named for their location and the part of the body they drain. These include the *left* and *right jugular trunks*, the *left* and *right subclavian* (sub-KLAY-vee-an) *trunks*, the *left* and *right bronchomediastinal* (BRAHN-koh-MEE-dee-as-tin-al) *trunks*, the *intestinal trunk*, and the *left* and *right lumbar trunks*. The two lumbar trunks and the intestinal trunk converge at the *cisterna chyli* (sis-TER-na KIGH-ligh), an enlarged chamber located just in front of the vertebral column, at the diaphragm level (**Figure 12.3A** on the next page).

The thoracic duct carries lymph superiorly, or upward, from the cisterna chyli. At its superior end, the thoracic duct receives the left jugular, subclavian, and bronchomediastinal

Memory Tip

The term *interstitial* comes from the Latin root word *-stit-* ("standing") and the prefix *inter-* ("between" or "among"). Thus, interstitial fluid occupies the spaces between cells, or the *interstitial space*. Interstitial fluid is also sometimes called *extracellular fluid*, which simply means "fluid outside of cells."

The bronchomediastinal trunks are so named because they receive lymph from the lungs and from the mediastinum, the collection of thoracic organs and tissues between the lungs, including the heart, trachea, esophagus, and thymus. The root word *bronch/o-* means "airway" (into the lungs). The word *mediastinum* comes from the Latin word meaning "middle." The organs and tissues that make up the mediastinum lie in the middle of the chest cavity, between the lungs.

The subclavian trunks, veins, and arteries all lie beneath the clavicle, or collarbone. The word *subclavian* comes from the Latin prefix *sub-* ("under") and the Latin word *clavicula* ("little key"). Ancient Roman physicians thought the clavicle resembled a small door key.

trunks. These trunks drain lymph from the head, left arm, and left side of the chest and lower neck, respectively (**Figure 12.3B**). Ultimately, the thoracic duct drains into the left subclavian vein.

The right lymphatic duct receives contributions from the right jugular, subclavian, and bronchomediastinal trunks. These trunks drain lymph from the right arm and the right side of the thorax and head (**Figure 12.3B**). The right lymphatic duct drains into the right subclavian vein. Lymph rejoins the blood via the lymphatic duct and the thoracic duct, and it once again becomes blood plasma.

Check Your Understanding

1. What two vital functions does the lymphatic system perform in the body?
2. What other body system does the lymphatic system most resemble? Why?
3. How does lymph formation begin?
4. How is lymph moved throughout the lymphatic vessels?
5. How did the different lymphatic trunks get their names?

Lymphatic Cells, Tissues, and Organs

The lymphatic system is made up of a complex network of cells, tissues, and organs that play a vital role in the body's nonstop battle against invasion by disease-causing agents. In this section, we will discuss the structure and function of the lymphatic cells, tissues, and organs.

Lymphatic Cells

Lymphocytes (lymphatic cells) are the distinctive cells of the lymphatic system. Lymphocytes make up about 20% to 30% of the white blood cells in whole blood and are abundant in lymphatic tissues, such as lymph nodes and the spleen.

All lymphocytes, along with other white and red blood cells, begin their lives in bone marrow. Some lymphocytes migrate to the thymus, an

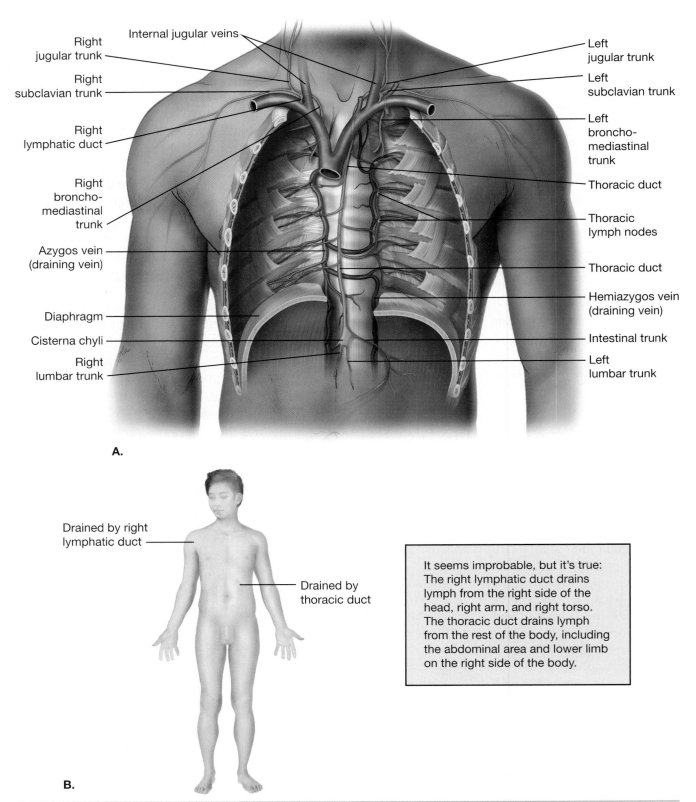

A.

B.

Figure 12.3 Lymphatic ducts and vessels. The right lymphatic duct collects lymph from the right jugular, subclavian, and bronchomediastinal trunks and drains into the right subclavian vein. The thoracic duct collects lymph from the left jugular, subclavian, and bronchomediastinal trunks and drains into the left subclavian vein. *How are lymphatic ducts named?*

organ in the thorax, where they complete their maturation before they move out to the blood and the rest of the body. These lymphocytes are called **T lymphocytes**, or simply *T cells*. (The *T* stands for *thymus*.) The lymphocytes that remain in the bone marrow become **B lymphocytes**, or *B cells*, as well as **natural killer (NK) cells**.

Natural killer cells play an important role in the nonspecific defense system of the body. They recognize and destroy virus-infected cells and cancer cells. By contrast, B and T cells are the main "soldiers" in the specific defense system. For example, B cells provide antibody-mediated immunity. This means that when they are activated, B cells produce antibodies, proteins involved in immune function. Antibodies circulate as free proteins in the bloodstream.

T cells include the cytotoxic T cells, which provide cell-mediated immunity. They also include helper and suppressor T cells, which regulate the activity of B cells and T cells.

Although they are not lymphocytes, **macrophages** (MAK-roh-fay-jehz) are important cells in lymphatic tissues. They start out as white blood cells called *monocytes*. When a monocyte migrates out of lymphatic circulation into the surrounding tissue, it develops into a macrophage. Macrophages phagocytize (surround and destroy) foreign cells and substances, and they help to activate T lymphocytes.

Memory Tip

It is helpful to remember that B cells mature in <u>b</u>one marrow—although their name comes from the fact that they were first discovered in the bursa (a fluid-filled sac involved in joint or muscle movement) of a chicken. Some people like to remember that B cells make anti<u>b</u>odies.

Lymphatic Tissues

Lymphatic tissue is loose connective tissue that contains many lymphocytes. Lymphatic tissue is present in mucous membranes and certain organs throughout the body. Mucous membranes, which line passageways open to the outside world (including the respiratory, gastrointestinal, urinary, and reproductive tracts), are potential routes of entry for infectious agents. Inside these passageways, **mucosa-associated lymphatic tissue (MALT)** keeps lymphocytes ready and waiting to stop the invaders (**Figure 12.1**).

The tonsils—small, almond-shaped masses of lymphatic tissue—form a ring of MALT around the pharynx (throat). A single **pharyngeal** (fa-RIN-jee-al) **tonsil** (sometimes called the *adenoid*) lies at the back of the nasopharynx (NAY-zoh-FAIR-inks), the part of the throat above the palate, and opens into the nasal cavity. The left and right **palatine tonsils** lie at the back of the mouth. The palatine tonsils are the largest and the most commonly infected. The **lingual** (LING-gwal) **tonsils** are located on either side of the base of the tongue.

In some parts of the body, lymphocytes and macrophages form small, localized clusters of dense tissue called **lymphatic nodules**. These nodules develop in areas often exposed to foreign microorganisms and help protect those areas against invasion.

Clusters of MALT in the small intestine are called *Peyer's patches*. MALT also protects the *appendix*, a small, worm-shaped tube at the junction of the large and small intestines.

Lymphatic Organs

Let's take a close look at three organs of the lymphatic system. They are the lymph nodes, spleen, and thymus.

Lymph Nodes. Small, bean-shaped organs called **lymph nodes** are located along the lymphatic vessels throughout the body (**Figure 12.4** on the next page). Lymph nodes serve a dual purpose. They cleanse the lymph by trapping bacteria, viruses, and other harmful substances, which in turn are destroyed by white blood cells. Lymph nodes also store and produce T cells and B cells that help fight infection.

Lymph nodes vary in size from smaller than a pea to the size of a lima bean (1 to 25 mm, or .04 to .98 in., in diameter). They have a fibrous

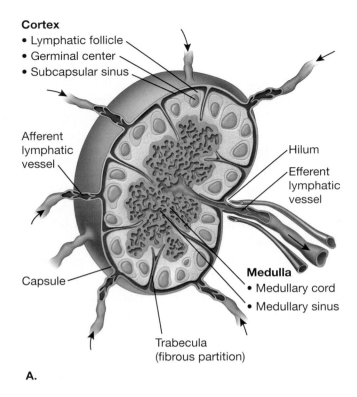

Cortex
- Lymphatic follicle
- Germinal center
- Subcapsular sinus

Afferent lymphatic vessel

Hilum

Efferent lymphatic vessel

Capsule

Medulla
- Medullary cord
- Medullary sinus

Trabecula (fibrous partition)

A.

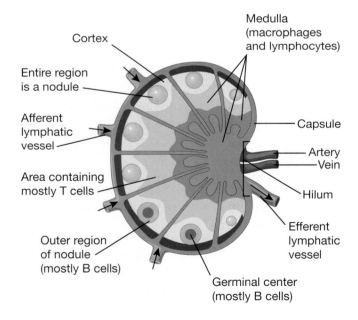

Cortex

Medulla (macrophages and lymphocytes)

Entire region is a nodule

Afferent lymphatic vessel

Capsule

Artery
Vein

Area containing mostly T cells

Hilum

Outer region of nodule (mostly B cells)

Efferent lymphatic vessel

Germinal center (mostly B cells)

B.

Figure 12.4 Lymph nodes. A—Cross section through a lymph node and associated lymphatic vessels. B—Simplified diagram distinguishing the cortex and medulla of a lymph node. *What important activities occur inside a lymph node? Do the lymph nodes in your neck become larger or smaller when you have a throat infection? Why?*

capsule and a spongy interior, packed with lymphocytes and macrophages.

Afferent lymphatic vessels carry lymph *into* the lymph nodes. The lymph moves slowly from the *cortex*, or outer portion of the lymph node, to the deeper *medulla*.

One or two *efferent lymphatic vessels* emerge from the *hilum* (HIGH-lum), a small indentation on one side of the node, and carry lymph to the next node. Efferent lymphatic vessels carry lymph *away from* the lymph nodes.

Most lymph passes through several lymph nodes on its way from a lymphatic capillary to the subclavian vein. Because lymph flows slowly, foreign particles such as bacteria or viruses are quickly detected. When a foreign particle is detected, it may be "eaten" by a macrophage, or it may activate an immune response.

When an immune response is activated, the lymphocytes quickly multiply, causing the lymph nodes to enlarge. When you have a throat infection, for example, the lymph nodes in your neck may become swollen. If you go to a doctor, she or he will examine your neck for "swollen glands"—a common description for enlarged lymph nodes.

Spleen. The **spleen**, located in the abdomen below the diaphragm, is the largest lymphatic organ in the human body (**Figure 12.5**). It measures 10 to 12 cm (4 to 5 in.) long and weighs 150 to 200 g (5 to 7 oz). Yet its size can vary considerably, even among healthy people. The spleen is located between the stomach and the body wall in the upper left quadrant of the abdomen.

One could say that lymph nodes filter lymph, and the spleen filters blood. There is some truth to this simple statement, although "scan, clean, and, if necessary, activate the immune response" more accurately describes the cleansing process than does the term "filter."

Like a lymph node, the spleen has a thin capsule and a spongy interior. It is dark red due to its large blood supply, which enters and leaves via the splenic artery and vein. The functional tissue inside the spleen contains red pulp and white pulp. The white pulp is rich in lymphocytes, which monitor blood flowing

Figure 12.5 A—Diagram of the spleen, anterior view. B—Simplified diagram of the histology (tissue structure) of the spleen. *Explain why you would* not *want to have your spleen removed even if you knew you could live a normal life without it.*

through the spleen for infectious cells and viruses. When the spleen detects an infectious agent, an immune response is activated, and lymphocytes begin to multiply.

Within the red pulp of the spleen, macrophages destroy old and worn-out red blood cells. The macrophages also remove old blood platelets and **pathogens**, or disease-causing agents, from the blood. Like lymph nodes, the spleen often becomes enlarged during an infection.

Because the spleen has a thin capsule and a soft interior, it may tear during a traumatic blow to the abdomen. This can happen during contact sports or a motor vehicle accident, for example. It may surprise you to learn that when the spleen has been surgically removed, a person can still lead a normal life, but with increased susceptibility to infection.

Thymus. The thymus (THIGH-mus) is a lymphatic organ that extends from the base of the neck downward into the thorax. It lies in front of the heart, trachea, and esophagus (**Figure 12.1**). The thymus is also an endocrine gland. (See chapter 8.) When compared to body size, the thymus is largest during childhood. It slowly but steadily shrinks after puberty.

All lymphocytes first develop in bone marrow from lymphatic stem cells. Some lymphocytes then migrate to the thymus, where they complete their maturation into T cells. Unlike lymph nodes, MALT, and the spleen, the thymus is *not* a site where lymphocytes lie in wait to ambush infectious agents. Rather, the thymus functions as a nursery for T cells.

 Check Your Understanding

1. Which two cells are the "soldiers" of the body's specific defense system?
2. Where are lymphatic tissues found in the body?
3. What two purposes do lymph nodes serve?
4. What is the largest lymphatic organ in the human body?
5. Where in the body do all lymphocytes first develop?

Lesson 12.1 Review and Assessment

Mini Glossary
Make sure that you know the meaning of each key term.

 Build vocabulary with e-flash cards and games

B lymphocytes lymphocytes that mature in the bone marrow before moving out to the blood and the rest of the body; also called *B cells*

endothelial cells cells that form the walls of lymphatic capillaries; their overlapping structure helps fluid enter the lymphatic capillaries and makes it hard for the fluid to leave

interstitial fluid fluid in the spaces between cells

lingual tonsils two masses of lymphatic tissue that lie on either side of the base of the tongue

lymph clear, transparent, sometimes faintly yellow fluid that is collected from tissues throughout the body and flows in the lymphatic vessels

lymph nodes small, bean-shaped structures found along the lymphatic vessels throughout the body

lymphatic nodules small, localized clusters of dense tissue formed by lymphocytes and macrophages

lymphatic trunks large lymphatic vessels that drain lymph from different parts of the body

lymphatic valves tissue flaps that act as one-way valves inside the lymphatic vessels

lymphatic vessels vessels that carry lymph

lymphocytes white blood cells that are abundant in lymphatic tissue

macrophages cells that phagocytize (surround and destroy) foreign cells, such as bacteria and viruses

mucosa-associated lymphatic tissue (MALT) lymphatic tissue found in mucous membranes that line passageways open to the outside world; these include the respiratory, gastrointestinal, urinary, and reproductive tracts

natural killer (NK) cells lymphocytes that play an important role in the nonspecific defense system of the body by killing virus-infected cells and cancer cells

palatine tonsils two masses of lymphatic tissue that lie in the back of the mouth, on the left and right sides; the largest and most commonly infected tonsils

pathogens disease-causing agents

pharyngeal tonsil lymphatic tissue that lies at the back of the nasopharynx, the part of the throat above the palate, and opens into the nasal cavity; commonly called the *adenoid*

spleen the largest lymphatic organ in the body, located in the abdomen below the diaphragm; filters blood and activates an immune response if necessary

T lymphocytes lymphocytes that complete their maturation in the thymus before they move out to the blood and the rest of the body; also called *T cells*

Know and Understand

 Assess

1. List the differences between lymphatic fluid, blood plasma, and interstitial fluid.

2. Explain what role the lymphatic system plays in maintaining blood pressure.

3. Identify the type of cells that form the walls of the lymphatic capillaries.

4. Identify the point at which blood plasma becomes lymphatic fluid.

5. List the lymphatic trunks and identify the parts of the body in which they are located.

6. Distinguish between T lymphocytes and B lymphocytes.

Analyze and Apply

7. In a sense, the lymphatic system is a plumber and a soldier. Which role do you think is more important? Build a case to support your choice.

8. Explain why lymphatic fluid, which usually has a clear color, takes on a milky appearance when it has drained from the small intestine.

9. Summarize the process by which lymphatic fluid moves through the lymphatic system.

In the Lab

10. As you know, the lymphatic system is similar to the cardiovascular system. Create simple models of both systems that clearly show one or two of the major differences between the systems.

11. Create your own figure of the human body. Label the lymphatic trunks and identify the organs associated with each trunk:
    A. Left and right jugular trunks
    B. Left and right subclavian trunks
    C. Left and right bronchomediastinal trunks
    D. Intestinal trunk
    E. Left and right lumbar trunks

Before You Read

Try to answer the following questions before you read this lesson.

What are phagocytes, and what role do they play in the defense systems of the body?

Why does inflammation occur in the body? What important purpose does it serve?

Lesson Objectives

1. Describe the role of the skin in protecting the body against infectious agents.
2. Define the complement system and explain the main difference between the classical pathway and the alternative pathway of this system.
3. Describe the inflammatory response and explain its purpose.
4. Explain what happens during a fever.

Key Terms

E-Flash Cards

alternative pathway
classical pathway
complement proteins
complement system
exocytosis
fever
inflammatory response
interferons

mast cells
monocytes
neutrophils
opsonins
phagocytes
phagocytosis
prostaglandins
pyrogens

We have seen how the lymphatic system works to keep fluids in balance and to activate immune responses against foreign substances. We will now examine the body's arsenal of defense against diseases that do *not* involve recognition of the precise identity of pathogens. These defensive "weapons" of the body include physical barriers, cellular and chemical defenses, inflammation, and fever.

Physical Barriers

The defense against infectious agents begins with physical barriers to their entry. The skin is quite effective as a barrier, as long as it is intact (**Figure 12.6** on the next page). Its outer layer, the epidermis, is a stratified squamous epithelium. That is, the epithelial, or surface, cells of the skin are flattened (squamous) and arranged in layers (stratified). The protein keratin, a major constituent of hair and nails, fills the flattened keratinocytes (keratinized cells) in the top layer of the epidermis. This keratin layer is flexible, strong, and hard to penetrate, due in part to the desmosomes (DEHZ-moh-sohms) that bind the deeper epithelial cells together.

Hair on the skin provides additional protection from chafing, sunburn, and insects. The acidic secretions of sweat glands and sebaceous glands (which produce sebum, a fatty lubricating substance) contain toxic chemicals that thwart bacterial growth. When the integrity of your skin is breached—by cuts or punctures, for example—you are at a much greater risk for infection. Burns also compromise—and can destroy—the protective function of the skin. For this reason, patients with serious burns are at a high risk for infection.

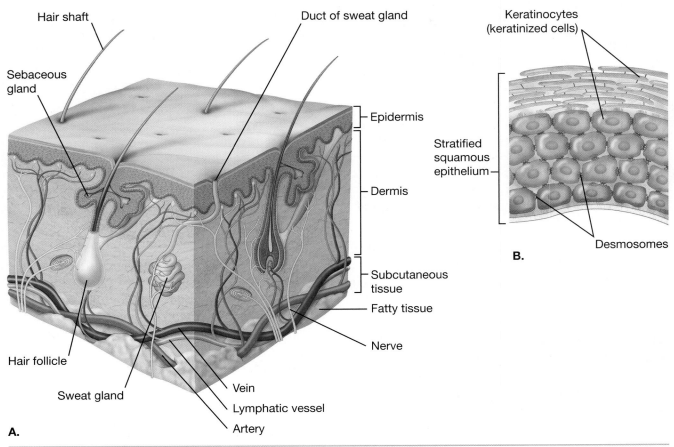

Figure 12.6 A—The skin and its structures help protect the body by serving as physical barriers against infectious agents. B—A layer of flattened cells filled with keratin, and deeper cells connected by desmosomes, make the skin strong and tough. Hair and the secretions of sweat glands and sebaceous glands provide additional protection. *When is the skin not an effective barrier to infectious agents?*

As stated in the previous lesson, protective mucous membranes line the respiratory, digestive, urinary, and reproductive tracts. Such protective linings are important because these tracts are open to the outside world and, therefore, vulnerable to invasion. The mucus they secrete forms a sticky layer that can trap microorganisms. Underlying mucosa-associated lymphatic tissue increases the chances that the microorganisms will be quickly recognized and destroyed.

The cells in the mucous membranes of the respiratory tract contain cilia, tiny hair-like structures that continually sweep the mucus upward to the throat, where it is swallowed. Bacteria caught in the respiratory mucus are then likely to be destroyed in the acidic environment of the stomach.

Cellular and Chemical Defenses

When pathogens penetrate the physical barriers, they face an array of cellular and chemical defenses. Within these defense systems, cells such as **phagocytes** (FAG-oh-sights) and NK cells work hard to protect the body against foreign invaders. In addition, interferons and antimicrobial proteins in the form of complement proteins act as chemical defenders against pathogens.

Each of these defense systems prevents or fights infection in its own way. These systems also interact to produce an inflammatory response. The inflammatory response is important because it speeds up tissue repair and boosts the body's ability to fight infection.

Phagocytosis

The process by which cells engulf and destroy foreign matter and cellular debris is called **phagocytosis** (**Figure 12.7**). Phagocytosis begins when a phagocyte recognizes its target and binds to it.

For example, **neutrophils** (NOO-troh-fils), the most common type of leukocytes (LOO-koh-sights), or white blood cells, can slip out of capillaries and into surrounding tissue. There they phagocytize (FA-goh-sigh-tighz) bacteria and cellular debris. Some **monocytes**, another class of leukocytes, develop into macrophages when they leave the bloodstream and enter tissues to phagocytize pathogens.

How does phagocytosis work? The phagocyte wraps its cytoplasm (the membrane surrounding the cell nucleus) around the target and encloses it in a membrane-bound compartment. This compartment protects the cell from damaging itself with the chemicals that it uses to destroy the engulfed material.

A lysosome (LIGH-soh-sohm), which contains acid and lysosomal enzymes, fuses with the material engulfed by the phagocyte. The lysosomal enzymes and acid usually destroy the target, and the debris is released from the cell through **exocytosis** (EHK-soh-sigh-TOH-sis). Exocytosis is a process in which the cell membranes fuse together and then push the debris from the cell vesicles to the outside of the cell.

Natural Killer Cells

Natural killer (NK) cells are lymphocytes that recognize and destroy abnormal body cells. Virus-infected cells and cancer cells often display unusual proteins on their surface, or they fail to display the usual proteins. In either case, they attract NK cells.

NK cells bind to cells that appear abnormal. The NK cells then release *perforins* (PER-for-ins)—proteins that destroy foreign cells—by exocytosis into the narrow space between the cells. The perforins embed themselves in the target cell membrane and self-assemble into doughnut-shaped pores. This process causes

perforations in the target cell. The target cell, now full of holes, soon dies. Cytotoxic T cells (discussed in the next lesson) use the same technique to kill their targets.

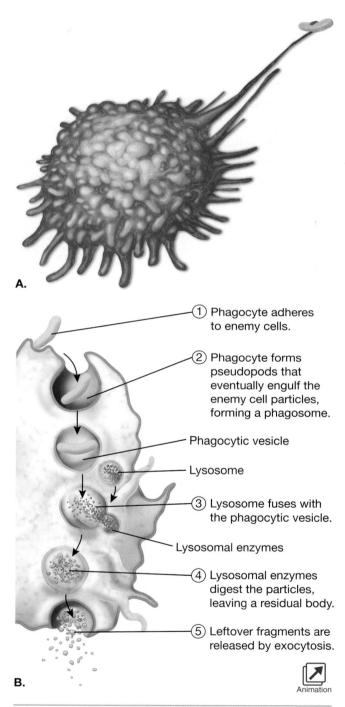

A.

1. Phagocyte adheres to enemy cells.

2. Phagocyte forms pseudopods that eventually engulf the enemy cell particles, forming a phagosome.

Phagocytic vesicle

Lysosome

3. Lysosome fuses with the phagocytic vesicle.

Lysosomal enzymes

4. Lysosomal enzymes digest the particles, leaving a residual body.

5. Leftover fragments are released by exocytosis.

B.

Animation

Figure 12.7 A—Illustration of a phagocyte (purple) extending its cytoplasm to engulf a bacterium (yellow). B—The events of phagocytosis. *In your own words, describe what happens during phagocytosis.*

Complement System

The **complement system** is a set of more than 30 proteins that circulate in the blood plasma through the body and work together to destroy foreign substances. The complement system is so named because it *complements*, or balances out, the effects of antibodies.

The complement system can be activated in two primary ways: via the **classical pathway** or the **alternative pathway**. The route to the classical pathway begins when one of the circulating **complement proteins**, usually inactive, recognizes antibodies bound to a target. The complement protein "doesn't care" whether a particular antibody is bound to a target; any

bound antibody will activate the complement protein. The activated protein kicks off a cascade of complement-protein activation.

The alternative pathway is initiated when another circulating, normally inactive complement protein recognizes foreign materials, such as bacterial cell walls. The classical and alternative pathways converge at complement protein C3. Activation of either pathway causes C3 to split into C3a and C3b (**Figure 12.8**). C3b sticks to target cells and makes them more attractive to phagocytes. Proteins that make cells more attractive to phagocytes are called **opsonins** (AHP-soh-nins). The process of making cells attractive to phagocytes is called *opsonization*.

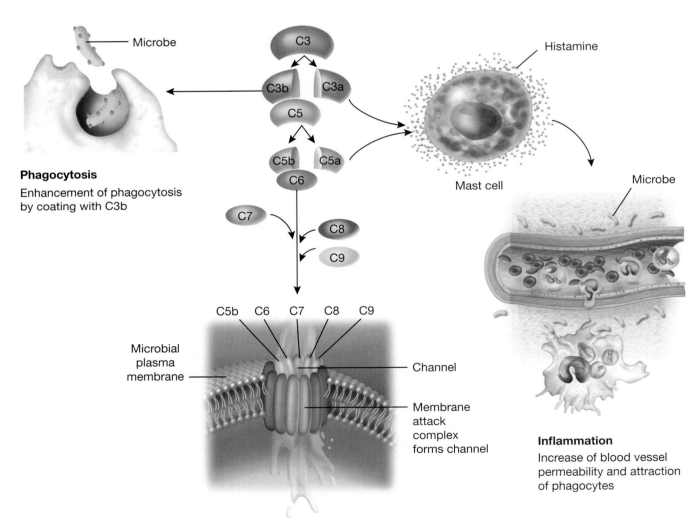

Phagocytosis
Enhancement of phagocytosis by coating with C3b

Microbe

C3

C3b   C3a

C5

C5b   C5a

C6

C7   C8

C9

Histamine

Mast cell

Microbe

C5b   C6   C7   C8   C9

Microbial plasma membrane

Channel

Membrane attack complex forms channel

Inflammation
Increase of blood vessel permeability and attraction of phagocytes

Figure 12.8 The classical and alternative pathways converge at the complement protein identified as C3. Activation of either pathway causes the protein to split, as you see here. The proteins then attack bacteria or viruses in different ways. *How many complement proteins are there, and why are they called "complement" proteins?*

Antibodies can also act as opsonins. C3a and another complement protein, C5a, cause **mast cells**, a type of cell found in connective tissue, to release histamine, a compound that activates an inflammatory response. (Mast cells and the inflammatory response will be discussed in more detail in the next section.) Additional proteins in the complement cascade are converted from inactive to active form. Once activated, complement proteins insert themselves into the bacterial cell membrane and form a *membrane attack complex (MAC)*, which creates a large, lethal hole in the cell membrane. The process by which complement proteins penetrate the cell membrane is similar to the way in which perforin molecules, produced by NK cells, make holes in their targets.

 Check Your Understanding

1. Where do defenses against infectious agents begin?
2. What protein makes the epidermis flexible, strong, and hard to penetrate?
3. What is the name for the process by which cells engulf and destroy foreign matter and cellular debris?
4. How many proteins make up the complement system?
5. What do NK cells and MACs have in common?

Interferons

A virus, unlike a bacterium, is not a cell. A virus is tiny, even when compared with the smallest bacterium. In short, a virus is a little bundle of nucleic acids with a protein coat. Because a virus cannot reproduce itself, it enters a cell and takes over the intracellular machinery. This process enables the virus to make many copies of itself. When the newly reproduced copies of the virus are released, they invade nearby cells. Thus, an infection is borne and spread.

Interferons (IN-ter-FAIR-ahns) are proteins released by cells that have been infected with viruses. Interferons are so named because they *interfere with* viral replication and spreading. They do not help the already-infected cells. They

do, however, help neighboring cells to resist viral infection.

There are several classes of interferons, and each class has multiple members. *Alpha interferons* are produced by virus-infected leukocytes. *Beta interferons* are produced by virus-infected fibroblasts (connective tissue cells). Both types of interferons can bind to receptors on neighboring cells, causing those cells to express proteins that slow down protein synthesis and hinder the reproduction of viral particles. *Gamma interferons* are produced by NK cells and T cells that have been activated by detection of foreign materials. Gamma interferons help macrophages to resist viral infection and attack virus-infected cells more quickly.

Because interferons help to block protein synthesis, they tend to hinder cell growth and division, including the rapid growth and division of cancer cells. When interferons were first discovered, the scientific community held high hopes that these antiviral proteins would be able to halt or cure many types of cancer. Although these hopes have not been fully realized, interferons have turned out to be useful therapeutic agents for treating certain diseases, including hepatitis C, some forms of leukemia (a cancerous disease of the white blood cells), and certain types of lymphoma (cancer that affects lymphatic tissue).

Inflammatory Response

The **inflammatory response**, also called *inflammation*, occurs when tissues have been injured by bacteria, toxins, trauma, or another cause. Although inflammation often is uncomfortable, its purpose is to promote the repair of damaged tissue.

Key steps in the inflammatory response are illustrated in **Figure 12.9** on the next page. When cells are damaged, they release proteins and chemicals that are usually stored within the cells. The appearance of these unusual chemicals in the interstitial fluid causes mast cells in the area to *degranulate*. This means that the mast cells release their intracellular stores of histamine granules, **prostaglandins** (PRAHS-ta-GLAN-dins), and other chemicals.

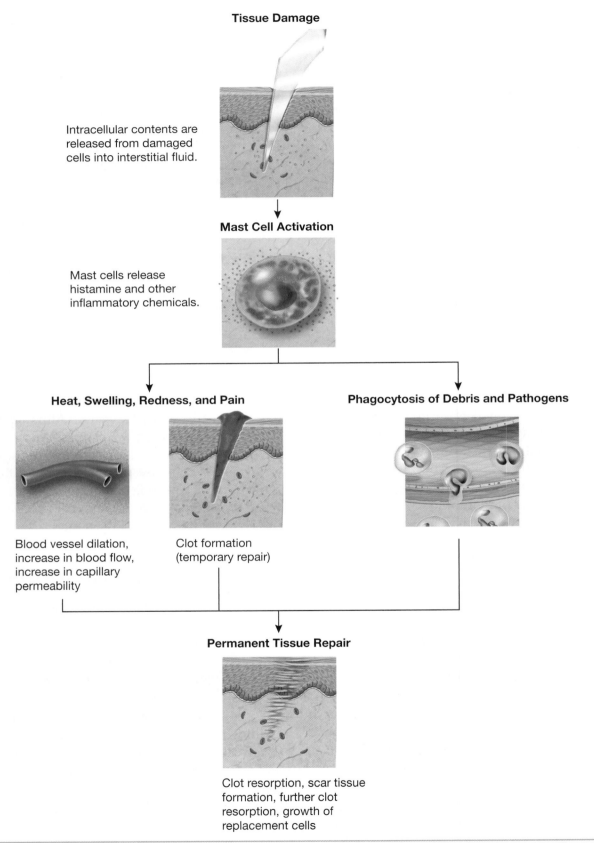

Tissue Damage

Intracellular contents are released from damaged cells into interstitial fluid.

Mast Cell Activation

Mast cells release histamine and other inflammatory chemicals.

Heat, Swelling, Redness, and Pain

Blood vessel dilation, increase in blood flow, increase in capillary permeability

Clot formation (temporary repair)

Phagocytosis of Debris and Pathogens

Permanent Tissue Repair

Clot resorption, scar tissue formation, further clot resorption, growth of replacement cells

Figure 12.9 The development of inflammation. The hallmarks of inflammation are heat, redness, swelling, and pain. *What important purpose does inflammation serve in the body?*

Histamine and the other chemicals attract phagocytes and lymphocytes to the injured or diseased area. The phagocytes consume cellular debris and pathogens, making the capillaries more permeable and causing the arterioles to dilate (increase their diameter). With the increase in capillary permeability comes more fluid leakage from the capillaries, which causes the interstitial fluid to increase in volume. The result: *swelling* of tissues in that area of the body.

The increased permeability inside the capillaries allows clotting proteins to move from the blood into the tissues, where they are activated to form a clot. The stretching of tissue from swelling, and the direct effect of histamine on nerve fibers, causes *pain*. The dilation of arterioles in the affected region causes more blood to flow to that region, which produces *redness* and localized warming, or *heat*. Heat, redness, swelling, and pain are the signs of inflammation.

The chemical processes involved in the inflammatory response cause an increase in local temperature, which boosts the metabolic rate of cells in the area. The accompanying increase in blood flow means that plenty of nutrients will be available for repair processes. You have probably noticed that when you experience swelling and pain from an injury or infection, you instinctively protect the part of your body that is affected. Taken together, the events of the inflammatory response lead to faster tissue cleanup and repair.

Fever

Fever is the maintenance of body temperature at a higher-than-normal level. Neurons in the hypothalamus of the brain work to regulate body temperature. The neurons in this area compare actual body temperature to its "set point," the ideal or desired body temperature. If the actual temperature is higher or lower than the set point, the hypothalamic neurons fire commands throughout the body to make adjustments that will bring the temperature to the desired level (**Figure 12.10**).

If the body is warmer than the desired temperature, sweat glands are activated and

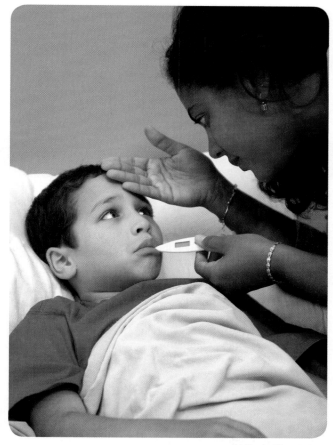

Rob Marmion/Shutterstock.com

Figure 12.10 Fever. *What part of your body regulates your body temperature?*

blood flow is redirected toward the skin to help dissipate heat. If the body is cooler than the desired temperature, blood flow to the skin and extremities is reduced to minimize heat loss. If the reduction in blood flow doesn't fix the problem, shivering begins.

Think of temperature control in a building, which works similarly: a thermostat compares the actual temperature to the set-point temperature. If the building is colder than desired, the thermostat turns on the heater. If the building is too warm, the thermostat turns on the air conditioner.

As you probably know, the normal set point for body temperature is about 98.6°F (37°C). But activation of leukocytes and macrophages can cause the cells to release **pyrogens** (PIGH-roh-jehns), chemicals that raise the set-point temperature of the neurons in the hypothalamus. The hypothalamic neurons then cause reflex adjustments that raise body temperature. The increase in temperature boosts the rate of biochemical reactions in cells by about 10% for every 1°C (1.8°F) rise in temperature. A severe fever is a dangerous side effect of infection and should be treated immediately.

 Check Your Understanding

1. What are the three classes of interferons?
2. What are the four signs of inflammation?
3. In which part of the brain do neurons work to regulate body temperature?

Lesson 12.2 Review and Assessment

Mini Glossary   Make sure that you know the meaning of each key term.

 Build vocabulary with e-flash cards and games

alternative pathway   one of the two primary ways in which the complement system can be activated; this pathway is triggered when the C3b complement protein binds to foreign material

classical pathway   a mode of complement system activation in which a circulating complement protein recognizes an antibody bound to foreign material

complement proteins   proteins in the blood that work with immune system cells and antibodies to defend the body against infection

complement system   a system of more than 30 proteins that circulate in the blood plasma through the body and work together to destroy foreign substances; complements, or balances out, the specific and nonspecific defense systems of the body

exocytosis   the process in which cell membranes fuse together and then push debris from the cell vesicles to the outside of the cell

fever   the maintenance of body temperature at a higher-than-normal level

inflammatory response   physiological response to tissue injury or infection, also called *inflammation*; the four signs of inflammation are heat, redness, swelling, and pain

interferons   proteins released by cells that have been infected with viruses; interfere with virus reproduction

mast cells   connective tissue cell with granules (particles) that contain histamine, a compound which, when released into surrounding fluid, activates an inflammatory response

monocytes   leukocytes that develop into phagocytizing macrophages

when they migrate out of lymphatic circulation into surrounding tissue

neutrophils   the most common type of white blood cell; can slip out of capillaries and into surrounding tissue, where they destroy bacteria and cellular debris

opsonins   proteins that make cells more attractive to phagocytes

phagocytes   cells that engulf and consume bacteria, foreign material, and debris

phagocytosis   the process by which a cell engulfs and destroys foreign matter and cellular debris

prostaglandins   fatty acids involved in the control of inflammation and body temperature

pyrogens   chemicals that tend to cause fever by raising the set-point temperature of the neurons in the hypothalamus

Know and Understand

 Assess

1. Describe how the skin acts as a physical barrier against infectious agents.

2. Explain how the skin thwarts bacterial growth and reduces the risk of infection.

3. Identify the structures of the respiratory tract that are responsible for sweeping bacteria to the stomach to be destroyed.

4. Summarize the process by which cells engulf and destroy foreign matter and cellular debris.

5. Describe the role of histamine in the inflammatory response.

Analyze and Apply

6. After reading the section on the complement system, describe in detail the two primary ways in which the complement system can be activated.

7. Explain how an infection caused by a virus develops and spreads. Be sure to include the characteristics of a virus.

8. Explain why someone with an injury or illness might say that the affected part of his or her body feels as though it is "on fire."

In the Lab

9. Using any materials available, make a model of each of the following structures associated with the lymphatic system. Be sure to include a detailed description of each structure.
   A. neutrophil   C. lysosome
   B. monocyte   D. natural killer cell

Before You Read

Try to answer the following questions before you read this lesson.

Why is the specific immune system also called the adaptive immune system?

What is an antibody, and what function does it serve?

Lesson Objectives

1. Explain the differences between humoral immunity (antibody-mediated immunity) and cellular immunity (cell-mediated immunity).

2. Describe the role of antigen-presenting cells (APCs) in immune system function.

3. Define the term *antibody* and explain its role in the specific defense system of the body.

4. Explain the difference between the primary and secondary immune responses.

Key Terms

E-Flash Cards

active immunity
antigen-presenting cells (APCs)
apoptosis
cellular immunity
clonal selection
humoral immunity
immune system
immunoglobulins

major histocompatibility complex glycoproteins (MHCs)
memory cells
passive immunity
precipitation
primary immune response
secondary immune response

Of the human body's defenses against disease, its specific defense systems are the most remarkable and complicated. The cells and chemicals that contribute to these specific defenses make up the **immune system**. The immune system is also called the *specific immune system*, or *adaptive immune system*. These terms are used because the immune system is highly specific in its responses to foreign substances. It is able to recognize new challenges, adapt to those challenges, and "remember" what it has learned. The lymphatic organs and tissues are the physical "home" of the immune system.

As with many body functions, we don't notice or appreciate our immune system as it works. The immune system is constantly finding, targeting, and eliminating bacteria and viruses. It even kills the body's own cells when they show signs of infection or cancerous development.

Patients with a compromised immune system are susceptible to diseases that never trouble those with a normal immune system. For example, babies born with severe combined immune deficiency (SCID), a genetic immune system deficiency, have a tragically poor prognosis unless they receive a successful bone marrow transplant. SCID, also known as the "bubble boy disease," gained global attention in the 1970s with news reports of David Vetter, a boy with SCID who had to live in a sterile, plastic bubble to avoid contact with bacteria and viruses. An infection that is minor for a person with a healthy immune system is potentially fatal for a person with SCID (**Figure 12.11** on the next page).

The many cells and chemicals of the immune system interact with one another in complex ways that are still not completely understood. This complexity makes the immune system challenging to study. We do, however, know a great deal about this fascinating system.

Figure 12.11 Severe combined immune deficiency (SCID), also known as "bubble boy disease," results in a poor prognosis unless the patient receives a bone marrow transplant that is successful. *How would a SCID diagnosis affect the way you live your life?*

Antigens

Antigens, as you learned in chapter 10, are large molecules, such as proteins, polysaccharides, glycolipids, or nucleic acids, on the surface of cells. Antigens identify cells as either "self" or "nonself" cells, thereby making it possible for the body to distinguish between its own cells and any nonself, or foreign, cells. This makes it possible for the immune system to recognize foreign cells and respond, which it does by producing antibodies that bind to and mark the foreign antigens. The foreign antigens may be parts of bacteria, viruses, or abnormal cells, but they are not necessarily pathogens. For example, substances that we are allergic to are foreign antigens, but they are not pathogens.

A single complex antigen molecule can have multiple foreign parts, or *antigenic determinants*. Larger molecules, especially proteins, are more likely to provoke an immune response than small ones because they have more antigenic determinants.

The antigens on the surfaces of our own cells (the "self" antigens described above) do *not* provoke an immune response. Why not? Any immature lymphocytes that *do* respond to "self" molecules are killed off early in the development process.

Immune System Cells

You read earlier that lymphocytes are the signature cells of the immune system. Other cells, such as **antigen-presenting cells (APCs)**, are also essential for proper immune function. Macrophages, dendritic cells (immune system cells in the skin and lymphatic organs), and B cells all can act as APCs (**Figure 12.12**).

Lymphocytes

Remember from lesson 12.1 that lymphocytes initially develop from stem cells in red bone marrow. Some travel to the thymus to complete their maturation; these are called *T* (for *thymus*) *lymphocytes*. Some lymphocytes complete their maturation in bone marrow; these are called *B* (for *bone*) *lymphocytes*.

All lymphocytes go through a screening process. If, during the screening process, a lymphocyte responds to the body's self-antigens as foreign matter, which it is not supposed to do, it undergoes **apoptosis** (AP-ahp-TOH-sis). Apoptosis, a programmed process of cellular self-destruction, ensures that the surviving lymphocytes do not attack the body's own tissues. (As we will see in lesson 12.4, this weeding-out process does not always work with 100% success. When it does not work perfectly, autoimmune disease, in which the immune system attacks the body's own tissue, can result.)

Each lymphocyte has many antigen receptors in its membrane. All the receptors in a lymphocyte membrane recognize one—and only one—antigen. Our bodies have millions of lymphocytes, and each one recognizes a particular antigen. So, you can see why this lesson is entitled "Specific Defenses."

Once the lymphocytes have matured, they travel throughout the blood to all parts of the body. Some lymphocytes circulate continuously while others "settle down" in lymph nodes, the spleen, or other lymphatic tissues.

Over the course of a lifetime, only a fraction of our lymphocytes will ever "meet" the antigen that binds to its particular antigen receptor. Lymphocytes that do not meet their antigen remain *quiescent*, or inactive.

When a lymphocyte does meet its antigen, the binding of the antigen to the antigen receptor stimulates the lymphocyte to *differentiate*. The lymphocyte divides repeatedly, making many copies of itself. Each copy is an exact genetic duplicate, or clone, of the original cell that was stimulated. This process is called **clonal selection**.

Most of the clones produced by lymphocytic differentiation become short-lived *effector cells* that fight an infectious invader. A few of the clones become **memory cells** that reside in lymphatic tissues, ready to respond if the same antigen reinvades the body.

MHC Proteins

For an immune response to be activated, it is not enough for antigens to be present—the antigens must be presented in a particular way. Antigens are displayed on the surfaces of cells by **major histocompatibility complex glycoproteins**, or *MHC proteins*.

There are two main classes of MHC proteins. The *class I MHC proteins* are found on the surfaces of *all* cells that contain nuclei. *Class II MHC proteins* are found only on the surfaces of antigen-presenting cells (APCs) and lymphocytes.

The class I MHC proteins, which are found on cell surfaces, display fragments of the many different proteins found inside the cells. This means that a normal body cell displays normal protein fragments (*self-antigens*) on its surface. When the immune system is working properly, passing lymphocytes ignore these self-antigens.

Just as the class I MHC proteins display fragments of normal proteins, they display fragments of abnormal, undesirable proteins that might be inside the cell. So, if a cell is infected or cancerous, it will display parts of the infectious agent, or cancer-related proteins, on its surface.

When a passing cytotoxic T (T_C) cell "sees" a cell that displays an unfamiliar antigen (for example, cancer-related proteins) on a class I MHC protein, it goes into "attack" mode. As **Figure 12.13** on the next page shows, an APC internalizes and breaks down a foreign particle, and it displays on its surface the particle fragments of class II MHC proteins.

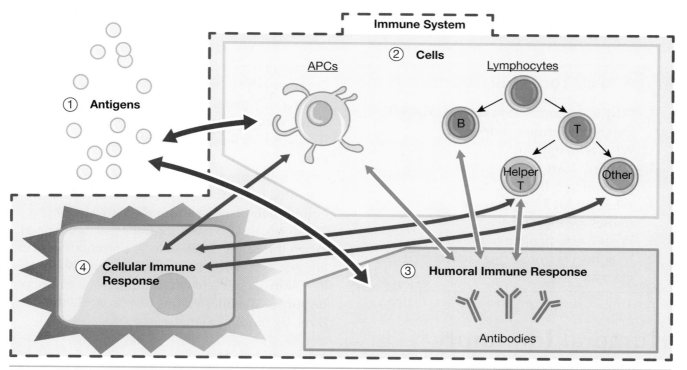

Figure 12.12 Diagram of the immune system. Helper T cells play a significant role in both the humoral and cellular immune responses. Other T cells are associated mainly with the cellular response. B cells are associated with the humoral response. APCs (antigen-presenting cells) are involved in both types of responses. *In general, how do humoral and cellular responses differ from the immunity provided by interferons or inflammation?*

1 Phagocytic APCs engulf the extracellular pathogens.

2 Lysosomal action produces antigenic fragments.

Plasma membrane

5 Antigenic fragments are displayed by class II MHC proteins on the plasma membrane.

4 Antigenic fragments are bound to class II MHC proteins.

3 The rough endoplasmic reticulum produces class II MHC proteins.

Rough endoplasmic reticulum

Lysosome

Nucleus

Phagocytic cell

Figure 12.13 Diagram of antigen presentation by an antigen-presenting cell. Antigen-presenting cells (APCs) use class II MHC proteins to display fragments of foreign molecules (antigens) on their surface. (1) The process begins when the APC phagocytizes the foreign object, such as a bacterium. (2) A lysosome, which contains digestive enzymes, fuses with the engulfed object and breaks it down into many pieces. (3) Meanwhile, the cell is also producing class II MHC proteins packaged in vesicles. (4) A vesicle containing class II MHC proteins fuses with the vesicle containing digested antigenic fragments. (5) These digested fragments bind to the class II MHC proteins, which are then displayed on the cell membrane.

 Check Your Understanding

1. Why is the immune system also called the *specific immune system*?
2. What is an antigen?
3. Name at least three types of antigen-presenting cells (APCs).
4. What are MHC proteins, and how many classes are there?
5. What has to happen to prevent a lymphocyte from being characterized as *inactive*?

Humoral Immunity

Humoral immunity, also called *antibody-mediated immunity*, is effective against pathogens located outside of cells—such as extracellular viruses, bacteria, and bacterial toxins. Humoral immunity begins when a B cell encounters the antigen that binds to its antigen receptors. During this encounter, the B cell undergoes clonal selection, as described previously. The B cell divides repeatedly, making many copies of itself.

B cell reproduction is most strongly activated when the B cell, with an antigen bound to it, presents the antigen to a helper T cell, which also has a receptor for that antigen. When the helper T cell detects presentation of an antigen by a B cell, it releases *interleukins* (IN-ter-LOO-kins), chemicals that stimulate an immune response. The interleukins fully activate the B cell by binding to it.

Plasma Cells

Some of the daughter cells produced by clonal selection become *memory helper B cells*, but most become plasma cells. The plasma cells have a cytoplasm full of *rough endoplasmic reticulum* (*RER*), a membranous network that is involved in protein synthesis.

In plasma cells, large quantities of antibodies are made in the RER and are secreted into the interstitial fluid. The antibodies made by the plasma cell "recognize" and bind to the same antigen that stimulated the original B cell. Thus, the clonal selection process for B cells produces an army of B cells, all of which make antibodies specifically directed at the invading antigen.

Antibodies

Antibodies are proteins that recognize particular antigens with great specificity. Antibodies are also called **immunoglobulins** (IM-yoo-noh-GLAHB-yoo-lins) because they are involved with immune function and originally were thought of as globular in shape.

An antibody is a Y-shaped protein made up of four *polypeptide chains* (**Figure 12.14**). The tips of the Y are the parts that can bind to an antigen. The antigen-binding portions have a variable amino acid sequence that determines the antigen's specific target. The variable regions on the two arms of the Y match each other, so that each arm binds to the same antigen. The stem and lower parts of the arms of the Y do not vary; they are the same for all antibodies of a given class.

There are five classes of antibodies, which are described in **Figure 12.15** on the next page. Antibodies do not directly destroy antigens. However, they interfere with antigen function and mark the antigens for destruction. The formation of an *antigen-antibody complex* can eliminate the threat of an antigen through multiple mechanisms. These mechanisms are described below:

- An antibody can *neutralize* a virus or bacterial toxin (a toxic chemical secreted by a bacterium) by occupying the binding site that the virus or toxin would use to attach to a target cell.
- **Precipitation** causes small, soluble (dissolvable) antigen molecules, rather than whole cells, to clump together. The resulting antigen complexes are too big to remain dissolved (soluble) in the bloodstream.
- Agglutination (a-gloo-ti-NAY-shun) is similar to precipitation, except that the antigens lie on the surface of a cell or virus; thus, the clumping process involves cells, viruses, or bacteria rather than small molecules.
- Binding of an antibody to its target causes a slight change in shape along the stem of the Y. Binding sites on the antigen are exposed, activating the complement system (described earlier). Antibodies and complement proteins on a pathogen make it more appealing to phagocytes.
- Antibody-antigen complexes also stimulate inflammation by causing mast cells and basophils (a type of white blood cell) to release histamine and other chemicals.

Figure 12.14 An antibody is a Y-shaped protein composed of four polypeptide chains. The tips of the arms of the Y have a variable amino acid sequence and are the sites at which antigens bind. *An antibody is a protein that recognizes certain pathogens and targets them specifically. What would be the effect on human health if antibodies did not display such specificity in targeting pathogens?*

Primary and Secondary Immune Responses

When an antigen enters the body for the first time, the immune system response is neither fast nor widespread. Because memory cells for the new antigen do not yet exist in the

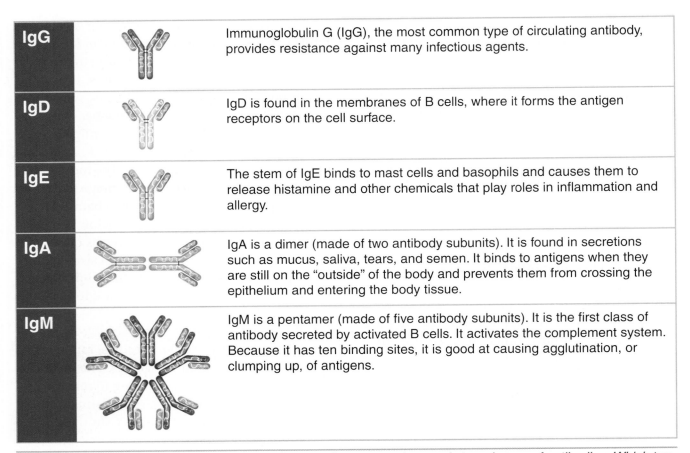

IgG	Immunoglobulin G (IgG), the most common type of circulating antibody, provides resistance against many infectious agents.
IgD	IgD is found in the membranes of B cells, where it forms the antigen receptors on the cell surface.
IgE	The stem of IgE binds to mast cells and basophils and causes them to release histamine and other chemicals that play roles in inflammation and allergy.
IgA	IgA is a dimer (made of two antibody subunits). It is found in secretions such as mucus, saliva, tears, and semen. It binds to antigens when they are still on the "outside" of the body and prevents them from crossing the epithelium and entering the body tissue.
IgM	IgM is a pentamer (made of five antibody subunits). It is the first class of antibody secreted by activated B cells. It activates the complement system. Because it has ten binding sites, it is good at causing agglutination, or clumping up, of antigens.

Figure 12.15 Different classes of antibodies. *Assume that you can have only two classes of antibodies. Which two would you pick? Based on your reading, make a case for why you would pick these two classes of antibodies.*

body, detection of the threat may take a while. When the threat is detected, the immune system response is limited. However, if the antigen returns, the immune system response will be faster and much stronger.

The **primary immune response** occurs when the body is first exposed to a foreign invader, such as a virus or bacterium. The **secondary immune response** occurs when the virus or bacterium enters the body for a second or subsequent time, with a stronger response to a lesser amount of antigen. The secondary immune response mainly involves memory cells, which developed during the body's initial exposure to the potentially harmful invader.

The difference between the primary and secondary immune responses, shown in **Figure 12.16**, is the reason that *vaccination* works. The word *vaccine* comes in part from the Latin word *vacca*, which means "cow." In the

late 1700s Edward Jenner, an English doctor, noticed that milkmaids were much less likely than other people to contract smallpox, a disease characterized by rash and raised blisters on the skin. At the time it was known that the disease cowpox, which could infect people as well as cows, was similar to smallpox but less severe.

Jenner believed that the exposure of milkmaids to cowpox made them resistant to smallpox. He tested his idea by injecting pus from the blisters of people infected with cowpox into healthy individuals. He then tried to give those healthy individuals smallpox by injecting them with pus from patients infected with smallpox. (Such experiments would be prohibited, with good reason, by the human subjects protection board of a modern hospital.) Jenner's series of careful experiments showed that a substance in the cowpox pus gave people a long-lasting immunity to smallpox.

The antibody-mediated immunity described earlier is also called **active immunity** because the antibodies are actively produced by the blood plasma cells of the body. **Passive immunity**, by contrast, is antibody-mediated immunity that comes from antibodies received from an outside source. In the case of infants, for example, the outside source of antibodies can be from breast milk, which is rich in antibodies. Another outside source is an injection of antibodies purified from the plasma of a blood donor.

Cellular Immunity

Cellular immunity, or *cell-mediated immunity*, is mediated by (that is, facilitated, or assisted, by) T cells. Cell-mediated immunity is not only *mediated by* cells; it is also *directed at* cells. When body cells are infected by a bacterium or virus, or when they become cancerous or precancerous, they display abnormal proteins on their surface. Cells of transplanted tissue also display foreign antigens. If the tissue is not well matched from donor to recipient, it will provoke a cell-mediated immune response.

Figure 12.17 on the next page illustrates how the cellular immune response is activated and how a specific T cell is selected for clonal reproduction. The cellular immune response begins when an antigen-presenting cell (APC) presents an antigen on its surface with a class II major histocompatibility (MHC) protein (**Figure 12.17A**). The APC encounters a T cell whose receptor matches the antigen. A glycoprotein known as CD4, which is found on the surface of helper T cells, "recognizes" and binds to part of the class II MHC protein on the APC (**Figure 12.17B**). This simultaneous binding of an antigen receptor to an antigen, and of a CD4 protein to a class II MHC protein, is a "double handshake" that activates the helper T cell. The helper T cell then divides rapidly, making many genetically identical copies (clones) of itself.

During the clonal selection process, the rapid cellular division of the helper T cell generates *active helper T cells* and some long-lived *memory helper T cells* (**Figure 12.17C**). An active helper T cell now helps activate another type of T cell: *cytotoxic T cells*, sometimes called *killer T cells*. Cytotoxic T cells have a CD8 glycoprotein that recognizes class I MHC molecules. (Recall that all nucleated cells use class I MHC proteins to display antigens.) When a cytotoxic T cell detects an antigen bound to its antigen receptors, *and* it detects with its CD8 molecule that the antigen is presented by a class I MHC protein, then the cytotoxic T cell is partially activated for clonal selection.

Complete activation of the cytotoxic T cell requires assistance from an activated helper T cell.

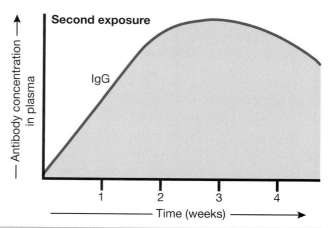

Figure 12.16 Primary and secondary immune responses. These graphs show the levels of immunoglobulin G (the most common antibody) in the blood plasma during an initial infection (left) and during a second infection (right). The response to the second exposure is larger and faster than the response to the first exposure. *Why is a secondary immune response to infection larger and faster than the primary response to the first exposure?*

Figure 12.17 Activation and clonal selection of T cells. A—Antigen presentation. B—Double recognition. C—Clone formation. *Now that the helper T cells (the blue cells in C above) have been cloned, what will they do?*

Once the cytotoxic T cell is fully activated, it divides repeatedly, producing three types of cells: *active cytotoxic T cells*, *memory cytotoxic T cells*, and *suppressor T cells*. Active cytotoxic T cells seek out and destroy antigen-displaying cells that initiated the immune response. Both memory cytotoxic T cells and suppressor T cells prevent the cellular response from being too strong or too long lasting.

An activated cytotoxic T cell binds to a cell displaying the foreign antigen recognized by that T cell. One way in which the activated cytotoxic T cell kills the target cell is by stimulating intracellular pathways that lead to apoptosis (programmed cell destruction). Another way in which the activated cytotoxic T cell kills the target cell is by releasing perforin molecules. Natural killer (NK) cells also use perforins to kill their targets, as we learned in lesson 12.2. Perforin molecules insert themselves into the target cell membrane and assemble to form a relatively large opening, or perforation, in the cell. This large hole is lethal to the target cell.

Lesson 12.3 Review and Assessment

Mini Glossary   Make sure that you know the meaning of each key term.

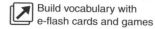 Build vocabulary with e-flash cards and games

active immunity immunity in which the blood plasma cells in the body make antibodies as a result of previous exposure to a disease or a vaccine

antigen-presenting cells (APCs) cells that process protein antigens and present them on their surface in a form that can be recognized by lymphocytes (white blood cells)

apoptosis a programmed process of cellular self-destruction (cell suicide)

cellular immunity immunity that arises from the activation of T lymphocytes (T cells) by antigen-presenting cells; cell-mediated immunity

clonal selection repeated division of a lymphocyte that produces many exact genetic copies (clones) of itself

humoral immunity immunity associated with free antibodies that circulate in the blood; antibody-mediated immunity

immune system the cells and chemicals that contribute to the body's specific defenses against disease

immunoglobulins antibodies; proteins that recognize particular antigens with great specificity

major histocompatibility complex glycoproteins (MHCs) family of proteins found on the surfaces of lymphocytes and other cells; help the immune system recognize foreign antigens and ignore "self" tissues

memory cells B lymphocytes and T lymphocytes in lymphatic tissues that can respond if a previously

encountered antigen invades the body again

passive immunity immunity that comes from antibodies received from an outside source, such as breast milk

precipitation the formation of an insoluble complex, such as a clump of antigen molecules joined together by antibodies

primary immune response the initial immune system response to a foreign invader such as a virus or bacterium

secondary immune response immune system response to an infectious agent that it has encountered before

Know and Understand

 Assess

1. Describe the genetic immune system deficiency that is more commonly known as "bubble boy disease."

2. Identify the types of cells that can act as antigen-presenting cells.

3. Explain the importance of the thymus to the body's immune system.

4. What two types of cells have antigen receptors, making humoral immunity possible?

5. Explain why T lymphocytes and B lymphocytes are so named.

Analyze and Apply

6. Explain why only a fraction of lymphocytes will ever "meet" the antigen that binds to their specific antigen receptor.

7. Describe the sequence of events that occurs when a lymphocyte meets an antigen.

8. Using the knowledge that you have learned about humoral immunity, list the steps that occur when a B cell undergoes clonal selection.

In the Lab

9. After reading lessons 12.2 and 12.3, you should have a good understanding of the difference between the nonspecific and specific defense systems of the body. Create a model, draw a picture with labels, or write an essay or a story in which you describe something that is protected or defended by both nonspecific and specific defenses. A garden, for example, might have a fence around it to keep out many different kinds of "invaders," yet the gardener might sprinkle snail bait in the garden for the specific purpose of preventing snails from eating his vegetables. Identify as many nonspecific and specific defenses as possible. In your model, picture, or written composition, compare your different defense mechanisms to the corresponding immune defenses studied in lessons 12.2 and 12.3.

10. Using the Internet and your knowledge of the lymphatic system, write a 250-word essay about David Vetter, the "bubble boy." Describe in detail the genetic disease with which he was affected.

Disorders and Diseases of the Immune System

Lesson Objectives

1. Explain what cancer is and what happens during metastasis.

2. Define the term *allergy* and explain the role of an antigen-presenting cell in an allergic response.

3. Explain what an autoimmune disorder is and give one example.

4. Describe how HIV is related to AIDS.

Key Terms

E-Flash Cards

acquired immune
    deficiency syndrome
    (AIDS)
allergen
anaphylaxis
autoimmune disorder

human
    immunodeficiency
    virus (HIV)
immunotherapy
lymphedema
metastasis
opportunistic infection
tolerance

From allergies to AIDS, many health problems can be linked to a compromised immune system. In the following section, we will explore some common disorders and diseases of the body's defense systems, along with their mechanisms.

Cancer and Lymph Nodes

Cancer is a disease in which the normal control of cell division (mitosis) fails, and a cell starts to divide too fast and without limit. As a solid tumor grows, cancerous cells sometimes break free from the tumor and migrate to other areas of the body. The process of cancer spreading from its initial location to another part of the body is called **metastasis** (meh-TAS-ta-sis). A cancer that has spread is said to be *metastatic*.

Metastatic cells can spread by entering a lymphatic vessel and traveling in the lymph to the nearest lymph node. When the cells reach the lymph node, they may get caught in the reticular tissue within the lymph node and continue growing. When some types of cancer have been diagnosed, it is standard for an oncologist (a doctor who specializes in cancer treatment) to get a sample of nearby lymph node tissue to determine whether the cancer has spread. The sample may be obtained by surgically removing one or more lymph nodes or by performing a needle biopsy using a syringe.

If cancer has metastasized to lymph nodes, then more lymph nodes may be removed to reduce the chances of further metastasis. Lymph node removal has risks. The biggest risk is that it disrupts the lymphatic drainage in the affected area of the body. As a result, fluid that leaks out of blood capillaries builds up in the interstitial space, causing tissue swelling and damage. This buildup of extracellular fluid is called **lymphedema** (LIMF-eh-DEE-ma).

Breast cancer often metastasizes to axillary (underarm) lymph nodes. Removal of axillary lymph nodes increases the risk of lymphedema of the arm—the most common type of lymphedema. Treatment options include a compression sleeve, physical therapy, and carefully designed, light exercise.

 Check Your Understanding

1. How is cancer spread?
2. What is the cause of lymphedema?

Allergies

Do you sneeze, cough, or suffer from itchy, watery eyes when you are exposed to dust, pollen, or animal dander? If so, you are not alone. Some 55% of Americans have an allergy to one or more substances in the environment.

An *allergy* is an inappropriately strong response of the immune system to an environmental antigen, such as dust mites, pet dander, pollen, or certain foods (**Figure 12.18**). In such cases, the antigen is not really a threat; the problem is an overreactive immune system.

Allergies arise when an antigen-presenting cell presents the antigen—an **allergen**—to a helper T cell in a person susceptible to allergies.

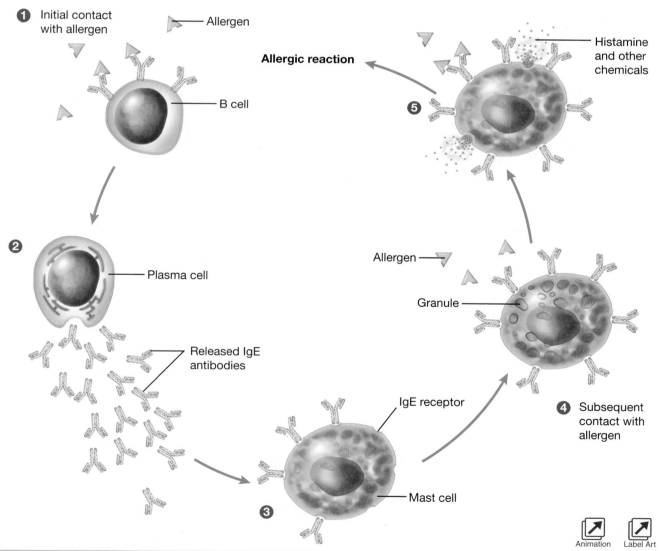

Figure 12.18 Diagram of an allergic reaction. *Why do you think some people have allergies and others don't?*

This allergen presentation activates the helper T cell, which in turn activates B cells, causing them to produce a class of antibodies called *IgE antibodies*. The IgE antibodies interact with mast cells and basophils, which become sensitive to the allergen. The next time the allergen is encountered, basophils and mast cells respond by secreting large amounts of histamine.

Histamine causes an inflammatory response, which can lead to symptoms such as a runny nose and watery, itchy eyes. In severe cases, such as with bee-sting allergies and certain nut allergies, exposure to the antigen causes large quantities of histamine to be released throughout the body. Excessive histamine in the body can lead to life-threatening symptoms. These include pulmonary obstruction due to inflammation and swelling of the airways and low blood pressure due to leakage of blood plasma into the interstitial space, through excessively leaky capillaries. Such a severe allergic reaction is called **anaphylaxis** (AN-a-fi-LAK-sis).

Anaphylaxis can be treated with an injection of epinephrine (EHP-i-NEHF-rin), a hormone that opens up the airways and constricts (narrows) the blood vessels. Antihistamine drugs, which block the effects of histamine, can be used to treat anaphylaxis as well as less severe allergic reactions.

Allergy shots, or allergen **immunotherapy**, are a longer-term treatment, aimed at preventing allergic reactions before they occur. In allergy-shot treatment, a specific allergen is injected underneath the skin, starting with tiny amounts and gradually building up to larger amounts. This gradual approach often leads to the development of immune system **tolerance** of the antigen. As a result, the allergic response may be reduced or eliminated.

Autoimmune Disorders

An **autoimmune disorder**, like an allergy, is a condition in which the immune system overreacts to an antigen that, in and of itself, does not pose an actual threat. In an allergy, the antigen is a substance outside the body (that is, in the environment). In an autoimmune disorder, the antigen is part of the body's own tissue.

When the immune system perceives the body's own tissue as foreign, it attacks that tissue as it would attack an invading organism. The cause of autoimmune disorders is often unclear. An autoimmune disorder sometimes develops when a genetically susceptible person is exposed to an environmental antigen that resembles one of the body's own molecules. The immune response to the outside antigen produces collateral damage (unintended harm) to the body's own cells.

More than 80 different types of autoimmune disorders have been identified. Examples include rheumatoid (ROO-ma-toyd) arthritis, in which the immune system attacks the synovial membrane that lines joint cavities; multiple sclerosis, in which the immune system attacks the myelin sheath that surrounds nerve cells; and type I diabetes. Multiple sclerosis is discussed in more detail in chapter 6; rheumatoid arthritis, in chapter 4; and type I diabetes (mellitus), in chapter 8.

In type I diabetes, cytotoxic T cells attack the cells in the pancreas that manufacture insulin, a hormone that metabolizes carbohydrates and fats and regulates glucose levels in the blood. Unfortunately, the cytotoxic T cell attacks are usually very effective; they destroy all or most of the insulin-producing cells. Once the insulin-producing cells are gone, they do not grow back. Type I diabetes is also called insulin-dependent diabetes because individuals with this autoimmune disease require regular insulin injections from an outside source.

 Check Your Understanding

1. What causes itchy, water eyes from exposure to dust, pollen, or animal dander?
2. What can excessive amounts of histamine do to the body?
3. Name two treatments for anaphylaxis.
4. What are some common autoimmune disorders?

HIV and AIDS

As its name indicates, **human immunodeficiency virus (HIV)** is a virus that

WHAT RESEARCH TELLS US

...*about* **Antibody-Based Drugs**

Many drugs have side effects that limit their usefulness because the drugs affect processes other than the specific disease mechanisms for which they are intended. Because antibodies bind very specifically, it has long been thought that they could make good drugs.

In the past 15 years, a growing number of antibody-based drugs have made it to market. They are made by fusing a B lymphocyte with a cultured cell derived from a cancerous lymph cell. The fused cell can divide without limit because it is derived from a cancer cell, and it makes one specific antibody because it is also derived from a B lymphocyte. The cell is allowed to divide, grow, and secrete its antibody product, which is harvested from the fluid bathing the cells. The antibody product is then packaged as a drug. Because the cells are genetic copies of the original fused cell, they

Figure 12.19 Micrograph of lymphocytes.

are called *clones*; the antibodies they make are called *monoclonal antibodies* because they come from a single clone. You can recognize many drugs that are monoclonal antibodies because they usually have the word segment *-mab* (for "monoclonal antibody") in their generic name.

Infliximab (sold as Remicade®) is an antibody to tumor necrosis factor, a protein that plays an important role in rheumatoid

arthritis, the disease for which it is most often prescribed. Trastuzamab (sold as Herceptin®) is an antibody to the human epidermal growth factor receptor 2 (HER2), which is found on the surface of some kinds of breast cancer cells. It is given as a chemotherapeutic agent to patients with HER2-positive breast cancer. Many more monoclonal antibody drugs exist, and the list continues to grow with advances in research.

Taking It Further

1. Working with another student or in a group, research monoclonal antibody drugs for cancer treatment. How do these drugs work? Why are they typically used? How are they given to patients? What are common side effects of these drugs? Prepare a report and share your findings with the class.

causes immune deficiency only in humans. HIV is the virus that can lead to **acquired immune deficiency syndrome (AIDS)**. HIV is commonly transmitted sexually, through sharing of needles during illegal drug use, or from mother to child during pregnancy, birth, or breastfeeding. Less common modes of transmission include blood transfusions or being accidentally "stuck" with a contaminated needle. The latter is a risk for healthcare workers.

Within a few weeks of infection, a person with HIV may develop flu-like symptoms that last one or two weeks. Others may not experience any symptoms at all. Although individuals infected with HIV may feel perfectly healthy, the virus is at work inside their bodies. Because HIV damages the immune system, it compromises the body's ability to fight disease-causing organisms.

As shown in **Figure 12.20**, the HIV virus infects lymphocytes that have the CD4 protein on their surface (CD4+ cells). Most CD4+ cells are helper T cells, and most helper T cells are CD4+. After the virus uses the intracellular machinery to make copies of itself, it breaks open the cell, killing the cell and releasing new, infectious virus particles.

Of all the immune cells, the helper T cells are probably the cells that the body can least afford to lose. The helper T cells are essential for strong activation of both the humoral and cellular immune responses. When the concentration level of helper T cells drops below 200/mm³, the immune system is seriously weakened, and the patient is said to have AIDS.

AIDS patients are highly susceptible to developing rare forms of cancer and

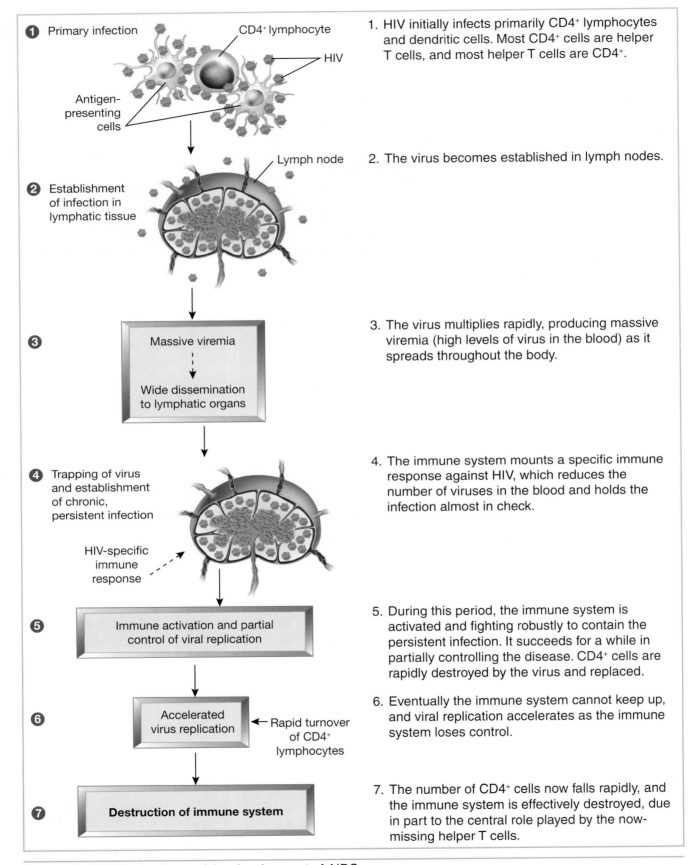

1 Primary infection

CD4⁺ lymphocyte

HIV

Antigen-presenting cells

1. HIV initially infects primarily CD4⁺ lymphocytes and dendritic cells. Most CD4⁺ cells are helper T cells, and most helper T cells are CD4⁺.

2 Establishment of infection in lymphatic tissue

Lymph node

2. The virus becomes established in lymph nodes.

3

Massive viremia

Wide dissemination to lymphatic organs

3. The virus multiplies rapidly, producing massive viremia (high levels of virus in the blood) as it spreads throughout the body.

4 Trapping of virus and establishment of chronic, persistent infection

HIV-specific immune response

4. The immune system mounts a specific immune response against HIV, which reduces the number of viruses in the blood and holds the infection almost in check.

5 Immune activation and partial control of viral replication

5. During this period, the immune system is activated and fighting robustly to contain the persistent infection. It succeeds for a while in partially controlling the disease. CD4⁺ cells are rapidly destroyed by the virus and replaced.

6 Accelerated virus replication

Rapid turnover of CD4⁺ lymphocytes

6. Eventually the immune system cannot keep up, and viral replication accelerates as the immune system loses control.

7 Destruction of immune system

7. The number of CD4⁺ cells now falls rapidly, and the immune system is effectively destroyed, due in part to the central role played by the now-missing helper T cells.

Figure 12.20 HIV infection and the development of AIDS.

opportunistic infection—an unusual infection that is never seen in people with healthy immune systems. Multidrug treatments for HIV are effective at suppressing viral reproduction for many years. However, these drugs can have serious side effects, such as nausea, vomiting, weight loss, and fatigue. Also, AIDS antiviral drugs are expensive and must be taken for life. Therefore, the scientific community continues its effort to create an HIV vaccine.

Lesson 12.4 Review and Assessment

Mini Glossary
Make sure that you know the meaning of each key term.

 Build vocabulary with e-flash cards and games

acquired immune deficiency syndrome (AIDS) a disease in which the immune system is greatly weakened due to infection with HIV, making a person more susceptible to rare cancers and opportunistic infections

allergen antigen that causes an inappropriately strong immune system response

anaphylaxis a severe and potentially life-threatening allergic reaction that may include airway obstruction and very low blood pressure

autoimmune disorder a condition in which the immune system attacks the body's own tissue

human immunodeficiency virus (HIV) the virus that causes AIDS

immunotherapy a long-term, preventive treatment for allergies; "allergy shots"

lymphedema a buildup of extracellular fluid in the body because of disruption in lymphatic drainage

metastasis the spreading of cancerous cells from their original location to another part of the body

opportunistic infection an infection that rarely or never occurs in people with a healthy immune system but that may occur in a person with a damaged immune system, such as from AIDS

tolerance reduction or elimination of the allergic response, which may occur after immunotherapy

Know and Understand

Assess

1. Describe the surgical procedure that is used to determine whether cancer has spread from its initial location to another part of the body.
2. List the potential risks associated with having a lymph node removed.
3. State the treatment options for a patient with lymphedema of the arm as a result of having an axillary lymph node removed.
4. Define IgE antibodies and describe how they are produced.
5. Identify the two cells responsible for secreting large amounts of histamine in response to an allergen.
6. Summarize the purpose of allergen immunotherapy.
7. Explain the difference between HIV and AIDS.
8. Describe the process by which an antibody-based drug is made.

Analyze and Apply

9. Breast cancer can metastasize, or spread. Identify the area of the body where breast cancer often metastasizes, and label it on a diagram of the human body.

10. Based on what you have learned about severe allergies, describe two ways in which histamine could cause life-threatening symptoms.

In the Lab

11. You are a doctor who has just seen the following patients. What is your diagnosis for each patient? Use information that you learned in this lesson, as well as information from previous chapters.

   Patient A: tests show very high cell counts in certain lymph nodes; the patient is not currently experiencing any pain or fatigue.

   Patient B: severe pain in the hands and feet; severe inflammation and swelling in the hands; fatigue

   Patient C: excessive sneezing, coughing, and watery eyes; symptoms began during a recent hiking trip

   Patient D: has two different infections; standard tests have failed to identify the cause of either infection; patient reports that she has been very healthy for the past two years

12. Using the Centers for Disease Control (CDC) website as a source, research anaphylaxis. Then create a poster illustrating the proper steps to follow when using an epinephrine injection pen for anaphylactic shock.

Career Corner
Anatomy and Physiology at Work

Careers in immunology and oncology involve extensive study of and work with the immune system. These careers in bioscience (that is, the scientific study of the body) require a high level of motivation, a great deal of education, and a lot of hard work. They can be highly challenging, rewarding, and profitable.

Immunologist

An immunologist may be a doctor, researcher, and/or college professor. Strong skills in mathematics, biology, and chemistry, along with a deep interest in scientific inquiry or human well-being, are important for success in the field of immunology.

Research immunologists typically work in a lab, performing scientific research in an effort to better understand the anatomy, physiology, and pathological conditions of the human immune system (**Figure 12.21**). Research immunologists study cells and genes in the body and conduct tests to determine how different chemicals interact with these cells and genes.

A career as a research immunologist requires a PhD from a university with an accredited program in immunology. The PhD degree, which may take five or more years to complete, involves extensive coursework and study in the areas of molecular and cellular biology, biochemistry, bacteriology, virology, and biostatistics, as well as ethical issues in scientific research.

Some medical doctors specialize in caring for patients with diseases of the immune system. Allergists and rheumatologists are two examples of this kind of medical specialist. Allergists treat patients with allergies. Rheumatologists treat patients with connective tissue diseases, many of which are autoimmune diseases. Both allergists and rheumatologists are medical doctors who, after completing four years of college and four years of medical school, have also completed a residency in pediatrics or internal medicine (three years) plus a fellowship in allergy or rheumatology (usually another two years).

Eduard Kyslynskyy/Shutterstock.com

Figure 12.21 Research immunologists study immune systems and associated diseases, often with the goal of finding vaccines and drugs to cure or lessen the damage done by certain diseases. *Given what you now know about immunity, do you think this is a field of study that you would like to make part of your career? Why or why not?*

Some immunologists forge a career in academia. These individuals continue to participate in research while teaching students enrolled in medical school or in an advanced immunology degree program at a college or university. To serve as a faculty member or administrator in higher education, an immunologist must have either a PhD or medical doctor (MD) degree.

Oncologist

An oncologist has an extraordinarily difficult job: diagnosing cancer and treating patients throughout the course of their disease, from diagnosis to recovery or death. While medical and surgical oncologists have similar responsibilities, surgical oncologists are qualified to perform operations on patients.

Typical job duties for both the medical oncologist and the surgical oncologist include making cancer diagnoses, preparing case histories, keeping records of physical examinations and test results, writing prescriptions, and monitoring treatment plans (**Figure 12.22**). Usually, the oncologist coordinates a cancer treatment team, which may include nurses, physician assistants, radiologists, rehabilitation therapists, dieticians, and social workers. Oncologists explain cancer development stages to patients, help educate them about their disease, discuss treatment options, and assist in pain management.

A career as an oncologist requires an MD degree from an accredited medical school, followed by an internal medicine residency and an oncology fellowship. In addition, oncologists may obtain board certification from an appropriate organization to demonstrate professional competence in their field.

Planning for a Health-Related Career

Do some research on the career of an immunologist or oncologist, or select a profession from the list of **Related Career Options**. Using the Internet or resources at your local library, find answers to the following questions:

1. What are the main responsibilities of the career that you have chosen to research?
2. What is the outlook for this career? Are workers in demand, or are jobs dwindling? For complete information, consult the current edition of the *Occupational Outlook Handbook*.
3. What special skills or talents are required? For example, do you need to be good at subjects such as biology, chemistry, and anatomy and physiology? Do you need to enjoy interacting with other people?
4. What personality traits do you think are needed to be successful in this job? For example, some characteristics of an effective oncologist are compassion, excellent analytical and problem-solving skills, and the ability to make sound clinical judgments under emotional pressure.
5. Does this career involve a great deal of routine, or is there variety among the day-to-day responsibilities?

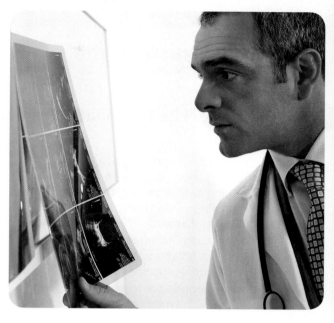

Auremar/Shutterstock.com

Figure 12.22 An important aspect of an oncologist's work is making a diagnosis. *What would be some advantages and disadvantages of a career in oncology?*

6. Does the work require long hours, or is it a standard, "9-to-5" job?
7. What is the salary range for this job?
8. What do you think you would like about this career? Is there anything about it that you might dislike?

Related Career Options

- Biochemist
- Biologist
- Epidemiologist
- Geneticist
- Hematologist
- Histologist
- Medical Physicist
- Medical Scientist
- Microbiologist
- Oncology Nurse
- Palliative Care Specialist
- Pathologist
- Pediatric Immunologist
- Pediatric Oncologist
- Radiation Therapist
- Radiologist
- Toxicologist
- Virologist

Chapter 12 Review and Assessment

Chapter Summaries

Build vocabulary with e-flash cards and games

Lesson 12.1 The Lymphatic System

Key Points

- The lymphatic system performs two vital functions in the human body: (a) it reabsorbs fluid from leaking capillaries and returns it to the cardiovascular system; and (b) it provides protection against disease.
- The lymphatic system includes lymphocytes, lymphatic vessels, lymphatic fluid, and lymphatic organs—lymph nodes, the spleen, and the thymus.
- There are two categories of lymphocytes: T lymphocytes and B lymphocytes.
- Natural killer cells and macrophages are important cells in maintaining the body's defenses.
- Lymph nodes cleanse the lymph by trapping harmful substances. Lymph nodes also produce and store T and B cells to help fight infection.

Key Terms

B lymphocytes
endothelial cells
interstitial fluid
lingual tonsils
lymph
lymph nodes
lymphatic nodules
lymphatic trunks
lymphatic valves
lymphatic vessels
lymphocytes

macrophages
mucosa-associated lymphatic tissue (MALT)
natural killer (NK) cells
palatine tonsils
pathogens
pharyngeal tonsil
spleen
T lymphocytes

Lesson 12.2 Nonspecific Defenses

Key Points

- The skin functions as a physical barrier against infectious agents, so when the integrity of your skin is breached, you are at a much greater risk for infection.
- Phagocytosis is the process by which cells engulf and destroy foreign matter and cellular debris.
- The complement system is made up of more than 30 proteins that circulate in the blood plasma and work together to destroy bacteria.
- Interferons are proteins released by cells that are infected with viruses. These proteins "interfere with" viral replication and spreading.

Key Terms

alternative pathway
classical pathway
complement proteins
complement system
exocytosis
fever
inflammatory response
interferons

mast cells
monocytes
neutrophils
opsonins
phagocytes
phagocytosis
prostaglandins
pyrogens

Lesson 12.3 Specific Defenses

Key Points

- The immune system is a complex system that is constantly finding, targeting, and eliminating bacteria, viruses, and other pathogens.

Key Terms

active immunity
antigen-presenting cells (APCs)
apoptosis

cellular immunity
clonal selection
humoral immunity
immune system

- Human immunity begins when a B cell encounters an antigen—anything that the immune system cells consider to be foreign—and binds to its specific antigen receptors.
- If a lymphocyte meets an antigen that matches its specific receptor cell, the lymphocyte binds with the antigen receptor to stimulate differentiation and clonal selection.
- Antibodies eliminate antigen threats with mechanisms such as neutralization, precipitation, agglutination, binding, and inflammation.
- A primary immune response occurs when the body is first exposed to a foreign invader. A secondary response occurs when the invader enters a second or subsequent time.
- In active immunity, antibodies are actively produced by the body's plasma cells. In passive immunity, antibodies are received from an outside source.

immunoglobulins
major histocompatibility complex glycoproteins (MHCs)
memory cells
passive immunity

precipitation
primary immune response
secondary immune response

Lesson 12.4 Disorders and Diseases of the Immune System

Key Points
- The process by which cancer spreads from its initial location to another part of the body via the lymphatic system is called *metastasis*.
- Allergies are caused by an inappropriately strong immune response.
- Some common autoimmune disorders are rheumatoid arthritis, multiple sclerosis, and type I diabetes.
- Human immunodeficiency virus (HIV) damages the immune system and compromises the body's ability to fight disease-causing organisms.

Key Terms
acquired immune deficiency syndrome (AIDS)
allergen
anaphylaxis
autoimmune disorder

human immunodeficiency virus (HIV)
immunotherapy
lymphedema
metastasis
opportunistic infection
tolerance

Chapter Assessments

Assess

Lesson 12.1

The Lymphatic System

Learning Key Terms and Concepts

1. What two vital functions does the lymphatic system perform in the human body?

2. *True or False?* The normal leakage rate of blood plasma across the entire body is 2 to 3 mL per minute.

3. *True or False?* Lymph formation begins with fluid that leaks out of blood vessel capillaries.

4. *True or False?* The human body has a pump similar to the heart that helps propel lymph through the network of lymph vessels.

5. Lymph from the thoracic duct drains into the _____ vein.

6. *True or False?* During the process of lymph drainage, lymphatic fluid never rejoins the blood to once again become blood plasma.

Thinking Critically

7. Assume you are a doctor talking to the parents of a high school football player with a ruptured spleen. Evaluate the causes and effects of this trauma in an explanation they could understand.

8. Explain the process that causes your lymph nodes to become swollen in response to exposure to an infection.

Lesson 12.2

Nonspecific Defenses

Learning Key Terms and Concepts

9. *True or False?* When skin has been cut or punctured, you are at a much greater risk for infection.

10. The process by which cells engulf and destroy foreign matter and cellular debris is called _____.
    A. exocytosis   C. inflammation
    B. phagocytosis   D. opsonization

11. _____ develop into macrophages when they leave the bloodstream and enter tissues.

12. The process by which cell membranes fuse together and then push debris from the cell vesicles to the outside of the cell is called _____.

13. The _____ is a set of more than 30 proteins that circulate in the blood plasma and work together to destroy bacteria.

14. The process by which complement proteins make cells more attractive to phagocytes is called _____.
    A. opsonization   C. phagocytosis
    B. activation   D. precipitation

15. *True or False?* A virus spreads by reproducing itself.

Thinking Critically

16. The complement system can be activated in two primary ways. Identify the two pathways and describe how each one is initiated.

Lesson 12.3

Specific Defenses

Learning Key Terms and Concepts

17. Where is the physical "home" of the immune system?

18. A(n) _____ is a large molecule on the surface of a cell that helps the body distinguish between "self" and "nonself" cells.

19. Which of the following *cannot* act as an antigen-presenting cell?
    A. macrophages   C. dendritic cells
    B. histamines   D. B cells

20. Where do T lymphocytes travel to complete their maturation?

21. A programmed process of cellular self-destruction is called _____.
    A. differentiation   C. apoptosis
    B. clonal selection   D. metastasis

22. *True or False?* Antibodies, also known as *immunoglobulins*, are Y-shaped.

23. How many classes of antibodies exist?

24. What do body cells display on their surface when they are infected by viruses or bacteria?

Thinking Critically

25. Explain how the immune system uses a vaccine to build a defense through the primary and secondary immune response.

26. Explain how clonal selection, or cloning of lymphocytes, works and what becomes of the clones.

Lesson 12.4

Disorders and Diseases of the Immune System

Learning Key Terms and Concepts

27. A cancer that has spread is said to be _____.

28. About what percentage of Americans have an allergy to one or more substances in the environment?

29. _____ is a hormone that opens up the airways and constricts the blood vessels.
    A. antihistamine   C. immunoglobulin
    B. anaphylaxis   D. epinephrine

30. A condition in which the immune system overreacts to an antigen that, in and of itself, does not pose an actual threat is called a(n) _____.

31. Which virus can lead to the development of AIDS?

32. Development of an immune system _____ of an antigen may reduce or eliminate an allergic response.

33. A severe allergic reaction that may include pulmonary obstruction and low blood pressure is called _____.

Thinking Critically

34. Describe the process by which a patient transitions from HIV-positive status to a diagnosis of AIDS.

Building Skills and Connecting Concepts

Analyzing and Evaluating Data

This chart gives the percentages of the population (between 15 and 49 years of age) infected with HIV in selected countries. Use the chart and your knowledge of geography (do some research if necessary) to answer the following questions.

35. What percentage of people between 15 and 49 years of age in the U.S. have contracted HIV? (Round your answer to the nearest whole number.)

36. List, in descending order, the six countries in the Western Hemisphere with the highest incidence of HIV, based on percentage of HIV infections.

37. Of the countries listed in the chart, is the average incidence of HIV greater in Asia or Europe?

38. What is the ratio of people in South Africa who have HIV compared to those in Japan, Germany, or China who have HIV?
    A. 64 to 1   C. 180 to 1
    B. 18 to 1   D. 22 to 1

Percentages of Age 15 to 49 Population with HIV in Select Countries			
Country	%	Country	%
Argentina	0.5	Japan	0.1
Canada	0.2	Mexico	0.3
Chile	0.4	Mozambique	11.5
China	0.1	Nigeria	3.6
Colombia	0.5	South Africa	17.8
France	0.4	United Kingdom	0.2
Germany	0.1	United States	0.6
India	0.3		

Communicating about Anatomy and Physiology

39. **Speaking** Debate the topic of vaccines for children. Divide into two groups. Each group should gather information in support of either the "pro" argument (children should be vaccinated) or the "con" argument (children should not be vaccinated). Use definitions and descriptions from this chapter to support your side of the debate and to clarify word meanings as necessary. You will want to do further research to find expert opinions, costs associated with vaccines, and other relevant information.

40. **Listening** As classmates deliver their presentations, listen carefully to their arguments. Take notes on important points and write down any questions that occur to you. Later, ask questions to obtain additional information or clarification from your classmates as necessary.

Lab Investigations

41. Using the information in your textbook and from websites approved by your instructor, create a tool for the parent(s) of a newborn child that offers a recommended vaccination schedule and allows the parent(s) to keep track of vaccinations. Be sure to add a calendar or other tracking method that could be helpful. Print out the tool and give a copy to each student in the class.

42. In addition to creating the tracking tool described above, prepare an information sheet that lists and describes each vaccine, the disease that the vaccine prevents, the potential side effects of the disease, and the potential side effects of the vaccine. Be sure to cite the research sources that you used to prepare your information sheet. Print out copies and share them with your classmates.

Expand your learning with additional online resources
- Supplemental Lab Activities
- Interactive Exercises
- Animations

www.g-wlearning.com/healthsciences

How does the food you eat become the energy you need?

The Digestive System and Nutrition

Chapter 13

 our body needs energy to function. Believe it or not, the source of that energy—the sun—is about 93 million miles away. The energy from sunlight is converted into chemicals by plants. The chemicals, including sugars such as glucose, fructose, and sucrose, store the energy. By eating plants and animals (that also eat plants), your body obtains the fuel it needs.

However, you need more than just energy to survive and thrive. You also need certain molecular building blocks that enable your body to grow and maintain itself. This is where your digestive system comes in. The digestive system brings all the molecules that you need into your body—including energy molecules.

Eating is the first step of the digestive process. Many more steps are involved in breaking down bite-sized fragments of food into microscopic pieces. These microscopic pieces are eventually absorbed into the blood. The digestive system also disposes of the parts of our food that cannot be absorbed by the body. In this chapter, we will learn how the structures and functions of the digestive system work together to process and store the energy and nutrients needed for a healthy body.

Chapter 13 Lessons

Lesson 13.1
Nutrition

Lesson 13.2
Anatomy and Physiology of the Digestive System

Lesson 13.3
Disorders and Diseases of the Digestive System

While studying, look for the online icon [↗] **to:**

- **Practice** with e-flash cards and vocabulary games
- **Review** with interactive art labeling
- **Assess** with online exercises
- **Expand** with interactive activities and animated videos
- **Listen** to pronunciations of key terms in the audio glossary

www.g-wlearning.com/healthsciences

Study on the Go

Use a mobile device to practice vocabulary terms, listen to pronunciations, and review with self-assessment quizzes.

www.m.g-wlearning.com

Nutrition

You may wonder why a chapter about the digestive system begins with a section about nutrition. The answer is that the digestive system exists to provide nutrients to the body. Earlier in this text, you read about the composition and function of blood before you studied the cardiovascular system. In this chapter, we will take a similar approach, studying the nutrients found in the food we eat, before examining the digestive system itself.

Energy

As you read this paragraph, your body is growing, moving, breathing, pumping blood, and staying warm. To perform these activities (and many others), your body needs **energy**, which is the ability of a physical system to do work.

Energy takes many forms. Heat is a form of energy, for example. Chemical energy, which is released during a chemical reaction, is the energy stored in the bonds of atoms and molecules. Kinetic energy is the energy of motion present in a moving object. Potential energy is stored energy, such as the energy stored in a stretched spring.

Measuring the Body's Energy Use

Just as there are many forms of energy, there are many ways to measure energy. For example, electric companies use a unit of measure called the *kilowatt hour* (*kWh*) to calculate energy usage by their customers. Energy is also measured in BTUs, or British thermal units.

Food scientists are interested in the potential energy found in foods. Food energy is often measured in terms of an item's capacity to produce heat. Heat energy is measured in

Calories or joules. In the metric system, the joule is the standard unit for measuring energy.

You're probably familiar with the term *calorie*. The type of calorie used by food scientists is written with a capital C. The **Calorie**, also called the *kilocalorie* (*kcal*), is used to measure the potential energy in foods. A single Calorie is equal to the amount of heat required to raise the temperature of 1 kilogram of water by 1°C.

Basal Metabolic Rate

The beating of your heart is an example of metabolic activity. The inspiration and expiration of air by your lungs is another example. Metabolic activities are the chemical and physical reactions that occur in an organism and that serve to keep it alive. The sum of these activities is referred to as *metabolism* (meh-TAB-oh-lizm).

To perform metabolic activities, your body needs energy. The amount of energy it needs varies. Not surprisingly, your body requires more energy when you are physically active than when you are asleep, reading, or watching television (**Figure 13.1**).

Scientists use a measure called the **basal metabolic rate (BMR)** to identify the amount of energy required to sustain a person's metabolism for one day if he or she is at complete rest.

BMR is expressed as Calories. For example, an average adult who weighs 150 pounds (68 kg) and has a body fat percentage of 25% (the fraction of body mass that is fat) will have a BMR of just under 1,500 Calories per day. If this person introduced any amount of activity into his or her day, a higher number of calories would be required.

BMR can differ significantly from one individual to the next. Factors that influence BMR include a person's age, gender, height, body mass, and body fat percentage. Because very few of us are inactive all day, our bodies require 20% to 70% more Calories than indicated by our BMR. The more active we are, the more energy and Calories we need. If you walk a mile, for example, your body will use about 50 Calories above your BMR.

Moderately active boys between 14 and 18 years of age need between 2,400 and 2,800 Calories a day. Girls in this age range need about 2,000 Calories per day. However, teenagers who are physically active need more energy. Each day, active boys need up to 3,200 Calories, whereas active girls need about 2,400 Calories.

Macronutrients, Vitamins, and Minerals

Nutrients are substances that the body needs for energy, growth, and maintenance. Water is a

A.

B.

Figure 13.1 One of the factors in BMR is activity level. A—At rest, the body needs less energy, or fewer Calories. B—The body needs more energy as activity level increases.

nutrient. Nutrients include **macronutrients**—the carbohydrates, proteins, and fats that you read about in chapter 2.

Vitamins and minerals are essential nutrients. Vitamins are organic compounds—carbon-based chemicals—that the body needs in small amounts to help regulate its processes. Minerals are elements, such as calcium and iron, that are required to maintain good health.

The *Dietary Guidelines for Americans* was created by the United States Department of Agriculture (USDA) and the US Department of Health and Human Services, with input from advisory panels of doctors and nutritionists. The guidelines state the levels of nutrients that you need to achieve a healthful diet. The *Dietary Guidelines* document is available online. Nutrition information can also be found by visiting the USDA's Food and Nutrition Information Center online, or by talking to the health and wellness teachers at your school.

Carbohydrates

Sugars and starches are foods, or ingredients in foods, that are classified as carbohydrates. Examples of sugar include fructose, which is found in fruits, and sucrose, more commonly known as table sugar. Some sources of starches include pasta, bread, and cereal (**Figure 13.2**). Once it has been fully digested, a gram of carbohydrate provides about 4 Calories of energy.

According to the USDA, about half of our energy should come from carbohydrates that are part of a healthful diet. No more than 25% of carbohydrate calories should come from sugars such as those found in soft drinks and other sweet foods. For example, if you consume a total of 2,000 Calories a day, about half of them should come from carbohydrates. This would equal about 250 grams (8 or 9 ounces) of carbohydrates per day. This does not mean that you should eat only 8 or 9 ounces of food. Remember that the 8 or 9 ounces is the weight of the carbohydrates alone. This measurement does not include, for example, the food's water weight, which is a significant part of the weight of most foods.

Tischenko Irina/Shutterstock.com

Figure 13.2 Bread is an example of a carbohydrate. *In a well-balanced diet, what percentage of energy comes from carbohydrates?*

 Check Your Understanding

1. How is kinetic energy different from potential energy?
2. What unit is used to count and measure energy in nutrition science?
3. How many Calories do moderately active teenage boys and girls need each day?
4. Which nutrients are classified as macronutrients?
5. Identify a food or ingredient that is a carbohydrate.

Proteins

Current dietary recommendations suggest that about a quarter of our energy be derived from proteins. As you learned in chapter 2, proteins are made of amino acids. There are 20 common amino acids in the human body. A protein contains varying amounts of the 20 amino acids. Nine of the amino acids are considered essential for adults, and twelve are considered essential for children. The body can produce nonessential amino acids if sufficient amounts of essential amino acids are present.

Meat, which is composed mostly of protein, provides a well-balanced mix of all 20 amino acids (**Figure 13.3**). You can also obtain sufficient protein, with all the essential amino acids, by eating a healthful vegetarian diet that includes legumes (beans, peas, or soy) and grains (rice, corn, or wheat).

Each gram of protein provides about 4 Calories of energy. In a diet of 2,000 Calories per day, this translates to 500 Calories, or 125 grams (about 4½ ounces) of protein per day.

Fats (Lipids)

Fats, or *lipids*, include oils and solid fats. As you learned in chapter 2, fats contain combinations of different types of fatty acids— saturated and unsaturated. Most saturated fatty acids come from animal sources, such as meats and dairy products. Some oils that come from plants, such as coconut oil and palm oil, are high in saturated fatty acids.

Most unsaturated fatty acids come from plant sources. Unsaturated fatty acids are classified as **monounsaturated fats**, **polyunsaturated fats**, or **trans-unsaturated fats**. Corn and soybean oils are high in polyunsaturated fatty acids (**Figure 13.4**). Canola oil and olive oil are high in monounsaturated fatty acids. The majority of trans-unsaturated fats, or *trans fats*, are artificially produced.

Most fats that contain a high percentage of saturated and trans fats are solid at room temperature. Fats that contain a high percentage of monounsaturated and polyunsaturated fatty acids tend to be liquid at room temperature.

Many scientific studies have shown that diets high in saturated fatty acids and trans fats are unhealthful, especially for the cardiovascular system. Several studies have established the benefits of replacing saturated fats and trans fats in the diet with naturally unsaturated fats, especially monounsaturated fats.

Each gram of fat delivers about 9 Calories of energy—or about twice as much energy per

Figure 13.3 Meat is one of the best dietary sources of protein and amino acids. *What are good sources of protein and amino acids for vegetarians?*

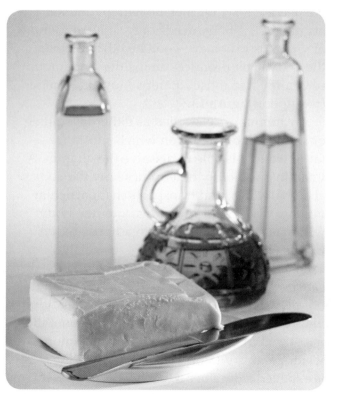

Figure 13.4 Oils and fats are a necessary part of a healthy diet, but they should be used sparingly. *Which types of fats should be avoided to maintain a healthy diet?*

Memory Tip
Saturated fats are called *saturated* because their hydrocarbon chains are fully loaded, or *saturated*, with hydrogen atoms. Unsaturated fats are not fully loaded, or saturated, with hydrogen atoms.

gram as a carbohydrate or protein. The *Dietary Guidelines for Americans* suggest that people between 4 and 18 years of age obtain a maximum of 25% to 35% of their total calories in the form of fats. Therefore, if you consume 2,000 Calories a day, you should limit your intake of fats to 55.5 grams, or about 2 ounces. The guidelines also state that people who eat a healthful diet overall should keep their intake of saturated fats and trans fats to a minimum.

Vitamins

Vitamins are organic chemicals that are needed for your metabolism to function normally. The body needs only small amounts of vitamins to achieve good health. However, the body itself produces an insufficient amount of vitamins, so most vitamins must be obtained from food (**Figure 13.5**).

Vitamins are classified as either fat soluble or water soluble based on which substance—fat or water—is able to dissolve the vitamin. A vitamin's solubility determines how the body absorbs, stores, and transports that particular vitamin. Fat-soluble vitamins enter the body with fats and can be stored in adipose tissue. Excess fat-soluble vitamins are not easily excreted from the body; they can be toxic, causing infection or disease. By contrast, fat does not play a role in the absorption of water-soluble vitamins. Water-soluble vitamins are generally not stored in the body. If you consume more water-soluble vitamins than you need, the excess is expelled from the body in urine.

Most water-soluble vitamins are **coenzymes** (koh-EHN-zighmz). A coenzyme is a molecule that combines with a protein to make a working enzyme. This coenzyme-protein combination can catalyze a chemical reaction.

Brian Chase/Shutterstock.com

Figure 13.5 Fruits and vegetables contain many of the vitamins and minerals that your body needs.

The table in **Figure 13.6** lists and describes the functions of some of the vitamins that your body needs. Your recommended daily vitamin intake depends on your age, gender, and health status. Long-term lack of a particular vitamin is called a **vitamin deficiency**. Certain health problems are related to vitamin deficiency. For example, a vitamin D deficiency can cause osteoporosis, muscle weakness, or high blood pressure.

Minerals

Like vitamins, **minerals** are elements that the body needs in relatively small amounts; yet they are essential for the proper functioning of the body. Both vitamins and minerals are classified as **micronutrients**.

The average daily recommended intake for different minerals varies. For example, about 4,700 mg of potassium is recommended each day. However, other minerals have daily recommended doses of only fractions of a milligram.

Figure 13.6 Micronutrients and Their Functions*

Water-Soluble Vitamins

Thiamine (B_1)	Coenzyme that works in multiple body systems; needed for many biochemical reactions including ATP-generating reactions; needed for the synthesis of acetylcholine, a chemical used by nervous system cells
Riboflavin (B_2)	Coenzyme that works in multiple body systems; needed for cellular reactions in eyes, skin, intestinal epithelia, and blood cells
Niacin (B_3)	Coenzyme that works in multiple body systems; needed for breakdown of fats and for skin cell metabolism
B_6	Coenzyme that works in multiple body systems; needed for chemical reactions involving amino acids (the building blocks of proteins)
B_{12}	Plays a role in the formation of red blood cells and in chemical reactions involving nucleic acids (the building blocks of DNA and RNA)
Folate (Folic acid, B_9)	Needed for chemical reactions involving amino acids and nucleic acids
Pantothenic acid (B_5)	Coenzyme that works in multiple body systems; used in the creation of several hormones; needed for biochemical processing of carbohydrates, lipids, and amino acids
Ascorbic acid (C)	Promotes protein synthesis, including collagen formation; an antioxidant that neutralizes free radicals, highly reactive chemicals that could otherwise cause damage

Fat-Soluble Vitamins

A	Helps form a light-sensitive chemical in the eyes; helps epithelial cells grow normally
D	Aids calcium and phosphorous absorption in the intestine, and prevents loss of those elements in the urine; needed for bone growth
E	Inhibits the breakdown of cell membranes; needed for red blood cell formation and for formation of DNA and RNA; an antioxidant that neutralizes free radicals
K	Plays a major role in blood clotting

Minerals

Calcium (Ca)	Helps form and maintain healthy bones and teeth; decreases the risk of developing some cancers; plays a role in regulation of blood pressure and immune system function
Fluoride (F)	Supports the deposition of calcium and phosphorus in bones and teeth; helps prevent cavities
Iodine (I)	A component of thyroid hormones that controls the regulation of body temperature, BMR, growth, and reproduction
Iron (Fe)	Part of hemoglobin and myoglobin, which transport oxygen in the body; component of many enzymes; essential for brain growth and function
Phosphorus (Ph)	An essential component of ATP; helps form and maintain healthy bones; helps activate and deactivate enzymes; a component of DNA and RNA
Potassium (K)	Plays a role in muscle contractions and the transmission of nerve impulses; helps regulate blood pressure
Sodium (Na)	Helps regulate water distribution and blood pressure; involved in nerve transmission and muscle function; aids in the absorption of some nutrients

*The functions listed for each micronutrient do not represent a complete list.

Minerals that are vital for good health include calcium and phosphorus, which are major components of bone. Iron helps red blood cells transport oxygen. Sodium is another required mineral, although the amount of sodium that the body needs is a subject of debate in the medical community.

Adults require about 1,000 mg of sodium per day. Government health organizations recommend that most people keep their sodium intake below 1,500 mg per day. However, most Americans consume an average of 3,400 mg of sodium each day because their diets are high in salt, or *sodium chloride*. Many Americans frequently eat high-salt foods, such as processed foods and meals from fast-food restaurants.

Strong evidence links a high-sodium diet to high blood pressure. People with high blood pressure have an increased risk of developing cardiovascular disease. The American Heart Association recommends that we strive to reduce our sodium intake.

 Check Your Understanding

1. What are the building blocks of proteins?
2. What are sources of saturated fatty acids?

Lesson 13.1 Review and Assessment

Mini Glossary   Make sure that you know the meaning of each key term.

 Build vocabulary with e-flash cards and games

basal metabolic rate the amount of energy required to sustain a person's metabolism for one day if he or she is at complete rest; also known as *BMR*

Calorie the unit that food scientists use to measure the potential energy in foods; the amount of heat required to raise the temperature of 1 kilogram of water by 1°C; also called *kilocalorie*

coenzymes molecules that are necessary for the action of enzymes

energy the capacity of a physical system to do work

fats substances found in foods that include oils and solid fats; can be classified either as saturated or unsaturated; also called *lipids*

macronutrients substances such as carbohydrates, proteins, and fats that the body requires in relatively large quantities

micronutrients vitamins and minerals that are essential to the body in small amounts

minerals elements that the body needs in relatively small amounts

monounsaturated fats one category of unsaturated fatty acids; sources include canola oil and olive oil

nutrients chemicals that the body needs for energy, growth, and maintenance

polyunsaturated fats one category of unsaturated fatty acids; sources include corn oil and soybean oil

trans-unsaturated fats one category of unsaturated fatty acids that are artificially produced; also called *trans fats*

vitamin deficiency the long-term lack of a particular vitamin in one's diet; may result in certain health problems

vitamins organic chemicals needed by the body for normal functioning and good health

Know and Understand

 Assess

1. List four different forms of energy.
2. List some of the factors that affect a person's basal metabolic rate (BMR).
3. Explain why some nutrients are called *micronutrients*.
4. Why should people limit their intake of sodium?
5. According to current dietary recommendations, how much of a person's energy should be obtained from protein?

Analyze and Apply

6. Explain why people need more energy each day than indicated by their BMR.

7. Compare and contrast saturated and unsaturated fats.
8. Explain why a person requires only small amounts of vitamins in his or her diet.

In the Lab

9. Suppose that you are a dietitian and one of your patients recently suffered a heart attack. Tests show that your patient, who eats a high-fat diet, has significant plaque buildup in his arteries. Research low-fat diets and create a diet plan for your patient. Include healthful options for each meal (breakfast, lunch, and dinner), as well as for snacks.

Lesson 13.2 Anatomy and Physiology of the Digestive System

Lesson 13.2

Before You Read

Try to answer the following questions before you read this lesson.

Can you live without a gallbladder?

What role does the liver play in digestion?

Lesson Objectives

1. Identify the organs of the digestive system and explain their functions.
2. Describe how food is digested and absorbed.

Key Terms

E-Flash Cards

absorption
alimentary canal
chemical breakdown
chyme
colon
defecation
emulsification
esophagus
gallbladder

gastrointestinal tract
gingiva
ingestion
large intestine
mechanical breakdown
propulsion
rectum
small intestine
stomach

The digestive system consists of a tube running through the body with organs alongside it. Most of these organs secrete substances into the tube. Food goes in one end, is broken down, and is partly absorbed. The portions that are not absorbed exit through the other end of the tube.

This may be a very simple view of the digestive system, but it's a starting point. By the time you finish this lesson, you will be able to describe the structure and function of the digestive system in much greater detail.

The tube that runs through the body is called the **alimentary** (al-i-MEHN-ter-ee) **canal**, also known as the **gastrointestinal** (GAS-troh-in-TEHS-tin-ahl) **tract** (*GI tract*). The GI tract begins with the mouth and ends with the anus. The primary organs of the digestive system located between the mouth and anus include the pharynx (commonly known as the *throat*), esophagus, stomach, small intestine, and large intestine.

Besides these primary organs, the digestive system includes accessory organs of digestion, such as the salivary glands, pancreas, liver, and gallbladder. These accessory organs are connected to the GI tract by ducts. The accessory organs secrete substances through the ducts that aid in chemical breakdown and absorption of food. **Figure 13.7** on the next page shows an overview of the alimentary canal and accessory organs of digestion. In total, the GI tract is approximately 9 meters (30 feet) long.

Activities of Digestion

There are different ways of looking at how the digestive system processes food. To help you understand how the system works, we'll divide the digestion process into six different activities. **Figure 13.8** on page 461 depicts these activities.

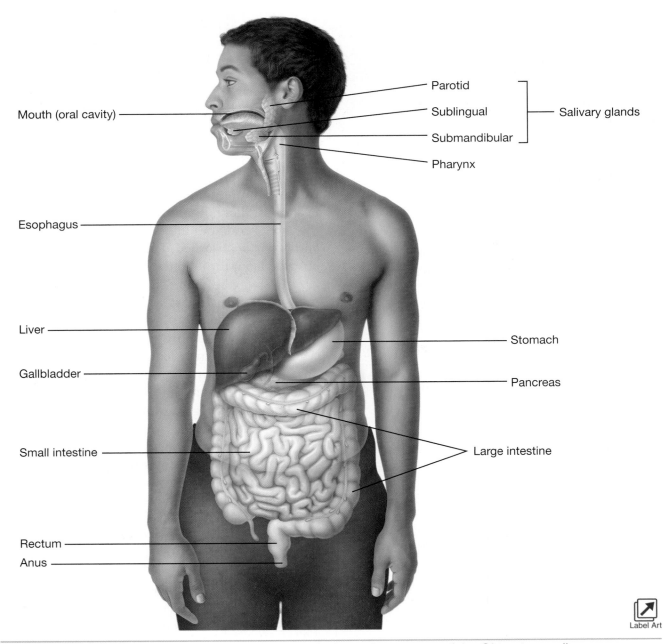

Figure 13.7 The organs of the digestive system include those that are part of the GI tract as well as accessory, or helper, organs that aid in digestion and nutrient absorption. *Which organs shown here are considered accessory organs, and are not part of the alimentary canal?*

The first activity in the process of digestion is **ingestion**—getting the food into the body. Ingestion involves the mouth, including the teeth, lips, and tongue.

Propulsion begins after ingestion and continues all the way along the GI tract. Propulsion is initiated by swallowing at the pharynx and peristalsis (PER-i-STAHL-sis), the symmetrical contraction of muscles that moves food along the remainder of the GI tract.

The actual "digesting," or breaking down of the food particles, occurs in two ways: mechanical and chemical breakdown. **Mechanical breakdown** reduces food into smaller pieces and increases the surface area of the food. Chewing, churning in the stomach, and

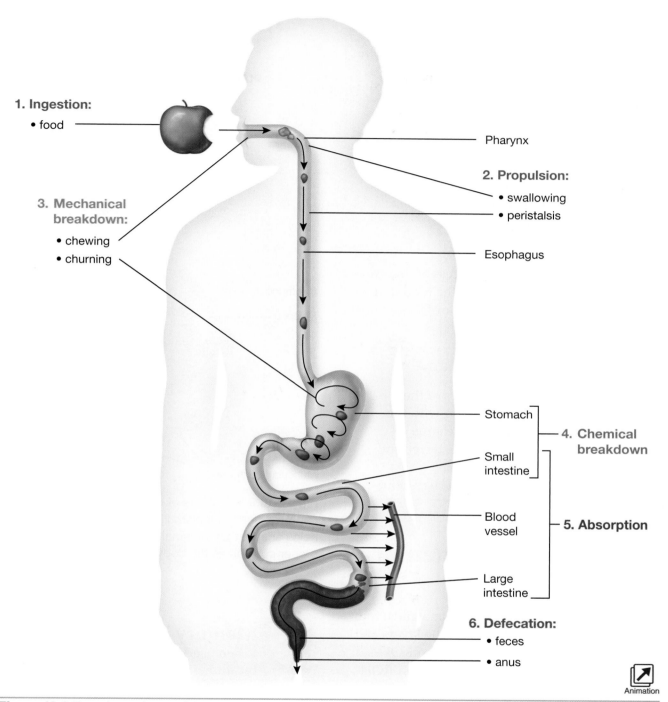

1. Ingestion:
- food

3. Mechanical breakdown:
- chewing
- churning

Pharynx

2. Propulsion:
- swallowing
- peristalsis

Esophagus

Stomach

Small intestine

4. Chemical breakdown

Blood vessel

5. Absorption

Large intestine

6. Defecation:
- feces
- anus

Animation

Figure 13.8 From ingestion to defecation, there are six activities involved in digestion. *What process moves food into and through the GI tract during the propulsion stage?*

further churning by muscular contraction in the small intestine all contribute to the mechanical breakdown of food.

The **chemical breakdown** of food is the part of the process that historically has been referred to as *digestion*. Enzymes in the lumen—the central opening of the alimentary canal into the stomach—and on the walls of the GI tract break large food molecules into smaller molecules.

Absorption, the fifth step in digestion, involves the movement of small food molecules from the lumen of the small intestine into the blood. Once absorption has occurred, the blood carries the food to other parts of the body.

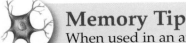

Memory Tip

When used in an anatomical sense, the word *lumen* means "the open space inside a hollow tubular structure," such as the intestine or a blood vessel. At the hardware store, you will see the word *lumens* listed on a lightbulb package. In this context, the number of lumens indicates the brightness of the bulb. *Lumen* is Latin for "light." If the alimentary canal is a tunnel, then you could say there is light at the end of the tunnel—the lumens at the end of the lumen!

The final activity in the process of digestion is **defecation**—the expulsion of the food that was not absorbed. This waste matter, or feces, exits the body via the anus.

✔ Check Your Understanding

1. List the organs or structures of the alimentary canal, beginning with the mouth and ending with the anus.
2. Approximately how long is the entire GI tract?
3. List the accessory organs of digestion.

Layers of the Alimentary Canal

The walls of the alimentary canal have four basic layers. From the inside out, the layers are the *mucosa*, the *submucosa* (SUB-myoo-KOH-sa), the *muscularis externa*, and the *serosa* (seh-ROH-sa). These layers are shown in **Figure 13.9**.

Mucosa

The mucosa, or *mucous membrane*, is layered as well. The mucosa has an innermost layer of epithelial tissue, whose surface is covered by mucus secreted by cells or glands. The mucosa also has a slightly deeper layer of areolar connective tissue. This tissue contains blood vessels, lymphatic vessels, nerves, and, in some areas of the body, mucus-secreting glands.

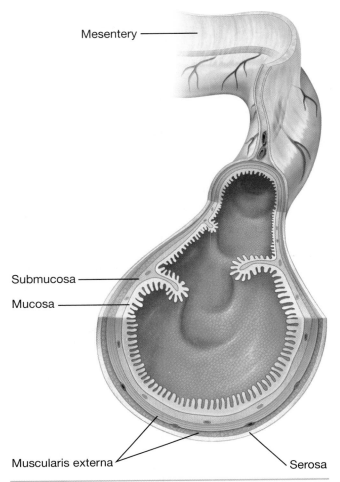

Figure 13.9 The layers of the walls of the alimentary canal, as seen in the small intestine. The mesentery helps ensure that the small intestines maintain their proper position as the body twists and moves.

Memory Tip

When used to describe the layers of the alimentary canal walls, the word *deeper* means "farther away from" the lumen. The submucosa, whose name means "under the mucosa," is deeper than the mucosa. Thus, the submucosa is farther from the lumen than the mucosa.

A surgeon who has entered the abdominal cavity and is cutting into the alimentary canal will first slice into the serosa, then the muscularis externa, followed by the submucosa, and finally the mucosa. After cutting the mucosa, the surgeon will have reached the lumen.

Submucosa

Below the mucosa lies the submucosa, a layer of irregular, dense connective tissue containing blood vessels, lymphatic vessels, and nerves. Lymphatic tissue and glands in some parts of the submucosa in the alimentary canal secrete substances that aid in digestion and absorption.

Muscularis Externa

The muscularis (MUS-kyoo-LAH-ris) externa surrounds the submucosal layer. In most of the alimentary canal, the muscularis externa has two layers of smooth muscle. The muscularis externa propels food through the alimentary canal by means of peristalsis. Mechanical breakdown of the food is also done by the muscularis externa as it churns and segments the food.

The inner muscle layer (closer to the lumen) has fibers that run in a circular manner around the lumen. The outer layer of muscle has fibers that run longitudinally, or lengthwise, along the canal. The layer of nerve fibers between the two layers regulates the activity of each layer.

Serosa

The outermost layer of the alimentary canal is the serosa. The serosa is so named because it is a serous membrane. Serous membranes are thin, slippery membranes that help minimize friction between organs and between organs and the body cavity wall (**Figure 13.10**).

In the abdominopelvic cavity, which contains most of the organs of digestion, the serous membrane is also known as the *peritoneum* (PER-i-toh-NEE-um).

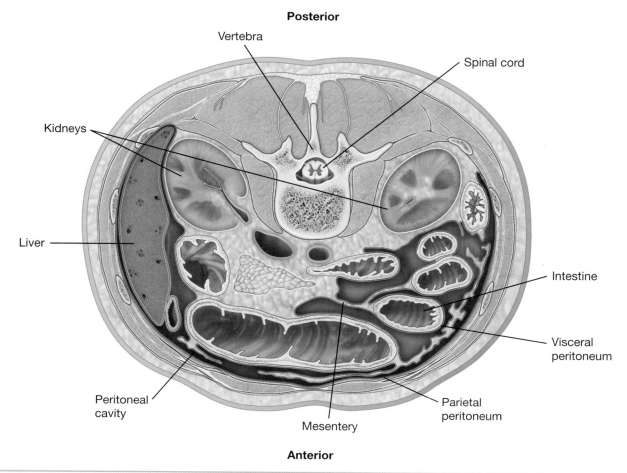

Figure 13.10 Transverse view of the abdominopelvic cavity. Some abdominal organs, such as the kidneys and pancreas are retroperitoneal; that is, they lie behind the peritoneum.

The peritoneum is divided into two layers—the parietal and visceral peritoneum. The parietal peritoneum is the part of the peritoneum that lines the body wall. The visceral peritoneum wraps around the organs and forms the outer layer of those organs.

The parietal and visceral peritoneum are connected to each other by the *mesentery* (MEHS-ehn-TER-ee), a double layer of peritoneum (**Figure 13.10** on the previous page). Blood and lymphatic vessels and nerves travel in the mesentery between the dorsal body wall and the organs of digestion. The mesentery also helps hold the abdominopelvic organs in their proper place, particularly the small intestine.

The "empty space" between the parietal and visceral peritoneum is called the *peritoneal* (PER-i-toh-NEE-al) *cavity*. It is filled with a watery fluid that allows the organs to move with minimal friction. Some organs—the kidneys and pancreas, for example—lie against the dorsal wall of the abdominopelvic cavity. These organs are said to be *retroperitoneal* (or "behind the peritoneum"), as **Figure 13.10** shows.

Digestive Organs and Their Functions

The digestive process involves several organs throughout the body. Some organs play a major role, while others aid in the process of digesting and absorbing nutrients. Let's take a closer look at the major organs of the digestive system.

The Oral Cavity

The mouth is also called the *oral cavity* (**Figure 13.11**). The mouth helps accomplish four of the six key activities of digestion:
- *ingestion* of food;
- *mechanical breakdown* of food (by chewing);
- *chemical breakdown* of food (by enzymes in the saliva); and
- *propulsion* of food (by pushing food back to the pharynx for swallowing).

The epithelial lining of the mouth is a mucous membrane called the *mucosa*, which you learned about earlier in this lesson.

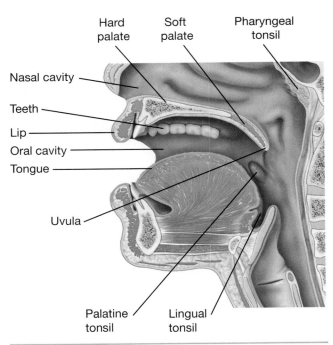

Figure 13.11 The oral cavity houses many digestive "tools" that begin the chemical and mechanical breakdown of food.

The lips assist with ingestion by grabbing food and pulling it into the mouth. The lips also keep food and liquids from leaking out of the mouth. The lips contain the *orbicularis* (or-BIK-yoo-LAH-ris) *oris* muscle. Like all skeletal muscles, this muscle is under voluntary control.

Anyone who has ever lost function in the lips understands the importance of this seemingly small body part. Loss of lip function can happen to a patient who has had a stroke. Strokes sometimes affect the nerves that control the lip muscles.

The tongue, like the lips, contains skeletal muscles. It has bumps, or *papillae*, on its surface. Some papillae house taste buds, whereas other papillae simply help the tongue grip food better. Besides providing us with our sense of taste, the tongue aids digestion in a couple of ways. It manipulates food in the mouth and moves chewed food to the back of the mouth for swallowing.

The cheeks form the lateral (side) borders of the oral cavity. The palate is the roof of the oral cavity. The front part of the palate, which is formed from parts of the maxillae (plural of maxilla) and palatine bones, is called the *hard palate*. The more posterior portion of the palate is called the *soft palate*. The soft palate is formed from a fold of mucous membrane.

The Nasal Cavity

The nasal cavity, the passageway for air entering and leaving via the nose, is located above the palate. When you look in your mouth, you can see the *uvula* (YOO-vyoo-la) hanging from the soft palate in the back. The uvula helps prevent food from entering the nasal cavity when we swallow.

Teeth and Gums

We use our teeth to begin the mechanical breakdown of food. When food is mechanically broken down into smaller pieces, its surface area is increased. The enlarged surface area helps digestive enzymes chemically break down the food. The gum, or **gingiva** (JIN-ji-vuh), is a soft tissue that covers the necks of the teeth and the maxilla (upper jaw) and mandible (lower jaw).

Children have 20 deciduous (temporary) teeth, which start to appear at around six months of age and are usually all visible by approximately two years of age. Starting around six years of age, 32 permanent teeth begin to form in the jawbones—16 in the mandible and

16 in the maxilla. As permanent teeth grow, they push out the deciduous teeth. The last permanent teeth, the wisdom teeth, usually do not appear until the late teens or early twenties.

The front four teeth on the top and bottom of the mouth are called *incisors*. Just lateral and posterior to the incisors, on each side of the mouth, are the canine teeth. Two molars follow each canine and complete a child's deciduous set of teeth, or *dentition*.

The permanent dentition adds two premolars, or *bicuspids*, between the canines and the molars. A third molar, commonly known as a *wisdom tooth*, is also added to each side of the mouth (**Figure 13.12**).

The incisors are shaped to be good at cutting. The molars are good at crushing and grinding. The canines and premolars are

Deciduous teeth

- Central incisor
- Lateral incisor
- Canine
- First molar
- Second molar

Permanent teeth

- Central incisor
- Lateral incisor
- Canine
- First premolar (bicuspid)
- Second premolar (bicuspid)
- First molar
- Second molar
- Third molar (wisdom tooth)

Figure 13.12 Deciduous teeth are eventually replaced by permanent teeth. The same permanent teeth appear on both the maxilla and mandible bones. *At what age do the permanent teeth begin to appear?*

Memory Tip

Many structures in and around the mouth contain the root word *-glosso-* or *-lingua-*, both of which refer to the tongue:

- The hypoglossal (HIGH-poh-GLAHS-al) and glossopharyngeal (GLAHS-oh-fah-RIN-jee-al) nerves go to the tongue region.
- The genioglossus (JEH-nee-oh-GLAHS-us) and hyoglossus (HIGH-oh-GLAHS-us) muscles form part of the tongue.
- The lingual frenulum (LING-gwahl FREHN-yoo-lum) is the thin band of tissue under the tongue that helps anchor it in the oral cavity.
- The lingual tonsil is at the back of the base of the tongue.

intermediate, with the canines more adapted for cutting and the premolars more adapted for grinding and crushing.

The Anatomy of the Tooth. The part of the tooth that projects out of the jawbone is called the *crown*. The part embedded in the jawbone is the *root*. The middle part, located between the crown and the root, is the *neck* (**Figure 13.13**).

The crown of each tooth has a coating of *enamel*. Enamel is the hardest material in the body, considerably harder than bone. The body of the tooth is made of *dentin*, a material that is similar to but harder and denser than bone. The *pulp cavity* is a hollow central region containing soft tissue, nerves, and blood vessels. The hollow *root canal* provides a passageway for nerves and blood vessels to reach the pulp cavity from the mandible (lower jaw) or maxilla (upper jaw). The nerves that occupy the pulp cavity alert us to oral pain or sensitivity by sending these signals via the nervous system.

Each tooth is securely anchored in its bony socket by the *periodontal* (PER-ee-oh-DAHN-tal) *ligament*, a meshwork of collagen fibers surrounding each root. Each incisor and canine has a single root; each premolar has one or two roots; and each molar has two or three roots.

Check Your Understanding

1. List the layers of the walls of the alimentary canal, starting with the innermost layer.
2. How do the lips assist with ingestion?
3. What are *papillae*?
4. To which digestive organ do the root words *-glosso-* or *-lingua-* refer?
5. How many permanent teeth are found in a healthy adult mouth?

Salivary Glands

The first accessory organs of digestion that contribute to the chemical breakdown of food are the three pairs of salivary glands (**Figure 13.7**).

Figure 13.13 The structure of a tooth. *What material is harder than bone and protects the crown of a tooth?*

Memory Tip

Many enzymes have names that end with the suffix *-ase*. These enzymes usually break down a molecule into smaller parts. *Proteases* break down proteins (long chains of amino acids) into short amino acid chains. *Lipases* break down lipids into free fatty acids and glycerol. *Amylases* break down starches (long chains of sugar subunits) into progressively shorter chains, ultimately producing chains that are two or three subunits long.

The salivary glands are located within the tissues surrounding the oral cavity. They secrete saliva into the mouth via connecting ducts.

The parotid (pa-RAHT-id) glands, the largest salivary glands, lie under the skin just below and in front of the ears. The submandibular (SUB-man-DIB-yoo-lar) salivary glands lie on the medial side of the lower back part of the mandible. The sublingual salivary glands are under each side of the tongue.

Saliva is composed mostly of water. It also contains mucus, antibodies, and several enzymes, including salivary amylase (AM-il-ays) and lingual lipase (LIGH-pays). The water and mucus help moisten food, while the antibodies protect the mouth against bacterial infection. Salivary amylase breaks down complex carbohydrates (also called *starches*) into shorter chains of sugar subunits. Lingual lipase initiates the chemical breakdown of fats.

The functions of saliva include
- moistening and lubricating food, making it easier to taste and swallow;
- protecting the mouth against bacteria; and
- initiating the chemical breakdown of food.

Pharynx

The pharynx (FAIR-ingks) is the region that connects the mouth and the nasal cavity to the trachea and the esophagus (**Figure 13.14**). As you learned in chapter 9, the pharynx plays an important role in respiration as well as digestion. From top to bottom, the pharynx is composed of three main parts:
- The nasopharynx (NAY-zoh-FAIR-ingks) connects the nasal cavity to the oropharynx. Only air passes through the nasopharynx.
- The oropharynx (OR-oh-FAIR-ingks) lies at the back of the mouth. Food, liquids, and air pass through the oropharynx.

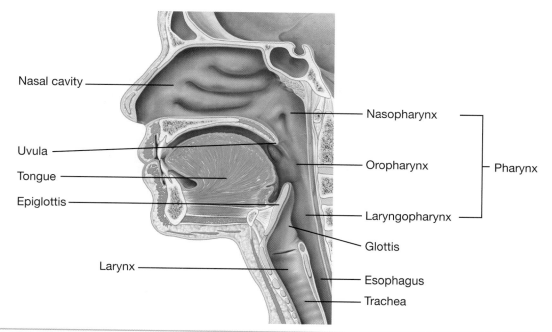

Figure 13.14 The pharynx is divided into three sections—the nasopharynx, oropharynx, and laryngopharynx. *The pharynx connects the mouth and nasal cavity to which structures?*

- The laryngopharynx (la-RING-goh-FAIR-ingks) includes the *glottis* (GLAHT-is)—the opening to the larynx and trachea—and extends down to the top of the esophagus.

The epiglottis is a fold of tissue on the front side of the oropharynx and laryngopharnx. Food, liquids, and air pass through the oropharynx and laryngopharynx. During the act of swallowing, coordinated contractions of the longitudinal and circular muscle layers in the walls of the pharynx push food through the pharynx and on to the esophagus. As food or liquid is swallowed, the epiglottis contracts downward to cover the glottis so that neither the food nor the liquid enters the trachea, or *airway*.

Figure 13.11 shows the tonsils, small bundles of lymphatic tissue. Like fortresses full of guards, the tonsils are full of lymphocytes that protect us from infection. The pharyngeal tonsil, located on the posterior wall of the nasopharynx, is often referred to as the *adenoid*. A palatine tonsil lies on each side of the entrance to the oropharnyx. The lingual tonsil is located at the base of the tongue, in the oropharynx.

Esophagus

The **esophagus** (eh-SAHF-a-gus) is a muscular tube that connects the pharynx to the stomach (**Figure 13.7**). It lies posterior to the trachea and heart and passes through an opening in the diaphragm, the muscle that separates the thoracic (chest) and abdominal cavities.

Just below the diaphragm, the esophagus reaches the stomach. When food enters the top of the esophagus during the act of swallowing, a wave of peristalsis begins. This wave of muscular contraction pushes food downward and into the stomach.

Stomach

The **stomach** is a reservoir in which food is broken down both mechanically and chemically before it enters the small intestine (**Figure 13.15**). Major regions of the stomach include the *cardia*, the *fundus*, the *body*, and the *pyloric region*.

The cardia (a term meaning "near the heart") is the region closest to the opening of the esophagus.

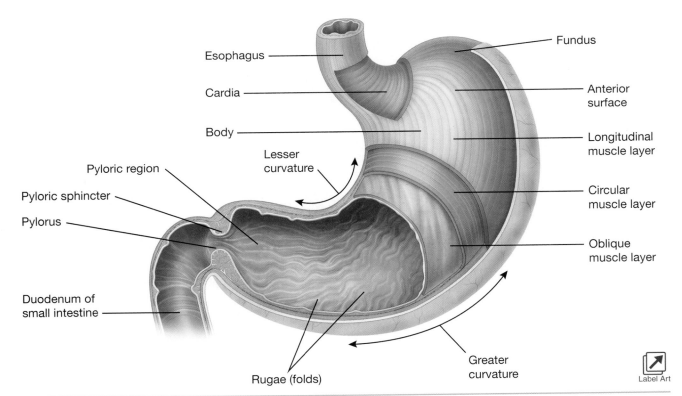

Figure 13.15 The stomach contains three layers of muscle, unlike most of the GI tract, which only has two layers. *What is the purpose of the oblique muscle layer in the wall of the stomach?*

The fundus is the upper end of the stomach, the body is the middle part, and the pyloric region is at the lower end.

The empty stomach has an internal volume of about 50 ml (1⅔ oz.). However, the folds of the inside wall, called *rugae* (ROO-gee), are able to flatten. As the stomach stretches, the rugae flatten, increasing the stomach's volume. When full, the stomach can hold two liters or more, and the rugae flatten until they almost disappear.

The wall of the stomach contains three layers of muscle, unlike most of the GI tract, which has only longitudinal and circular muscle. The extra layer, called the *oblique* (ahb-LEEK) muscle layer because its fibers run diagonally, sits beneath the circular and longitudinal muscle layers. The oblique muscle layer helps the stomach churn food and remains strong even when stretched.

The *pylorus* (pi-LOR-us) is the opening from the stomach into the small intestine. The wall of the pylorus contains the pyloric sphincter, a ring of circular, smooth muscle that must relax to allow food to pass into the small intestine.

Lining of the Stomach. The lining of the stomach is a simple columnar epithelium made of mucus-secreting cells. (For a review of columnar epithelial tissue, see chapter 2.) A microscopic view of the stomach lining reveals millions of tiny openings called *gastric pits* (**Figure 13.16**). Each opening leads to a tubular *gastric gland* that secretes *gastric juice*. Gastric juice is also secreted as part of a parasympathetic nervous system response—seeing, smelling, and tasting food alerts the nervous system that digestion is about to begin.

The cells lining the gastric pits secrete mucus. The cells lining the gastric gland include mucus-secreting cells, parietal cells, chief cells, and enteroendocrine cells. The parietal

Figure 13.16 The lining of the stomach contains gastric pits and gastric glands. A gastric pit is a tubular opening in the stomach lining that connects to a deeper tubular gastric gland.

cells secrete hydrochloric acid (HCl) and a glycoprotein called *intrinsic factor* that helps the body absorb vitamin B_{12}. The chief cells secrete the protein pepsinogen (pehp-SIN-oh-jehn). Enteroendocrine cells produce the hormone *gastrin* (GAS-trin), which stimulates the secretion of more gastric juice.

Hydrochloric acid secreted by the parietal cells makes the stomach contents very acidic, with a typical pH of 1.5 to 2.5. This acidic environment helps kill bacteria and aids in the conversion of inactive pepsinogen to active pepsin, a protein-digesting enzyme.

Chemical Reactions in the GI Tract and Stomach. The secretion of protein-digesting enzymes in the GI tract creates a potentially dangerous situation: the enzymes could start digesting, or breaking down, the body's own tissues. Our bodies are able to avoid this dangerous situation as long as adequate mucus is produced. The mucus lines the stomach wall and protects it from the eroding effects of hydrochloric acid and other protein-digesting enzymes such as pepsin.

When food enters the stomach, it mixes with the acidic gastric juice to form **chyme** (kighm). Active contractions of the muscular wall keep the mixture well stirred. Pepsin breaks down proteins in the food into shorter amino acid chains. Intrinsic factor binds to any vitamin B_{12} molecules present, enabling the vitamin to be absorbed when it later reaches the small intestine. The hormone gastrin, and nerve impulses on the vagus nerve, both stimulate secretion of gastric juice and churning activity of the stomach muscles. Relaxation of the pyloric sphincter allows chyme to enter the small intestine.

✔ Check Your Understanding

1. Which pair of salivary glands is the largest?
2. List the functions of saliva.
3. Which anatomical structures are connected by the pharynx?
4. What are *rugae*?
5. How much can the stomach hold when it is full?

Small Intestine

The **small intestine** gets its name from its diameter, which is much smaller than that of the large intestine. If intestines were named for their length, the small intestine would be called the *long* intestine. The small intestine is the longest segment of the GI tract, with a length of 6 or 7 meters (about 7 or 8 yards) when relaxed. Most chemical breakdown of food occurs in the small intestine. It is also the site of all food absorption and most water absorption.

Segments of the Small Intestine. The small intestine has three segments: the *duodenum* (DOO-ah-DEH-num), the *jejunum* (jeh-JOO-num), and the *ileum* (IL-ee-um), all shown in **Figure 13.17**. The duodenum is the first and shortest segment. It begins at the pyloric sphincter and continues for about 25 centimeters (about 10 inches).

The secretions of the liver, gallbladder, and pancreas enter the duodenum via the duodenal ampulla (DOO-ah-DEH-nal am-POOL-la), a small chamber in the wall of the duodenum. The duodenal papilla, a small cone of tissue on the wall of the duodenum, contains the opening of the duodenal ampulla.

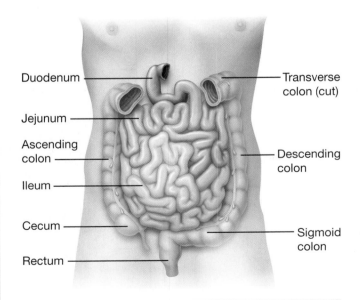

Figure 13.17 The small intestine is divided into three segments—the duodenum, jejunum, and ileum. *Which of the three segments of the small intestine is the shortest?*

The jejunum follows the duodenum and is about 2.5 meters (about 8 feet) long. The ileum is the last and longest segment of the small intestine, measuring between 3.5 and 4 meters (12 to 13 feet) long. Chemical digestion, absorption, and propulsion by peristalsis occur in all three segments of the small intestine.

The Lining of the Small Intestine. The surface area of the small intestine's lining is greatly increased by several structural features. The inner surface of the small intestine has circular folds, which are large enough to see with the naked eye (**Figure 13.18A**). The surface of each fold is covered with finger-like projections called *villi*, and with tubular indentations called *intestinal crypts*, which are similar to gastric pits in the stomach (**Figure 13.18B**).

> **Memory Tip**
> Recall that a villus is made up of many cells and has lacteal and blood capillaries in its core. A microvillus, on the other hand, is much smaller than a single cell. It contains little more than cytoplasm and a few protein filaments for stiffening. The basic cellular information in chapter 2 may also help you remember the difference between villi and microvilli.

Each villus (the singular form of *villi*) contains a lymphatic capillary called a *lacteal* (LAK-tee-al), as well as blood capillaries. The epithelial cells of the villi have tiny, finger-like projections on the exposed surfaces of the cells,

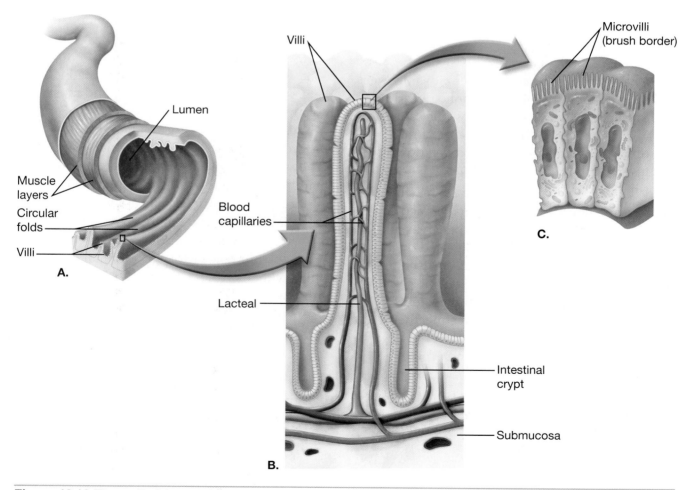

Figure 13.18 The wall of the small intestine. A—The lining of the small intestine contains circular folds. B—The surfaces of the folds are covered with villi and intestinal crypts. C—The epithelial cells covering the villi have microvilli on the part of the cell membrane that faces the lumen of the intestine.

which face the lumen of the intestine. These microscopic projections are called *microvilli* (**Figure 13.18C** on the previous page). The microvilli are collectively called the *brush border* because, when viewed with a microscope, they resemble a fuzzy edge on one side of the cell.

Chemical Breakdown in the Small Intestine. Chyme enters the duodenum from the stomach, where it mixes with bile and pancreatic juice. Bile plays an important role in **emulsification**, the breakdown of large fat particles into smaller, more evenly distributed particles.

Pancreatic juice contains several chemicals, such as *bicarbonate, pancreatic amylase, pancreatic lipase*, and *inactive pancreatic proteases*. These chemicals break down the chyme and food particles in the duodenum.

- *Bicarbonate* is an alkaline molecule that neutralizes acidic chyme.
- *Pancreatic amylase* breaks down starches into chains that are as short as two sugar molecules (disaccharides).
- *Pancreatic lipase* breaks down lipids into their constituent fatty acids and monoglycerides. The emulsification of lipids by bile salts greatly increases the surface area of the lipids, allowing them to be broken down faster by lipase.

When *inactive pancreatic proteases* reach the duodenum, they are converted to their active forms. This happens because the pancreas, like the stomach, must avoid being digested by its own proteases. The pancreas protects itself by secreting proteases in an inactive form.

By the time carbohydrates and proteins approach the end of the small intestine, their chemical breakdown is nearly complete. The final stage of carbohydrate and protein breakdown occurs with brush border enzymes attached to the surfaces of the microvilli. Sucrase, for example, is a brush border enzyme that breaks sucrose (table sugar) into the single sugar molecules glucose and fructose.

Absorption from the Small Intestine into the Blood. Absorption of food molecules into the blood occurs in all three segments of the small intestine. This process is enhanced by the large surface area created by the intestinal folds, villi, and microvilli.

Monosaccharides, such as glucose, and most amino acids are actively transported into the epithelial cells of the small intestine. The monosaccharides move from the epithelial cells into the blood capillaries within each villus. The blood in these capillaries, now rich in nutrients, is collected by the portal vein, which delivers the blood to the liver. The blood serves as a transport system for oxygen and carbon dioxide, and it helps the body absorb nutrients.

Free fatty acids and monoglycerides also enter the epithelial cells. The epithelial cells repackage these lipid subunits with proteins to form chylomicrons (KIGH-loh-MIGH-krahnz). The chylomicrons are too large to enter the blood capillaries, but they can and do enter the lacteals (**Figure 13.18** on the previous page). The lymph in the lacteals eventually enters the bloodstream, as you learned in chapter 12.

Most of the water that is absorbed into the blood is also absorbed in the small intestine. Water-soluble vitamins (vitamin C and most B vitamins) enter with the water.

Vitamin B_{12} is too large and electrically charged, though, to be absorbed on its own. So how does it make its way into the blood? Vitamin B_{12} binds to intrinsic factor, which is produced by the parietal cells of the stomach. Epithelial cells in the ileum have receptors for intrinsic factor, which enable them to actively take in the intrinsic factor-B_{12} combination. Fat-soluble vitamins (A, D, E, and K) are absorbed with lipids.

Liver and Gallbladder

The liver and the gallbladder are accessory organs of digestion. The **gallbladder** is the digestive organ that stores bile and delivers it to the duodenum when needed.

You can live without a gallbladder (many people do), but you can't live without a liver. The digestive function of the liver and gallbladder is to make bile, deliver it in a timely manner to the duodenum, and store it there. The duodenum uses bile to aid in the chemical breakdown of lipids.

Figure 13.19 shows the shape and position of both the liver and the gallbladder. The liver is the largest organ, by weight, in the abdominopelvic or thoracic cavity. It lies just under the diaphragm, primarily on the right side of the body.

Functions of the Liver. The liver has many functions. Most of its functions are metabolic, which means that they are related to the synthesis and processing of various chemicals. These functions fall under the general category of maintaining a stable, healthy internal body environment—in other words, maintaining homeostasis. The specific metabolic functions of the liver include the following:

- maintenance of normal blood concentrations of glucose, lipids, and amino acids
- conversion of one nutrient type to another—for example, conversion of carbohydrates to lipids or, if necessary, amino acids to glucose
- synthesis and storage of glycogen and secretion of cholesterol, plasma proteins (such as albumin), and clotting factors

- storage of iron, lipids, and fat-soluble vitamins
- absorption and inactivation of toxins, hormones, immunoglobulins, and drugs

The Liver's Blood Supply. As you learned in chapter 11, the liver has a very unusual blood supply. You know that the liver receives oxygenated blood from the hepatic artery, which branches off the aorta. You also know that blood leaves the liver via the hepatic vein, which drains into the inferior vena cava. So far, these circulatory processes are not unusual.

What is unusual is that the liver also receives deoxygenated, nutrient-rich blood from the stomach and intestines via the hepatic (heh-PAT-ik) portal vein. This blood makes its way through the capillaries of the stomach, the small intestine, or the large intestine. In these organs, the blood loses its oxygen and absorbs whatever nutrients are present. Then it travels to the liver via the hepatic portal vein, and on through the liver capillaries.

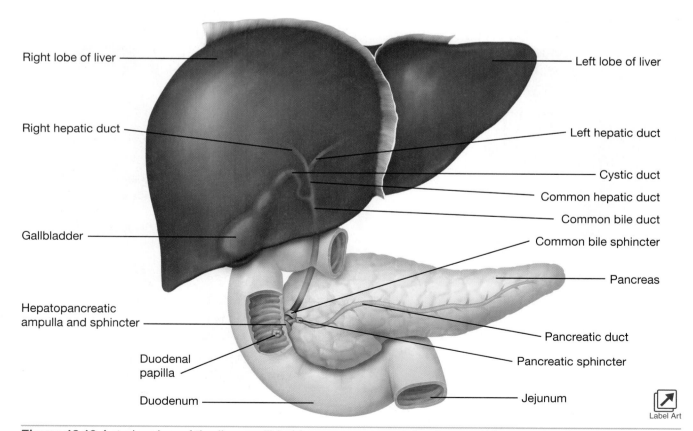

Figure 13.19 Anterior view of the liver, gallbladder, pancreas, and duodenum. *What are the digestive functions of the liver and gallbladder?*

Memory Tip

The root word *hepato-* means "liver." *Hepatocytes* are liver cells. *Hepatitis* is an inflammation of the liver. *Hepatic* blood vessels go to and from the liver.

Portare is a Latin word meaning "to carry." *Portal* veins *carry* blood from one capillary bed to another. The hepatic portal system is by far the largest portal system in the body. There is also a tiny, but important, portal circulation system between the hypothalamus and the pituitary gland in the brain.

Usually, blood goes through only one set of capillaries on its way from the arterial to the venous side of the circulatory system. In this case, however, it goes through two sets of capillaries.

The liver capillaries, called *sinusoids* (SIGH-nuh-soyds), are "leakier" than most capillaries (**Figure 13.20**). Sinusoids contain fenestrations, or holes, in their walls, and lack a surrounding basement membrane, which is present in most capillaries. This leakiness makes it easy for nutrients to diffuse (spread out) from the capillaries to the hepatocytes (HEHP-a-toh-sights), or liver cells, and for proteins secreted by the hepatocytes to enter the capillaries.

Hepatic portal circulation serves an important function—delivering concentrated nutrients to the liver. Without this system, the nutrients from the stomach and intestines would be diluted, mixing with blood from the rest of the body. This would make the liver's job of processing and storing nutrients much harder.

Figure 13.20 Detailed anatomy of a liver lobule. Blood flows from the triads "in" toward the central vein, through sinusoids (leaky capillaries), as indicated by the solid white arrows. Bile produced by hepatocytes is collected in bile canaliculi and flows "out" to the bile duct branches at the triads.

Liver Lobules. At a microscopic level, the liver is made up of a million or so functional units called *liver lobules* (**Figure 13.20**). A lobule is about one millimeter (a fraction of an inch) across. Each lobule includes hepatocytes, blood vessels, and *bile canaliculi* (kan-a-LIK-yoo-ligh)—"little canals"—and ducts that collect bile.

At each corner of each liver lobule is a portal triad that consists of a bile duct, a small hepatic artery, and a small portal vein. Blood enters the lobule through the portal vein and the hepatic artery. The blood flows through the sinusoids, exchanging nutrients, oxygen, and other substances with the hepatocytes. The blood is collected in the central vein, and from there it flows to the hepatic vein. The hepatic vein carries the blood from the liver to the vena cava.

Bile. While blood is flowing rapidly from the portal triads to the central vein, *bile* is moving slowly in the opposite direction. Bile is a watery solution containing *bile salts*, which are derived from cholesterol. When bile salts combine with fat droplets in chyme, the bile salts emulsify, or break apart, the fats. Detergents, like bile salts, are emulsifying agents. Emulsification greatly increases the total surface area of fats, thus aiding their breakdown by lipases.

Bile is made and secreted by hepatocytes, or liver cells. Bile is moved into the bile canaliculi, which carry it to the bile ducts at the triads. Small bile ducts join together to form the right and left hepatic ducts, which travel from the right and left lobes of the liver. These two ducts merge to form the common hepatic duct (**Figure 13.19**). The hepatic duct then joins with the cystic duct, coming from the gallbladder, to form the common bile duct. The common bile duct and the pancreatic duct meet at the wall of the duodenum to form a small chamber, the duodenal ampulla, which opens into the duodenum at the duodenal papilla (DOO-ah-DEH-nal pa-PIL-a).

Bile Storage. The liver makes bile at a fairly steady rate of about one liter per day. However, the body does not need the bile at a steady rate. Bile is needed only after a meal, when there is chyme in the duodenum.

This mismatch between the liver's steady supply of bile and the body's intermittent demand for it is why we have a gallbladder. The gallbladder releases bile after a meal that contains fat. Several sphincters work together to control bile outflow. These include the common bile sphincter, pancreatic sphincter, and the hepatopancreatic sphincter, which encircles the duodenal papilla.

When the body's demand for bile is low, bile coming down the hepatic duct travels up the cystic duct to be stored in the hollow gallbladder (**Figure 13.19**). Bile stored in the gallbladder becomes somewhat more concentrated because some of its water has been absorbed. When chyme—especially chyme containing a lot of fat—enters the duodenum, the muscular wall of the gallbladder contracts, squeezing out stored bile. At the same time, the common bile duct and hepatopancreatic sphincter relax, so that the bile can flow into the duodenum to emulsify the fat.

People with gallstones may have their gallbladder removed surgically. A person without a gallbladder still produces and secretes bile at a modest rate, but does not get the surge of bile that is needed to help digest a particularly fatty meal. Therefore, a person without a gallbladder should avoid large, fatty meals to prevent steatorrhea, the presence of excess fat in feces, which can cause fecal incontinence.

 Check Your Understanding

1. Name the three segments of the small intestine.
2. What is the function of bile in the small intestine?
3. Describe the digestive functions of the liver and the gallbladder.
4. List the metabolic functions of the liver.
5. Where is bile stored?

Pancreas

Like the liver and the gallbladder, the pancreas is an accessory organ of digestion. As **Figure 13.7** shows, the pancreas is nestled behind and underneath the stomach.

The pancreas is also part of the endocrine system and functions as both an endocrine and an exocrine gland. It secretes products into the blood (endocrine function) and into the lumen of the small intestine (exocrine function).

Like the liver, the pancreas has both digestive and metabolic functions. Its digestive function is to make and secrete pancreatic juice into the duodenum. Its metabolic function is to make the hormones insulin and glucagon and secrete them into the bloodstream.

Pancreatic Juices. Pancreatic juices contain digestive enzymes that break down all the major classes of nutrients: proteases, amylases, and lipases. Pancreatic proteases are produced and secreted in an inactive form, to prevent self-digestion of the pancreas and its ducts. These inactive proteases are converted in the duodenum into the active proteases trypsin, chymotrypsin, and carboxypeptidase.

Pancreatic juice also contains pancreatic amylases that break down starches and pancreatic lipases that break down lipids. Pancreatic juice is alkaline due to the presence of bicarbonate. The bicarbonate in pancreatic juice neutralizes the hydrochloric acid in the chyme that comes from the stomach.

Glucose Regulation. The metabolic function of the pancreas is to secrete hormones that regulate the concentration of glucose in the blood. This is a classic example of hormonal regulation of the internal environment, for the purpose of maintaining homeostasis.

A high concentration of glucose in the blood causes beta cells in the pancreas to synthesize, or produce, insulin and secrete it into the blood. The blood transports insulin, which binds to receptors on cells throughout the body. In the liver, insulin causes hepatocytes to extract more glucose from the blood and store it by converting it to glycogen. The binding of insulin to adipocytes (AD-i-poh-sights) causes greater glucose uptake and conversion of glucose to fat for storage. These actions cause the concentration of glucose in the blood to fall.

Glucagon is a hormone that is made and secreted by alpha cells in the pancreas when

Memory Tip

To help you distinguish *glucagon* from terms such as *glucose* and *glycogen*, remember that "glucagon is secreted when glucose is gone."

blood glucose levels are low. Like insulin, glucagon binds to receptors on cells throughout the body. However, its effects are opposite to those of insulin. For example, glucagon *promotes* conversion of glycogen to glucose in liver cells. Its actions have the overall effect of causing the concentration of glucose in blood to rise.

Large Intestine

The **large intestine** has a larger diameter than the small intestine, but a shorter length; it measures about 1.5 meters (5 feet) when relaxed (**Figure 13.7**). The major segments of the large intestine are the cecum (SEE-kum), colon, rectum, and anal canal. The anal canal terminates at the anus. The colon is the longest section of the large intestine. The main functions of the large intestine are propulsion and elimination of waste. Absorption of water, electrolytes, and some vitamins are additional, but limited, functions.

A distinctive feature of the large intestine is the presence of large colonies of bacteria. These bacteria perform some helpful tasks, including synthesis of some B vitamins and vitamin K. The bacteria are usually not harmful, although the smelly gas they produce, which is occasionally expelled through the anus, is annoying.

The Cecum. The *cecum* is the first part of the large intestine to receive food from the small intestine. The end of the ileum connects to the cecum at the *ileocecal* (IL-ee-oh-SEE-kal) *valve*. This valve is usually closed, but it opens in response to gastrin released by the stomach. It is also partially controlled by the nervous system. When the ileocecal valve opens, digested remnants of food travel from the ileum into the cecum.

The appendix hangs off of the lowest part of the cecum. The appendix contains lymphocytes that help protect the body from infectious organisms in digested food. Unfortunately, these lymphocytes do not protect the appendix itself from blockage, inflammation, and infection—appendicitis. The treatment for appendicitis is surgical removal of the appendix.

The Colon. The **colon** has four major segments: the ascending, transverse, descending, and sigmoid colons. The *ascending colon* extends upward from the cecum to the right kidney, where it takes a 90-degree turn. Here the *transverse colon* begins. It crosses from right to left, and when it reaches the left edge of the abdominopelvic cavity, it turns down and becomes the *descending colon.* The descending colon leads to the *sigmoid* (SIG-moyd) *colon,* which twists around and ends at the rectum (**Figure 13.21**).

When what remains of food reaches the large intestine, almost all of its extractable nutrients have been harvested. During the 12 to 24 hours that the residue spends in the colon, additional

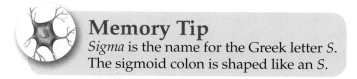

Memory Tip
Sigma is the name for the Greek letter *S.* The sigmoid colon is shaped like an *S.*

water, some electrolytes (sodium and chloride), and water-soluble vitamins are absorbed. The colon absorbs less of these substances than the small intestine does.

Rectum, Anal Canal, and Anus

We have now arrived at the final parts of the alimentary canal: the rectum, anal canal, and anus. The sigmoid colon turns into the **rectum,** a short segment whose lower end comprises the anal canal. The *anus,* the opening to the outside world, is usually closed due to constriction of the internal and external anal sphincters. The internal anal sphincter is made of smooth muscle. The external anal sphincter is composed of skeletal muscle.

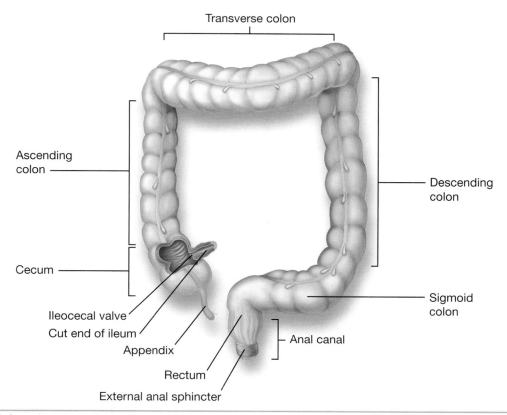

Figure 13.21 Anterior view of the large intestine. The small intestine has been removed. *The large intestine contains colonies of what substance?*

Defecation, the elimination of solid waste, begins when waste reaches the rectum. The waste stretches the rectal wall, initiating reflex contractions of muscles in the sigmoid colon and rectum. These reflex contractions push the waste toward the anus, causing the internal anal sphincter to relax. As a skeletal muscle, the external anal sphincter is under voluntary control. It relaxes when the time is appropriate, allowing defecation to occur.

Lesson 13.2　Review and Assessment

Mini Glossary　Make sure that you know the meaning of each key term.

 Build vocabulary with e-flash cards and games

absorption　the movement of food molecules from the small intestine into the blood

alimentary canal　the passage leading from the mouth to the anus through the pharynx, esophagus, stomach, and intestine; gastrointestinal tract

chemical breakdown　the breakdown of large food molecules into smaller molecules by enzymes; historically referred to as *digestion*

chyme　the mixture of food and digestive juice in the stomach and duodenum

colon　longest segment of the large intestine

defecation　the discharge of feces from the rectum

emulsification　the breakdown of large fat particles into much smaller particles, aided by bile

esophagus　the muscular tube that connects the pharynx and stomach

gallbladder　the digestive organ that stores bile and delivers it to the duodenum when needed

gastrointestinal tract　the stomach, small intestine, and large intestine; alimentary canal

gingiva　soft tissue that covers the necks of the teeth, the mandible, and the maxilla; also called the *gum*

ingestion　the intake of food and liquids via the mouth

large intestine　the portion of the digestive tube between the small intestine and the anus; its major segments are the cecum, colon, rectum, and anal canal

mechanical breakdown　the breakdown of food into smaller pieces, thus increasing its surface area

propulsion　the movement of food through the gastrointestinal tract that is stimulated by swallowing at the pharynx and peristalsis, muscular contractions that move food through the rest of the GI tract

rectum　the short, final segment of the digestive tube whose lower end is the anal canal

small intestine　the portion of the digestive tract where most of the chemical breakdown of food, food absorption, and water absorption occurs; the longest segment of the GI tract

stomach　the reservoir in which food is broken down mechanically and chemically before it enters the small intestine

Know and Understand

 Assess

1. List the six activities of digestion.
2. The oral cavity helps to accomplish which four activities of digestion?
3. What is the difference between the hard palate and the soft palate?
4. How do the salivary glands secrete saliva into the mouth?
5. What substances combine to form saliva?
6. Where in the alimentary canal is the pyloric sphincter located?
7. List the chemicals found in pancreatic juice.
8. What does the root word *hepato-* mean?
9. What are the main functions of the large intestine?

Analyze and Apply

10. Evaluate the ways in which the structures and functions of the digestive system contribute to the processing and storage of energy in the body.

11. Explain the functions of the water, mucus, antibodies, and enzymes found in saliva.
12. Describe the purpose of the acidic environment in the stomach.
13. Explain why a person cannot live without a liver.
14. Describe how the pancreas regulates the concentration of glucose in the blood.

In the Lab

15. Using different colors of clay, create all the organs of the alimentary canal, as well as the accessory organs of digestion. On a piece of poster board or other heavy paper, assemble your digestive system by placing the organs that you created in the proper anatomical positions. Beside each organ, write its name and function (digestive and/or metabolic).

Before You Read

Try to answer the following questions before you read this lesson.

What is the source of the discomfort commonly known as heartburn?

What is an ulcer?

Lesson Objectives

1. Describe some of the common disorders and diseases of the digestive system.

2. Explain the damage that gingivitis can do in the oral cavity as well as throughout the entire body.

3. Describe lifestyle changes that would lessen the symptoms of gastroesophageal reflux disease.

Key Terms

E-Flash Cards

cholecystectomy
constipation
Crohn's disease
diarrhea
gallstones
gastroenteritis
gastroesophageal reflux
gastroesophageal reflux
  disease (GERD)

hepatitis
inflammatory bowel
  disease
pancreatitis
periodontal disease
ulcer
ulcerative colitis

Digestive ailments are some of the most common reasons that people of all ages seek medical attention. Each time we eat, we ingest nonsterile foreign material, some of which contains potential pathogens. The digestive environment itself is harsh, with strong acids and enzymes that can be very damaging. Considering the state of the digestive environment, you might expect digestive illnesses to be even more common than they are.

Gingivitis and Periodontal Disease

Diseases of the digestive system are not limited to stomachaches. The health of the oral cavity, which is part of the GI tract, can affect the entire body. Gingivitis is an inflammation of the gingiva, or *gum tissue* (**Figure 13.22** on the next page). Gingivitis is the most common form of **periodontal disease**—disease that affects the supporting structure of the teeth.

Gingivitis is caused by long-term plaque accumulation on the teeth. *Plaque* is a sticky mixture of bacteria, food particles, and mucus that hardens to form *tartar* if it is not regularly removed by brushing and flossing. Buildup of plaque and bacteria activates an inflammatory response from the immune system. If not treated, gingivitis can cause damage to the jawbone around the tooth and weakening of the periodontal ligament that holds the tooth in its socket. Untreated gingivitis can eventually lead to tooth loss.

People with gingivitis are at an increased risk of developing cardiovascular disease. The inflammation of oral tissue is thought to shift the entire body into a pro-inflammatory state,

Figure 13.22 Gingivitis is an inflammation of the gum tissues, caused by plaque buildup on the teeth. *What is the name of the disease that affects the supporting structure of the teeth as well as the gums?*

increasing the likelihood of atherosclerosis, or hardening of the arteries. Gingivitis can usually be treated by professional teeth cleaning and improved oral hygiene.

Gastroesophageal Reflux Disease (GERD)

Gastroesophageal (GAS-troh-eh-SAHF-a-JEE-al) **reflux** is the movement of chyme from the stomach into the lower esophagus. The stomach wall is protected from the harmful effects of the acids in chyme by a thick layer of mucus, but the esophagus is unprotected. As a result, gastroesophageal reflux can cause a painful burning sensation commonly known as *heartburn*, due to its location in the esophagus near the heart.

If heartburn occurs regularly, the lower esophagus can become chronically inflamed. This condition is called **gastroesophageal reflux disease (GERD)**. Pregnancy can cause GERD because the growing uterus pushes other abdominal organs up and out of their usual positions. GERD can also be caused by a hiatal (high-AY-tal) hernia, in which part of the stomach protrudes through the hiatus, or opening in the diaphragm that normally accommodates the esophagus.

Treatment for GERD includes eating smaller, more frequent meals. It is also wise to avoid eating before bedtime because lying down after a meal worsens symptoms. If necessary, surgery can be done to fix a hiatal hernia, thereby reducing GERD symptoms.

Ulcers

An **ulcer**, or more specifically a *peptic ulcer*, is a break in the protective lining of the stomach, duodenum, or lower esophagus. Ulcers can be extremely painful because the break in the lining causes the deeper structures of the body to be exposed to, and damaged by, the acidic chyme and protein-digesting enzymes.

Most cases of peptic ulcer are caused by infection from the bacterium *Helicobacter pylori* (HEHL-i-koh-BAK-ter pigh-LOR-igh), or *H. pylori*. The name of this bacterium reflects its helical shape and its discovery in tissue samples from the pyloric region of the stomach.

The long-held belief that stress or spicy food can cause ulcers is not supported by scientific evidence. Some evidence does suggest, however, that stress or spicy food can make an existing ulcer worse. Ulcer treatment includes antibiotics to kill the infectious bacterium. Drugs that slow down the release of acid in the stomach are often prescribed to reduce the painful symptoms.

Gastroenteritis

Gastroenteritis (GAS-troh-ehn-ter-IGH-tis) is an inflammation of the stomach or intestine that produces some combination of nausea, vomiting, diarrhea, and abdominal pain. Gastroenteritis is often contagious and is sometimes called "stomach flu," although it is unrelated to influenza. The most common cause of gastroenteritis in children is infection with rotavirus. The goal of treatment is to reduce symptoms through restoration of lost fluid and electrolytes, preferably through oral rehydration therapy.

Inflammatory Bowel Disease

Inflammatory bowel disease is a disease in which the walls of either the small or large intestine become chronically inflamed. Inflammatory bowel disease often results in diarrhea and pain. The cause of this condition is not clear.

Ulcerative colitis (koh-LIGH-tis) is a form of inflammatory bowel disease that usually affects only the colon and the mucosal layer of the intestinal wall.

Crohn's disease can affect all four layers of the digestive tract wall. Inflammation from Crohn's disease usually affects the small intestine or colon.

Patients with Crohn's disease and ulcerative colitis also suffer from malabsorption. This can result in weight loss when the illness flares up, and require high-calorie supplements.

Each of these inflammatory diseases is often characterized by alternating periods of pain and remission during which symptoms are mild. Treatment may include steroids to reduce inflammation during flare-ups. Lifestyle changes such as reduction of fiber in the diet also help.

Constipation and Diarrhea

Constipation and diarrhea are digestive ailments that are often symptoms of other diseases. **Constipation**, or difficulty with defecation, usually occurs when waste spends too much time in the colon. So much water is absorbed from the waste that the remaining waste becomes nearly solid, and therefore, more difficult to pass. Causes of constipation include weakness of the bowel muscle, lack of fiber, lack of exercise, and some prescription drugs.

Diarrhea is characterized by abnormally frequent, watery bowel movements. It occurs when waste does not spend enough time in the colon where excess water would be absorbed.

As a result, the waste contains more water than usual. Diarrhea also occurs when unusually large amounts of water are left in the waste despite normal travel time through the intestine.

Causes of diarrhea include dysentery (an infection of the intestines or stomach by a bacterium, virus, or parasites), food poisoning, inflammatory bowel disease, or milk consumption by a person with lactase deficiency. Lactase deficiency is the inability to break down lactose, or milk sugar. This condition is common in people who are not of European descent. Lactase deficiency causes no problems if milk and other dairy products are avoided.

Treatment for diarrhea and constipation depends on the cause. In cases of diarrhea, lost water and electrolytes may be replaced orally or by intravenous infusion.

Hepatitis

Hepatitis is a disease characterized by inflammation of and damage to the liver. Hepatitis has many possible causes, treatments, and prognoses (or likely outcomes). Liver damage is the common feature among all types of hepatitis.

Causes of hepatitis include viral infection, excessive use of alcohol or drugs (prescription or illegal), and poisoning (such as from certain mushrooms). Acute hepatitis, which lasts for less than six months, may result in healing of the liver and a return to normal liver function. Unfortunately, acute hepatitis may also lead to progressive liver damage and death. Chronic hepatitis lasts longer than six months, and its symptoms are usually less severe.

Because the liver is the site of many biological and chemical processes, damage to this vital organ can cause a wide variety of symptoms. One common symptom of hepatitis is jaundice, or yellowed skin and whites of the eyes. A damaged liver is unable to discharge bilirubin, a product of red blood cell destruction, into the bile. As a result, people with hepatitis sometimes develop jaundice as bilirubin accumulates in the body.

Another symptom of hepatitis is the inability of blood to clot normally. The liver produces the clotting proteins that circulate in the blood, but a damaged liver does not produce enough of these proteins. One sign of hepatitis visible during laboratory analysis of blood samples is the presence of liver enzymes in the blood. These enzymes are released from dying liver cells.

At least five viruses are known to cause acute hepatitis; these are labeled *A* through *E*. Hepatitis viruses vary in severity and ease of spread. Proper hygiene is key for preventing the spread of viral hepatitis. Vaccines are available that provide immunity to hepatitis A and B.

Pancreatitis

Pancreatitis (PAN-kree-a-TIGH-tis) is an inflammation of the pancreas. It occurs when the pancreatic enzymes, especially proteases, become active while they are still in the pancreas. When this occurs, the pancreas starts to break down its own tissues, resulting in severe abdominal pain.

In the United States, most cases of pancreatitis are linked to alcoholism. There is no cure for pancreatitis; however, medication to reduce pain is often prescribed, and lost fluids are replenished.

Occasionally, pancreatitis is caused by a gallstone that lodges in the common outflow tract of the pancreas and gallbladder. This blockage prevents the release of pancreatic juice. Eventually, the enzymes in the juice become active and start damaging the tissue.

Gallstones

Gallstones are solid crystals that form from substances in bile (**Figure 13.23**). Gallstones are usually created in the gallbladder and then get stuck in the cystic duct or common bile duct. This blockage prevents further secretion of bile, resulting in pain and inability to digest fat.

Special drugs may be used to dissolve the gallstones, but usually the gallbladder is removed in a procedure called a **cholecystectomy** (KOH-leh-sis-TEHK-toh-mee). This surgical procedure

Roblan/Shutterstock.com

Figure 13.23 Gallstones affect the ability of the gallbladder to secrete bile.

is often done laparoscopically (through a few small openings). The loss of the gallbladder means that one should eat smaller, more frequent, and less fatty meals.

Cancer

Cancers of the digestive system are among the most common forms of cancer. They can also be among the deadliest. In the United States, for example, colon cancer is the third most common cancer in men and women and the second leading cause of cancer-related deaths. Only lung cancer causes more deaths than cancers of the digestive system.

Typically, cancers of the digestive system grow slowly. In some cases, they are not detected until they have entered nearby body tissues. These cancers usually originate in the epithelial cells of the GI tract or the accessory organs of digestion. Primary tumors (tumors that are new and did not spread from another site) can arise anywhere in the system. Besides colon cancer, cancers of the rectum, the mouth, and the tissues surrounding the mouth are the most common. Cancers of the esophagus, stomach, pancreas, and liver are less common, but they result in high mortality rates.

Cancers of the digestive system can be serious, but screening and early detection play a big role in improving treatment outcomes. Currently, the intestines are the only organ in the digestive system that can be screened for cancer or precancerous growths (polyps). The colonoscopy, for example, is a common screening test for cancers of the colon and rectum. During a colonoscopy, a doctor looks at the entire length of the large intestine and rectum with a long, flexible scope called a *colonoscope*. A small video camera attached to the colonoscope enables the doctor to take pictures or video of the colon. Special instruments can be passed through the colonoscope to biopsy (remove and examine) tissue samples, if necessary. Colonoscopies are typically done in a hospital outpatient department, clinic, or doctor's office.

 Check Your Understanding

1. What is gingivitis?
2. Which bacterium causes most peptic ulcers?
3. What effect does malabsorption have on patients with Crohn's disease?
4. What is the usual cause of constipation?
5. What procedure is performed to remove gallstones?

Lesson 13.3 Review and Assessment

Mini Glossary   Make sure that you know the meaning of each key term.

 Build vocabulary with e-flash cards and games

cholecystectomy   surgical removal of the gallbladder

constipation   condition characterized by difficulty in defecating

Crohn's disease   a chronic, inflammatory bowel disease that usually affects the small intestine or colon

diarrhea   the occurrence of frequent, watery bowel movements

gallstones   solid crystals that form from substances in the bile of the gallbladder

gastroenteritis   an inflammation of the stomach or intestine that produces some combination of nausea, vomiting, diarrhea, and abdominal pain

gastroesophageal reflux   the movement of chyme from the stomach into the lower esophagus

gastroesophageal reflux disease (GERD)   chronic inflammation of the esophagus caused by the upward flow of gastric juice

hepatitis   a disease characterized by inflammation of and damage to the liver

inflammatory bowel disease   a condition in which the wall of the small and/or large intestine becomes chronically inflamed

pancreatitis   inflammation of the pancreas

periodontal disease   a disease that affects the supporting structure of the teeth and the gums

ulcer   a break in the lining of the stomach, duodenum, or lower esophagus

ulcerative colitis   an inflammatory bowel disease that usually affects the colon and the mucosal layer of the intestinal wall

Know and Understand

 Assess

1. What causes gingivitis?
2. What is a hiatal hernia?
3. Why are ulcers painful?
4. Which digestive disorder is often called the "stomach flu" although it is unrelated to influenza?
5. Why is pancreatitis so painful?
6. Why do people with gallstones have a difficult time digesting fat?
7. Where do most cancers of the digestive system originate?

Analyze and Apply

8. Explain why the buildup of plaque on the teeth and gums can be dangerous, potentially leading to heart disease.
9. Explain why GERD is common during pregnancy.

10. Why are ulcers commonly treated with antibiotics?
11. Explain the relationship between constipation and water absorption in the large intestine.

In the Lab

12. Create an informational pamphlet on the digestive system disorder of your choice. Research the following to address in your pamphlet:
    A. definition and description of the disorder
    B. symptoms of the disorder
    C. causes of the disorder
    D. age groups affected
    E. tests or scans used to diagnose the disorder
    F. treatments
    G. prognosis
    When finished, present your pamphlet to the class.

Career Corner
Anatomy and Physiology at Work

The digestive system brings into your body the molecules that you need from nutrients in food. By eating a healthful and well-balanced diet, your body gets the molecules that it needs the most. Many people have found challenging and fulfilling careers in promoting good nutrition and oral health, and in diagnosing and treating diseases of the digestive system.

Nutritionist or Dietitian

Nutritionists and dietitians are experts in food and nutrition. They advise people about the foods that they can eat to stay healthy, get healthy, or cope with disease. They work in many settings, including schools, cafeterias, nursing homes, hospitals, and companies that make prepared food.

One of the responsibilities of a nutritionist or dietitian is to educate people about proper nutrition and healthful lifestyles. Nutrition and lifestyle information and advice may be delivered in a one-on-one setting with individual patients, or it may be presented to small or large groups of people (**Figure 13.24**).

Some dietitians work with a variety of patients; others focus on helping people with a specific disease or disorder. For example, people with renal failure, or kidney disease, may be better able to manage their disease by adopting a particular diet. A dietitian specializing in patients with kidney disease would create a diet plan to meet the specific nutritional needs of these patients.

Most nutritionists and dietitians attend four years of college to obtain their bachelor's degree in nutrition, dietetics, or a related field. Many students are required to complete supervised, hands-on training during a postgraduate internship. Most states require that nutritionists and dietitians be licensed and state certified. These qualifications can be obtained by passing an exam.

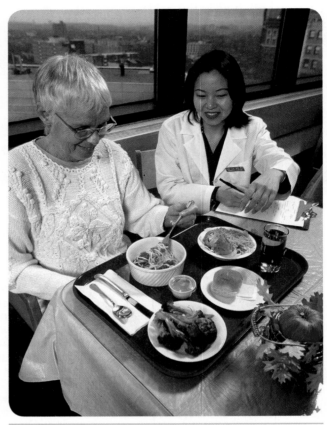

Figure 13.24 Dietitians educate patients about healthful nutrition and lifestyles.

Dental Hygienist

Dental hygienists clean teeth, examine teeth and gums, and provide preventive dental care. During a typical teeth cleaning, a dental hygienist will focus on removing plaque and tartar from the patient's teeth. This is done to help prevent cavities and gum diseases such as gingivitis. Dental hygienists may also take X-rays of the teeth (**Figure 13.25**).

One of the most important responsibilities of a dental hygienist is to educate patients on how to care for their teeth and gums. A dental hygienist might demonstrate the most effective way to brush teeth or the proper method of flossing, skills that are both necessary for achieving good oral health.

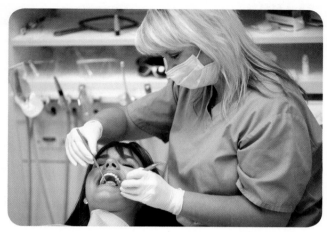

Figure 13.25 Dental hygienists work closely with dentists to monitor and help improve the oral health of their patients.

Dental hygienists work under the supervision of dentists. To become a dental hygienist, you must complete a two-year associate's degree program. High school coursework in biology, anatomy and physiology, and nutrition provides a good base of knowledge for future dental hygienists. In the United States, dental hygienists must pass a certification exam after they have earned their degree. The certification exam may include both written and practical portions.

Planning for a Health-Related Career

Do some research on the career of a dietitian, nutritionist, or a dental hygienist. You may choose instead to research a profession from the list of **Related Career Options**. Using the Internet or resources at your local library, find answers to the following questions:

1. What are the main tasks and responsibilities of a person employed in the career that you chose to research?

2. What is the outlook for this career? Are workers in demand, or are jobs dwindling? For complete information, consult the current edition of the *Occupational Outlook Handbook*, published by the US Department of Labor. This handbook is available online or at your local library.

3. What special skills or talents are required? For example, do you enjoy research? Do you need to be good at biology and anatomy and physiology? Do you need to enjoy communicating with other people?

4. What personality traits do you think are necessary for success in the career you have chosen to research? For example, a dental hygienist works closely with patients. Would you mind touching another person's face and mouth?

5. Does the work involve a great deal of routine, or are the day-to-day responsibilities varied?

6. Does the career require long hours, or is it a standard, "9-to-5" job?

7. What is the salary range for this job?

8. What do you think you would like about this career? Is there anything about it that you might dislike?

Related Career Options

- Chemical Technician
- Dental Assistant
- Dental Laboratory Technician
- Dentist
- Food Science Technician
- Food Scientist
- Gastroenterologist
- Health Educator
- Operating Room Technician
- Orthodontist
- Periodontist
- Urologist

Chapter Summaries

Lesson 13.1 Nutrition

⬈ Build vocabulary with e-flash cards and games

Key Points

- In nutrition, the Calorie, also called the *kilocalorie*, is used to measure energy.
- Your body needs energy to perform metabolic activities.
- The more active you are, the more energy and Calories you need.
- Your body needs many different nutrients, or chemicals, for energy, growth, and maintenance.
- Nutrients include water, macronutrients (carbohydrates, proteins, and fats), vitamins, and minerals.
- Carbohydrates include sugars and starches.
- Proteins are composed of amino acids.
- Fats, also called *lipids*, are composed of fatty acids that may be saturated or unsaturated.

Key Terms

basal metabolic rate (BMR)
Calorie
coenzymes
energy
fats
macronutrients
micronutrients

minerals
monounsaturated fats
nutrients
polyunsaturated fats
trans-unsaturated fats
vitamin deficiency
vitamins

Lesson 13.2 Anatomy and Physiology of the Digestive System

Key Points

- The alimentary canal, or GI tract, is about 9 meters (30 feet) long.
- The accessory organs of digestion include the salivary glands, pancreas, liver, and gallbladder.
- Digestion begins with the mechanical and chemical breakdown of food in the mouth.
- The uvula, which hangs from the soft palate, helps prevent food from entering the nasal cavity.
- Three pairs of salivary glands aid in digestion— the parotid glands, submandibular glands, and sublingual glands.
- The pharynx connects the mouth and nasal cavity to the trachea and esophagus.
- The esophagus connects the pharynx to the stomach.
- The stomach breaks food down mechanically and chemically.
- The small intestine connects to the stomach and consists of three segments–the duodenum, jejunum, and ileum.

Key Terms

absorption
alimentary canal
chemical breakdown
chyme
colon
defecation
emulsification
esophagus
gallbladder

gastrointestinal tract
gingiva
ingestion
large intestine
mechanical breakdown
propulsion
rectum
small intestine
stomach

- Bile, used to digest fats, is made by the liver.
- The digestive function of the gallbladder is to store bile and deliver it to the duodenum when needed.
- The pancreas is an accessory digestive organ with both digestive and metabolic functions.
- The large intestine is connected to the small intestine and consists of four major segments: the cecum, colon, rectum, and anal canal.

Lesson 13.3   Disorders and Diseases of the Digestive System

Key Points

- Gingivitis is an inflammation of the gingiva, or gum tissue, caused by long-term plaque accumulation on the teeth.
- Most peptic ulcers are caused by the bacterium *Helicobacter pylori*, or *H. pylori*.
- Gastroenteritis is an often contagious inflammation of the stomach that produces nausea, vomiting, diarrhea, and/or abdominal pain.
- Cancer of the digestive system organs usually originates in the epithelial cells of the GI tract or accessory digestive organs.

Key Terms

cholecystectomy
constipation
Crohn's disease
diarrhea
gallstones
gastroenteritis
gastroesophageal reflux
gastroesophageal reflux
   disease (GERD)

hepatitis
inflammatory bowel
   disease
pancreatitis
periodontal disease
ulcer
ulcerative colitis

Chapter Assessments

Lesson 13.1

Nutrition

Learning Key Terms and Concepts

1. Growing, moving, and breathing are activities that require the body to use _____.

2. Food scientists use the kilocalorie, or _____, to measure the potential energy in food.

3. The sum of all the chemical and physical reactions that occur in the body is called _____.

4. If you changed your daily routine from an inactive to an active lifestyle, your BMR would _____.
   A. go up   C. remain the same
   B. go down   D. fluctuate

5. Moderately active teen girls typically need to consume about how many Calories per day?
   A. 2,000   C. 2,800
   B. 2,400   D. 3,200

6. *True or False?* Protein delivers about twice as much energy as carbohydrates and fats.

7. Which of the following is not a nutrient?
   A. proteins   C. bacteria
   B. vitamins   D. water

8. Which of the following foods is classified as a carbohydrate?
   A. chicken breast   C. olive oil
   B. rice   D. butter

9. Proteins are made up of varying amounts of 20 different_____.
   A. vitamins   C. chromosomes
   B. lipids   D. amino acids

10. _____ fatty acids are derived mainly from animal sources.

11. Unsaturated fatty acids may be either _____ or _____.

12. *True or False?* Fat-soluble vitamins can be stored in the body.

13. *True or False?* Water-soluble vitamins can be stored in the body.

Thinking Critically

14. Why is basal metabolic rate (BMR) an insufficient method of calculating the required daily intake of an active teenager?

15. Using what you have learned about the different kinds of fats—saturated, unsaturated, and trans fats—explain which are healthful and which are unhealthful.

Lesson 13.2

Anatomy and Physiology of the Digestive System

Learning Key Terms and Concepts

16. The alimentary canal is also called the _____.

17. The _____ breakdown of food reduces food into smaller pieces through chewing and stomach churning.

18. The process of muscles contracting for the purpose of moving food particles along the GI tract is called
    A. absorption
    B. peristalsis
    C. ingestion
    D. churning

19. Which of the following accurately lists the layers of the walls of the alimentary canal, starting from the innermost layer?
    A. submucosa, mucosa, serosa, and muscularis externa
    B. mucosa, submucosa, muscularis externa, and serosa
    C. serosa, submucosa, mucosa, and muscularis externa
    D. mucosa, serosa, submucosa, and muscularis externa

20. The mouth is also called the _____.

21. There are _____ pairs of salivary glands in the mouth.
    A. three
    B. five
    C. seven
    D. nine

22. The muscular tube that connects the pharynx to the stomach is the _____.
    A. trachea
    B. small intestine
    C. esophagus
    D. colon

23. *True or False?* The folds in the wall of the stomach are called *rugae*.

24. The three segments of the small intestine, beginning with the segment closest to the stomach, are the _____.
    A. ileum, jejunum, and cecum
    B. duodenum, jejunum, and ileum
    C. cecum, colon, and ileum
    D. jejunum, ileum, and duodenum

25. Bile is made by _____ and stored in the _____.

26. The purpose of bile is to digest _____.

27. The pancreas produces two hormones, insulin and _____, and secretes them into the bloodstream.

28. The four major segments of the large intestine, starting with the segment closest to the small intestine, are the _____.
    A. cecum, rectum, colon, and anal canal
    B. cecum, anal canal, rectum, and colon
    C. anal canal, rectum, colon, and cecum
    D. cecum, colon, rectum, and anal canal

Thinking Critically

29. Using what you have learned about propulsion and peristalsis in the GI tract, explain what reverse peristalsis is and what might cause it.

30. Recalling what you learned about the layers of the alimentary canal, why would it be important for a surgeon to know and understand these layers, particularly their order?

Lesson 13.3

Disorders and Diseases of the Digestive System

Learning Key Terms and Concepts

31. Gingivitis is an inflammation of the _____, or gum tissue.

32. Gingivitis results from long-term buildup of _____ on the teeth.

33. Plaque is a sticky mix of bacteria, food particles, and _____ that hardens to form tartar if not removed by brushing and flossing.

34. Because of its location, GERD is commonly called _____.

35. Which bacterium causes most peptic ulcers?

36. Gastroenteritis in children is commonly caused by infection with _____.
    A. salmonella
    B. hepatitis
    C. rotavirus
    D. staphylococcus

37. _____ is a digestive disease that affects all four layers of the digestive tract wall.
    A. Inflammatory bowel disease
    B. Gastroesophageal reflux disease
    C. Crohn's disease
    D. Ulcerative colitis

38. _____ can be caused by waste spending too much time in the colon.

39. _____ occurs when waste does not spend enough time in the colon.

40. _____ is an inflammation of the pancreas.

41. _____ are solid crystals that form from bile and can block the secretion of bile into the small intestine.

42. Cancer of the digestive system organs usually originates in _____ cells of the GI tract.
    A. squamous
    B. blood
    C. nerve
    D. epithelial

Thinking Critically

43. Evaluate the cause and effect of periodontal disease on the structure and function of the cardiovascular system.

44. Why might chyme harm the esophagus but not the stomach?

Building Skills and Connecting Concepts

Analyzing and Evaluating Data

This bar graph from the Centers for Disease Control shows the incidence of colon cancer, by race/ethnicity and gender, in the United States in a particular year. Use the graph to answer the following questions.

45. How many black females per 100,000 had colon cancer?

46. Which group had the highest incidence of colon cancer?

47. What is the difference in the number of cases of colon cancer between Hispanic males and white males per 100,000?

48. Which group had the lowest number of colon cancer diagnoses? Do some research to find out why this particular group has the lowest incidence of this disease.

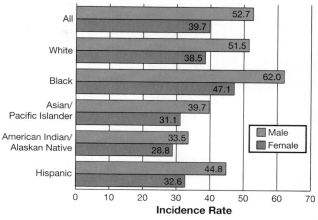

Colon Cancer Incidence Rates*
by Race/Ethnicity and Gender

	Male	Female
All	52.7	39.7
White	51.5	38.5
Black	62.0	47.1
Asian/Pacific Islander	39.7	31.1
American Indian/Alaskan Native	33.5	28.8
Hispanic	44.8	32.6

Incidence Rate

*Per 100,000 persons; age-adjusted to 2000 U.S. standard population. Not mutually exclusive from the other groups.

Communicating about Anatomy and Physiology

49. **Listening** With a group of three other students, research one of the following disorders or diseases: gingivitis, GERD, hiatal hernia, Crohn's disease, pancreatitis, or peptic ulcer. Each student investigates one of these topics: signs and symptoms, diagnostic tests, treatment options, or prognosis. Then each group presents their findings to the class, and the other class members take notes on the presentation.

50. **Speaking** Working in groups of three students, create flash cards for the key terms in this chapter. Each student chooses a lesson and makes flash cards for the key terms in that lesson. On the front of the card, write the term. On the back of the card, write the pronunciation and a brief definition. Use your textbook and a dictionary for guidance. Then take turns quizzing one another on the pronunciations and definitions of the key terms.

Lab Investigations

51. Analyze nutrient data on food labels of various snack foods.

    Materials: Snack food labels from potato and tortilla chips, crackers, pretzels, cookies, candy, granola bars, fruit snacks, and packaged cakes or doughnuts

    The latest recommendations for "healthy" snacks include the following nutritional information: 7 g or less of fat, 2 g or less of saturated fat, 0 g trans fat, 15 g or less of sugar, 250 mg or less of sodium, and artificial sweeteners.

    Create a spreadsheet that lists nutritional information for each snack food. Include the total

amount of fat, saturated fat, trans fat, sugar, sodium, and any artificial sweeteners in your spreadsheet. Then create a report identifying the snacks that you evaluated to be the "healthiest" based on the data.

Expand your learning with additional online resources
- Supplemental Lab Activities
- Interactive Exercises
- Animations

Companion Website

www.g-wlearning.com/healthsciences

How are wastes filtered from your blood and flushed from your body?

The Urinary System

A stable chemical environment inside the human body is essential for life and health. The biochemical reactions of life require watery surroundings and a stable level of salt in the body fluids. Proteins will not fold properly—and enzymes will not work—if the fluid that bathes, or surrounds, them is too salty or not salty enough.

The urinary system adapts to changing conditions so that the body's internal environment stays constant. The key organs in the urinary system are the kidneys. These two bean-shaped organs are remarkable for the number of tasks they accomplish. The other organs of the urinary system—two ureters, the bladder, and the urethra—are also essential, but their functions are much simpler than those of the kidneys.

We will explore the anatomy and physiology of the kidneys in lessons 14.1 and 14.2. In lesson 14.2, which covers urine formation, storage, and excretion, we will learn about the ureters, bladder, and urethra. In the last lesson of this chapter, we will discuss tests of kidney function and disorders and diseases of the kidneys.

Chapter 14 Lessons

Lesson 14.1
Anatomy of the Kidney

Lesson 14.2
Urine Formation, Storage, and Excretion

Lesson 14.3
Diseases and Disorders of the Urinary System

While studying, look for the online icon to:

- **Practice** with e-flash cards and vocabulary games
- **Review** with interactive art labeling
- **Assess** with online exercises
- **Expand** with interactive activities and animated videos
- **Listen** to pronunciations of key terms in the audio glossary

www.g-wlearning.com/healthsciences

Companion Website

Study on the Go

Use a mobile device to practice vocabulary terms, listen to pronunciations, and review with self-assessment quizzes.

www.m.g-wlearning.com

G-W Mobile

Anatomy of the Kidney

Before You Read

Try to answer the following questions before you read this lesson.

Where in the body are the kidneys located?

Which blood vessels and nerves go to and from the kidneys?

What does the inside of the kidney look like, to the unaided eye?

Lesson Objectives

1. Describe the location and size of the kidney.
2. Know the basic anatomy of the kidney.
3. Describe the anatomy of the nephron.
4. Trace the flow of blood through the kidney.

Key Terms

E-Flash Cards

collecting duct
distal convoluted
  tubule
glomerulus
nephron
nephron loop
proximal convoluted
  tubule (PCT)

renal corpuscle
renal cortex
renal medulla
renal pelvis
renal tubule
urinary system
vasa recta

The **urinary system** is composed of structures that excrete liquid waste in the form of urine, retain water and salt, and maintain homeostasis. The kidneys, the main players in the urinary system, purify many times their weight in fluid each day, eliminating waste from the blood while retaining valuable chemical compounds. The kidneys control the volume of water in the body, and in doing so they control blood volume and blood pressure.

The kidneys also regulate the pH and saltiness of blood. Physiologists and healthcare providers use the term *osmolality* (AHZ-moh-LAL-i-tee) as a more precise term for saltiness. The osmolality of fluid is the number of dissolved molecules per unit volume of fluid. The kidneys control the concentration of various ions in the blood, including sodium, chloride, potassium, magnesium, and calcium. They make the hormones erythropoietin (eh-RITH-roh-POY-eh-tin) and renin. And they convert vitamin D to its active form. In short, no human-engineered device comes close to doing what a kidney does, especially in such a small package.

Kidney Location and Size

The kidneys are located on either side of the spinal column, high in the lumbar (lower back) region (**Figure 14.1**). They are *retroperitoneal* (REHT-roh-PER-i-toh-NEE-al); that is, they lie behind the peritoneum, the membrane that lines the abdominopelvic cavity. (The prefix *retro-* means "back" or "located behind.") The two lowest ribs offer some protection to the kidneys against physical blows from behind.

Each kidney is about 11 centimeters long, 6 centimeters wide, and 3 centimeters thick—somewhat larger than a deck of cards. A kidney

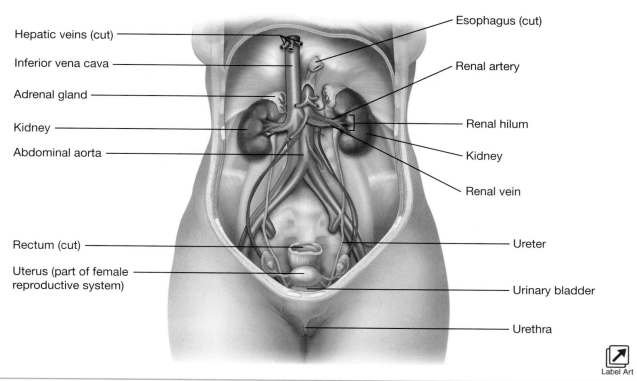

Hepatic veins (cut)

Inferior vena cava

Adrenal gland

Kidney

Abdominal aorta

Rectum (cut)

Uterus (part of female reproductive system)

Esophagus (cut)

Renal artery

Renal hilum

Kidney

Renal vein

Ureter

Urinary bladder

Urethra

Label Art

Figure 14.1 Urinary system anatomy. The kidneys lie against the posterior body wall, on either side of the spinal column. *Which vessel supplies blood to the kidneys? From which vessel does purified blood exit the kidneys?*

weighs about 150 grams (one-third of a pound). The liver, located above the kidneys, pushes the right kidney to a slightly lower position than the left. Each kidney has a convex (outward-curving) lateral edge and a concave (inward-curving) medial surface. The indentation on the medial surface, where blood vessels and nerves enter the kidney, is called the renal hilum (REE-nal HIGH-lum). The kidney usually is cushioned by some fat. The small adrenal gland, an endocrine system organ, sits on top of the kidneys.

Anatomy of the Kidney

A frontal section through the kidney separates it into a "front half" and a "back half" (**Figure 14.2**). The lighter-colored, outer part of the kidney is called the **renal cortex**. The darker inner part, the **renal medulla**, is divided into *renal pyramids*. The "base" of each pyramid faces outward, toward the cortex. The rounded tip of the pyramid, the *papilla* (pa-PIL-a), faces the

center of the kidney. The pyramids are separated by *renal columns*, inward extensions of cortex-like tissue. The **renal pelvis** is the deepest part of the kidney. Urine produced in the cortex and medulla seeps into the renal pelvis, which drains into the *ureter* (YOOR-eht-er), a tube that leads from the kidney to the *bladder* (**Figure 14.1**).

Nerve and Blood Supply

The kidneys make up about 0.5% of total body weight, but they receive 20% to 25% of the blood pumped by the heart, under resting conditions. Therefore, the renal artery and renal vein, which connect each kidney to the nearby abdominal aorta, have a large diameter (**Figures 14.1** and **14.2**). The renal artery supplies blood to the kidneys. The renal vein drains purified blood from the kidneys.

The renal nerve fibers, which are mostly from the sympathetic division of the autonomic nervous system (ANS), discussed in chapter 6, form an irregular mesh on the outside of the

Renal cortex

Renal medulla

Papilla of pyramid

Renal pyramid
in renal medulla

Renal column

Fibrous capsule

Hilum

Renal pelvis

Ureter

Label Art

Figure 14.2 Frontal section through the kidney. The kidney has a light-colored cortex around the outside and a darker renal medulla inside. *Where are the "base" and the "tip" of a renal pyramid?*

renal artery. The renal artery, vein, nerves, and ureter all connect to the kidney at the hilum.

 Check Your Understanding

1. Where are the kidneys located in the abdominopelvic cavity?
2. What is the name of the outer part of the kidney, which is lighter in color than other parts?
3. What is the function of the ureter?

The Nephron

The basic working unit of each kidney is the **nephron** (NEH-frahn), shown in **Figure 14.3**. Each kidney contains about one million nephrons. Each nephron has its own blood supply and creates urine, which passes through a collecting duct to the renal pelvis. **Figure 14.3** shows the structure of a nephron. Each nephron has two main parts: the **renal corpuscle** (KOR-puh-suhl), shown in **Figure 14.3A**, and the **renal tubule** (TOO-byool), shown in **Figure 14.3B**.

The renal corpuscle has a tuft of capillaries called the **glomerulus** (glah-MER-yuh-lus) and a surrounding, cuplike *glomerular capsule*. Blood enters the glomerulus through an *afferent arteriole*, passes through the "ball" of capillaries, and exits via the *efferent arteriole*.

Memory Tip
Afferent comes from the Latin verb phrase *ad ferro*, which means "to carry toward." *Efferent* comes from the Latin *ex ferro*, which means "to carry away." The word *ferry* has the same origin.

The glomerular capsule has an outer surface and an inner surface, and a hollow space in between called the *glomerular capsule space*. The inner surface of this space is formed by *podocytes* (PAHD-oh-sights)—literally, "foot cells"—that wrap around the capillaries. The podocytes have finger-like processes that interdigitate (interlock) with one another. Between the processes of the podocytes are tiny *filtration slits*.

To understand the relationship between the glomerulus and the glomerular capsule, imagine

Figure 14.3 Structure of a nephron. A—Renal corpuscle. B—Renal tubule and surrounding capillaries. The renal tubule includes the proximal convoluted tubule, the nephron loop, and the distal convoluted tubule. *Through which arteriole does blood enter the corpuscle? Through which arteriole does blood leave the corpuscle?*

punching your fist into a big water balloon—softly enough that you don't pop the balloon. Your fist is like the ball of capillaries, and the balloon, now wrapped around your fist, is the capsule. The layer of the balloon against your fist is like the podocytes, and the space inside the balloon is like the glomerular capsule space.

As blood passes through the capillaries, a lot of the blood plasma leaks through the endothelial cells of the capillaries (which are much leakier than capillaries in most of the body), and through the filtration slits of the surrounding podocytes, into the glomerular capsule. After much processing, some of this fluid becomes urine.

The *renal tubule* and the capillaries that surround the tubule are shown in **Figure 14.3B**. The renal tubule has three main parts: the proximal convoluted tubule, the nephron loop, and the distal convoluted tubule.

The **proximal convoluted tubule (PCT)** begins at the glomerular capsule. The fluid in the glomerular capsule space passes into the PCT. The fluid then enters the **nephron loop** (also called the *loop of Henle*), first through the *descending limb* and then through the *ascending limb*. The descending limb and the lower part of the ascending limb have much thinner walls than the rest of the ascending limb and the proximal and distal convoluted tubules.

After the fluid reaches the end of the thick part of the ascending limb of the nephron loop, it enters the **distal convoluted tubule**. The fluid that reaches the end of the distal convoluted tubule enters the **collecting duct** (**Figure 14.3B**). Each collecting duct receives fluid from the distal convoluted tubules of several nephrons. The collecting ducts merge into larger ducts, which ultimately drain into the hollow renal pelvis.

The renal corpuscle and the proximal and distal convoluted tubules lie in the renal cortex. The nephron loops enter the renal medulla. The parallel nephron loops and surrounding capillaries give the renal cortex a striated (finely striped) appearance. Some nephrons, called *cortical nephrons*, have short nephron loops that penetrate only slightly into the medulla. Other nephrons, called *juxtamedullary* (JUKS-ta-MEHD-yoo-LAIR-ee) *nephrons*, have long nephron loops that penetrate deeply into

the renal medulla. The juxtamedullary nephrons are the only nephrons that can produce highly concentrated urine.

Memory Tip

The word *juxtamedullary* is made up of the prefix *juxta-* (which means "next to" or "nearby") and the word *medullary*. The corpuscles of juxtamedullary nephrons lie *next to* the medulla.

The efferent arteriole, which carries blood out of the glomerulus, connects to a second set of capillaries called the *peritubular* (per-i-TOO-byuh-lar) *capillaries*. The peritubular capillaries surround the proximal and distal convoluted tubules. Many efferent arterioles from juxtamedullary nephrons give rise to capillaries that run parallel—first down and then up—with the long nephron loops. These capillaries are called **vasa recta** (Latin for "straight vessels").

✓ Check Your Understanding

1. What are the two main parts of a nephron?
2. Where are podocytes located?
3. What are the three main parts of the renal tubule?

Blood Flow through the Kidney

We can now summarize the path taken by blood as it flows through the kidney. First, blood enters the kidney via the renal artery and, after passing through a series of progressively smaller arteries, reaches the afferent arteriole at the entrance to the glomerulus. The blood then flows through the glomerular capillaries, and as it does, a significant fraction of the blood plasma (the noncellular, or fluid, part of blood) enters the glomerular capsule space. The blood then exits the glomerulus, passes through the efferent arteriole, and enters a second set of capillaries—either the peritubular capillaries or the vasa recta. Finally, as the blood passes through the second set of capillaries, it reabsorbs most of the fluid—but not the waste—that it lost in the glomerulus. The blood, now largely free of waste, collects into *venules*, which merge to form larger veins, and exits the kidney via the renal vein.

In most parts of the body, blood passes from arteriole to capillary to venule, and then into larger veins. Kidney circulation is unusual because it does not follow this pattern. In the kidney, blood passes from afferent arteriole to capillaries to efferent arteriole to another set of capillaries, and only then to a venule and larger veins.

Lesson 14.1 Review and Assessment

Mini Glossary

Make sure that you know the meaning of each key term.

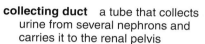 Build vocabulary with e-flash cards and games

collecting duct   a tube that collects urine from several nephrons and carries it to the renal pelvis

distal convoluted tubule   the last part of a nephron through which urine flows before reaching the collecting duct

glomerulus   a cluster of capillaries around the end of a renal corpuscle

nephron   the fundamental excretory unit of each kidney

nephron loop   the U-shaped part of the nephron that is between the proximal convoluted tubule and the distal convoluted tubule; has a descending limb and ascending limb; *loop of Henle*

proximal convoluted tubule   the part of the nephron between the glomerular capsule and the nephron loop; minerals, nutrients, and water are reabsorbed from the filtrate here

renal corpuscle   the part of a nephron that consists of a glomerular capsule with its included glomerulus

renal cortex   the lighter-colored, outer layer of the kidney that contains the glomeruli and convoluted tubules

renal medulla   the darker, innermost part of the kidney

renal pelvis   a funnel-shaped cavity in the center of the kidney where urine collects before it flows into the ureter

renal tubule   the part of a nephron that leads away from a glomerulus and empties into a collecting tubule; consists of a proximal convoluted tubule, nephron loop, and distal convoluted tubule

urinary system   the organs involved in the formation, storage, and excretion of urine; includes the kidneys, ureters, bladder, and urethra

vasa recta   thin-walled blood vessels that begin and end near the boundary between the renal cortex and the renal medulla, and which extend deep into the renal medulla, running parallel to the nephron loops; play a role in the formation of concentrated urine

Know and Understand

 Assess

1. What is meant by the description of the kidneys as *retroperitoneal*?

2. What happens to urine that is produced in the renal cortex and the renal medulla?

3. Where do the renal artery, renal vein, nerves, and ureter connect to the kidney?

4. What is the basic working unit of the kidney?

5. What are the names of the arteries that lead into and out of the glomerulus?

6. Which part of the renal tubule begins at the glomerular capsule?

7. Which type of nephron has long nephron loops that penetrate deeply into the renal medulla?

8. What happens to blood as it passes through the peritubular capillaries or the vasa recta?

Analyze and Apply

9. The kidneys, which make up about 0.5% of total body weight, receive 20% to 25% of the blood pumped by the heart (under resting conditions). What can you conclude about the kidneys based on this fact?

10. How does the flow of blood through the kidneys differ from the flow of blood through other parts of the body?

In the Lab

11. Build a three-dimensional kidney. You will need clay in several colors (brown, red, blue, yellow, orange, and white), pins, paper, tape, and textbook illustrations for reference. Include and then label each of the following: fibrous capsule, renal hilum, renal cortex, renal medulla, renal pyramids, papilla, renal columns, renal pelvis, renal artery, renal vein, and ureter. Keep the following points in mind as you construct your 3-D model:

A. Build your model so that it opens like a book, with the hilum serving as the "spine."

B. Include arterioles and venules that branch off the renal artery and vein and go up between the renal pyramids into the renal cortex.

C. Use brown clay for the majority of the kidney, red for the artery/arterioles, blue for the vein/venules, yellow for the ureter, white for the nerve, and orange for the adrenal gland.

Urine Formation, Storage, and Excretion

Before You Read

Try to answer the following questions before you read this lesson.

What are the three key steps involved in the formation of urine?

How does urine get from where it is made to where it is stored?

How does the nervous system control the excretion of urine, and which muscles play a role?

Lesson Objectives

1. Explain how the kidneys produce urine.
2. Explain how both hydrostatic and osmotic pressure contribute to urine production.
3. Describe the reabsorption and secretion steps in the formation of urine.
4. Describe how urine is stored and excreted from the body.
5. List the steps in micturition.

Key Terms

E-Flash Cards

aldosterone
angiotensin
antidiuretic hormone (ADH)
atrial natriuretic peptide (ANP)
detrusor
diuresis
external urethral sphincter
glomerular filtration rate (GFR)
hydrostatic pressure

internal urethral sphincter
micturition
osmosis
osmotic pressure
reabsorption
renin
secretion
trigone
ureter
urethra
urinary bladder

To better understand how the body disposes of wastes, let's first consider two different ways that you could design a system for removing chemical wastes and toxins from fluid. Approach 1 would be to create a filter that allows wastes and toxins to pass through and does not allow anything "good" to pass through. Then you simply dispose of whatever substances pass across the filter.

Approach 2 would be to make a leaky filter whose pores allow water and other substances to pass through. Many good substances, as well as wastes, will pass through this nonselective filter. Therefore, you would need to pass the *filtrate* (fluid that has crossed a filter) through another stage of processing, in which the good substances, and most of the water, are pumped back into the body. After that stage, only wastes, toxins, and a little bit of water would remain on the filtered side. At that point the remaining water and waste would be excreted.

Approach 1 sounds like it would be simpler and maybe more efficient than Approach 2. However, the body uses Approach 2 for removing chemical wastes and toxins from fluid. Why?

It is impossible to predict all the different kinds of wastes and toxins that an individual might need to excrete during his or her lifetime. Even if you did know exactly what you would need to excrete ahead of time, it probably would be impossible to make the hypothetical filter described in Approach 1 above. Why? In short, wastes and toxins sometimes are not very different from "good" molecules in size, electrical charge, and other properties.

Approach 2 presumably was favored by the human body because it works well even when the wastes and toxins are not known ahead of time. In Approach 2, one simply "throws out everything" and then selectively reclaims the good molecules, whose identity is known in advance.

Urine Formation

The first step in removing wastes and toxins from the body is the formation of urine. Three processes are involved in urine formation: filtration, **reabsorption**, and **secretion**. **Figure 14.4** shows a simplified view of where these processes occur in the nephron. Notice the renal corpuscle with a capillary in the glomerular capsule, and the renal tubule and collecting duct with a capillary running next to it. Filtration occurs at the corpuscle, where water and small, dissolved molecules diffuse (spread) into the glomerular capsule. Water, ions, glucose, and other "good" substances are later reabsorbed into the capillary from the tubule. Some waste molecules, ions, and other molecules are secreted from the capillaries into the tubule and collecting duct. Let's now take a more detailed look at these three urine formation processes.

Filtration

Glomerular filtration, which occurs in the renal corpuscle, is the first step in urine formation. Glomerular filtration is the movement of water and solutes (dissolved substances) from the capillaries into the glomerular capsular space. The water that reaches the capsule is called the *glomerular filtrate*. To reach the glomerular capsular space, water and solutes must cross the capillary endothelial cells, the basement membrane (a layer of extracellular protein), and the podocytes of the glomerular capsule. These three structures are collectively known as the *filtration membrane*.

Red and white blood cells are too large to cross the filtration membrane. Large and medium-sized proteins, such as albumin—the most common protein in blood plasma—are also prevented from crossing the filtration membrane. But water and small molecules and ions can cross this membrane. The list of substances that do cross the filtration membrane includes water, glucose, sodium, potassium, chloride, amino acids, urea (a waste product of metabolism), many kinds of prescription and over-the-counter drugs, and other molecules smaller than about 3 nanometers in diameter.

The total amount of water filtered in a unit of time is called the **glomerular filtration rate (GFR)**. A normal GFR value is about 125 milliliters per minute in males and

Figure 14.4 Formation of urine in the nephron—a functional view. 1. Filtration from the glomerular capillaries into the glomerular capsule (brown arrow) occurs in the renal corpuscle. 2. Reabsorption is the movement of water, ions, glucose, and other substances back into the capillaries (pink arrow). 3. Wastes and some ions, drugs, and toxins are secreted from the capillaries into the tubule (orange arrow). *What substances are filtered from the blood in step 1? What are some substances that are not filtered at that point?*

105 milliliters per minute in females. Laboratory tests are used to determine GFR, one of the most important benchmarks for assessing kidney health. If you multiply the normal GFR (the amount filtered per minute) by the number of minutes in a day, you get about 150 to 180 liters of glomerular filtrate per day! Because our urine output is (fortunately) nowhere close to 180 liters a day, this tells us that the majority of the filtrate eventually will be reclaimed by the body. The driving force for glomerular filtration is pressure: hydrostatic pressure and osmotic pressure.

Hydrostatic Pressure. You know **hydrostatic pressure** as "regular" pressure. It is the pressure of water in a balloon that makes the balloon swell. It is the pressure in pipes that makes water come out when you turn on the faucet. Water is pushed by hydrostatic pressure from where the pressure is high to where it is low.

In a glomerulus, the hydrostatic pressure in the capillaries is the blood pressure there—about 55 mmHg (millimeters of mercury). This figure is considerably higher than the pressure of about 20 to 25 mmHg found in most capillaries. The pressure in the glomerular capsular space is only 15 mmHg, so there is a hydrostatic pressure difference of 40 mmHg pushing water from the capillaries into the capsule.

Osmotic Pressure. Unlike hydrostatic pressure, **osmotic** (ahs-MAHT-ik) **pressure** is a kind of pressure that we do not notice in our everyday lives. Osmotic pressure is created by the presence of dissolved substances in water. High osmotic pressure "pulls in" water from areas of low osmotic pressure. Hydrostatic pressure, by contrast, "pushes" water from areas of high to low pressure.

The more dissolved substances in a fluid, the higher its osmotic pressure. Therefore, water is drawn in to "salty" areas (ones that are full of dissolved substances) from areas where the water is "purer" (areas that have fewer dissolved substances). The movement of water from an area of low osmotic pressure to an area of high osmotic pressure is called **osmosis** (ahz-MOH-sis).

In the renal corpuscle, the blood has a higher osmotic pressure than the filtrate because the

proteins, which are too big to cross the filtration membrane, are present only on the "blood" side of the membrane. The molecules that are small enough to cross the membrane are present in equal concentrations on both sides, so they do not create an osmotic pressure difference. The osmotic pressure is about 30 mmHg higher in blood than in filtrate.

We can compare the size and direction of the pressure differences to determine the net amount and direction of pressure across the filtration membrane. We have seen that the hydrostatic pressure is 40 mmHg higher in the capillary than in the glomerular capsular space, and the osmotic pressure is 30 mmHg higher in the capillary than in the capsular space. These pressures act in opposite directions: High hydrostatic pressure *pushes*, and high osmotic pressure *pulls*. Thus, there is a net filtration pressure of 10 mmHg pushing water from the capillary into the capsule (**Figure 14.5**).

Pressure Controls. The high blood pressure in the glomerular capillaries is due in large part to the efferent arteriole, which acts as a constricting

Figure 14.5 Pressures driving filtration. Hydrostatic pressure in the glomerular capillary (HP$_{gc}$) pushes water out of the capillary. Hydrostatic pressure in the capsular space (HP$_{cs}$) pushes back, from the capsule to the capillary. Osmotic pressure in the glomerular capillary (OP$_{gc}$) pulls water into the capillary. *What is the net filtration pressure of water being pushed out of the capillary?*

agent that limits the outflow of blood from the glomerulus. The more constricted the efferent arteriole is, the higher the glomerular pressure will be, and the greater the glomerular filtration will be. By contrast, constriction of the afferent arteriole, which lies upstream of the glomerulus, limits inflow to the glomerulus and causes glomerular pressure—and therefore glomerular filtration—to drop. The presence of both an afferent and an efferent arteriole provide the body with the ability to control glomerular pressure and glomerular filtration.

Hormones and sympathetic nerves to the kidney both have the ability to regulate the renal arterioles. The sympathetic nerves have a greater effect on the afferent arterioles than on the efferent arterioles. Sympathetic nerve activity rises during exercise and during stressful situations that evoke a fight-or-flight response.

When sympathetic nerve activity increases, the afferent arterioles constrict more than the efferent arterioles. This constriction causes a drop in glomerular capillary pressure and a decrease in glomerular filtration rate, for the reasons described above. The decrease in glomerular capillary pressure and GFR helps the body to reduce urine output and keeps blood volume high, which is useful during exercise. These physiological effects probably gave us an advantage in surviving some fight-or-flight situations in our past.

✔ Check Your Understanding

1. Two approaches to removing wastes and toxins from fluids were described in this lesson. Why do we think the body uses the second approach rather than the first?
2. Name at least three substances that are too large to cross the filtration membrane; name three that can cross the membrane.
3. Why is glomerular filtration rate important?
4. Is the hydrostatic pressure in the capillaries of the glomerulus higher or lower than in other capillaries throughout the body?
5. Do *more* dissolved substances in a fluid mean higher or lower osmotic pressure?

Reabsorption

The filtrate from the glomerular capsule flows into the renal tubule. As it flows through the tubule, and then into the collecting duct, most of the water and dissolved substances are reabsorbed into the blood in the capillaries surrounding the tubule. Most reabsorption occurs in the proximal convoluted tubule (PCT). The remainder occurs in the distal convoluted tubule and the collecting duct.

The epithelial cells that form the wall of the PCT have microvilli on their luminal (lumen-facing) side. These microvilli increase the surface area of the PCT, enhancing its reabsorptive ability. The major steps involved in reabsorption are shown in **Figure 14.6** on the next page.

Sodium. Sodium is the most abundant ion in the filtrate, and it is actively pumped out of the tubular epithelial cells by sodium-potassium pump proteins. These carrier proteins use adenosine triphosphate (ATP) to move sodium from the cell into the interstitial space that surrounds the peritubular capillary.

The active excretion of sodium from the cell by the sodium-potassium pump leaves the cytoplasm (the inside of the cell) with little sodium. Since there is a high concentration of sodium in the tubular fluid, sodium spreads into the cell from the tubule. The sodium that has been pumped out of the cells and into the space surrounding the capillaries then diffuses into the capillaries.

Cotransport proteins in the part of the cell membrane that faces the tubule bring sodium into the cell. Using the energy from this sodium entry, the cotransport proteins pump various desirable substances from the lumen into the cell. This is an example of secondary active transport, which was discussed in chapter 2.

Secondary Active Transport. In secondary active transport, the energy of one substance going "downhill" is used by a protein to pump another substance "uphill." Glucose, amino acids, some ions, and vitamins enter the cell from the tubule by means of secondary active transport with sodium. These valuable substances then spread

Figure 14.6 Reabsorption in the proximal convoluted tubule. The lumen of the tubule is at the far left, and the peritubular capillary is at the right. The cells lining the tubule have been enlarged to show details, and the microvilli on the luminal side of the cell have been omitted for clarity. 1. Sodium-potassium pumps (the green transport proteins shown above) actively pump sodium (Na^+) out of the tubule cell and potassium ions (K^+) into the cell. 2. Sodium flows down its energy gradient into the cell. 3. Glucose and amino acids are cotransported into the cell with sodium, by secondary active transport. 4. Water enters the cell from the tubule through aquaporin channels, and it leaves the cell on the capillary side through aquaporin channels. *Are the substances being reabsorbed into the blood "good" molecules or "bad?" Explain.*

out of the cell on the other side, and diffuse into the peritubular capillary.

Osmotic Pressure. The positive charge on the sodium ions tends to draw negatively charged chloride out of the tubule and into the peritubular capillaries. The active pumping of sodium into the interstitial space, and its diffusion into the peritubular capillaries, creates a relatively high osmotic pressure in the capillaries and in the interstitial space. The high osmotic pressure draws water by osmosis out of the tubule, through the cell, and into the interstitial space and the capillary. Aquaporin (ak-kwa-POR-in) channels in both sides of the cell give water an easy way to enter and exit the cell. Thus, the active pumping of sodium provides the driving force for reabsorption of glucose, amino acids, vitamins, chloride and some other ions, and water.

Secretion

At the same time that the "good" substances are being reabsorbed by the blood, wastes still in the blood are being actively secreted (pushed) from the capillaries. Waste products, such as urea, that were not fully removed during filtration are actively pumped out of the capillaries and into the renal tubule by the cells that form the walls of the tubules. This active "pumping" of wastes from capillary blood into the tubules is called *secretion*. Unlike filtration, which is a passive process, secretion is active; that is, it uses chemical energy, often in the form of ATP, to move molecules.

Tubular epithelial cells—cells in the walls of the proximal and distal convoluted tubules and collecting duct—actively push certain molecules, such as urea and uric acid, into the lumen, or hollow central part, of the renal tubule. The lumen of the tubule contains the fluid that will eventually be eliminated from the body as urine. Pushing unwanted molecules into the lumen of the renal tubule is the body's way of getting rid of them. This active pushing of molecules into the lumen is called *tubular secretion*.

The tubular epithelial cells can also secrete hydrogen ions (acid, H+) or bicarbonate ions (base, HCO_3^-) to maintain the pH of arterial blood at about 7.4. The renal tubule epithelial cells also secrete, or push out, some drugs, if they are present in the blood. Penicillin and aspirin are examples of drugs that are eliminated from the body by the kidneys in this manner.

The Renal Medulla

So far, we have discussed mainly the reabsorption and secretion that take place in the proximal and distal convoluted tubules, both of which are located in the renal cortex. Let's now look at what happens to the wastes and the "good" substances as they travel down and then back up through the renal medulla (**Figure 14.7**).

The descending limb of the nephron loop is thin because its finely structured epithelial cells lack the active pumping capability or intracellular machinery (such as mitochondria) of the PCT cells. Thus, no active reabsorption or secretion occurs in either the descending limb

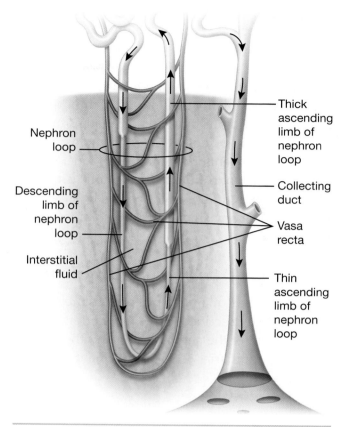

Figure 14.7 The renal medulla. Notice the change in thickness of the descending and ascending limbs. *Why are these changes significant?*

or the thin ascending limb of the nephron loop. Water can leave the filtrate in the descending limb but not in the ascending limb, whose cells lack aquaporin channels. The thick portion of the ascending limb, which *does* have pumping capability, actively reabsorbs sodium, but water cannot follow due to the lack of aquaporin channels in the ascending limb.

The reabsorption of sodium in the thick, ascending limb of the nephron loop, where water cannot be reabsorbed, and the permeability to water of the descending limb of the nephron loop, work together to create very salty interstitial fluid in the renal medulla.

Limited amounts of urea are intentionally allowed to reenter the interstitial space as urine travels down the collecting duct. Reentry of urea within the interstitial space contributes to the high osmolality of the interstitial fluid in the renal medulla. As you will recall from lesson 14.1, osmolality is a measure of the number of dissolved molecules (in this case sodium molecules) per unit volume of fluid. The net result of these processes, whose complexity is beyond the scope of this chapter, is that the deepest parts of the renal medulla can have an interstitial osmolality of about 1,200 milliosmoles (mOsm), about four times higher than normal interstitial fluid osmolality. (Milliosmoles are a measurement of the number of ions, or particles, that contribute to the osmotic pressure of a solution. A milliosmole is equal to one-thousandth of an osmole per unit volume of fluid.)

The Countercurrent Mechanism

A key to the maintenance of the state of affairs just described is the geometric arrangement of the nephron loop and the parallel vasa recta capillaries. This arrangement is shown in **Figure 14.8**.

Capillary blood grows highly concentrated as it goes down the vasa recta into the renal medulla because osmosis draws water out of the capillary. As the blood ascends in the vasa recta, osmosis causes water to re-enter the capillaries. As a result, the blood leaving the vasa recta is no more and no less concentrated than it was when it entered, despite having passed through an area of very high interstitial fluid concentration. Thus, the deep parts of the renal medulla are allowed to get the blood flow they need with no destruction to the high concentration of interstitial fluid, which is necessary for the production of highly concentrated urine.

The geometric arrangement that makes this process possible is called a *countercurrent mechanism*. It is called *countercurrent* because the blood flows "down" the vasa recta, then back past itself in the opposite direction.

The flow of filtrate in the nephron loop is also a countercurrent arrangement because the

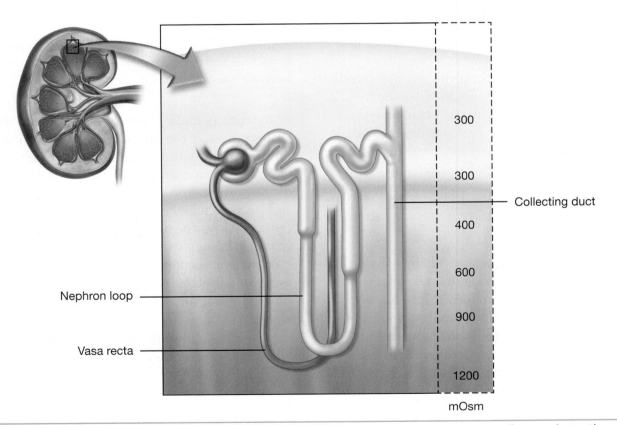

Figure 14.8 Water permeability of the descending limb of the nephron loop, and active sodium reabsorption from the ascending limb, establish the high osmolality of the deep renal medulla. The numbers on the right show the osmolality of the interstitial fluid, represented in milliosmoles (mOsm), in the renal medulla. *Does higher osmolality mean more or less "saltiness"?*

filtrate flows down the descending limb, then up the ascending limb, adjacent to where it is going down. As is the case with the vasa recta, the close proximity of these parallel pathways helps the kidney create and maintain high osmolality of the interstitial fluid in the deep parts of the renal medulla.

When urine travels down the collecting duct, through the deepest parts of the medulla, water can be reabsorbed from the collecting duct by osmosis into the highly concentrated interstitial fluid. When this occurs maximally, the urine can reach, as stated previously, an osmolality of 1,200 milliosmoles because the water in the collecting duct reaches osmotic equilibrium with the interstitial space.

 ### Check Your Understanding

1. Where does most of the reabsorption of water and dissolved substances take place in the kidneys?
2. Active pumping of which ion provides the force for reabsorption of glucose and amino acids?
3. What substances are reabsorbed and secreted in the ascending and descending limbs of the nephron loop?
4. Why does the blood become highly concentrated as it travels down the vasa recta?
5. How would you compare the concentration of blood leaving the vasa recta to that of blood entering the vasa recta?

Hormonal Regulation of Urine Volume and Composition

By the time the filtrate reaches the distal convoluted tubule, about 80% of the water and 90% of the sodium and chloride that entered the glomerular capsular space have been reabsorbed. The amount of reabsorption in the proximal convoluted tubule and nephron loop is relatively constant. The reabsorption in the distal convoluted tubule and collecting duct, however, is adjusted by hormones to maintain homeostasis.

In other words, the "fine tuning" of urine volume and composition occurs in the distal convoluted tubule and collecting duct. Three key hormones that control this fine tuning are aldosterone, atrial natriuretic peptide, and antidiuretic hormone.

Aldosterone. A steroid hormone called **aldosterone** (al-DAHS-ter-ohn) is produced in the adrenal cortex. A drop in blood sodium concentration or a rise in blood potassium concentration directly stimulates the secretion of more aldosterone. A decrease in blood pressure also stimulates more aldosterone secretion, but by an indirect mechanism: decreased blood pressure causes greater secretion of the hormone **renin** (REE-nin), a protein, by the kidney.

Renin circulates in the blood and binds to the circulating protein angiotensinogen. Renin acts on angiotensinogen to produce **angiotensin** (an-jee-oh-TEHN-sin), a polypeptide hormone in the blood that constricts blood vessels and increases blood pressure. After binding to angiotensinogen, the renin cuts the angiotensinogen into two fragments, one of which is angiotensin I. An enzyme in the lungs, appropriately named *angiotensin-converting enzyme*, converts angiotensin I into angiotensin II by removing two amino acids. Angiotensin II stimulates adrenal cortical cells to secrete more aldosterone.

Aldosterone acts on the distal convoluted tubule cells and collecting duct to increase the amount of sodium reabsorption and potassium secretion. Because more sodium is reabsorbed than potassium is secreted, water follows the sodium and also is reabsorbed more when a greater amount of aldosterone is present. As a result, aldosterone causes a decrease in the volume and sodium content of urine, and an increase in its potassium content. The decreased urine volume means that more water is retained in the circulation, which causes blood pressure to rise. Thus, the decrease in blood pressure that led—via the renin-angiotensin mechanism—to more aldosterone secretion is corrected.

Atrial Natriuretic Peptide. A hormone made by the atria of the heart, **atrial natriuretic** (NA-tree-yoo-REHT-ik) **peptide (ANP)** is released in response to increased stretching of the atria, which occurs when blood volume is high. ANP inhibits sodium reabsorption in the collecting ducts, which causes decreased water reabsorption due to osmotic pressure effects. As a result, urine volume and sodium excretion increase, which tends to correct the high blood volume that stimulated ANP production.

Antidiuretic Hormone. A peptide hormone secreted by the pituitary gland, **antidiuretic** (AN-tee-digh-yoo-REHT-ik) **hormone (ADH)** is also known as *vasopressin*. ADH is secreted more when blood osmolality increases.

Blood osmolality increases when we become dehydrated because our water intake has not kept up with water loss. Antidiuretic hormone causes collecting duct cells to produce more aquaporin molecules and insert them in their own membranes. As a result, more reabsorption of water occurs in the collecting ducts, which produces more concentrated urine.

When we are strongly dehydrated and ADH levels are high, reabsorption of water in the collecting ducts is so effective that the urine leaving the collecting duct is extremely concentrated, with an osmolality of about 1,200 milliosmoles. If we are well hydrated, ADH levels are low. As a result,

little water is reabsorbed in the collecting duct, and urine osmolality can drop to between 50 and 100 milliosmoles.

✔ Check Your Understanding

1. Does the "fine tuning" of urine volume and composition occur in the proximal or the distal convoluted tubule?
2. Does an increase in secretion of renin lead to higher or lower blood pressure?
3. If you become dehydrated, will your body secrete more or less ADH?
4. What hormone goes into action when blood volume is too high?

Urine Storage

Urine is made continuously by the kidney. Unlike the respiratory system, which excretes waste (carbon dioxide) continuously, the urinary system excretes waste intermittently. Therefore, we need a place to store the urine until the time and place for elimination are appropriate. We also need plumbing—structures to take the urine from where it is made to where it is stored, and from where it is stored to the outside.

Ureters

Each kidney is connected by a **ureter** (YOOR-et-er) to the bladder (**Figure 14.1**). The renal pelvis connects to the hollow ureter, as shown in **Figure 14.2**. Each ureter is lined with epithelium and contains smooth muscle in its wall. The ureters connect to the bladder via the posterior wall of the bladder.

Urinary Bladder

The **urinary bladder**, or *bladder*, is a hollow, muscular organ that stores urine. It sits on the floor of the pelvic cavity (**Figure 14.1**). The bladder lies under the peritoneum, and its superior surface is directly covered by the peritoneum. In men, it is positioned directly in front of the rectum and above the prostate gland. In women, it is positioned in front of the vagina and uterus.

Memory Tip

The word **diuresis** (DIGH-yoo-REE-sis) is made up of the prefix *di/a-* meaning "through," the combining form *-ur/o-* meaning "urine," and the suffix *-sis*, which means "state of" or "condition." *Diuresis* literally means "state or condition of urine passing through"—in short, "urine production."

Antidiuretic hormone reduces diuresis. *Diuretic drugs*, which increase diuresis, are widely prescribed, both to reduce blood pressure and to reduce the buildup of fluid in the body (edema) that occurs in patients with weak or failing hearts. "Loop diuretics," such as furosemide (trade name Lasix®) reduce sodium reabsorption in the ascending limb of the nephron loop. Other blood pressure-lowering agents work by inhibiting angiotensin-converting enzyme, by blocking the receptors for angiotensin, or by other mechanisms.

The bladder wall is made of smooth muscle, the **detrusor** (dee-TROO-zer), with a layer of epithelial cells on its interior. When the bladder is empty, it collapses, causing folds to develop in the walls and lining. A moderately full bladder may contain 500 milliliters of urine. An extremely full bladder can contain as much as 1,000 milliliters.

The bladder has three openings: one *ureteric orifice* for each of the two ureters, plus the opening of the urethra. The urethra connects to the bladder at the *bladder neck*. The imaginary triangle formed by the two ureteric openings and the urethra is the **trigone** of the bladder.

Urethra

The **urethra** (yoo-REE-thra) is a thin tube that connects the urinary bladder to the outside (**Figure 14.9**). It begins at the neck of the bladder, in its midline. A layer of smooth muscle that encircles the urethra where it exits the bladder is called the **internal urethral sphincter**.

In men, the prostate gland lies directly below the bladder. The prostatic urethra is the portion of the urethra that passes right through the prostate gland. As we will see in Chapter 15: The Male and Female Reproductive Systems, the prostate gland contains tiny ducts that deliver its secretions into the prostatic urethra.

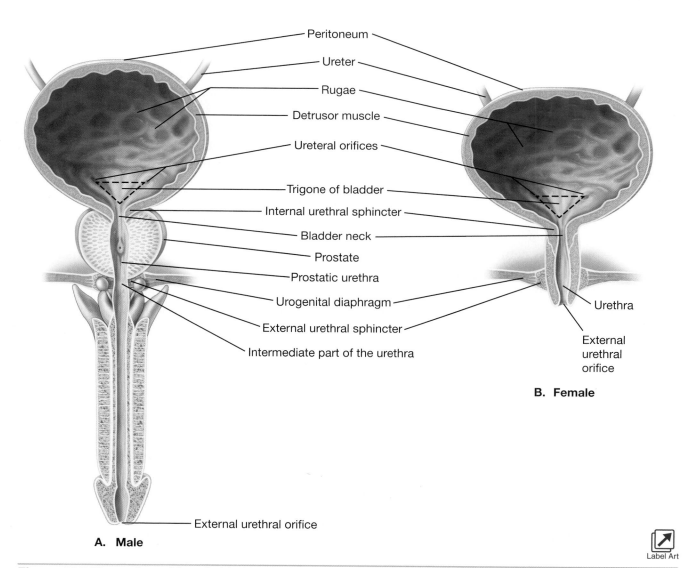

Peritoneum
Ureter
Rugae
Detrusor muscle
Ureteral orifices
Trigone of bladder
Internal urethral sphincter
Bladder neck
Prostate
Prostatic urethra
Urogenital diaphragm
External urethral sphincter
Intermediate part of the urethra
External urethral orifice

A. Male

Urethra
External urethral orifice

B. Female

Label Art

Figure 14.9 The male and female bladder and urethra. *Where is the bladder positioned in the male? Where is it positioned in the female? For both males and females, how many openings does the bladder have? (Note: the trigone is a clue.)*

The next part of the male urethra, the intermediate part, passes through the muscles of the pelvic floor, which make up the *urogenital* (yoor-oh-JEHN-i-tal) *diaphragm*. A ring of skeletal muscle, the **external urethral sphincter**, surrounds the intermediate part of the urethra where it passes through the urogenital diaphragm. The intermediate part continues to the base of the penis and becomes the *spongy urethra* as it passes down the length of the penis, finally opening to the outside at the *external urethral orifice*.

The total length of the male urethra is about 20 centimeters (8 inches). The intermediate part of the urethra and the spongy urethra also carry seminal fluid, as we will learn in the next chapter.

The female urethra is only 3 to 4 centimeters (1.5 inches) long. Like the male urethra, it is surrounded by the external urethral sphincter as it passes through the urogenital diaphragm; its external opening is also called the *external urethral orifice*.

 Check Your Understanding

1. Why would the bladder be unnecessary if the urinary system functioned more like the respiratory system?
2. Is urine stored in the ureters or the bladder?
3. Which tube in the urinary system, the ureter or the urethra, leads to the outside of the body?
4. Is the urethra longer in males or females?

Urine Excretion

Thousands of collecting ducts in each kidney produce a steady trickle of urine into the renal pelvis. As fluid from the kidney enters the ureter, the ureter stretches. This stretching causes a wave of contractions to develop in the smooth muscle wall of the ureter. The wave of muscle contractions travels down the ureter, pushing the urine ahead of it. You may recognize this process of contractions pushing materials down a tube as *peristalsis*. You read about peristalsis in

earlier chapters, such as Chapter 5, *The Muscular System* and Chapter 13, *The Digestive System and Nutrition*.

The release of urine from the bladder is called *urination*, *voiding*, or **micturition** (mik-choo-RISH-un). Micturition requires contraction of the detrusor to force urine out of the bladder, and simultaneous relaxation of both the internal and external sphincters to open the pathway for release.

Because the internal sphincter is made of smooth muscle, it is controlled subconsciously by the autonomic nervous system. By contrast, the external urethral sphincter is made of skeletal muscle. This means that the external urethral sphincter is consciously controlled by somatic motor nerve fibers. (The autonomic and somatic branches of the nervous system are described in chapter 6.) In short, the autonomic reflexes of micturition occur in the spinal cord, while conscious control of the external urethral sphincter originates in the brain.

Figure 14.10 shows the pathways and actions involved in micturition. The numbers in the following description correspond to the numbers in the figure.

1. As the bladder fills, it stretches. Stretch receptors in the wall generate action potentials that excite sensory neurons in the bladder wall. These neurons send impulses to the sacral portion of the spinal cord.
2. Interneurons in the spinal cord signal motor neurons in the sacral cord that the bladder is stretched.
3. The sacral cord neurons send impulses back out to the bladder via parasympathetic nerve fibers.
4. The impulses sent to the bladder through the parasympathetic nerve fibers cause the detrusor to contract and the internal urethral sphincter to relax.
5. While the detrusor is contracting and the internal urethral sphincter is relaxing, the spinal cord sends a signal to the brain, "telling" it that the bladder is stretched (from step 1).
6. The sensory message from the spinal cord activates the micturition reflex center in the

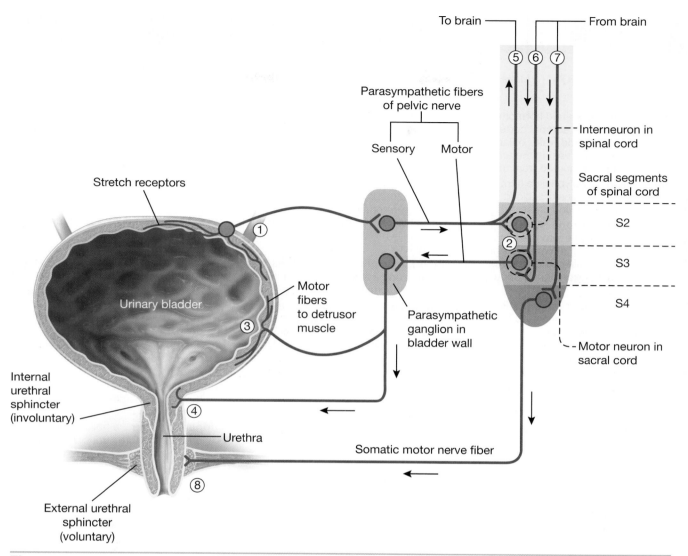

Figure 14.10 The pathways and actions involved in micturition. *Based on what you see in the drawing, do you think any nerve impulses go directly to the brain from the bladder, or do they all go through the spinal cord? How would you describe the brain's involvement in the micturition process?*

brain stem, which sends impulses to the sacral cord.

7. The detrusor contracts, and the internal urethral sphincter relaxes. At the same time that this happens, the person becomes consciously aware that the bladder is full. If the time is not right for urination, there is no change in the steady signal to the external urethral sphincter that causes it to stay contracted. If the time is right for urination, nerve impulses are sent from the brain stem to the sacral spinal cord.

8. From the sacral spinal cord, the nerve impulses travel to the external urethral

sphincter, signaling it to relax. As a result, the pathway for micturition becomes fully open, the detrusor contracts, and the urine is expelled.

Early in childhood, we unconsciously learn that we can aid the expulsion of urine. We do this, without realizing it, by contracting the respiratory diaphragm and the skeletal muscles of the abdomen. This muscle contraction raises pressure in the abdominal cavity, which pushes down on the top of the bladder, thus helping to force urine out. This voluntary effort to raise intra-abdominal pressure is called the *Valsalva maneuver*, and can also be useful in aiding defecation.

Lesson 14.2 Review and Assessment

Mini Glossary   Make sure that you know the meaning of each key term.

Build vocabulary with
e-flash cards and games

aldosterone   a steroid hormone produced in the adrenal cortex that regulates salt and water balance in the body by increasing the amount of sodium reabsorbed from urine

angiotensin   a polypeptide hormone in the blood that constricts blood vessels and increases blood pressure

antidiuretic hormone (ADH)   a peptide hormone secreted by the pituitary gland that constricts blood vessels, raises blood pressure, and reduces excretion of urine; vasopressin

atrial natriuretic peptide (ANP)   a peptide hormone secreted by the atria of the heart that promotes excretion of sodium and water and lowers blood pressure

detrusor   the smooth muscle that forms most of the bladder wall and aids in expelling urine

diuresis   urine excretion

external urethral sphincter   a ring of skeletal muscle that surrounds

the intermediate part of the urethra where it passes through the urogenital diaphragm; this muscle is voluntarily controlled during release of urine from the body

glomerular filtration rate (GFR)   the total amount of water filtered from the glomerular capillaries into the glomerular capsule per unit of time; usually measured in milliliters per minute

hydrostatic pressure   the pressure exerted by a liquid as a result of its potential energy

internal urethral sphincter   a layer of smooth muscle located at the inferior end of the bladder and the proximal end of the urethra; this muscle, which prohibits release of urine, is under involuntary control

micturition   urination

osmosis   the movement of water molecules from a region of low osmotic pressure to a region of high osmotic pressure

osmotic pressure   a pressure created by the presence of dissolved substances in water

reabsorption   the movement of water and dissolved substances from the filtrate (in a renal tubule) back into the blood

renin   an enzyme made and secreted by the kidneys; aids in the production of angiotensin

secretion   the active movement of substances from the blood into the filtrate, which will become urine

trigone   the triangular region of the bladder formed by the two ureteric orifices and the internal urethral orifice

ureter   a duct through which urine travels from the kidney to the bladder

urethra   a thin tube that connects the urinary bladder to the outside environment

urinary bladder   a hollow, muscular organ that stores urine; bladder

Know and Understand   Assess

1. What are the three major processes involved in urine formation?

2. During filtration in the glomerular capsule, water and solutes move from where to where? What is the water called after this movement?

3. What two types of pressure are involved in the filtration process that creates urine?

4. Name four substances that diffuse into the capillaries as a result of secondary active transport.

5. For proper urine formation, should the osmolality levels of the interstitial fluid in the renal medulla be normal or higher than normal?

6. List the three key hormones involved in "fine tuning" urine volume and composition.

7. How does the urinary system differ from the respiratory system in eliminating waste?

8. Which structure(s) contract and which structure(s) relax during micturition?

Analyze and Apply

9. Compare and contrast hydrostatic pressure and osmotic pressure.

10. Explain how and why the nervous system is involved in excreting urine from the body.

11. Explain the relationship between antidiuretic hormone and dehydration.

In the Lab

12. Conduct a simple experiment to see how osmosis works. Place a few cherries in a bowl of water and then put a lid on the bowl. Take the lid off the bowl the next day and examine the cherries. How have the cherries changed? How do you explain these changes? In your explanation, use terms that you learned in this lesson.

Diseases and Disorders of the Urinary System

Before You Read

Try to answer the following questions before you read this lesson.

What are the two forms of diabetes, and how does each affect the urinary system?

What is renal dialysis and who needs it?

Why do women experience more urinary tract infections than men?

Lesson Objectives

1. Explain how different tests of renal function work, and what these tests tell us.

2. Describe urinary system disorders, diseases, and treatment options.

Key Terms

E-Flash Cards

chronic kidney disease
creatinine
hemodialysis
kidney stone
osmotic diuresis
peritoneal dialysis

renal dialysis
urine specific gravity
urinalysis
urinary tract infection (UTI)

Many illnesses, of both renal and nonrenal origin, cause changes in the urine. Therefore, the analysis of urine—**urinalysis**—is a standard part of a complete physical examination. In this lesson, we'll discuss some medical conditions of nonrenal origin that create abnormalities in the urine and eventually lead to kidney damage. We'll also identify the causes and symptoms of several disorders and diseases of the urinary system, along with treatment options.

Assessing Renal Function

The amount, appearance, smell, and chemical content of urine can reveal clues to abnormalities in kidney function. Because the kidneys regulate the composition of blood, analysis of blood is essential for evaluation of kidney function.

Physical Characteristics of Urine

Urine is normally clear and yellow (**Figure 14.11**). Cloudy urine may indicate a urinary tract infection. A color other than yellow may result from the presence of blood in the urine—which is never normal—or from certain vitamin supplements, drugs, or foods.

The pH of urine can vary from 4.5 to 8.0 under normal conditions. A urine pH of 6.0 is quite typical. The **urine specific gravity** is a measure of the urine's mass per unit volume, divided by the density of pure water. Normal urine has a specific gravity of 1.003 to 1.035, with higher numbers indicating more concentrated urine—that is, urine that contains more dissolved substances. A typical daily volume of urine is 0.5 to 2.0 liters (1 pint to ½ gallon).

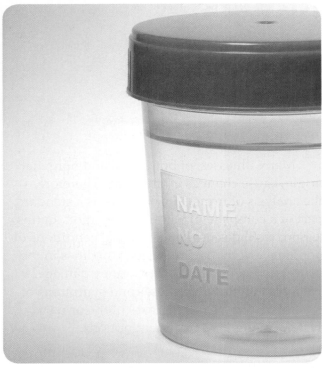

HSNphotography/Shutterstock.com

Figure 14.11 A sample of urine. Urine that is cloudy instead of clear indicates a possible urinary tract infection. *If the color of urine is not yellow, as it should be, what are some possible causes?*

Chemical Composition of Urine

Urine is about 95% water. Urea is the most abundant solute in urine. It is a type of *nitrogenous* (nitrogen-containing) *waste* produced by the normal chemical breakdown of proteins. Potassium, chloride, sodium, and other ions are typically present in urine. The presence of red or white blood cells, protein, or glucose in urine is abnormal and usually will lead to further testing to determine the cause.

Inexpensive test kits allow rapid measurement of many compounds in urine. The kits contain small plastic strips with chemicals that change color in response to the presence or concentration of various compounds in urine. A microscope is also essential for checking a urine sample for blood cells, bacteria, and other abnormalities.

Glomerular Filtration Rate

As was mentioned in lesson 14.2, the measurement of glomerular filtration rate (GFR)

is a key part of assessing kidney function. One approach to measuring GFR is based on the following idea: if a substance in blood plasma is easily filtered by the glomerulus, and is neither reabsorbed nor secreted by the renal tubules, then the rate at which that substance collects in the urine should be an indicator of GFR. If one can measure the concentration of this substance in blood and in urine, one can estimate GFR by an equation.

Inulin, a nontoxic polysaccharide derived from plants, meets these requirements, and has been used by physiologists and clinicians to estimate GFR in research studies. Although inulin is considered an excellent way to measure GFR, it is not routinely used because it requires an infusion of inulin into the patient's blood.

The most common way to estimate GFR is by measuring blood concentration of **creatinine** (kree-AT-in-een), a normal by-product of muscle metabolism that is produced at a steady rate. Creatinine is freely filtered by the glomerulus. (To a small extent, creatinine is also secreted by the tubule, which means that it is not a perfect compound for measuring GFR.) If the GFR is high, creatinine will be removed rapidly from the blood by glomerular filtration, and the creatinine blood concentration will be low. If GFR is low, creatinine will not be removed rapidly from the blood, and the creatinine blood concentration will be high.

Equations have been developed and tested that allow one to estimate GFR based on a patient's blood creatinine level. The most widely used equation includes correction factors to adjust for the age, gender, and race of the patient.

 Check Your Understanding

1. Why is the analysis of urine a standard part of a complete physical examination?
2. What pH range is considered normal for urine?
3. When urine has a high specific gravity, what does this indicate?
4. What is the most common method of measuring glomerular filtration rate?

Diabetes

Diabetes, which means "passing through" in Greek, refers to conditions in which urine output is abnormally elevated—in other words, too much water is passing through the body. The two types of diabetes, as you know from reading chapter 8, are diabetes mellitus and diabetes insipidus. (When the term *diabetes* is used alone, it refers to *diabetes mellitus*.)

Diabetes Mellitus

Diabetes mellitus is characterized by the production of large amounts of urine that contains glucose, a sweet, colorless sugar. (The Latin word *mellitus* means "sweet.") Diabetes mellitus develops in one of two ways: when the body fails to produce insulin (a hormone produced in the pancreas) and when the body's cells fail to respond to insulin.

Diabetes mellitus can be considered a malabsorption disorder (unable to absorb nutrients) because cells do not absorb glucose across their membranes effectively. This results in the need for patients to match their caloric intake with their energy needs throughout the day. They need to choose calories carefully to avoid large peaks and valleys in blood glucose.

Type I diabetes mellitus is an autoimmune disease in which the body's immune system attacks and destroys the insulin-producing cells of the pancreas. Type II diabetes mellitus is less well understood. Both types of diabetes involve an inability to metabolize glucose properly after carbohydrate digestion. As a result, blood glucose levels can soar.

Figure 14.12 on the next page illustrates carbohydrate digestion and blood glucose regulation in a healthy person. Because a person with type I diabetes cannot make insulin, the blood glucose level can soar after a carbohydrate-rich meal. This is because muscle cells and fat cells are not stimulated by insulin to take up and store glucose.

As we discussed in lesson 14.2, glucose normally is filtered by the glomerulus and fully reabsorbed in the renal tubule, due to cotransport with sodium in the tubule. In diabetes mellitus, so much glucose enters filtrate from the glucose-rich plasma that the tubule cannot reabsorb it all—which is why the urine of patients with diabetes mellitus may have a sweet odor.

The excess glucose in the filtrate creates osmotic pressure, which interferes with normal water reabsorption in the tubule and collecting duct. The result is less water reabsorption and more urine production. This is an example of **osmotic diuresis**, an increase in urine production due to abnormally high osmolality of the filtrate.

One of the most serious, long-term consequences of diabetes mellitus is kidney damage, or *diabetic nephropathy* (neh-FRAHP-a-thee). Diabetes mellitus is the most common cause of chronic kidney disease and renal failure, both of which are discussed later. Excessive protein in the urine (*proteinuria*) is often the first sign of kidney damage, followed by a gradual decrease in glomerular filtration rate. The kidneys are more likely to function for a longer period of time in diabetic patients who control their blood glucose well.

Memory Tip

The word *nephropathy* in the term *diabetic nephropathy* comes from the Greek words *nephros*, which means "kidney," and *pathos*, which means "disease" or "suffering."

Diabetes Insipidus

Diabetes insipidus is characterized by the production of large amounts of urine (more than 12 liters a day in severe cases) that is highly diluted. The urine specific gravity is less than the normal lower limit of 1.002, and the urine osmolality is also low, indicating that the urine is mostly water with very few substances dissolved in it.

Diabetes insipidus is usually caused by failure of the pituitary gland to produce normal amounts of antidiuretic hormone (ADH). In a minority of cases, the disease is caused by unresponsiveness of the kidney to ADH.

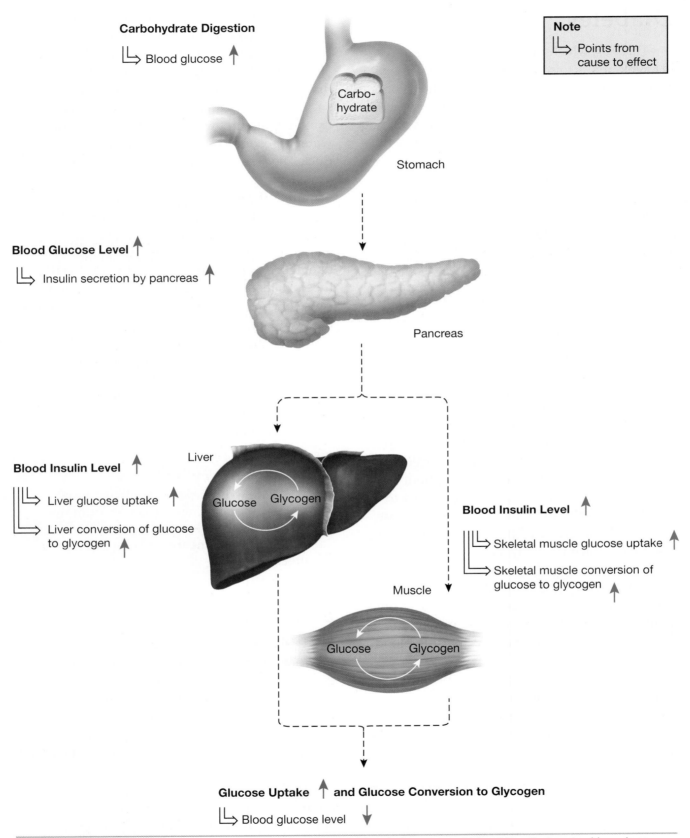

Figure 14.12 Effects of normal carbohydrate digestion on blood glucose and blood insulin levels. *How does diabetes mellitus cause a breakdown in the processes shown above?*

As we learned in lesson 14.2, ADH causes the collecting ducts to be permeable to water. The collecting ducts are the site for the final stage of water reabsorption; therefore, collecting duct reabsorption is critical for the formation of concentrated urine. The regulation of blood osmolality by ADH in a healthy person is shown in **Figure 14.13**. In the absence of ADH, or if the kidney cannot respond to ADH, little or no water is reabsorbed as the urine flows down the collecting duct.

For example, in a person with diabetes insipidus, the brain does not make ADH (central diabetes insipidus), or the kidney does not respond to it (nephrogenic diabetes insipidus), so the kidney does not reabsorb water as much as normal. As a result, urine output is much higher than normal, and the patient is always thirsty, due to the constant loss of fluid. Patients whose diabetes insipidus is caused by a failure to produce ADH often can be helped with a prescription for a synthetic form of ADH.

Memory Tip

In the term *diabetes insipidus*, the Latin word *insipidus* means "weak." The urine of a person with diabetes insipidus could be considered to be weak, because both its specific gravity and urine osmolality are low.

Chronic Kidney Disease

Chronic kidney disease is defined by evidence of kidney damage (usually proteinuria) or a glomerular filtration rate less than 60 milliliters per minute, for at least three months. Chronic kidney disease develops slowly. Diabetes mellitus is the most common cause, followed by hypertension (high blood pressure). Careful management of diabetes, and aggressive treatment of high blood pressure with drugs such as angiotensin-converting enzyme (ACE) inhibitors and angiotensin receptor blockers, may slow the progression of chronic kidney disease.

Reduced sodium concentration in blood

High sodium concentration in blood

Saved water dilutes sodium

ADH causes increased water reabsorption, less urine production

Hypothalamus

Pituitary gland

Pituitary releases ADH

Figure 14.13 Regulation of blood osmolality by ADH. In a healthy person, regulation of both blood sodium concentration and blood osmolality is roughly equivalent because sodium is the biggest contributor to blood osmolality. *What happens to urine output in a person with diabetes insipidus?*

When GFR decreases to 15 milliliters per minute or less, a patient is said to have renal failure—the most severe stage of chronic kidney disease. In renal failure, the kidneys are unable to adequately perform their task of maintaining homeostasis. Without treatment, a person cannot survive very long in this state. Waste products accumulate in the blood, and levels of pH and various ions are no longer well controlled. At this stage, the patient must receive renal dialysis, a medical technique in which the blood is filtered through a machine, or a kidney transplant.

Because the supply of donor kidneys is very limited, most patients with renal failure undergo dialysis. However, the process of dialysis compromises a patient's health and lowers his or her life expectancy. In short, filtering the blood through a machine is not as good for one's health or life span as having a real kidney.

Renal Dialysis

Renal dialysis (digh-AL-i-sis) is the removal of wastes from the blood by artificial means. The two types of dialysis are hemodialysis and peritoneal dialysis. Both forms of dialysis remove water, urea, and some sodium from the body.

Hemodialysis

In **hemodialysis** (HEE-moh-digh-AL-i-sis), blood is withdrawn from an artery, pumped through a dialyzer—a large machine positioned next to the patient—and then returned to the patient through a vein. The *dialyzer* (DIGH-a-LIGH-zer) acts as an artificial kidney, although it does not perform all the functions of a real kidney (**Figure 14.14**).

In the dialyzer, the blood passes through thin tubes whose semipermeable walls make up

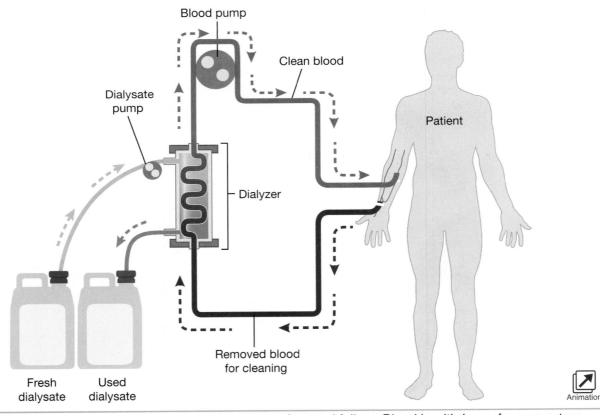

Figure 14.14 Hemodialysis is the most common treatment for renal failure. Blood is withdrawn from an artery, usually in the forearm, and is pumped through a dialyzer. In the dialyzer, a semipermeable membrane separates the blood from dialysate. Dialysate is a fluid with a chemical composition similar to blood plasma. Wastes including urea cross from the blood into the dialysate. The "cleaned" blood returns to the body. The used dialysate is discarded. *In the dialyzer, a semipermeable membrane separates the blood from dialysate. How is this process accomplished in the kidneys?*

WHAT RESEARCH TELLS US

...*about* Paired Kidney Transplants

The human kidney is one of the most commonly transplanted organs in the body. A kidney transplant is done when a person has chronic, or end-stage, renal failure. In the United States, the two leading causes of end-stage renal failure are diabetes and high blood pressure.

A transplanted kidney may come from a living donor or a recently deceased person. Research indicates that patients who get a kidney from a live donor have better health and life-expectancy outcomes than those who receive a cadaver kidney.

Unfortunately, there are far fewer kidneys available than there are patients who need them. We each have two kidneys and can donate one of them. Research shows that live donors do not have shorter or less healthful lives.

Live-donor transplants can be difficult to arrange. Often, a family member who is willing to donate a kidney is not immunologically compatible with the relative who needs a kidney. In other words, the kidney from the willing donor would be rejected by the recipient's body. To address this problem, doctors have sometimes performed "paired" kidney transplants.

For example, Bob is willing to donate a kidney to Mark, but Mark's blood type and body tissue are incompatible with Bob's. Meanwhile, Mallory is willing to donate a kidney to Pearl, but Pearl's blood type and body tissue are incompatible with Mallory's. Let's suppose that Bob is compatible with Pearl, and Mallory is compatible with Mark. If they all agree to make "crossed" donations, then both Mark and

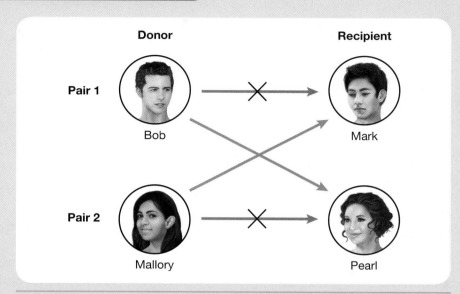

Figure 14.15 Paired kidney transplants with crossed kidney donation.

Pearl will get the kidneys they need (**Figure 14.15**).

Paired kidney transplants can work in even larger circles of donors and recipients. In 2011, a chain of 30 linked kidney transplants was completed—the largest paired-kidney transplant chain ever. This "pay-it-forward" chain took four months to complete and involved hospitals throughout the United States. Such a large chain of linked kidney transplants was possible due to significant advances in organ donor technology. For example, extremely precise and efficient methods were used to keep a kidney viable (healthy) while it was harvested at one hospital and then flown to a recipient in another location. Improved surgical techniques increased the odds of success for each operation. Also, computer technology played a key role in the linked-kidney transplant chain. Before the operations were arranged, a special software

program was used to identify possible matches between the patients and willing donors who had joined a national registry.

Taking It Further

1. Research the topic of kidney transplants in general or paired kidney transplants in particular. What is required of a donor? What are transplant risks for both the donor and the recipient? What does the procedure involve? What kind of medical care must the organ recipient continue to have after surgery? What happens when a person's body rejects a transplanted kidney?

2. Can you think of any ethical issues that a paired kidney transplant might present for donors and recipients? Prepare an argument with supporting research, and present your case in an oral report to the class.

the dialysis membrane. Dialysis fluid circulates around those tubes. Urea, other wastes, water, and some electrolytes diffuse out of the blood and into the dialysis fluid. The dialysis fluid is discarded, and the blood is returned to the body.

Peritoneal Dialysis

In **peritoneal dialysis**, dialysis fluid is added to the abdominopelvic cavity through a surgically implanted port in the abdomen. As the dialysis solution sits in the abdomen for an hour or more, it absorbs water and wastes from capillaries in the mesentery (the membrane that attaches the intestines to the wall of the abdomen) and elsewhere in the abdominopelvic cavity. The peritoneum itself serves as the dialysis membrane that separates the blood from the dialysis fluid.

Kidney Stones

A **kidney stone** is not really a stone. It is a solid crystalline mass that forms in the urine (**Figure 14.16**). Kidney stones are usually made of calcium-containing compounds, but they can also be composed of magnesium or uric acid.

Kidney stones usually form in the renal pelvis, but they may form in the ureter or bladder. Stones smaller than 5 millimeters in

Piotr Malczyk/Shutterstock.com

Figure 14.16 Kidney stones. *At what size can kidney stones become lodged in the ureter?*

diameter may pass from the body in the urine without difficulty. If a larger stone develops in the kidney, it will be carried by urine flow to the ureter, where it will get stuck. When a kidney stone gets lodged in the ureter, intense pain usually occurs.

Lithotripsy (LITH-oh-TRIP-see) is the use of intense, ultrasonic sound waves to break up a kidney stone into pieces small enough to be passed from the body in the urine. The risk of additional kidney stone development can be reduced by drinking a lot of fluids. Greater fluid intake increases the volume and flow rate of urine, reducing the likelihood of crystallization.

Urinary Tract Infections

A **urinary tract infection (UTI)** is usually caused by bacteria that enter the urethra at its outside opening. If the bacteria reach the bladder, the resulting infection can lead to *cystitis* (sis-TIGH-tis), an inflammation of the bladder epithelium. Urinary tract infections are more common in women than in men; women have a shorter urethra, so bacteria can more easily reach the bladder.

UTI symptoms include pain during urination, increased urinary frequency, fever, and sometimes cloudy or dark urine. If the bacteria travel up the ureters to the kidneys, the kidneys themselves can become infected. The resulting condition is *pyelonephritis* (PIGH-eh-loh-neh-FRIGH-tis). Besides the symptoms already described, patients often experience pain in the kidney region of the back.

> ✓ **Check Your Understanding**
>
> 1. What is renal failure?
> 2. What are two types of renal dialysis?
> 3. What substances does dialysis remove from the blood?
> 4. What is the ideal source of a kidney used for transplantation?
> 5. What are kidney stones composed of?
> 6. Which type of microorganism causes urinary tract infections?

Lesson 14.3 Review and Assessment

Mini Glossary
Make sure that you know the meaning of each key term.

 Build vocabulary with e-flash cards and games

chronic kidney disease a condition defined by evidence of kidney damage or a glomerular filtration rate less than 60 milliliters per minute for at least three months

creatinine a normal by-product of muscle metabolism; it is produced by the body at a fairly steady rate and is freely filtered by the glomerulus

hemodialysis a procedure for removing metabolic waste products from the body; blood is withdrawn from an artery, pumped through a dialyzer, and then returned to the patient through a vein

kidney stone a solid crystalline mass that forms in the kidney and that may become stuck in the renal pelvis or ureter; usually made of calcium, phosphate, uric acid, and protein

osmotic diuresis an increase in urine production caused by high osmotic pressure of the glomerular filtrate, which "pulls" more water into the filtrate

peritoneal dialysis a renal dialysis method that uses the patient's peritoneum to filter fluids and dissolved substances from the blood

renal dialysis the removal of wastes from the blood by artificial means

urine specific gravity the density (mass per unit volume) of urine, divided by the density of pure water

urinalysis laboratory analysis of urine to test for the presence of infection or disease

urinary tract infection (UTI) an infection of the urethra, bladder, ureters, and/or kidney, usually caused by bacteria that enter the urethra at its outside opening

Know and Understand

 Assess

1. Urine consists primarily of what substance? What is the most abundant solute in urine?

2. Why is blood creatinine concentration used to assess kidney function? Why is creatinine considered better than inulin for measuring GFR?

3. Why does the urine of many patients with diabetes mellitus have a sweet odor?

4. Why does the absence of antidiuretic hormone cause diabetes insipidus?

5. How is chronic kidney disease defined by glomerular filtration rate?

6. Which functions of the kidneys can be accomplished through renal dialysis? Which functions cannot be accomplished?

7. What are the two types of renal dialysis, and what is the difference between them?

8. How is lithotripsy used to treat kidney stones?

9. Why are urinary tract infections more common in women than in men?

Analyze and Apply

10. Compare and contrast the symptoms and the causes of diabetes mellitus and diabetes insipidus.

11. Suppose that you are a doctor or a nurse practitioner. One of your patients, a 24-year-old woman, complains of frequent, painful urination. She has a slight temperature. You request a urine sample from her. Her urine is dark and cloudy. What do you think is causing her symptoms?

In the Lab

12. In this activity you will measure pH and compare the pH measurements of several substances to that of urine.

Using litmus paper, a liquid pH indicator, or a pH meter and probe, measure the pH of the following substances: distilled water, juice squeezed from a lemon, black coffee, household ammonia, bleach, vinegar, a carbonated beverage, milk of magnesia, and a solution of baking soda and water.

Draw a pH "ruler" and mark it with the units 0 to 14. (Note: A neutral pH is 7. A solution with a pH below 7 is acidic. A solution with a pH above 7 is alkaline.) For each substance that you tested, determine whether the pH is neutral, acidic, or alkaline, and write its name in the corresponding area along the ruler.

A urine pH of 6.0 is typical. Compare the pH of the tested substances with that of urine.

Career Corner
Anatomy and Physiology at Work

The urinary system performs the critical work of filtering waste products from our blood and in maintaining a stable chemical environment inside our bodies. Many people have found fulfilling careers in the diagnosis and treatment of diseases and disorders of the urinary system. We will explore two of these careers.

Nephrologist

A nephrologist, or renal physician, is a medical doctor who specializes in the diagnosis and treatment of kidney diseases and disorders (**Figure 14.17**). Most nephrologists divide their time between seeing patients in office settings and in hospitals. Some work at kidney and dialysis centers. Renal patients usually see a nephrologist after being referred by their primary care physician.

Nephrologists diagnose kidney problems by ordering and interpreting tests, such as blood tests, urinalyses, ultrasound procedures, and biopsies, in which a small piece of tissue is removed from the kidney and examined for signs of disease. Nephrologists also manage the care of patients with chronic kidney disease, including patients on dialysis. Patients who need surgery—to remove kidney stones or to treat kidney cancer, for example—are referred to another type of doctor called a *urologist*.

A nephrologist's patients have a variety of illnesses and disorders, several of which are covered in this lesson. They may have infections or kidney stones. They may have kidney problems brought on by pregnancy or by a genetic condition. However, many of the nephrologist's patients have chronic kidney disease caused by conditions such as hypertension or diabetes. After assessing the seriousness of the renal disease, nephrologists may prescribe medication to lower blood pressure, prescribe renal dialysis, or refer patients for kidney transplantation.

In the United States, a nephrologist has a bachelor of science degree and a medical doctor (MD) degree. Medical school is followed by three years of training in internal medicine, and then by a nephrology fellowship lasting two or three years. A physician who has completed this training is eligible to take the examination to become a board-certified nephrologist.

Renal Dialysis Technician

Renal dialysis technicians perform and monitor the dialysis treatment of kidney patients. They work under the supervision of a registered nurse. Most renal dialysis technicians are employed in dialysis facilities, most of which are located in hospitals and outpatient facilities.

Following a prescription written by a doctor, renal dialysis technicians prepare the

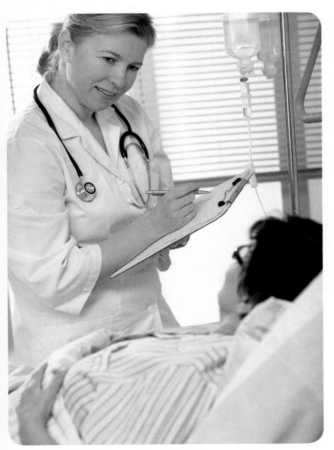

Alexander Raths/Shutterstock.com

Figure 14.17 A nephrologist talks with a patient in the hospital.

dialysate, the solution that is used in the dialysis treatment. They test and prepare the dialysis equipment. They also prepare patients for dialysis, which involves inserting needles for access to an artery and a vein (**Figure 14.18**).

While patients are undergoing treatment, renal dialysis technicians monitor and adjust the dialysis machinery. They monitor patients and measure blood-flow rates and fluid removal rates. They must be prepared for dialysis-related emergencies. Renal dialysis technicians are responsible for maintaining dialysis machines in proper working order. Because they work directly with patients, renal dialysis technicians must have good communication skills and be able to respond to their patients' emotional needs.

To become a renal dialysis technician, you must have a high school diploma and certification. Certification requirements vary by state, but usually involve passing an examination and successfully completing up to 18 months of on-the-job training.

Planning for a Health-Related Career

Do some research on the career of a nephrologist or a renal dialysis technician.

Figure 14.18 A renal dialysis technician prepares a patient for dialysis.

Alternatively, select a profession from the list of **Related Career Options**. Using the Internet or resources at your local library, find answers to the following questions:

1. What are the main tasks and responsibilities of a person employed in the career that you chose to research?
2. What is the outlook for this career? Are workers in demand, or are jobs dwindling? For complete information, consult the current edition of the *Occupational Outlook Handbook*, published by the US Department of Labor. This handbook is available online or at your local library.
3. What special skills or talents are required? For example, do you need to be good at biology and anatomy and physiology? Would you be able to master the operation of complex machinery used to treat patients?
4. What personality traits do you think are necessary for success in the career that you chose to research? For example, renal dialysis technicians must have excellent interpersonal, communication, and problem-solving skills.
5. Does the work involve a great deal of routine, or are the day-to-day responsibilities varied?
6. Does the career require long hours, or is it a standard, "9-to-5" job?
7. What is the salary range for this job?
8. What do you think you would like about this career? Is there anything about it that you might dislike?

Related Career Options

- Diabetes Educator
- Home Health and Personal Care Aide
- Renal Dietitian
- Renal Nurse
- Renal Social Worker
- Transplant Surgeon
- Urologist

Chapter Summaries

Lesson 14.1 Anatomy of the Kidney

Build vocabulary with
e-flash cards and games

Key Points

- The main functions of the urinary system are to excrete wastes, retain water and salt, and maintain homeostasis.
- The kidneys are the key organs in the urinary system. They are located on either side of the spinal column, behind the peritoneum.
- The nephron, the basic working unit of the kidney, has two main parts: the renal corpuscle and the renal tubule.
- The glomerulus, one of the major structures in the nephron, is a small, ball-shaped mass of capillary vessels that filter blood to make urine.
- The renal tubule, another key structure in the nephron, contains the fluid that has been filtered by the glomerulus.
- Fluid from distal convoluted tubules enters collecting ducts. The collecting ducts merge into larger ducts, which drain fluid into the renal pelvis.
- The renal pelvis is the deepest part of the kidney. Urine produced in the cortex and medulla of the kidney seeps into the renal pelvis. Fluid then drains from the renal pelvis into the ureter, a tube leading from the kidney to the bladder.

Key Terms

collecting duct
distal convoluted tubule
glomerulus
nephron
nephron loop
proximal convoluted
   tubule (PCT)

renal corpuscle
renal cortex
renal medulla
renal pelvis
renal tubule
urinary system
vasa recta

Lesson 14.2 Urine Formation, Storage, and Excretion

Key Points

- Three steps are involved in urine formation: filtration, reabsorption, and secretion.
- The first step in urine formation is glomerular filtration, which occurs in the renal corpuscle.
- Glomerular filtration rate (GFR) is the total amount of water filtered in a unit of time. GFR is an important benchmark for assessing kidney health.
- Osmosis is the movement of water from an area of low osmotic pressure to an area of high osmotic pressure.
- Hormones and sympathetic nerves to the kidney both regulate the afferent and efferent arterioles, which in turn control urine output.

Key Terms

aldosterone
angiotensin
antidiuretic hormone
   (ADH)
atrial natriuretic peptide
   (ANP)
detrusor
diuresis
external urethral sphincter
glomerular filtration rate
   (GFR)
hydrostatic pressure

internal urethral sphincter
micturition
osmosis
osmotic pressure
reabsorption
renin
secretion
trigone
ureter
urethra
urinary bladder

- Three hormones—aldosterone, atrial natriuretic peptide, and antidiuretic hormone—are key to "fine tuning" urine volume and composition.
- Urine is stored in the bladder, which stretches as it fills. The stretching generates actions in the nervous system that eventually signal the detrusor to contract and the internal urethral sphincter to relax. When the "time is right," the brain sends signals that cause the external urethral sphincter to relax, and the urine is expelled.

Lesson 14.3 — Diseases and Disorders of the Urinary System

Key Points
- The amount, color, pH, and specific gravity of urine are characteristics that can indicate abnormalities in kidney function.
- Urine typically contains 95% water, urea, and ions. The presence of red or white blood cells, protein, or glucose in urine is abnormal.
- Glomerular filtration rate (GFR) is estimated by measuring the concentration of creatinine in the blood.
- Diabetes mellitus and hypertension are the two main causes of chronic kidney disease.
- Patients who have renal failure must receive renal dialysis or a kidney transplant.
- Kidney stones are small crystalline masses that can form in the kidney, ureter, or bladder.
- Urinary tract infections are caused by bacteria that enter the urethra at its outside opening.

Key Terms
chronic kidney disease
creatinine
hemodialysis
kidney stone
osmotic diuresis
peritoneal dialysis
renal dialysis
urine specific gravity
urinalysis
urinary tract infection (UTI)

Chapter Assessments

Assess

Lesson 14.1

Anatomy of the Kidney

Learning Key Terms and Concepts

1. Which of the following is the name of the lighter-colored, outer part of the kidney?
   A. renal cortex
   B. renal medulla
   C. renal pelvis
   D. renal pyramids

2. Which organ of the endocrine system sits on top of each kidney?
   A. adrenal gland
   B. pituitary gland
   C. thyroid gland
   D. pancreas

3. Approximately how many nephrons does each kidney contain?
   A. 1,000
   B. 100,000
   C. 1 million
   D. 10 million

4. Which blood vessel is connected to the kidney and carries blood into it?
   A. renal vein
   B. abdominal aorta
   C. glomerular capillaries
   D. renal artery

5. What is the name of the tube that leads from the kidney toward the bladder?
   A. PCT
   B. vasa recta
   C. ureter
   D. urethra

6. What are the three main parts of the renal tubule?

7. *True or False?* Cortical nephrons are the only nephrons that produce highly concentrated urine.

8. Where are the peritubular capillaries located?

Thinking Critically

9. Compare and contrast the cortical nephrons and the juxtamedullary nephrons.

10. Why do you think the descending limb and the lower part of the ascending limb have thinner walls than the rest of the ascending limb and the proximal and distal convoluted tubules?

Lesson 14.2

Urine Formation, Storage, and Excretion

Learning Key Terms and Concepts

11. Which of the following is *not* a process in the formation of urine?
    A. absorption   C. secretion
    B. reabsorption   D. filtration

12. The endothelial cells, basement membrane, and podocytes combine to form the _____.

13. Which of the following is an important benchmark in assessing kidney health?
    A. PCT   C. ADH
    B. ADP   D. GFR

14. *True or False?* Hydrostatic pressure is influenced by the amount of dissolved substances in water.

15. In the renal corpuscle, does the blood or the filtrate have a higher osmotic pressure?

16. What important purpose is served by the microvilli on the wall of the proximal convoluted tubule?

17. Which of the following allow water to easily enter and exit cells during reabsorption?
    A. sodium-potassium pump proteins
    B. aquaporin channels
    C. cotransport proteins
    D. renal tubules

18. Are the proximal and distal convoluted tubules located on the same side of the nephron loop or on different sides?

19. Which of the following is *not* an accurate description of the interstitial fluid in the renal medulla?
    A. watery   C. concentrated
    B. salty   D. higher than normal osmolality

20. Which substances are reabsorbed from the renal tubule? Which are secreted into it?

21. A decrease in blood sodium or an increase in potassium results in secretion of _____.

22. *True or False?* The detrusor muscle must relax for urine to be excreted.

23. The external and internal sphincter muscles are controlled in different ways. Explain.

24. *True or False?* The brain plays a role in excretion of urine.

Thinking Critically

25. Explain why a GFR of 125 milliliters per minute tells us that the body reabsorbs most of the glomerular filtrate.

26. Compare and contrast the functions of the three key hormones involved in urine volume and composition.

Lesson 14.3

Diseases and Disorders of the Urinary System

Learning Key Terms and Concepts

27. Approximately what percentage of urine is water?

28. When GFR is high, creatinine concentration is _____; when GFR is low, creatinine concentration is _____.

29. Which of the following is normally present in urine?
    A. urea   C. glucose
    B. white blood cells D. protein

30. *True or False?* In diabetes, too much water is passing through the body.

31. *True or False?* Diabetes is a kidney disease.

32. *True or False?* Creatinine is a normal by-product of muscle metabolism.

33. An increase in urine production due to abnormally high osmolality of the filtrate is called _____.

34. A deficiency in which hormone is linked to the development of diabetes mellitus?

35. What is often the first sign of kidney damage?

36. What are the two main causes of chronic kidney disease?

37. What are the two types of renal dialysis, and how do they work?

38. What does dialysis remove from the blood?

39. What are kidney stones? How can they be treated and prevented?

40. A urinary tract infection may affect which organs of the urinary system?

Thinking Critically

41. Carbohydrate digestion is impaired in a person who has diabetes mellitus. What can you conclude about the ideal diet of a person with this disease? Which types of foods should be avoided?

42. Suppose that you are a patient with renal failure. Compare and contrast a kidney transplant with renal dialysis in terms of benefits and costs.

Building Skills and Connecting Concepts

Analyzing and Evaluating Data

Figure 14.18 shows selected urine measurements over a period of time for a 30-year-old adult male. Answer the questions using the data and what you have learned in this chapter.

Figure 14.18 Selected Urine Measurements				
Test	**1**	**2**	**3**	**4**
Specific gravity	1.023	1.031	1.027	1.046
Daily volume	1.25 L	1.20 L	1.15 L	1.0 L
GFR	125 mL/m	95 mL/m	80 mL/m	75 mL/m

43. Is the specific gravity of the patient's urine trending higher or lower?

44. Would the patient's urine be "saltier" in test 2 or test 4?

45. By what percentage did the patient's daily volume of urine production drop between test 1 and test 4?
    A. 80%   C. 8%
    B. 2%   D. 20%

46. How would you assess this patient's kidney health? Give specific reasons for your assessment.

Communicating about Anatomy and Physiology

47. **Writing and Speaking.** Create a picture book for preschool-aged children that describes the journey of grape juice through the urinary system. Use simple explanations about the urinary system. Include drawings with the text. Test your book by sharing it with a preschool-aged child, after getting a parent's permission.

48. **Speaking.** With a partner, role-play the following situation: A doctor must explain to a patient with renal failure why he or she must start renal dialysis. One student plays the role of the doctor; the other acts as the patient. Use your own words to explain how renal dialysis works. You may use the figures in this lesson for reference. As the doctor explains the dialysis process, the patient should ask questions if the explanation is unclear. Switch roles and repeat the activity.

Lab Investigations

49. Working with a partner, perform this observational experiment to observe, on a simplified scale, the inner workings of the human kidneys. Materials: Two clear glass jars, one regular coffee filter (basket style), large rubber band, chalk, water, red food coloring.

First, mix one-half spoonful of crushed chalk with one-half cup of water in a clear glass jar. Add a few drops of food coloring to the water. (The water represents blood; the chalk represents toxins in the blood.) Next, place the coffee filter over the top of the second glass jar and secure it with the rubber band. (The coffee filter represents the kidneys filtering toxins from the blood.) Finally, pour the chalk-and-water mixture through the coffee filter into the second jar.

Observe what happens to the chalk (toxins) as the colored water (blood) drips into the second jar. With your lab partner, develop a brief, written summary that explains how the results of this experiment help illustrate the glomerular filtration process in the kidneys. Be sure to use these terms in your summary: renal corpuscle, glomerular filtration, glomerular capsular space, glomerular filtrate, solutes, filtration membrane.

Expand your learning with additional online resources
- Supplemental Lab Activities
- Interactive Exercises
- Animations

Companion Website

Expand

www.g-wlearning.com/healthsciences

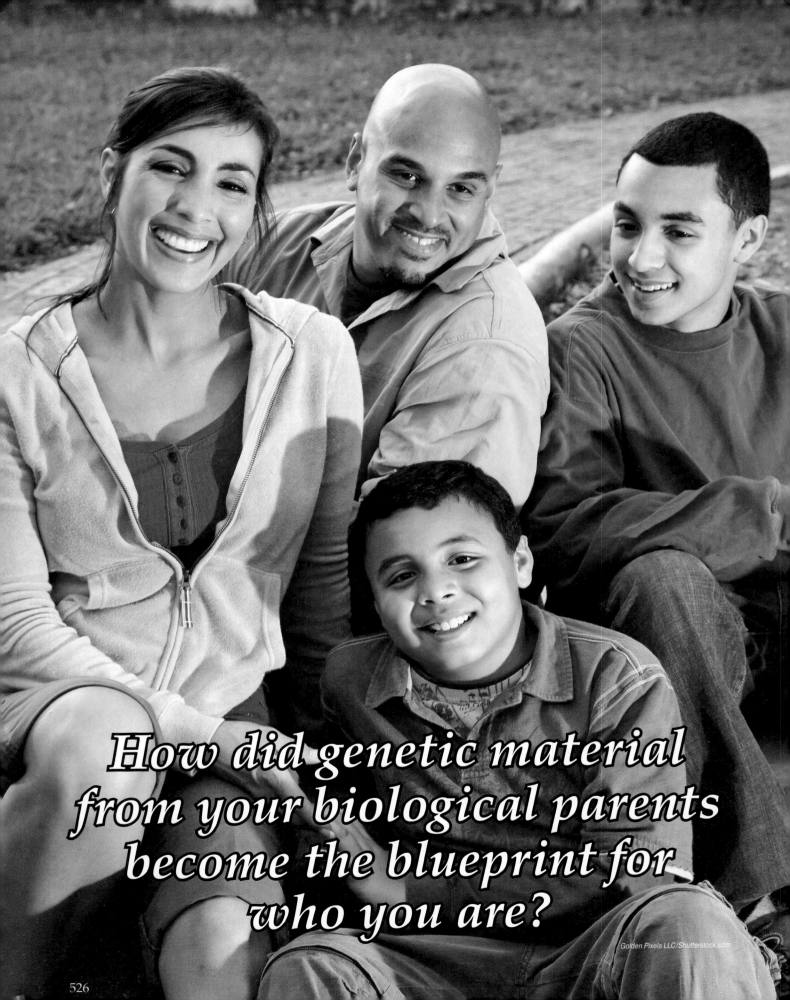

How did genetic material from your biological parents become the blueprint for who you are?

Chapter 15

The Male and Female Reproductive Systems

*R*eproduction, pregnancy, and childbirth are among the most significant, if not *the* most significant, of life's events. It is not unreasonable to say that all the other physiological systems in the body function in part to help ensure that we live long enough to reproduce and care for our young, until they can take care of themselves.

In the human reproductive system, major structural and functional differences exist between the sexes, unlike with the other anatomical systems. The male system has two principal functions, and the female reproductive system has five.

We will begin by reviewing the differences between meiosis and mitosis—important information to have in mind when we later discuss the generation of sperm and eggs. We will then explore the anatomy and physiology of the male reproductive system, followed by the anatomy and physiology of the more complicated and multifunctional female reproductive system. We will discuss pregnancy, childbirth, and lactation (the production and secretion of breast milk). Finally, we will review some of the more common disorders and diseases of the male and female reproductive systems.

While studying, look for the online icon to:

- **Practice** with e-flash cards and vocabulary games
- **Review** with interactive art labeling
- **Assess** with online exercises
- **Expand** with interactive activities and animated videos
- **Listen** to pronunciations of key terms in the audio glossary

Companion Website

www.g-wlearning.com/healthsciences

Study on the Go

Use a mobile device to practice vocabulary terms, listen to pronunciations, and review with self-assessment quizzes.

www.m.g-wlearning.com

Lesson 15.1

Reproduction and Development of the Human Reproductive Systems

Before You Read

Try to answer the following questions before you read this lesson.

What is sexual reproduction?

How is genetic diversity created during human reproduction?

When do the male and female reproductive systems develop?

Lesson Objectives

1. Describe the main difference between sexual reproduction and asexual reproduction.
2. Identify the stages of mitosis.
3. List the stages of meiosis.
4. Explain the differences between mitosis and meiosis.
5. Describe the development of the reproductive systems during the embryonic and fetal stages.
6. Describe the biological changes that occur during male and female puberty.

Key Terms

E-Flash Cards

centromere
chromatids
chromosomes
crossovers
diploid
fertilization
follicle-stimulating
  hormone (FSH)

gametes
haploid
luteinizing hormone
  (LH)
meiosis
menarche
zygote

In this lesson, we will examine both sexual and asexual reproduction. We will then compare the two different processes—mitosis and meiosis—involved in cell reproduction. Finally, we will learn about the development of the male and female reproductive systems.

Reproduction

When most animals, including human beings, reproduce, their offspring receive genetic material from both parents. Each parent contributes half of the genetic material for each offspring. This type of reproduction is called *sexual reproduction.*

Another way of reproducing involves only one parent. In this case, the offspring are *clones*, or genetic copies, of the parent. This method is called *asexual reproduction.*

Asexual reproduction is not uncommon in the plant kingdom. It occurs more rarely in a few animal species, including flatworms. Asexual reproduction is simple because only one parent is required and no "sorting" of genetic material is needed. Genetic diversity still occurs because of mutations that arise every now and then.

Sexual reproduction, which involves two parents, offers the advantage of producing individuals who are genetically different from their parents. Sexual reproduction is more complicated than asexual reproduction, and the additional steps required mean more opportunities for things to "go wrong."

Sexual reproduction requires that each parent produce **gametes** (GAM-eets), cells for reproduction that contain half as many **chromosomes** as a normal cell. Chromosomes are structures in the nuclei of our body cells that contain our individual DNA and genes. **Fertilization** is the formation of a single cell containing the genetic material from two gametes—one gamete from each parent. The fertilized cell produced by the combining of gametes is called a **zygote** (ZIGH-goht). The zygote is the single cell from which a new individual will develop.

Mitosis versus Meiosis

You learned about mitosis in chapter 2. In this section you will learn about a similar-sounding cell division process—**meiosis**. Mitosis occurs in all of the body's tissues, throughout life, as the body grows and renews itself. Meiosis, on the other hand, occurs only in the sex organs, and produces a special kind of cell. Let's look at these processes side by side so that you can understand them both better.

Mitosis

The development of a zygote into an adult requires that one cell give rise to trillions of cells. Mitosis (migh-TOH-sis) is the process of cell division by which this growth occurs. We will briefly review mitosis, which was discussed in greater detail in chapter 2.

In mitosis, one cell divides to make two "daughter" cells. The two daughter cells are genetically identical to the mother cell, except for the occasional mutation. The process of mitosis is shown in the left panel of **Figure 15.1** on the next page.

Before mitosis begins, the mother cell has 23 pairs of chromosomes—22 similar pairs, plus two X chromosomes if female, or an X and a Y chromosome if male. The two members of a chromosomal pair are called *homologous* (hoh-MAHL-uh-gus) *chromosomes*. For the purpose of explanation, only 2 of the 23 pairs are shown in the figure.

Homologous chromosomes are very similar, but they are not quite identical. The mother cell inherited one of each of 23 chromosomes

from each parent. Therefore, you can think of the purple chromosomes shown in the mother cell in **Figure 15.1** as chromosomes from the mother, and you can think of the green chromosomes as being from the father—or vice versa. As you know, a complete diagram would depict 23 purple chromosomes and 23 green chromosomes.

Because humans have two homologous versions of each chromosome, we have two versions of each gene in our genome—one gene from each parent. (A genome is an individual genetic code, the total amount of genetic information contained in a set of chromosomes.) The important exception to this general rule is that males have 22 homologous pairs, plus one X and one Y chromosome. The X and Y chromosomes are not homologous. This fact is important for understanding the inheritance patterns of certain genetic diseases that preferentially affect males. By contrast, females have 23 pairs of homologous chromosomes, including two X chromosomes.

In both mitosis and meiosis, DNA duplication occurs during the first stage of cell division, called *interphase* (see **Figure 2.20** on page 61). Interphase is essentially the normal, resting state of a cell.

In *prophase*, the stage during which the cell prepares for mitotic division, the nuclear membrane dissolves. The DNA, which had been diffuse (scattered or spread out), condenses into chromosomes. The duplicated chromosomes, called sister **chromatids** (KROH-ma-tids), remain attached to each other at a point along their length called the **centromere** (SEHN-troh-meer), as seen in **Figure 15.2** on page 531.

In *metaphase*, the chromosomes line up in the middle of the cell. A protein called *separase* splits the sister chromatids by cutting the centromeres in half.

In the remaining phases of mitosis each chromosome is pulled to one side of the cell or the other, and the cytoplasm divides (**Figure 2.21** on page 62). The result is two cells, each with 46 chromosomes that are identical to the 46 chromosomes in the mother cell.

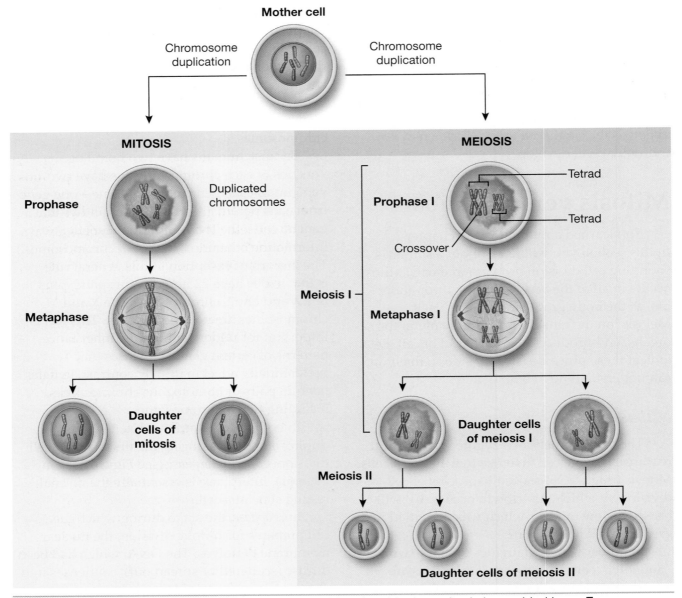

Figure 15.1 Comparison of mitosis with meiosis. An abbreviated look at mitosis is provided here. For a more complete look at the process, see **Figures 2.20** and **2.21** on pages 61 and 62. Also note that to more clearly illustrate the process only 2 of the 23 pairs of chromosomes are shown. *How many pairs of homologous chromosomes are in the genome of a male? a female? During which stage in mitotic division does DNA condense into chromosomes?*

✓ Check Your Understanding

1. Is genetic diversity possible in asexual reproduction? Explain.
2. Name an advantage of sexual reproduction over asexual reproduction.
3. How is a gamete different from normal cells in the human body?
4. What is the end result of mitosis?

Meiosis

A cell with two copies of each chromosome—in other words, a normal cell—is said to be **diploid** (DIP-loyd). A cell with just one version of each chromosome is **haploid** (HAP-loyd). Gametes, the cells for reproduction, are haploid cells.

In meiosis, the goal is to produce gametes, or haploid cells. In short, this is done by duplicating

Duplicated chromosome

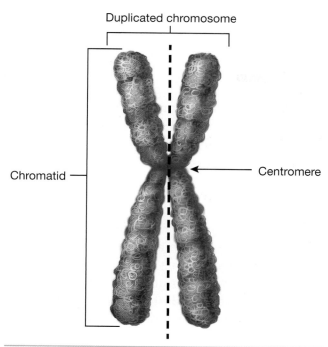

Chromatid

Centromere

Figure 15.2 Sister chromatids. *How are the chromosomes shown here different from those shown in the mother cell in* Figure 15.1?

the DNA once, and then dividing twice, to produce four haploid cells. Keep in mind that meiosis occurs only in the primary sex organs—the testes (TEHS-teez) and the ovaries.

DNA duplication is the first major task of meiosis. During prophase of the first meiotic division ("Meiosis I" in **Figure 15.1**), duplicated pairs of homologous chromosomes come together to form tetrads, clusters of four chromosomes. (The prefix *tetra-* comes from a Greek word meaning "four"). The clustering of homologous chromosomes in tetrads allows **crossovers** to form. A crossover is a connection that forms between homologous chromosomes, which results in the swapping of portions of chromosomes. Tetrads and crossovers form in meiosis but not in mitosis. Crossovers generate additional genetic diversity in the gametes.

When chromosomes separate in the first meiotic division, the sister chromatids are not separated as they are in mitosis (see **Figure 2.21** again). The daughter cells of the first meiotic division contain 23 *duplicated* chromosomes. (Due to crossing over, these duplicates are not exactly identical.) By contrast, the daughter

cells of mitosis contain 23 pairs of *homologous* chromosomes—in other words, 46 *different* chromosomes. Remember that homologous chromosomes consist of "one from dad and one from mom," whereas duplicated chromosomes are two copies of the same chromosome (from *either* mom or dad).

In the first meiotic division, the segregation of chromosomes to one or the other daughter cell is random. It is as though the mother cell "flips a coin" to decide whether to send the purple or the green version of chromosome 1 to the daughter cell on the left. (The other chromosome always goes to the other daughter cell.) Again, the mother cell "flips a coin" to determine whether the purple or the green version of chromosome 2 goes to the left. This process continues for all 23 pairs of chromosomes.

When you flip a coin 23 times, more than 8 million possible outcomes can occur. Therefore, each mother cell that undergoes meiosis can produce 8 million different, possible daughter cells in the first meiotic division. And that does not even take into account the additional genetic diversity generated by crossovers.

In the second meiotic division ("Meiosis II" in **Figure 15.1**), the two daughter cells of Meiosis I divide without chromosome duplication. Sister chromatids are cut apart, and the four resulting cells contain 23 chromosomes each. These haploid cells are the final product of meiosis.

 Check Your Understanding

1. Is a haploid cell associated with mitosis or meiosis?
2. What is the end result of meiosis?

Development and Puberty

The male and female reproductive systems, unlike the other organ systems, do not become functional until later in life. Let's now take a look at sexual organ development and the unique, final maturation process called *puberty*. In this section, we will briefly mention some parts of the reproductive system that will be described more fully in lessons 15.2 and 15.3.

The Y chromosome contains a gene called *SRY*, which stands for "*sex-determining region Y.*" The gene encodes a protein called a *transcription factor*, which controls when other genes are *transcribed*—in other words, when they are switched on or off. By regulating other genes, the SRY gene acts as a molecular switch that triggers a cascade of events leading to the development of male sex organs. A zygote *with* a normal Y chromosome, therefore, becomes a male. A zygote *without* a Y chromosome will develop into a female.

Embryonic and Fetal Development

During the first six to seven weeks of development, male and female embryos are visually indistinguishable. Reproductive organs begin to develop in the fifth week, and for the next two weeks they develop in the same way in both males and females.

In the seventh week of development, the SRY gene starts to take effect in embryos that have a Y chromosome. Male sex organs begin to develop, starting with the testes. The cells in the developing testes secrete testosterone, which causes the penis, scrotum, and male accessory organs to develop.

Embryos that do not have an SRY gene will start to develop ovaries in the eighth week. In the absence of testosterone, female accessory organs and external genitals develop. In the final two months of gestation, the testes descend from the pelvic cavity into the scrotum in males. In females, the ovaries descend somewhat, but they remain within the pelvic cavity.

The body's "default plan" is to develop female reproductive anatomy. The presence of a Y chromosome, and the resulting production of testosterone, causes male anatomical structures to develop. Embryos that cannot produce testosterone—or whose cells do not recognize and respond to testosterone—will develop the external genitals of a female, even if they have a Y chromosome.

At the time of childbirth, the blood levels of **follicle-stimulating hormone (FSH)** and **luteinizing** (LOO-tee-in-ighz-ing) **hormone (LH)** in the newborn are high. However, these levels decline rapidly and remain low for 8 to 14 years, until the onset of puberty. Because FSH and LH are low, the testes do not produce testosterone, and the ovaries do not produce estrogen or progesterone (proh-JEHS-teh-rohn). Thus, the reproductive organs remain nonfunctional for the first 8 to 14 years of life.

Puberty

The typical human life span includes a series of stages—from birth to death—that are collectively referred to as the human growth and development cycle. Certain physical, cognitive, and socioemotional milestones characterize each stage. The stages are: infancy (birth to age 1), toddlerhood (ages 1 to 3), early childhood (ages 3 to 5), middle childhood (ages 6 to 10), adolescence (ages 11 to 19), early adulthood (ages 20 to 39), middle adulthood (ages 40 to 65), and older adulthood (ages 66 and up).

Puberty is the final maturation of the reproductive system. Lasting several years, it marks the time when sexual reproduction becomes possible. Puberty normally starts between 8 and 13 years of age in females and between 9 and 14 years of age in males. Adolescence officially begins with the appearance of secondary sex characteristics (described below) and ends when adult height has been reached.

The initial stimulus for puberty is elevated secretion of gonadotropin-releasing (GOH-nad-oh-TROH-pin) hormone, or GnRH. This hormone is secreted by the hypothalamus in the brain. GnRH causes the pituitary to produce more follicle-stimulating hormone and luteinizing hormone. In turn, FSH and LH stimulate production of gonadal hormones—testosterone in males, and estrogen and progesterone in females. The rising levels of gonadal hormones stimulate maturation of the reproductive organs, and cause the appearance of secondary sex characteristics (**Figures 15.3A**).

Female development. In females, the first phase of puberty is marked by breast growth,

Figure 15.3 Secondary sex characteristics appear at puberty. Both males and females develop underarm and pubic hair; males develop facial hair. Females develop breasts and a wider pelvis that eventually aids in childbirth. *What additional secondary sex characteristics appear at puberty for males? What additional characteristics appear for females?*

followed by the development of secondary sex characteristics: growth of axillary (underarm) and pubic hair, and gradual changes in the width of the pelvis and the size of the pelvic outlet to facilitate pregnancy and childbirth. In addition, skeletal growth accelerates.

About two years after the beginning of puberty, **menarche** (MEHN-ar-kee)—the first menstrual bleeding—occurs. Ovulation cycles typically are irregular for the first one or two years. They become more regular as puberty reaches its conclusion. At this time, the epiphyseal plates in the long bones close, causing height growth to stop.

Male development. In males, the first visible phase of puberty is marked by growth of the scrotum and testes. As in females, secondary sex characteristics appear, with a key difference: besides pubic and axillary hair growth, an increase in the size of the larynx and the length of the vocal folds causes the voice to deepen. The penis grows larger in proportion to body size.

During the early years of puberty, males typically experience erections at unexpected times, as well as occasional emission of semen during sleep. (The discharge of semen during sleep is called a *nocturnal emission*.) By the end of puberty, mature sperm are present in semen. As in females, the epiphyseal plates close, and the long bones in the body stop growing.

 Check Your Understanding

1. Is the SRY gene associated with the development of males or females?
2. Elevated levels of which hormone initiate puberty: LH, FSH, or GnRH?
3. Name at least one secondary sex characteristic shared by males and females.
4. Summarize the human growth and development cycle.

Lesson 15.1 Review and Assessment

Mini Glossary   Make sure that you know the meaning of each key term.

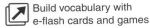
Build vocabulary with
e-flash cards and games

centromere   the point or region on a chromosome that divides the chromosome into two arms and functions as the point of attachment for the sister chromatids; provides movement during cell division

chromatids   paired strands of a duplicated chromosome that become visible during cell division and that are joined by a centromere

chromosomes   rod-shaped structures in the nuclei of our body cells that contain individual DNA and genes

crossovers   connections that form between homologous chromosomes during meiosis, resulting in the swapping of portions of chromosomes

diploid   a cell having two sets of chromosomes: one set from the mother and one set from the father

fertilization   the formation of a single cell that contains the genetic material from two gametes, one from each parent

follicle-stimulating hormone (FSH)   a hormone secreted by the anterior pituitary that stimulates the production of eggs in women and sperm in men

gametes   mature haploid male or female cells that unite with cells of the opposite sex to form a zygote; eggs and sperm

haploid   having a single set of unpaired chromosomes

luteinizing hormone (LH)   tropic hormone produced by the anterior pituitary that signals the egg's release from the follicle, stimulates the production of progesterone and small amounts of estrogen in women, and stimulates the interstitial cells of the testes to produce testosterone in men

meiosis   a type of cell division that produces eggs (in females) or sperm (in males), daughter cells with half the chromosome number of the parent cell

menarche   the first menstrual bleeding

zygote   a diploid cell produced by the fusion of a sperm with an egg; a fertilized egg

Know and Understand

Assess

1. What do we call the offspring of asexual reproduction?

2. Which is simpler—sexual or asexual reproduction?

3. Are there 22 or 23 pairs of chromosomes in a normal human cell?

4. How many pairs of homologous chromosomes do males have? How many do females have?

5. How many chromosomes are there in a mother cell as mitosis begins?

6. What is the difference between haploid and diploid cells?

7. What role do crossovers play in genetic diversity?

8. What is the first major event of meiosis?

9. What are the age ranges for the onset of puberty in males and in females? At what point does puberty end?

Analyze and Apply

10. Compare and contrast asexual and sexual reproduction, identifying and explaining as many differences as possible.

11. Compare and contrast mitosis and meiosis, explaining as many similarities and differences as possible.

12. Explain the differences between the embryonic and fetal development of the male sex organs as compared to the female sex organs.

In the Lab

13. In this activity, you will demonstrate how meiotic cell division creates a gamete with half the chromosomes of other cells, and how random assignment of chromosomes creates gametes with many different combinations of chromosomes. You will start with 46 chromosomes (23 from the mother and 23 from the father). **Materials:** small bowl, 23 pennies (chromosomes from the mother), 23 nickels (chromosomes from the father), 1 quarter, 2 sets of coin-sized labels numbered 1–23. **Procedure:** Place the pennies in a row across the desk, evenly spaced. Place a nickel next to each penny. Place a numbered label beside each penny-nickel pair. For example, the first penny and nickel should be labeled "1," the next penny and nickel should be labeled "2," and so forth, through the 23 pairs. Flip the quarter. If it lands heads up, place the penny from the first penny-nickel pair into the bowl. If it lands tails up, place the nickel from the first penny-nickel pair into the bowl. Continue flipping the quarter for each penny-nickel pair until you have 23 coins in the bowl. Record the numbers of the pennies and nickels in the bowl. Repeat 5 times. How many times did you get the exact same combination of coins? According to the lesson, how many combinations may occur if you repeated this forever? Plot the outcomes in a spreadsheet and share your findings with the class.

Lesson Objectives

1. Describe the anatomy of the male reproductive system.

2. Explain how sperm are created and delivered for reproduction.

3. Describe the phases of the male sexual response.

Key Terms

E-Flash Cards

bulbourethral glands
ductus deferens
ejaculation
epididymis
erection
gonads

penis
prostate gland
semen
seminal glands
seminiferous tubules
sperm

Male Reproductive Anatomy

In this lesson, we will first discuss the anatomy of the male reproductive system. We will then examine the physiology of the system, including the formation of sperm and the male sexual response.

For both males and females, the primary reproductive organs are the **gonads** (GOH-nads), the sites in which gametes are made. In males, the gonads are the testes, also called the *testicles;* the gametes are called *sperm.* **Sperm** are the male haploid cells that can fertilize an egg to make a zygote. In females, the gonads are the *ovaries* and the gametes are called *oocytes,* or eggs. You will learn more about the female reproductive organs in the next lesson.

The *accessory reproductive organs* in the male reproductive system are the other structures needed for sperm maturation and delivery of sperm to the female. These include the external genitals—the penis and scrotum—and the internal structures, including five accessory glands. These glands are the prostate, the two seminal glands, and the two bulbourethral (BUL-boh-yoo-REE-thral) glands.

Scrotum and Testes

The scrotum is a pouch of skin that hangs outside the body below the pelvic cavity, in the midline and anterior to the anus (**Figure 15.4** on the next page). The scrotum contains the two testes and associated ducts.

The external location of the scrotum causes the temperature of the testes to be about 34°C (93.2°F), which is cooler than the core body temperature of 37°C (98.6°F). Sperm formation

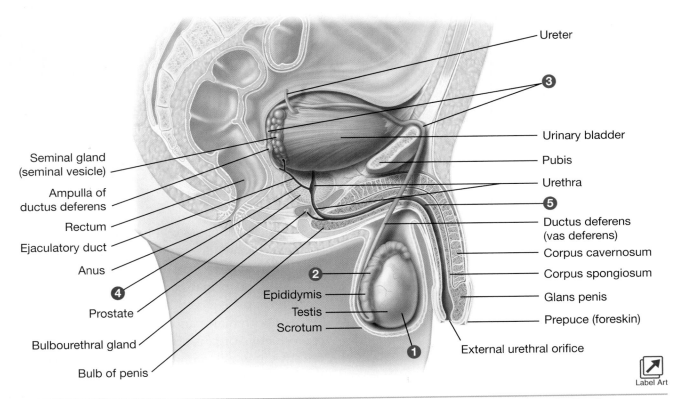

Figure 15.4 Sagittal view of the male reproductive organs. 1—Sperm form in the testes (one testis shown here). 2—Sperm spend 10 to 14 days in the epididymis before they reach full maturation. 3—Smooth muscle in the ductus deferens propels sperm toward the urethra. 4—Sperm from the ductus deferens and fluid from the seminal gland pass through the ejaculatory duct into the urethra. The prostate gland also secretes fluid into the urethra. 5—During ejaculation, semen moves through the urethra and out of the body. *How does the anatomy of the scrotum enhance the production of sperm?*

is most vigorous at this cooler temperature. Two muscles—the cremaster and the dartos—work together to maintain optimum temperature of the scrotum. When the scrotum is cold, the cremaster and dartos muscles contract to pull the organ closer to the body. When the scrotum is warm, the cremaster and dartos relax to allow the scrotum more freedom and greater surface area.

The testes (singular *testis*) are the two primary male reproductive organs inside the scrotum. **Figure 15.4** shows one testis and the **epididymis** (EHP-i-DID-i-mis), a structure that holds the testes in place.

The testis contains a dense network of small tubes in which sperm forms. These are called **seminiferous tubules**.

The seminiferous tubules connect to the tubules of the epididymis, which lies on the posterior side of the testis. The tubules in the upper part of the epididymis converge to form the

duct of the epididymis. This duct travels down, behind and to the side of the testis, to the bottom of the testis, where it bends back upward. As the duct runs upward, it is known as the **ductus deferens**, or the *vas deferens* (vas DEHF-eh-rehnz). The ductus deferens, and the arteries and veins that supply and drain the testis and epididymis, ascend in the spermatic cord and then enter the pelvic cavity (**Figure 15.5**).

Penis

The **penis** (**Figure 15.4**) is designed to deliver sperm to the female reproductive tract. The shaft of the penis leads to the *glans penis*, the enlarged end. The *prepuce* (PREE-pyoos), or foreskin, is a loose fold of skin that covers much of the glans penis.

Circumcision is the surgical removal of the prepuce. This practice may be done for religious,

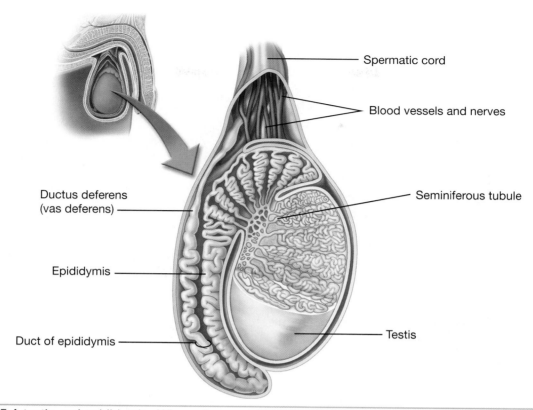

Figure 15.5 A testis and epididymis. *Where do sperm form, in the epididymis or the seminiferous tubules?*

cultural, or hygienic reasons. Circumcision has been shown to reduce the risk of certain sexually transmitted diseases. However, some cultures oppose infant circumcision as an unnecessary medical procedure.

The shaft of the penis contains *erectile tissue* and the *urethra* (yoo-REE-thra). The opening at the outer end of the urethra is the *external urethral orifice*. The erectile tissue in the shaft are separated into two *corpora cavernosa* (which lie parallel to each other and extend the length of the shaft) and one *corpus spongiosum* (spun-jee-OH-sum). These tissues contain spaces in which blood can pool. During sexual arousal, the erectile tissues become enlarged and rigid due to engorgement with blood.

Ducts of the Male Reproductive System

The male duct system (shown in both **Figure 15.4** and **15.5**) transports sperm from the testes, where it is formed, to the external urethral orifice at the tip of the penis. Sperm from the seminiferous tubules of each testis enter the epididymis. The duct of the epididymis carries sperm to the ductus deferens. The two ductus deferens carry sperm from the scrotum into the pelvic cavity, inside the body.

Each ductus deferens proceeds from front to back along the upper lateral border of the bladder. At the posterior side of the bladder, the ductus deferens turns downward and widens slightly to form a chamber called the *ampulla* (am-POO-la) of the ductus deferens. The outlet of the ampulla and the duct from the seminal gland merge to form the *ejaculatory duct*, which is much shorter than the ductus deferens. The ejaculatory duct from each side enters the prostate and, in the center of the prostate, joins the urethra. The urethra carries urine out of the body during micturition (urination), and it conveys sperm out of the body during sexual intercourse.

Accessory Glands and Semen

Semen is the fluid that contains sperm, which is delivered to the female during intercourse. Sperm cells make up only about 10% of the volume of semen. Most seminal volume comes from the *accessory glands* of the male reproductive system shown in **Figure 15.4**.

The two **seminal glands**, or *seminal vesicles*, produce up to 70% of the volume of semen. The **prostate gland** sits directly under the bladder. The urethra passes through the middle of the prostate gland as it descends from the bladder. The glandular tissue of the prostate secretes fluid that makes up one-quarter to one-third of seminal volume. Several ducts from the prostate join the urethra as it passes through the prostate. The two small **bulbourethral glands** lie below the prostate. Their ducts join the urethra and contribute a small amount of fluid to semen.

During ejaculation, the total volume of semen ejected typically is 2 to 5 milliliters. Semen contains 20 million to 150 million sperm cells per milliliter (**Figure 15.6**).

Check Your Understanding

1. In what part of the testes do sperm form?
2. Sperm make up what percentage of the total volume of semen?
3. Where do the ducts that carry sperm from the testes meet the urethra?

Male Reproductive Physiology

Let's now take a look at how the organs of the male reproductive system work. The male reproductive system has two principal functions: to create sperm and to deliver those sperm to the site of fertilization.

Sperm Formation

Sperm formation, or *spermatogenesis* (sper-mat-oh-JEHN-e-sis), occurs in the walls of the seminiferous tubules of the testes. Stem cells called *spermatogonia* (sper-mat-oh-GOH-nee-a) undergo mitosis. One of the two daughter cells remains as a stem cell for future division, and the other daughter cell becomes a *primary spermatocyte* (sper-MAT-oh-sight).

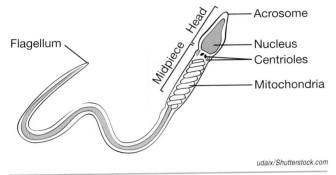

udaix/Shutterstock.com

Figure 15.6 A sperm cell. *What is the name of the fluid that contains sperm? Name the three types of glands that contribute to the development of this fluid.*

The primary spermatocyte is diploid—it has 46 chromosomes. The first meiotic division yields two secondary spermatocytes, and the second meiotic division produces four *spermatids* (SPER-mat-ids). The spermatids are gametes: they are haploid, with 23 chromosomes each.

Each immature spermatid develops a *flagellum* (fla-JEHL-um), or tail, which it will use to "swim" up the female reproductive tract. Once the spermatid has a flagellum, it is released into the lumen of the seminiferous tubule. At this stage it is referred to as a *sperm*, although it is not yet mature. From the development of a primary spermatocyte to the release of sperm into the seminiferous tubule, the process takes nine to ten weeks. Immature sperm move from the seminiferous tubules of the testes to the epididymis where it spends about three weeks achieving maturation.

Sexual Response

The male sexual response has two complementary components: erection and ejaculation. **Erection** permits the penis to gain entry to the female reproductive tract. **Ejaculation** is the discharge of sperm from the ejaculatory duct.

During erection, the penis enlarges and stiffens in response to sexual stimulation. Neural impulses travel along parasympathetic nerve fibers to the erectile tissues of the penis, triggering the production and release of nitric oxide (NO). Production and release of nitric oxide causes the arterioles in the penis to relax; as a result, more blood fills the tissue, and the penis becomes erect.

Ejaculation is the ejection of semen from the body. When sexual stimulation is sufficient, a burst of activity occurs on sympathetic nerves leading to the male reproductive tract. These nerve impulses cause peristaltic contractions of smooth muscle in the male duct system, and of smooth muscle in the male accessory glands. The nerve impulses also cause contraction of the urethral sphincter at the base of the bladder, which prevents mixing of urine with semen. The burst of nerve activity, ejaculation of semen, and the pleasurable sensation are called an *orgasm*.

Lesson 15.2 Review and Assessment

Mini Glossary   Make sure that you know the meaning of each key term.

 Build vocabulary with e-flash cards and games

bulbourethral glands two small glands at the base of the penis that secrete mucus into the urethra

ductus deferens the secretory duct of the testis, which extends from the epididymis and joins with the excretory duct of the seminal gland; vas deferens

ejaculation the discharge of sperm from the ejaculatory duct during the male sexual response

epididymis a system of small ducts in the testis, in which sperm mature

erection the condition of erectile tissue when filled with blood, which permits the penis to gain entry to the female reproductive tract

gonads the organs that produce gametes (oocytes and sperm): the ovaries in females and the testes in males

penis the reproductive organ that delivers sperm to the female reproductive tract

prostate gland the gland that sits directly under the bladder and surrounds the beginning of the urethra in the male; produces about one-third of the fluid volume of semen

semen the fluid that contains sperm, which is delivered to the female during intercourse; penile ejaculate

seminal glands glands that produce up to 70% of the volume of semen; seminal vesicles

seminiferous tubules small tubes in the testes in which sperm form

sperm (singular or plural) the male gamete; a haploid cell that can fertilize an egg to make a zygote

Know and Understand

 Assess

1. Where are gametes made?
2. From a reproductive standpoint, what is the penis designed to accomplish?
3. Are the seminiferous tubules inside the epididymis, or do they connect to the epididymis?
4. Trace the path of sperm from the testes to the external urethral orifice, naming each duct and organ through which the sperm travel.
5. What is the name of the fluid that contains sperm as they travel through the male reproductive system?
6. In which stem cells does the production of sperm cells begin?
7. What is the purpose of a flagellum?
8. What is the role of sympathetic nerves in stimulating ejaculation?

Analyze and Apply

9. Compare the structures and functions of spermatogonia, spermatocytes, and spermatids.
10. Explain how the anatomy of the male reproductive system makes erection possible.

In the Lab

11. When the temperature of the scrotum rises above the optimal level, the cremaster and dartos muscles relax. This causes the surface area of the scrotum to increase, which lowers its temperature. Demonstrate how surface area affects the transfer of heat and temperature.
   Materials: 2 disposable vinyl gloves; 2 large bottles, 2 large beakers (1,000 mL), string or rubber bands, warm water, ice, thermometer.
   Procedure: Fill a large bottle with water and ice. Fill the other bottle with warm water. Pour the ice water into the two beakers. Tie off the five fingers of one glove, decreasing its surface area, and pour 7 fluid ounces of the warm water into it. Immediately immerse the glove into a beaker, holding the open end out of the water. After 3 minutes, measure and record the temperature of the water inside the glove. Repeat the procedure with the other glove, but do not tie off the fingers. How do the water temperatures inside the gloves compare? What can you conclude about the relationship between surface area and heat transfer?

Female Reproductive System Anatomy and Physiology

Before You Read

Try to answer the following questions before you read this lesson.

What are the primary and accessory female reproductive organs?

How do the female reproductive organs and secondary sex characteristics develop during puberty?

What happens during the ovarian and the uterine cycles?

Lesson Objectives

1. Describe the anatomy of the internal structures of the female reproductive system.
2. Describe the female external genitalia.
3. List the steps in oogenesis.
4. Identify the monthly changes in the ovaries and the uterus, and the major hormones involved in the reproductive process. Explain how these changes prepare the body for fertilization and pregnancy.

Key Terms

E-Flash Cards

cervix
clitoris
labia majora
labia minora
lactiferous duct
mammary glands
oocyte

oogenesis
ovarian cycle
ovulation
uterine cycle
uterine tubes
uterus
vagina

Female Reproductive System Anatomy

We will now examine the primary and accessory reproductive organs of the female.

The Ovaries

The ovaries, shown in **Figure 15.7**, are the primary reproductive organs in the female—the organs in which gametes are made. Just as the testes produce sperm and secrete the hormone testosterone, the ovaries produce ova (eggs) and secrete the hormones estrogen and progesterone.

The two oval-shaped ovaries, which are about 3.0 centimeters long and 1.5 centimeters wide, are positioned against the posterior wall of the pelvic cavity. The ovaries, like the testes, have a fibrous outer covering, as the right ovary of **Figure 15.7** shows. Unlike the testes, however, the ovaries do not contain ducts. Instead, they contain many ovarian follicles.

Each follicle inside the ovaries contains a single **oocyte** (OH-uh-sight), or egg cell, and multiple surrounding cells. At any given time, the ovaries contain follicles in different stages of maturation. Primordial (prigh-MORD-ee-al) follicles are the most plentiful and least mature. They contain a single layer of cells surrounding the oocyte.

A primary follicle is slightly larger than a primordial follicle, but still has only a single layer of cells surrounding the oocyte. Secondary and vesicular follicles are larger and have more cells surrounding the oocyte. Each month one follicle reaches maturity, and the oocyte that it contains is released from its ovary during **ovulation**. Maturation of ovarian follicles and the details of ovulation will be discussed in the next section of this lesson.

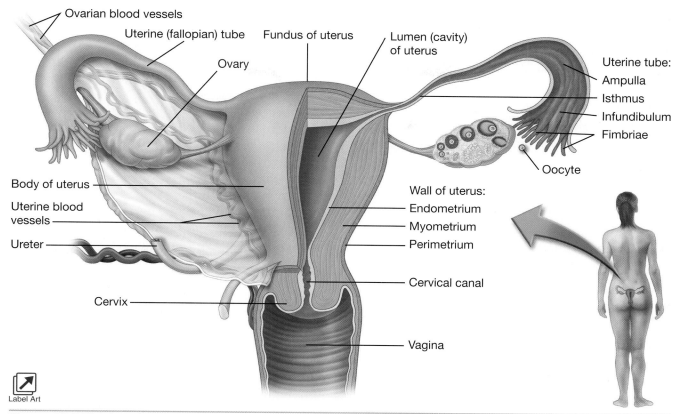

Figure 15.7 The female reproductive organs, posterior view. A cutaway view of one ovary shows development of an oocyte. *How are the ovaries similar to and different from the testes in the male?*

Ducts of the Female Reproductive System

There are a couple of significant differences between the female and male reproductive duct systems. One major difference is the open-ended design of the female system. In males, sperm are formed in the seminiferous tubules of the testes, which connect directly to the duct system that carries the sperm out of the body. In females, the duct system is open at the ovarian end (**Figure 15.7**).

Another significant difference is that the female reproductive system is completely separate from the urinary tract. The female urethra is not in any way a part of the reproductive tract. In males, by contrast, the urethra serves a dual purpose: it is both the outlet for the urinary system and the terminal portion of the reproductive tract.

Let's now take a closer look at the structure of the female duct system: the uterine tubes, the uterus, and the vagina.

Uterine Tubes. Each of the two **uterine** (YOOT-er-in) **tubes** begins at the lateral end of its ovary and curves up and around the ovary to terminate at the top lateral portion of the uterus (**Figure 15.7**). The hollow tube is open at the ovary. It has fringe-like projections called *fimbriae* (FIM-bree-igh), which wrap part of the way around the ovary. The cells lining the uterine tube, including the fimbriae, have vibrating cilia, which are short, microscopic, hair-like structures.

At the time of ovulation, the vibrating cilia of the fimbriae sweep fluid and, usually, the ovulated oocyte into the uterine tube. Cilia in the tube, and peristaltic contractions of the smooth muscle in the wall of the tube, move the oocyte toward the uterus. The uterine tube passes through the wall of the uterus and opens into the lumen, or cavity, of the uterus.

The open-ended design of the female duct system has one great benefit and several drawbacks. The benefit is that it provides an ovulated oocyte with a means of entry into the reproductive tract. Once in the reproductive tract, the oocyte can be fertilized, and it can develop into an embryo and then a fetus. The fetus evolves into a newborn human being, which emerges from the mother's body during childbirth.

On the other hand, because the female duct system is open at the ovaries, the oocyte released each month is not always captured by the fimbriae. The oocyte usually dies soon thereafter, but on rare occasions a sperm reaches the oocyte and fertilizes it while it sits in the pelvic cavity. If this happens, the fertilized egg may implant on the wall of the pelvic cavity. A fertilized egg that implants in the pelvic cavity, or in the uterine tube rather than in the uterus, is called an *ectopic pregnancy*.

An ectopic pregnancy cannot survive because the embryo is in an environment that is not designed to support development. Inevitably, a *spontaneous abortion* (naturally occurring premature termination of pregnancy) will end an ectopic pregnancy. This type of spontaneous abortion is a medical emergency that can involve significant internal bleeding.

✔ Check Your Understanding

1. Which reproductive organs in the female are the counterpart to the testes in the male?
2. At ovulation, how does the oocyte move to the uterus?
3. How does an ectopic pregnancy occur?
4. What are the two major differences between the duct systems of the male and female reproductive systems?

The Uterus. The **uterus** (YOOT-er-us), also known as the *womb*, is a hollow, muscular organ located in front of the rectum and behind the bladder. It usually lies with its upper end tipped forward over the bladder, as **Figure 15.8** shows. Its purpose is to receive and nourish a fertilized egg, and to expel the fetus by forceful, muscular contractions during childbirth about nine months later.

The wall of the uterus has three layers, which are visible in **Figure 15.7**. The *perimetrium*

Memory Tip

The word *uterus* comes from the Greek word *metra*, which means "womb." Ultimately, *metra* comes from the Greek word *meter*, which means "mother." The root word *metra* appears in the names for the walls of the uterus—*endometrium*, *myometrium*, and *perimetrium*.

The combining form *endo-* means "inside" or "within." Thus, the *endometrium* is the innermost layer of the uterine wall. The combining form *myo-* means "muscle." The *myometrium*, the middle layer of the uterine wall, is composed of muscle. Finally, the combining form *peri-* means "surrounding" or "enclosing." The *perimetrium* is the outer layer of the uterine wall—the layer that surrounds the myometrium and the endometrium.

(per-i-MEE-tree-um) is the thin, membranous outer layer. The *myometrium* (migh-oh-MEE-tree-um), which comprises the bulk of the uterine wall, is made of smooth muscle. The *endometrium* (ehn-doh-MEE-tree-um) is the mucosal tissue that forms the innermost layer of the uterus.

The endometrium is perhaps the most fascinating layer of the uterus for a couple of reasons. First, it undergoes significant changes on a four-week cycle. Second, it is the layer that receives, envelops, and nourishes a fertilized egg.

The layer of the endometrium that is closer to the lumen is called the *functional layer*. The functional layer grows thicker under the influence of hormones and is shed during menstruation (discussed later in this section). The basal layer is the deeper layer of the endometrium. The basal layer is not shed during menstruation.

The narrow, lower end of the uterus is called the **cervix** (SER-viks). The cervical canal is the narrow passageway that connects the lumen of the uterus to the lumen of the vagina.

The Vagina. The **vagina** is a thin-walled tubular structure below the uterus. It is sometimes called the *birth canal* because the infant passes through the vagina during birth. During intercourse, sperm are delivered to the lumen of the vagina. In normal, healthy adult women, the pH of the

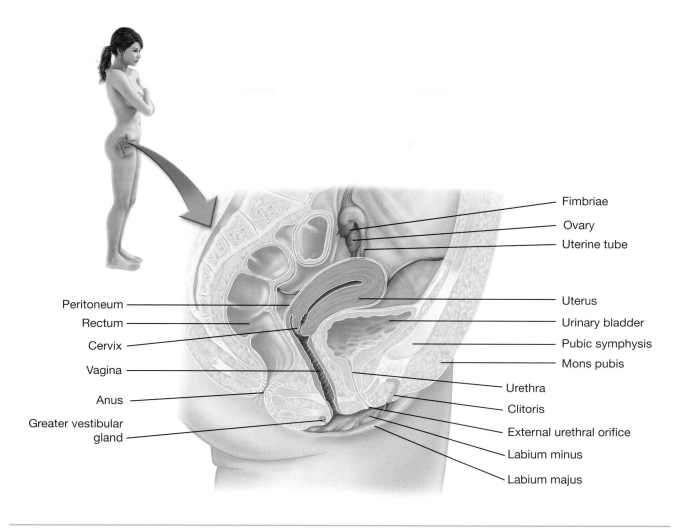

Figure 15.8 The female reproductive organs, midsagittal section. *What is the purpose of the uterus?*

vagina is rather acidic, which helps prevent bacterial infection. Apart from childbirth or intercourse, the walls of the vagina usually touch each another. This means that the lumen is a potentially open space rather than an actual open space.

 Check Your Understanding

1. Where is the uterus located inside the female body?
2. How many layers make up the wall of the uterus?
3. What is the name of the narrow passageway that connects the lumen of the uterus to the lumen of the vagina?
4. At which end is the female duct system open?

The External Genitalia

The reproductive structures on the outside of the body are the *external genitalia*. The *vulva* is another name for the external genitalia in females. The vulva includes the labia, mons pubis, clitoris, and vestibule. The female external genitalia are shown in **Figure 15.9**.

The *mons pubis* (pubic mound) is the region of skin and underlying fat in front of the vaginal opening on which pubic hair starts to grow during puberty. Just posterior to the mons pubis are the **labia majora**, two skin folds that lie parallel on either side of the vaginal opening. *Labia majora* is plural for *labium majus*.

Inside the labia majora are the **labia minora**, a smaller pair of skin folds. Both the labia majora and labia minora (singular *labium minus*) limit

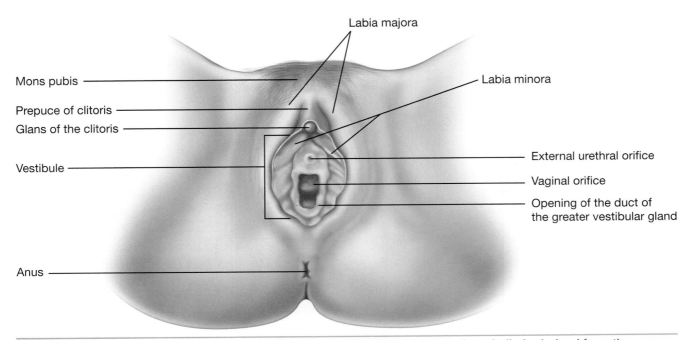

Labia majora

Mons pubis

Prepuce of clitoris

Glans of the clitoris

Vestibule

Anus

Labia minora

External urethral orifice

Vaginal orifice

Opening of the duct of the greater vestibular gland

Figure 15.9 The female external genitalia. *Which part of the female external genitalia is derived from the same embryologic precursor as the erectile tissue of the penis?*

entry of infectious material into the reproductive tract. Within the labia minora is the *vestibule*, the recessed area in which the vaginal and urethral openings lie. The two *greater vestibular glands* secrete lubricating mucus onto the epithelium of the vestibule.

The **clitoris** (KLIT-or-is), a small structure at the anterior end of the vestibule, is composed of erectile tissue. The clitoris is derived from the same embryologic precursor as the erectile tissue of the penis. The clitoris is covered anteriorly by a skinfold called the *prepuce*, and the exposed tip is called the *glans*. (As you can see, these terms echo the names of similar structures in the penis.) The clitoris is richly endowed with sensory nerve endings.

The Mammary Glands

The female **mammary glands** produce milk for the newborn baby. Increased estrogen in females during puberty stimulates maturation of the mammary glands. The mature mammary gland is capable of lactation, or milk production, but does not produce milk unless stimulated to do so by the hormone prolactin, which is released after childbirth. **Figure 15.10** shows the structure of a lactating mammary gland.

The mammary glands are modified sweat glands. Like sweat glands, they are part of the skin. Each mammary gland lies on top of the *pectoralis major*, the most superficial muscle of the anterior chest wall. On the surface of the breast is the protruding nipple, which is surrounded by a ring of pigmented skin called the *areola* (uh-REE-oh-la).

The mammary gland contains 15 to 20 lobes internally, each of which has many smaller lobules capable of producing milk. Each lobe secretes its milk into a **lactiferous** (lak-TIF-er-us) **duct** that opens at the nipple. When the breast is not lactating, the glandular tissue remains undeveloped and occupies very little space. The size of the nonlactating breast is determined by the amount of adipose (fat) tissue and interspersed glandular tissue.

✓ Check Your Understanding

1. What is the name of the external genitalia in females?
2. Which part of the female reproductive system is composed of erectile tissue?
3. Which gland of the female reproductive system is a modified sweat gland?

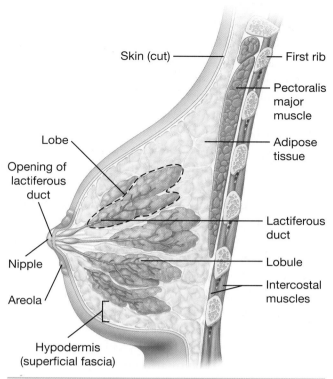

Figure 15.10 A lactating mammary gland.

Labels for figure:
- Skin (cut)
- Lobe
- Opening of lactiferous duct
- Nipple
- Areola
- Hypodermis (superficial fascia)
- First rib
- Pectoralis major muscle
- Adipose tissue
- Lactiferous duct
- Lobule
- Intercostal muscles

Physiology of the Female Reproductive System

The functions of the female reproductive system are to generate eggs, to deliver the eggs for fertilization, to nourish the developing embryo and fetus, to give birth, and to provide liquid nourishment after birth. We will now take a look at how the organs of the female reproductive system function.

Oogenesis

Oogenesis (oh-ah-JEHN-eh-sis) is the process by which oocytes, or egg cells, are generated. Because gametes must be haploid, the oogenetic process involves meiosis. Oogenesis is similar to spermatogenesis, but also differs from it.

Oogenesis begins in the ovaries of the female fetus before birth. *Oogonia*, diploid stem cells that correspond to spermatogonia in males, undergo mitosis and produce primary oocytes, which correspond to primary spermatocytes. Each primary oocyte is surrounded by a single layer of follicle cells, thus forming a *primordial follicle*.

The oocyte in the primordial follicle starts the process of meiosis before the female fetus is born; however, meiosis stops partway through the first meiotic division. About one to two million oocytes are present as primordial follicles at birth. About one-quarter to one-half million of these oocytes survive to puberty. This number is more than enough because only one oocyte is released per month for a period of 30 to 40 years, for a total of fewer than 500 oocytes over a lifetime.

At puberty, the increased level of follicle-stimulating hormone triggers a small number of follicles to develop further each month. One of these follicles becomes the dominant follicle and its oocyte completes the first meiotic division, producing two unequal daughter cells. The *secondary oocyte* gets half the chromosomes and almost all the cytoplasm and organelles. The other cell—a polar body (nonfunctional cell)—gets half the chromosomes and practically nothing more.

The secondary oocyte begins to undergo the second meiotic division, but meiosis stops partway through. The oocyte is released from the ovary—that is, ovulation occurs (discussed later). The second meiotic division of the oocyte resumes and is completed after ovulation, if and when the oocyte is fertilized.

The second meiotic division follows the same unequal pattern as the first, yielding a tiny polar body and a large haploid oocyte. Meanwhile, the first polar body may or may not complete the second meiotic division. The end result of the process is one haploid oocyte and two or three polar bodies.

 Check Your Understanding

1. What is oogenesis?
2. Approximately how many oocytes are released during a female's lifetime?
3. What event triggers the second meiotic division of the oocyte?

The Female Sexual Cycle

The "monthly" cycle of the female reproductive system, commonly referred to as the *menstrual cycle*, spans 28 days on average, but the actual duration of the cycle varies from about 21 to 40 days. During this cycle, the ovaries and the uterus undergo changes, as do several key hormones (**Figure 15.11**).

First, we will look at what happens in the ovaries during one cycle. We will then examine the changes taking place at the same time in the uterus. We will refer to these changes as the *ovarian cycle* and the *uterine cycle,* but keep in mind that all of these changes are occurring at the same time, as part of one monthly cycle.

The Ovarian Cycle. The **ovarian cycle** is the sequence of events associated with maturation and release of an oocyte. The cycle has two main phases: the *follicular phase*, which lasts from day 1 to day 14, and the *luteal phase*. Ovulation, the release of the oocyte, marks the end of the follicular phase and the beginning of the luteal phase. These changes in the ovary are also illustrated in **Figure 15.12** on page 548.

The Follicular Phase. Each month, several primordial follicles from each of the two ovaries develop into primary follicles. Gradually, one of the primary follicles becomes dominant. This means that only one follicle, from one ovary, develops fully and is released (ovulated) each month.

The maturation of the primordial follicles into one dominant *primary follicle* marks the initial stage of follicular development. The cells of the primary follicle surrounding the oocyte then divide. When these cells become more than one layer thick, they are called *granulosa* (GRAN-yoo-LOH-sa) *cells*; at this stage, the follicle is called a *secondary follicle.*

The secondary follicle grows and the oocyte develops a clear, extracellular glycoprotein coat called the *zona pellucida* (peh-LOO-si-da). Spaces filled with clear liquid begin to appear in the follicle, around the oocyte. The follicle is now called a *late secondary follicle.*

When the fluid-filled spaces in the follicle merge into a single, large, fluid-filled *antrum* (cavity), the follicle is called a *vesicular follicle.* As the follicle develops first into a late secondary follicle, and then into a vesicular follicle, the growing number of granulosa cells, triggered

by follicle-stimulating hormone, secrete greater amounts of estrogen.

Figure 15.11C shows the steady rise of estrogen from day 5 to day 14. The rising estrogen level inhibits release of FSH from the hypothalamus during this time, which is why the FSH level decreases slightly from about day 6 to day 12. The large vesicular follicle now bulges against the ovarian wall (**Figure 15.12**, step 4).

At about this time, the pituitary gland starts to secrete more FSH and luteinizing hormone. The high level of LH causes the primary oocyte to complete its first meiotic division, and the secondary oocyte begins its second meiotic division.

The surge in LH then causes the bulging vesicular follicle to rupture the ovarian wall (**Figure 15.12**, step 5). The result is ovulation—the release of the secondary oocyte and a layer of surrounding cells, called the *corona radiata*, into the pelvic cavity. This release concludes the follicular phase of the ovarian cycle, and the luteal phase begins.

The Luteal Phase. The oocyte normally will be swept into the uterine tube by the vibrating cilia of the fimbriae. The remaining cells of the follicle, which are still in the ovary, form the *corpus luteum* (Latin for "yellow body"). Luteinizing hormone, which surged during ovulation, helps stimulate formation of the corpus luteum. The disruption of the estrogen-secreting granulosa cells by ovulation causes blood estrogen levels to plummet after ovulation.

The cells of the corpus luteum begin to secrete progesterone, and the progesterone level in the blood rises steadily during the early part of the luteal phase, as the corpus luteum grows. The corpus luteum secretes modest amounts of estrogen, leading to a slight rebound of estrogen levels in the early part of the luteal phase. These changes in progesterone and estrogen levels are shown in **Figure 15.11C**.

After about ten days, the corpus luteum begins to disintegrate if the oocyte has not been fertilized. This disintegration causes the progesterone and estrogen levels to drop in the late luteal phase. The corpus luteum turns into a small bundle of scar tissue called the *corpus albicans* (Latin for "white body").

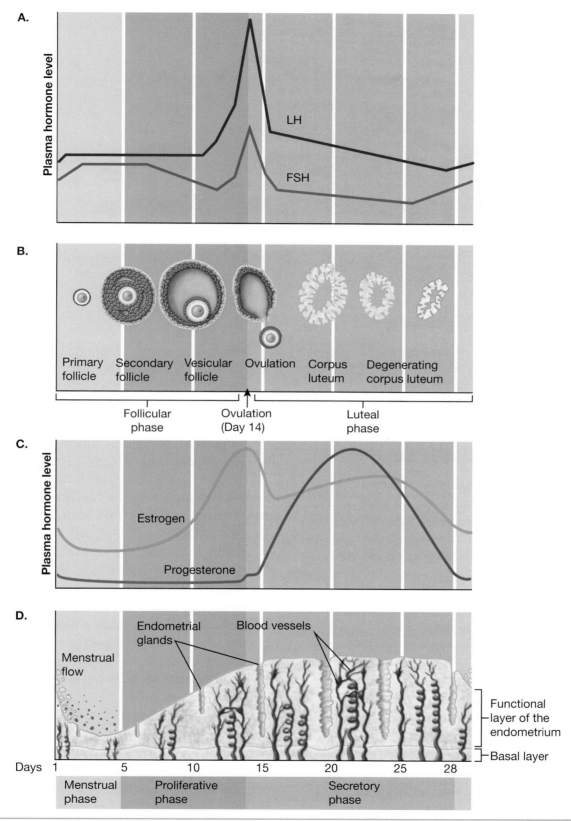

Figure 15.11 Hormonal and structural changes during the female sexual cycle. The events of one complete female cycle, lasting 28 days, are shown. The time scale, shown horizontally at the bottom, applies to all four panels of the figure. We assume for these drawings that the ovulated oocyte is *not* fertilized. If it *were* fertilized, then the events of the second half of the cycle would be quite different for all four panels.

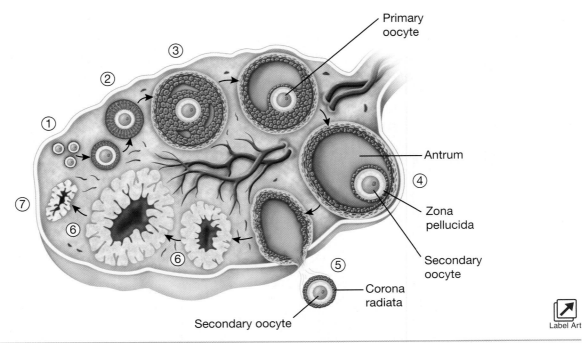

Figure 15.12 Changes in the ovary during the ovarian cycle. 1—Primary follicles. 2—Secondary follicle. 3—Late secondary follicle. 4—Vesicular follicle. 5—Ovulation. The secondary oocyte is released, along with surrounding corona radiata cells. 6—Remaining cells of the follicle turn into the corpus luteum (shown twice). 7—If fertilization does not occur, the corpus luteum turns into a small bundle of scar tissue.

Check Your Understanding

1. What is the duration of the monthly cycle of the female reproductive system?
2. What are the two main phases of the ovarian cycle?
3. Why does FSH level decrease from day 6 to day 12 of the ovarian cycle?
4. What happens to the corpus luteum if the oocyte has not been fertilized within 10 days of ovulation?

The Uterine Cycle. While the ovaries are undergoing their changes, the uterus is also changing (**Figure 15.11D**). The three phases of the **uterine cycle** are the menstrual phase, the proliferative phase, and the secretory phase.

The *menstrual phase* lasts for the first four to five days of the cycle. During this time, the outer layer of the endometrium, the *functional layer*, breaks down. The blood and tissue that are lost during this stage pass from the uterus, through the cervical canal, and out of the vagina, producing the *menstrual discharge*. By the end

of the menstrual phase, the functional layer has been completely shed.

The *proliferative phase* begins as soon as the menstrual phase ends. The functional layer of the endometrium rapidly grows back, aided by the rising level of estrogen.

During ovulation, the rapid regrowth of the endometrium slows down. Now the rising level of progesterone, which is being made by the corpus luteum in the ovaries, causes the functional layer of the endometrium to develop a dense network of blood vessels. The endometrium also develops nutrient-secreting glands that will nourish an embryo, if one implants. These events take place in the *secretory phase*.

If fertilization does not occur, the corpus luteum begins to disintegrate, and the progesterone level in the blood falls. As a result, the blood vessels in the functional layer deteriorate, leading to tissue breakdown and bleeding. Thus, a new cycle begins.

Female Sexual Response

As with males, sexual excitement in females activates neural reflexes from the sympathetic and parasympathetic divisions of the autonomic nervous system. Sexual stimulation, which can involve psychological and tactile (touch) stimuli, activates parasympathetic nerves to the erectile tissue of the clitoris, which becomes engorged with blood. In addition, autonomic nerves activate smooth muscle fibers in the nipple, causing it to become erect. Increases in both vestibular gland and vaginal wall secretions stimulate production of lubricating fluid that facilitates intercourse.

Orgasm is marked by intense pleasure and rhythmic contraction of smooth muscle in the reproductive tract that may help move sperm toward the oocyte. In females, orgasm is not required for conception. In males, however, orgasm and associated ejaculation are required for successful delivery of sperm and fertilization.

Lesson 15.3 Review and Assessment

Mini Glossary   Make sure that you know the meaning of each key term.

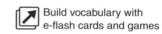 Build vocabulary with e-flash cards and games

cervix   the narrow, lower end of the uterus that has the opening through which a baby passes during childbirth

clitoris   a cylindrical body of erectile tissue that lies at the anterior end of the vulva

labia majora   two skin folds posterior to the mons pubis that lie parallel on either side of the vaginal opening

labia minora   a smaller set of skin folds inside the labia majora

lactiferous duct   a duct through which milk is secreted and which opens at the nipple

mammary glands   the milk-producing glands in the female

oocyte   egg cell

oogenesis   the process by which oocytes, or female gametes, are generated

ovarian cycle   the sequence of events associated with maturation and release of an oocyte

ovulation   the release of an oocyte, or egg, from the ovarian follicle

uterine cycle   the monthly cycle of changes that the uterus undergoes;

includes the menstrual, proliferative, and secretory phases

uterine tubes   tubes in which the oocyte is fertilized; begin at the lateral end of the ovary and go up and around the ovary to terminate at the top lateral portion of the uterus

uterus   a hollow, muscular organ located in front of the rectum and behind the bladder; the womb

vagina   a thin-walled, tubular structure below the uterus; birth canal

Know and Understand

 Assess

1. Explain how the female reproductive system is organized, including subdivisions of each component.
2. What does each follicle in an ovary contain?
3. Where does the uterine tube begin and end?
4. What is an ectopic pregnancy, and why is it a medical emergency?
5. What is the narrow lower end of the uterus called?
6. Describe the anatomy of the vulva. What are the parts of the vulva called, and where are they located in relation to each other?
7. What is the function of the female mammary glands?
8. What sequence of events occurs during the ovarian cycle?
9. List the names of the uterine cycle phases, and describe what occurs during each phase.

Analyze and Apply

10. Analyze the similarities and differences between the ovarian and uterine cycles.
11. Compare and contrast the three phases of the uterine cycle.

In the Lab

12. Since the female duct system is open at the ovary, what moves the oocyte from the ovary to the uterus where it must implant? Study **Figure 15.7**. Using four different colors of clay, create models of these four structures: uterus, uterine tube (with fimbriae), ovary, and oocyte. Arrange your models as they appear in the figure. Demonstrate how an oocyte is swept into the uterine tube and into the uterus. Explain what can happen to the oocyte when it is not captured by the fimbriae.

Fertilization, Pregnancy, and Birth

Before You Read

Try to answer the following questions before you read this lesson.

Where is an oocyte fertilized, and where does it go after it is fertilized?

What is the placenta, and how does it help the embryo and fetus develop?

What are the stages of labor?

Lesson Objectives

1. Describe how a zygote develops and implants in the uterus.
2. Describe the physiological changes that occur in the mother and developing child during pregnancy.
3. Explain the sequence of events involved in childbirth.
4. Explain how breast milk is produced and secreted.

Key Terms

E-Flash Cards

amniotic fluid
blastocyst
delivery of the placenta
dilation
embryo
expulsion
fetus
human chorionic
   gonadotropin (hCG)

implantation
lactation
let-down reflex
oxytocin
placenta
prolactin
umbilical cord

Fertilization of the Oocyte

Fertilization occurs when the chromosomes of the oocyte and the sperm unite to produce a zygote, the first cell of a new individual. As explained in lesson 15.1, each gamete—the oocyte and the sperm—has 23 chromosomes. Thus, fusion of the gametes produces a zygote with a "full set" of 46 chromosomes.

An ovulated oocyte can live for, at most, about 24 hours before it is fertilized. If the ovulated oocyte is not fertilized within this time frame, it will die. By contrast, sperm can live for up to five days in the female reproductive tract. This means that for fertilization to be successful, intercourse must occur no more than two days before ovulation and no more than 24 hours after ovulation.

The Journey of the Sperm

During a single act of intercourse, between tens of millions and several hundred million sperm are deposited in the vagina. If a sperm had a mind, there would be only one thing on it: find the egg and fertilize it.

Each sperm propels itself by wiggling its flagellum back and forth. The oocyte, if present, will be in the distal third of the uterine tube, which is as far as it will have advanced during its one day of viability. Thus, the sperm must travel from the vagina to the cervical canal, through the cervical canal to the uterus, through the uterus to the uterine tube, and then along the uterine tube to the oocyte.

Many sperm are lost at each stage of the journey. Some sperm leak out of the vagina, and many others do not find the cervical opening. Of those that do enter the uterus, most will not make it to the uterine tube that contains an oocyte at the other end. Eventually, a few thousand sperm may reach the oocyte. Although sperm can make this journey of 10 to 15 centimeters (4 to 6 inches) within 5 to 10 minutes, they require as much as 10 hours in the female reproductive tract for capacitation.

Capacitation (ka-pas-i-TAY-shun) is the process by which sperm becomes able to penetrate and fertilize an oocyte. Each sperm contains at the tip of its head a bundle of *acrosomal* (AK-roh-sohm-al) *enzymes* that allow it to digest the protective glycoproteins surrounding the oocyte. When sperm first arrive in the vagina, this package of enzymes is well shielded from accidental release by a cell membrane thickened with extra cholesterol. The sperm are unable to fertilize the oocyte until the protective cap is worn away by contact with the fluids of the female, a process that takes up to 10 hours.

Sperm Penetration

When sperm successfully find the oocyte, they wiggle between the surrounding cells of the corona radiata to reach the zona pellucida, the glycoprotein layer surrounding the oocyte (**Figure 15.13**). Contact with the zona pellucida induces release of the acrosomal enzymes,

Nejron Photo/Shutterstock.com

Figure 15.13 Sperm attempting to penetrate an oocyte. *What enables sperm to penetrate the cell membrane of an egg?*

which start to bore a hole toward the oocyte membrane. The acrosomal enzymes of hundreds of sperm are required to "drill" holes all the way through the zona pellucida. A late-arriving sperm, benefiting from the work of the earlier sperm, will make its way through the holes in the zona pellucida and bind to specific receptors on the oocyte membrane. This binding causes the membranes of the two cells to join together, and the nucleus of the sperm, which contains the sperm's chromosomes, enters the cytoplasm of the oocyte.

Protection against Polyspermy

Many sperm are trying to fertilize the oocyte at the same time. If more than one succeeds—an outcome called *polyspermy* ("many sperm")—the oocyte will have too many chromosomes and will not survive. The oocyte protects itself against this possibility by figuratively "closing the door" as soon as one sperm merges with it.

Sperm entry causes sodium channels in the cell membrane to open, which results in sodium entry to the oocyte and the release of stored calcium ions from the oocyte. The rise in calcium in the cell reactivates meiosis, which was arrested partway through the second meiotic division. The rise in calcium also triggers the release of chemicals into the space just outside the oocyte. These chemicals react with water to form a protective shield around the oocyte. The net effect of the sodium entry, the calcium release, and the chemical reaction is to prevent additional sperm from fertilizing the oocyte.

Completion of Meiosis and Fertilization

The second meiotic division of the oocyte is now complete. This second meiosis has generated two haploid daughter cells: a tiny, nonviable (nonfunctional) polar body, and the rest of the oocyte. The nuclear membranes of the sperm and the oocyte then dissolve, and their chromosomes intermingle. Fertilization is now complete. The oocyte and the sperm have become a zygote.

Check Your Understanding

1. What is the first cell of a new individual called?
2. When must intercourse occur for fertilization to be successful?
3. How does sperm propel itself?
4. How long can an unfertilized, ovulated oocyte live?
5. How far, in inches, does sperm travel to reach an oocyte?

Pregnancy

Pregnancy, or *gestation*, is the period from fertilization to birth. It lasts approximately 265 days. It is conventional to measure pregnancy duration from the first day of the last menstrual period because that is a date that the woman is likely to know. When measured this way, the typical duration of pregnancy is about 280 days, or 40 weeks, or 9 months plus 1 week.

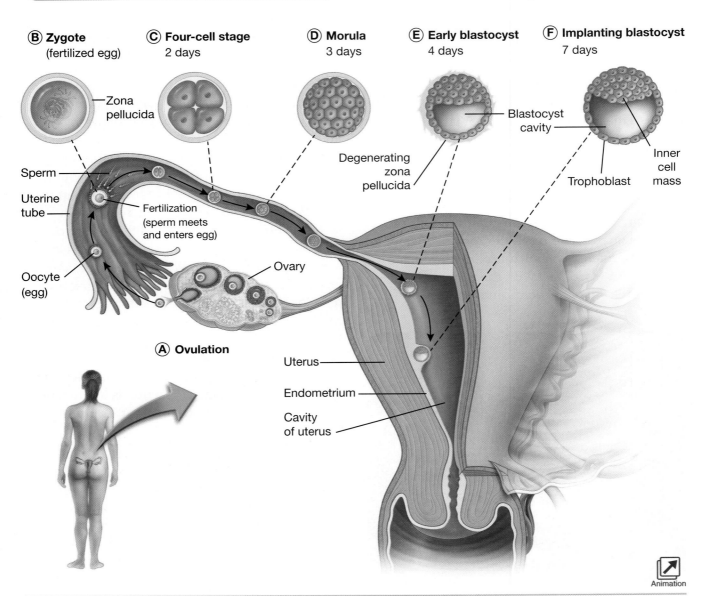

Figure 15.14 Ovulation to fertilization to implantation. A—An oocyte is released from the ovary. B—The egg is fertilized by a sperm. The zygote divides by mitosis. C—The embryo reaches the four-cell stage. D—The embryo becomes a morula, a solid ball of cells. E—A fluid-filled cavity develops in the embryo, now called a *blastocyst*. F—The blastocyst implants on the endometrium.

From Fertilization to Implantation

After the zygote has been formed (**Figure 15.14B**), it continues its slow movement toward the uterus. During its four- to five-day trip in the uterine tube, the zygote divides without changing its overall size. Thus, it develops a larger number of smaller cells.

As **Figure 15.14D** shows, 3 days after fertilization the zygote is a solid ball of 16 cells called a *morula*. By day 4, a **blastocyst** (BLAS-toh-sist), or fluid-filled cavity, develops inside the ball of cells. The blastocyst enters the uterine cavity and sheds the zona pellucida. Cell division continues, and by day 7 the blastocyst develops an *inner cell mass* and a thin layer of surrounding *trophoblast* (TROH-foh-blast) *cells.* At this point, the endometrium is at the peak of its development: it has grown thick and full of blood vessels to nourish an embryo and fetus.

As **Figure 15.11D** shows, peak development of the endometrium occurs around day 15 of the uterine cycle. **Implantation**, the binding of the blastocyst to the endometrium begins around this time. The blastocyst gradually burrows into the endometrium, and the nearby endometrial cells proliferate, or grow quickly in number. In 5 days (now 12 days after fertilization), the blastocyst is fully embedded in the endometrium. Implantation is complete.

Despite implantation, a potential problem awaits the blastocyst: the loss of the endometrial layer that is nourishing it. As we learned in our discussion of the uterine cycle in lesson 15.3—and as we saw in the illustration of endometrium structural changes in **Figure 15.11D**—the endometrial layer begins to degenerate around day 27 or 28 of the monthly cycle. This would be 13 or 14 days after fertilization, just after the completion of implantation.

Deterioration of the endometrium in a normal cycle (that is, a cycle without fertilization) results from a decline in the hormones estrogen and progesterone. The decline of estrogen and progesterone is due to the atrophy of the corpus luteum at the end of the month.

If the endometrial layer were to be shed, as it usually is during this phase of the cycle, then the blastocyst would be lost. This does not happen, however, because the trophoblast cells secrete a hormone called **human chorionic** (kor-ee-AHN-ik) **gonadotropin (hCG)**, which "rescues" the corpus luteum. Human chorionic gonadotropin prevents atrophy of the corpus luteum, which continues to secrete progesterone and estrogen so that the endometrium is not shed.

The levels of hCG, estrogen, and progesterone in the blood during pregnancy are shown in **Figure 15.15**. The rise in estrogen and progesterone after week 12 occurs because the placenta (which we will discuss in the next section) develops and starts to secrete these hormones. At the same time, hCG secretion diminishes and the corpus luteum, which has completed its mission, atrophies.

Pregnancy-test kits determine whether or not there is any hCG in the urine. Such tests work because hCG is present in pregnant women, but it is not present in nonpregnant women. When hCG is present, small amounts "spill over" from the blood into the urine.

Development of the Placenta, Embryo, and Fetus

As implantation progresses, the inner cell mass grows larger and more complex as its cells

Figure 15.15 Hormone levels in the mother's blood during pregnancy. *How do pregnancy-test kits work?*

divide and rearrange. When the **embryo** is tiny, it can get the nutrients it needs by simple diffusion from the tissue of the endometrium, which has a rich blood supply for this purpose. However, as the embryo grows, it needs more nutrients than the endometrium can supply.

The **placenta** is the organ that grows in the uterus to meet the nutritional needs of the embryo, which is called a **fetus** after 8 weeks of development. The placenta of a 13-week-old fetus, shown in **Figure 15.16**, contains cells of the fetus and cells of the mother. The placenta spreads out like a pancake on the wall of the uterus.

The placenta contains intertwining blood vessels from the cardiovascular systems of the fetus and the mother. The cardiovascular system is the first organ system of the embryo to

function in a meaningful way. Just three and one-half weeks after fertilization, when the embryo is only six millimeters (one-quarter inch) long, the immature heart begins to pump newly formed blood cells through newly formed blood vessels. Neither the embryo nor the fetus can receive oxygen (O_2) or expel carbon dioxide (CO_2) by breathing, and neither can obtain nourishment by eating. The placenta takes care of these needs.

Fetal vessels carry blood, pumped by the fetal heart, through the umbilical cord to and from the placenta. In the placenta, fetal capillaries are surrounded by cavities filled with maternal blood. The maternal and fetal blood do not actually mix; however, the thin layer of cells that separates them allows easy diffusion of nutrients from maternal blood to fetal blood, and diffusion of wastes in the reverse direction.

Figure 15.16 A 13-week-old fetus (end of first trimester). The fetus is about ten centimeters long (crown to rump). The placenta is attached to the wall of the uterus. The fetus is bathed in amniotic fluid contained in a sac whose layers are (from the inside going out) the amnion, the chorion, and the decidua capsularis. *The placenta takes over for what structure in providing nourishment to the embryo?*

Unfortunately, alcohol or drugs, if present in the mother's blood, will also reach the fetus by this pathway and will affect its development.

As **Figure 15.16** shows, the fetus fills up the uterine cavity by week 13. It is surrounded by a set of membranes and bathed in clear **amniotic** (am-nee-AHT-ik) **fluid**. The inner membrane of its sac is called the *amnion*. Outside the amnion is the *chorion*, which, like the amnion, is derived from the fetal tissue. The outermost membrane is called the *decidua capsularis* (Latin for "capsule that falls off, or sheds"); this membrane is derived from the mother's tissue. The *umbilical cord*, which contains two arteries and one vein, connects the fetus to the placenta.

 Check Your Understanding

1. How long is gestation when measured from the first day of the last menstrual period?
2. What is the term for the process by which the blastocyst binds to the endometrium?
3. Which organ system is the first to function in a meaningful way in an embryo?
4. At what point in its development does the embryo become a fetus?

Childbirth

Childbirth, also called *parturition* (part-uh-RISH-un), normally occurs 38 to 42 weeks after the first day of the last menstrual period. Toward the end of gestation, high levels of estrogen and progesterone cause the uterine muscle cells to become more sensitive to **oxytocin** (AHK-see-TOH-sin), a hormone that plays a key role in labor. Oxytocin is released by the pituitary glands of both the fetus and the mother.

Fetal oxytocin causes the placenta to release *prostaglandins*, lipid compounds that trigger uterine muscle contractions. Once the uterine muscle has started to contract, the baby's head is pushed into the cervical opening, causing mechanical receptors to be stretched there. These receptors send messages to the brain that stimulate maternal oxytocin release, causing even more vigorous contractions of the uterine

muscle and even greater stretching of the cervical receptors. This is an example of physiological *positive feedback*: an action triggers a response that, in turn, causes the original action to occur with greater strength and frequency.

Stages of Labor

The stages of labor are dilation, expulsion, and delivery of the placenta. When the time for birth arrives, most fetuses are in the head-down position, also called the *vertex presentation*. The vertex presentation, which causes the baby's head to exit the mother's body first, is shown in **Figure 15.17**. A rump-first position, or *breech presentation*, makes delivery much more difficult.

The **dilation** stage begins with uterine contractions and ends with a full widening of the cervical canal. In early dilation (**Figure 15.17A**), the cervix is several centimeters dilated, and the baby's head is "looking sideways" as it enters the pelvic outlet. In late dilation (**Figure 15.17B**), the cervix is fully dilated (10 centimeters), and the baby's head starts to rotate to a "looking-to-the-rear" orientation as it moves deeper into the pelvis. Dilation, which can last from 6 to 12 hours or longer, is usually the longest part of labor.

The **expulsion** stage (**Figure 15.17C**), the period from full dilation to delivery of the baby, lasts less than an hour in most cases. Strong contractions of the uterus, each lasting a minute or longer, occur at two- to three-minute intervals, forcing the baby's head out. Once the head has emerged, the rest of the body usually follows quickly. The baby is still connected to the mother by the **umbilical cord**, which is clamped and cut.

Delivery of the placenta (**Figure 15.17D**) is the last stage of birth. During this stage, strong uterine contractions continue, causing detachment of the placenta from the uterine wall and expulsion from the mother's body.

Lactation

Lactation is the production of milk by the mother. Breast milk is a uniquely important source of nutrition for the developing infant. It contains

Umbilical cord
Placenta
Uterus
Vagina
Cervix
A.

Pubic symphysis
Sacrum
B.

C.

Uterus
Placenta (detaching)
Umbilical cord
D.

Figure 15.17 The stages of labor. A—Early dilation. B—Late dilation. C—Expulsion. D—Delivery of the placenta. *How wide is the cervix when it is fully dilated?*

amino acids, fats, carbohydrates, and vitamins that are well absorbed by the infant's digestive system. Breast milk also contains antibodies from the mother that help protect the infant from infection while its own immune system is immature. Successful lactation requires activation of the normally inactive milk-producing cells of the mammary gland, as well as delivery of the milk through ducts to the baby. The two processes are regulated by two different hormones.

Late in pregnancy, high levels of estrogen and progesterone stimulate the hypothalamus in the brain to produce *prolactin-releasing factor*, a hormone that triggers the release of **prolactin** from the pituitary gland. Prolactin stimulates the secretory cells of the mammary glands to produce milk.

Following birth, the infant suckling at the nipple activates receptors that trigger the release of the hormone oxytocin from the mother's pituitary. Oxytocin, which was also important for labor and delivery, causes the **let-down reflex**—the contraction of smooth muscle cells in the mammary glands, which allows milk to be squeezed toward and out of the nipple.

 Check Your Understanding

1. What are the stages of labor?
2. Describe the difference between vertex presentation and breech presentation during the delivery of a baby.
3. What is the term for the production of milk by the mother?

WHAT RESEARCH TELLS US

...about Egg Freezing as a Solution for Infertility

More women than ever are waiting until their 30s or 40s to have children. As a result, age-related infertility has grown more common.

Aging can cause infertility for several reasons. A woman in her 30s or 40s has a smaller number of eggs in her ovaries, and the ovaries don't release eggs as often as they did when the woman was younger. Also, the eggs tend not to be as healthy. To complicate matters, only about 25% of all fertilized eggs implant in the uterus. Miscarriage, in which the fetus is spontaneously expelled from the body, is more common in women as they age.

New technologies are available to help women who, for medical, economic, or other reasons, are postponing childbirth until later in life. One of these technologies is *oocyte cryopreservation*, more commonly known as *egg freezing*. It is less controversial than embryo cryopreservation because the oocyte is not fertilized, and so is not, by itself, a potential person.

The road to egg freezing begins when a fertility specialist—a medical doctor—prescribes drugs that stimulate a woman's ovaries to produce multiple eggs. The doctor then uses a needle, and ultrasound imaging for guidance, to harvest eggs from the ovaries. The eggs and some surrounding fluid from the pelvic cavity are extracted and placed in a flat dish. A laboratory technician identifies individual eggs through a microscope and withdraws them from the dish for freezing.

If isolated eggs were simply placed in a freezer, ice crystals would form inside them, causing irreversible damage. For this reason, various strategies have been devised to limit ice crystal formation and preserve the viability of the eggs. The two broad strategies used are *dehydration* followed by slow freezing, and *vitrification*.

In dehydration followed by slow freezing, different chemicals are used to draw as much water as possible out of the eggs before they are slowly cooled. When the eggs reach approximately -30°C to -40°C (-20°F to -40°F), they are plunged into liquid nitrogen for long-term storage. Liquid nitrogen is simply nitrogen gas (the main component of air) that has been refrigerated to -321°F (-196°C) or cooler. At -321°F, nitrogen gas liquefies.

In vitrification, the eggs are placed in a very small volume of chemical preservative solution for less than a minute, after which they are quickly cooled by direct exposure to liquid nitrogen.

When a woman is ready to have children, the eggs are removed from the liquid nitrogen storage tank and thawed. In a procedure called *intracytoplasmic sperm injection (ICSI)*, each egg is fertilized by injection with a single sperm (**Figure 15.18**). When an egg has developed into an embryo, it is implanted into the uterus through a catheter, a flexible tube that is easily inserted into small openings in the body.

In October 2012, the American Society of Reproductive Medicine (ASRM) reclassified egg freezing— oocyte cryopreservation—as a proven treatment for infertility. Previously, the process was considered experimental. The ASRM based its decision on analyses of many scientific studies. The studies showed that rates of fertilization and birth, and the health

Figure 15.18 Light micrograph of a human oocyte about to be injected with sperm. This procedure, called *intracytoplasmic sperm injection*, is one type of *in vitro* fertilization.

outcomes of the resulting children, were just as good with eggs that had been frozen as they were with *in vitro* fertilization (IVF) of fresh eggs that had never been frozen.

Taking It Further

1. Desiree is a 36-year-old, single female undergoing chemotherapy treatment for breast cancer. She has always wanted to have a child. When Desiree's oncologist informs her that the chemotherapy drugs may cause sterility, Desiree decides to have her eggs frozen, which will allow her to postpone pregnancy until she is cancer free. Do research on the health and financial risks, as well as ethical considerations, associated with egg freezing. Develop a "pro" argument in favor of Desiree's decision or a "con" argument against it. Support your argument with facts from expert sources. Present your case to the class.

Lesson 15.4 Review and Assessment

Mini Glossary
Make sure that you know the meaning of each key term.

amniotic fluid   a clear fluid in which the embryo, and then the fetus, is suspended

blastocyst   a fluid-filled cavity

delivery of the placenta   the last stage of birth in which the placenta detaches from the uterine wall and is expelled

dilation   the stage of labor during which the opening of the cervix dilates, or widens

embryo   the developing human from the time of implantation to the end of the eighth week after conception

expulsion   the stage of labor that starts at full dilation and ends when the baby is delivered

fetus   a developing human from eight weeks after conception to birth

human chorionic gonadotropin (hCG)   a hormone secreted by the trophoblast cells of the embryo that prevents deterioration of the corpus luteum and stimulates progesterone production in the placenta

implantation   the binding of the blastocyst to the endometrium

lactation   secretion of milk by the mammary glands

let-down reflex   contraction of smooth muscle cells in the mammary glands that allows milk to be squeezed toward and out of the nipple

oxytocin   a hormone that stimulates uterine contractions during labor and milk secretion during breastfeeding

placenta   the organ that grows in the uterus to meet the nutritional needs of the embryo and fetus

prolactin   a hormone that stimulates the secretory cells of the mammary glands to produce milk

umbilical cord   the cord that connects the fetus to the placenta

Know and Understand

Assess

1. Describe what occurs during capacitation.

2. When is the second meiotic division of the oocyte complete, and what is the result?

3. How is sperm able to penetrate the zona pellucida of the oocyte?

4. What is polyspermy and how is it prevented?

5. How is menstruation prevented once a blastocyst has successfully implanted in the endometrium?

6. What is human chorionic gonadotropin hormone, and where does it come from?

7. Which hormones are secreted by the placenta?

8. How do the embryo and, later, the fetus receive oxygen and nutrients, and how do they expel carbon dioxide and waste?

9. What does breast milk contain that makes it a uniquely important source of nutrition for the developing infant?

10. What is the let-down reflex?

Analyze and Apply

11. How is childbirth—in particular, the roles of fetal and maternal oxytocin—an example of a positive feedback system?

12. You are a doctor with a patient who is reluctant to breast-feed her newborn infant. What would you say to convince her of the benefits of breast feeding?

In the Lab

13. Diffusion is movement of material from a place where it is concentrated to a place where it is less concentrated. This occurs in the placenta, when nutrients pass from maternal blood, through a layer of cells, and into fetal blood. Using the membrane that separates an eggshell from the egg white, demonstrate the process of diffusion through a membrane.

Materials: 2 raw eggs, 1 to 2 L of white vinegar, 3 beakers (1 of 1,000 mL and 2 at 250 mL), 100 mL of corn syrup, 100 mL of distilled water, a food scale, measuring tape, and plastic wrap

Procedure: Place uncracked eggs in the larger beaker and cover with vinegar. Set aside. After four days, very gently rinse the eggs with cool water until the shells dissolve. Measure and record the weight, length, and circumference of each egg. Then place each egg in a 250 mL beaker. Cover one with distilled water and the other with corn syrup. Set aside. After one day, rinse off the eggs and measure them again. Describe your observations about the change in the size of each egg before and after soaking. In which direction is diffusion occurring in each instance?

Before You Read

Try to answer the following questions before you read this lesson.

Why are some males infertile?

Why are some females infertile?

What types of cancer affect the reproductive system?

Lesson Objectives

1. Describe common causes of male infertility.

2. Describe common causes of female infertility.

3. Identify some common sexually transmitted diseases, and describe their symptoms and treatments.

4. Identify different types of cancer that affect the reproductive system.

Key Terms

E-Flash Cards

chlamydia
genital herpes
gonorrhea
human papillomavirus
 (HPV)

infertility
sexually transmitted
 disease

Disorders of the human reproductive system impair the ability to reproduce. Infertility is a common reproductive disorder. Because the male and female reproductive systems are open to the outside environment, they are vulnerable to infection and disease. Reproductive system diseases, such as those that are sexually transmitted, require immediate medical attention because they can easily be spread to healthy individuals. Cancers of the reproductive system are among the most prevalent of all cancers. In this lesson, we will learn about common disorders and diseases of the male and female reproductive systems, their signs and symptoms, and their treatments.

Infertility

Infertility is the inability to get pregnant. It is defined clinically as the inability of a couple to conceive after at least one year of unprotected intercourse. Infertility may be due to male or female causes (**Figure 15.19** on the next page).

Male Infertility

Two common causes of male infertility are insufficient healthy-sperm count and the inability of sperm to be released. An insufficient quantity of healthy sperm, often called "low sperm count," has numerous possible causes, many of which are treatable. These causes include abnormal levels of the hormones that regulate sperm production (luteinizing hormone and follicle-stimulating hormone); chronic, warm temperature of the testes, which need to be somewhat below normal body temperature for optimum sperm production; smoking; heavy use of alcohol, cocaine, or marijuana; use of anabolic steroids (body-building drugs); exposure to

Monkey Business Images/Shutterstock.com

Figure 15.19 Doctors may recommend that couples make lifestyle changes to increase their chances of pregnancy. *What recommendations might they make?*

environmental toxins; and older age. If infertility is related to low sperm count—as is frequently the case—further investigation often can help determine a cause, and, if applicable, appropriate treatment can be given.

The inability of sperm to be released can be caused by impotence or damage to the ducts that convey sperm and other components of semen. Impotence, or the inability to maintain an erection, is also called *erectile dysfunction* (ED). Causes of ED include damage to the nerves or blood vessels of erectile tissues, side effects of some medications, prostate surgery, older age, stress, and psychological factors. The male duct system can be damaged by injury or by scarring from disease.

Female Infertility

Causes of female infertility include failure to ovulate, inability of the egg to reach the uterine tube and travel to the uterus, and inability of the blastocyst to implant successfully on the endometrium.

Failure to ovulate is usually accompanied by abnormal menstrual periods—either a complete absence of menstrual periods, called *amenorrhea* (a-MEHN-oh-REE-a), or cycles of unusual or unpredictable length. Failure to ovulate is often associated with abnormal levels of follicle-stimulating or luteinizing hormone, or abnormal levels of both hormones. Causes

include polycystic ovarian syndrome (PCOS) and abnormalities of the pituitary (which secretes FSH and LH) or the hypothalamus, which secretes GnRH. Other causes of failure to ovulate include scarring of the ovaries, failure of the mature follicle to rupture, and premature menopause.

Inability of the oocyte to enter and make it through the uterine tube usually results from scarring and damage to the tube. Uterine tube damage can be caused by diseases of the reproductive tract (usually sexually transmitted diseases); abdominal cavity infection (appendicitis, for example); previous surgery, which can cause scarring, or *adhesions* (areas where tissues stick together inappropriately); ectopic pregnancy, discussed in lesson 15.3; or congenital abnormalities.

Failure of the blastocyst to implant on the endometrium can have multiple causes. These causes include scars or adhesions on the endometrium from previous infections or surgery; *endometriosis* (EHN-doh-MEE-tree-OH-sis), the growth of endometrial cells outside the uterus (usually in the abdominal cavity), which produces inflammation and alters the balance between progesterone and estrogen; *uterine fibroids*—benign tumors of the muscular layer of the uterus; and abnormalities of the blastocyst itself.

Treatment for Infertility

A variety of treatments are available for male and female infertility, and they depend on the identified cause. Treatments include

- lifestyle changes (less alcohol, drug, or tobacco use in men can help stabilize or increase sperm count, and reduced stress can be helpful for both sexes);
- drugs to induce ovulation; and
- surgery to correct anatomical issues.

When these treatments fail, a variety of assisted reproductive technologies is available, the most common of which is *in vitro fertilization (IVF)*. IVF requires harvesting one or more oocytes from the mother and combining them in a petri dish with sperm collected from the father. Fertilization occurs in the dish (*in vitro fertilization* literally means "fertilization in glass"); then the embryo is transferred into the uterus for implantation.

Check Your Understanding

1. What is the clinical definition of infertility?
2. What are the two most common causes of male infertility?
3. What are the three most common causes of female infertility?
4. How can male and female infertility be treated?

Sexually Transmitted Diseases

There are a wide variety of sexually transmitted diseases (STDs). A **sexually transmitted disease** is an infection that can be passed from one person to another by sexual intercourse or genital contact. In this lesson, we will discuss the most common sexually transmitted diseases: AIDS, gonorrhea, chlamydia, genital herpes, and human papillomavirus. Sexually transmitted diseases are also referred to as *sexually transmitted infections (STIs)*.

HIV and AIDS

Acquired immune deficiency syndrome (AIDS) is the most lethal sexually transmitted disease. It is caused by the human immunodeficiency virus (HIV), which is shown in **Figure 15.20**. See chapter 12 for a more detailed discussion of HIV/AIDS.

Gonorrhea

In the United States, **gonorrhea** (GAHN-oh-REE-a) infection rates have been falling for the past 35 years. Gonorrhea still is, however, a common infectious disease, especially among teenagers and young adults.

Gonorrhea may cause pain during urination, unusual discharge of fluid from the vagina

Figure 15.20 A simplified diagram of the virus that causes AIDS. *What is the name of the virus that causes AIDS?*

or penis, or no symptoms at all. In women, gonorrhea can damage the endometrium and uterine tubes and can lead to infertility, even if the infection produces no symptoms. Because gonorrhea is caused by a bacterium, it can be successfully treated with antibiotics.

Chlamydia

Chlamydia (kla-MID-ee-a) is the most commonly reported STD in the United States. Its incidence has been rising.

Chlamydia often causes no symptoms, but it can damage the female reproductive tract, leading to infertility and increased risk of ectopic pregnancy. Chlamydia can be easily and successfully treated with antibiotics. The CDC recommends that all sexually active young women get an annual screening test for chlamydia.

Genital Herpes

Genital herpes is caused by *herpes simplex virus type 1 (HSV-1)* or *herpes simplex virus type 2 (HSV-2)*. It is a common STD: genital HSV-2 infects about one out of six Americans between 14 and 49 years of age.

Genital herpes may cause blisters or sores in the genital or anal area or near the mouth, or it may cause no symptoms. In fact, most people with genital herpes are unaware that they have it. Pregnant women who have—or have been exposed to—genital herpes need to discuss this fact with their healthcare provider. This consultation is recommended because this STD can spread from a pregnant mother to her unborn child, with serious or fatal results. There is no cure for genital herpes, but the condition is manageable with antiviral drugs.

Human Papillomavirus

Human papillomavirus (HPV) causes genital warts and cervical cancer. The most common STD in the United States, human papillomavirus infects both men and women. Some 6 million new infections emerge each year, and one-half of all sexually active adults will be infected with HPV at some point in their lives.

In most people, the immune system eliminates HPV, but it takes about two years to do so. HPV may produce no symptoms.

Pelvic Inflammatory Disease

Pelvic inflammatory disease (PID) is an inflammation of the uterus, uterine tubes, ovaries and/or other organs of the peritoneal (abdominopelvic) cavity. PID is caused by a bacterial infection. It is a potentially serious complication of chlamydia and gonorrhea in females.

The symptoms of pelvic inflammatory disease may include mild to severe pelvic pain, fever, and painful urination. When the symptoms are mild, PID often goes unrecognized. PID can be effectively treated with antibiotics. Prompt treatment is important to prevent permanent damage to the reproductive organs, including scarring of the uterine tubes. Such damage can cause infertility and increase the risk of ectopic pregnancy.

Detection and Prevention

Sexually transmitted diseases can infect any sexually active person. A person with symptoms—such as a discharge of unusual fluid from the genitals, burning during urination, or unusual sores, growths, or a rash—should stop having sex and see a healthcare provider immediately. The use of a condom during sex helps prevent the spread of most STDs. However, abstinence from sexual activity is the only foolproof method of preventing STDs.

 Check Your Understanding

1. How do sexually transmitted diseases spread from one person to another?
2. What is the most commonly reported STD in the United States?
3. Which STD can cause infected women to develop cervical cancer?

Cancers of the Reproductive System

Cancers of the reproductive system in males and females are among the most common and among the deadliest cancers. When detected early, however, these cancers often can be successfully treated. Millions of people in the United States are cancer survivors. In discussions of cancer, you'll often see the words *incidence* and *mortality*. *Incidence* refers to the number of people who get the disease; *mortality* refers to the number of people who die from it.

Prostate Cancer

After skin cancer, the cancer with the highest incidence among men in the United States is prostate cancer. After lung cancer, prostate cancer is the second most frequent cause of cancer mortality among men. Older men and men with a family history of prostate cancer are among those with an increased risk of developing prostate cancer.

Most prostate cancers, which are slow-growing, originate in the gland cells that produce the fluid added to semen. Screening tests are available for prostate cancer, the most common of which is the *prostate-specific antigen (PSA) test*. The PSA test is valuable in the early detection and treatment of prostate cancer, and it saves lives. However, the test sometimes produces false-positive results, prompting a series of

WHAT RESEARCH TELLS US

...*about* Genetic Research and Cancer Treatment Breakthroughs

Cancers of the reproductive tract, like cancers of other organs and tissues, are diseases in which cells grow "out of control," as seen in **Figure 15.21**. In reading chapter 2, you learned that cancer cells have mutations in their DNA. Often, these mutations result from damage to the genes that regulate cell division. Cells become cancerous because the mechanisms that regulate cell division—which act as "brakes" on cell division—no longer work.

Advances in technology are making it possible for scientists to decipher more information about the genetic makeup of cancer cells. Likewise, this technology is enabling scientists to identify people who, because of their genetic constitution, are more likely to develop cancer. These advances are leading to earlier detection of cancer as well as potentially significant changes in cancer care.

Genes Associated with Cancer

Researchers have found that a person's genetic makeup can make him or her more likely to develop cancer. This information can be used to detect cancer at its earliest stage, when it can be successfully treated. For example, women who inherit a mutant form of the BRCA1 or BRCA2 gene have a significantly elevated risk of developing breast or ovarian cancer. These genes, named for their association with breast cancer, provide the genetic codes for proteins that repair damaged DNA. When the BRCA1

Paul Hakimata Photography/Shutterstock.com

Figure 15.21 Microscopic view of ductal breast cancer cells in a tissue culture.

and BRCA2 genes are damaged, cells are less able to repair the DNA damage that can occur as we grow and age. As a result, the risk of further gene mutation, and thus the risk of cancer, increases.

A woman can be tested for the mutant forms of the BRCA1 and BRCA2 genes. If she has the mutation, she can undergo periodic screenings to detect precancerous changes in cells.

Women with damage to the BRCA1 or BRCA2 genes account for only about 15% of breast cancer cases. The remainder of cases do not have a direct hereditary cause, and may arise from gene mutation that occurs randomly throughout life.

New Cancer Treatments

Besides alerting women to a potential genetic vulnerability to cancer, advances in technology are reducing the time and cost required to determine the DNA sequence of cancer cells from individual patients. These technological benefits can lead to improved cancer care. For example, some tumors have a genetic mutation that makes them responsive to certain anti-cancer drugs. A doctor and patient with this knowledge could choose drug therapy accordingly.

Currently, more information is available on cancer cell mutations than there are drug therapies to effectively target and treat these mutations. Medical researchers continue their efforts to develop drugs tailored to the specific DNA mutations identified in different types of cancer cells.

Taking It Further

1. Why does damage to genes that regulate cell division often cause cancer?

2. How can doctors use a patient's genetic information to detect cancer at its earliest stage?

3. How can doctors use genetic information about cancer cells to treat cancer patients?

follow-up tests and treatments that have risks of their own. Furthermore, the PSA test may not distinguish between rapidly growing, malignant tumors and slow-growing tumors that might safely be left alone.

Treatment of prostate cancer includes surgery to remove cancer cells, radiation therapy, and chemotherapy. Radiation therapy is the use of X-rays to kill cancerous cells. Radiation therapy for prostate cancer is sometimes "delivered" to the tumor by surgically implanting radioactive "seeds"—each about the size and shape of a grain of rice—into the prostate gland. This method, known as *brachytherapy*, may have fewer unwanted side effects than other treatment options.

Cancers of the Female Reproductive Tract

The three most commonly diagnosed cancers of the female reproductive tract—and the deadliest (not including breast cancer)—are uterine, ovarian, and cervical cancers. These cancers affect about 70,000 American women annually and cause more than 20,000 deaths each year.

Uterine Cancer. Cancer of the uterus is the most frequently diagnosed cancer of the female reproductive tract. Uterine cancer almost always develops in cells of the endometrium, the inner lining of the uterus. For this reason, *endometrial cancer* is another term for uterine cancer. Abnormal uterine bleeding often reveals the presence of uterine cancer before it spreads within the body. Surgical removal of the entire uterus (known as *hysterectomy*), uterine tubes, and ovaries is the standard initial treatment. More than 80% of uterine cancer patients survive for at least five years after diagnosis.

Ovarian Cancer. Cancer of the ovary is the fifth most common cause of cancer-related death among women in the United States. Ovarian cancer causes more deaths than any other cancer of the female reproductive tract. Unlike uterine cancer, ovarian cancer usually does not cause any symptoms until the disease has spread beyond its initial site. For this reason, the average five-year survival rate of ovarian cancer patients is about 40%. The standard initial treatment is surgical removal of the uterus, uterine tubes, and ovaries. In most cases, surgery is followed by chemotherapy. Currently, there are no effective screening tests for ovarian cancer.

Cervical Cancer. Among cancers of the female reproductive tract, cervical cancer is the third most commonly diagnosed, and it ranks third as a cause of death among US women, after uterine and ovarian cancers. (Although the cervix is part of the uterus anatomically, cervical cancer is considered a different type of cancer from uterine cancer.) The *Papanicolaou test*, or *Pap smear*, is a screening test that has significantly reduced cervical cancer mortality over the last 35 years. It is used not only to detect cervical cancer but also to detect precancerous conditions in the cervix. Cervical cancer develops slowly, and the Pap smear allows early detection and surgical treatment.

Most cervical cancers are caused by high-risk forms of human papillomavirus. HPV also causes most anal cancers and about half of all vaginal, vulvar, and penile cancers. Health professionals expect that over the next few years, the incidence and mortality rates of cervical cancer, and perhaps those of other reproductive system cancers, will drop because of widespread use of vaccines that protect against HPV infection.

Breast Cancer

Breast cancer is a type of cancer that forms in the tissues of the breast—usually in the ducts and lobules. Males can develop breast cancer, but females typically are affected. After skin cancer, breast cancer is the most commonly diagnosed cancer among women in the United States. More women die from breast cancer than from any other cancer, with the exception of lung cancer. However, the breast cancer death rate has been declining due to early detection and more effective treatment therapies.

Factors that raise a woman's risk of developing breast cancer include advanced age, a family history of breast cancer, menarche at an early age, late onset of menopause, being overweight, and never having given birth.

Early detection of breast cancer improves the odds of successful treatment. For this reason, regular clinical breast examinations and mammography are recommended. Mammography involves the production of an X-ray image (mammogram) of the breast to detect a tumor while it is still small. A yearly mammogram is recommended for women 40 years of age and older. In addition many women regularly examine their own breasts for lumps and other unusual changes. This is called a *breast self-exam*. If a woman discovers an abnormality during a breast self-exam, she should contact a doctor.

Breast cancer is treated with surgery to remove cancer cells and with radiation therapy and/or chemotherapy to kill cancer cells. Treatment options, such as what kind of surgery to have or which drugs to use, depend on the specific clinical details of each case. Surgery options range from a "lumpectomy," in which only a small region of cancer tissue is removed, to a radical mastectomy, in which all the breast tissue and surrounding lymph nodes are removed.

Lesson 15.5 Review and Assessment

Mini Glossary   Make sure that you know the meaning of each key term.

 Build vocabulary with e-flash cards and games

chlamydia   a sexually transmitted disease that often causes no symptoms, but can damage the female reproductive tract and lead to infertility and increased risk of ectopic pregnancy

genital herpes   a sexually transmitted disease that may cause blisters or sores in the genital or anal area

or near the mouth; may cause no symptoms

gonorrhea   a sexually transmitted disease that may cause pain during urination, unusual discharge of fluid from the vagina or penis, or no symptoms at all; can lead to infertility

human papillomavirus (HPV)   a sexually transmitted disease that

causes genital warts and that can cause cervical cancer

infertility   the inability of a couple to get pregnant

sexually transmitted disease   an infectious disease transmitted through sexual contact; also referred to as a *sexually transmitted infection*

Know and Understand

 Assess

1. What is meant by the phrase *low sperm count*?
2. What is another name for impotence?
3. Which hormones, when present at abnormal levels, can result in failure to ovulate?
4. What are some causes of uterine tube damage?
5. What are uterine fibroids?
6. What is the most lethal STD?
7. Which STD often causes no symptoms, but can cause infertility and an increased risk of ectopic pregnancy if left untreated?
8. Which STD is the most common in the United States, affecting 50% of all sexually active adults at some point in their lives?
9. How are cancer cells different from normal cells?
10. Which screening tests are used to detect cancers of the prostate, cervix, and breast respectively?
11. Which cancer of the female reproductive tract has the highest incidence among women in the United States? Which cancer has the highest mortality among women?

Analyze and Apply

12. Compare and contrast male and female infertility.
13. How can a sexually active lifestyle increase a person's risk of becoming infertile? What can people do to help ensure that their reproductive systems function normally when they want to have children?
14. Explain the meanings of the words *incidence* and *mortality* as they relate to discussions of cancer.

In the Lab

15. Working with a small group of students, pick one of the sexually transmitted diseases discussed in this lesson that is of particular interest to you and the members of your group. Create an educational presentation using presentation software or online tools that represents the causes, symptoms, and treatments for that condition. Share your presentation with the class.

Career Corner
Anatomy and Physiology at Work

The basic role of the male and female reproductive systems is to ensure that genes are passed on to a new generation through reproduction, pregnancy, and childbirth. Many people have found careers in the promotion of reproductive health and in the diagnosis and treatment of diseases and disorders of the reproductive system. We will explore two of these careers.

Diagnostic Medical Sonographer

A diagnostic medical sonographer uses ultrasonic imaging equipment to diagnose and monitor medical conditions. Ultrasonic imaging uses sound waves (ultrasound) to generate pictures of structures inside the body. The technique is called *ultrasound imaging* because it uses sound frequencies far beyond those that can be detected by the human ear. The pictures created by ultrasound imaging are called *sonograms*, and the procedure itself is sometimes called an *ultrasound*. An echocardiogram is one type of sonogram. These images are studied by diagnostic medical sonographers and doctors to diagnose health problems.

Diagnostic medical sonographers specialize in one or more parts of the body. For example, obstetric sonographers perform ultrasound imaging of organs and tissues of the female reproductive system. Their patients are often pregnant women who have ultrasounds to monitor the health and growth of the fetus. A video display screen allows the obstetric sonographer to share ultrasound images with expectant mothers.

Diagnostic medical sonographers work in hospitals, doctors' offices, and medical laboratories (**Figure 15.22**). They must be able to use complex, computerized imaging equipment and assess the images they produce to ensure that they are sufficiently clear and detailed. They are also responsible for maintaining the equipment they use. Because they work with patients, diagnostic medical sonographers must

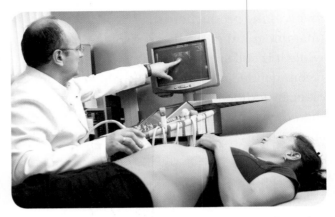

Dmitry Kalinovsky/Shutterstock.com

Figure 15.22 A diagnostic medical sonographer shows a patient ultrasound images of the fetus that she is carrying.

possess good communication and interpersonal skills. They explain ultrasound test procedures, answer patients' questions, and provide comfort and reassurance to nervous or distraught patients.

The minimum requirement to become a diagnostic medical sonographer is an associate's degree or a postsecondary certificate awarded by a community college. Many employers require that sonographers have professional certification. To be certified, they must earn a diagnostic medical sonography degree or complete a certificate program from an accredited college, or complete a health-related program and have appropriate clinical experience. They must also pass an examination. Certification examinations are given by the American Registry for Diagnostic Medical Sonography. Professional certification is also required in some states.

Job opportunities for diagnostic medical sonographers are plentiful. In fact, the demand for diagnostic medical sonographers is expected to grow faster than the average for many other professionals.

Obstetrician-Gynecologist

An obstetrician-gynecologist (ob-gyn) is a doctor who specializes in the healthcare of women, including the diagnosis and treatment of disorders of the female reproductive system. The ob-gyn also provides routine physical care to teenage girls and women. According to the American College of Obstetricians and Gynecologists, a teenage girl should make her first visit to a gynecologist between the ages of 13 and 15.

Ob-gyns examine patients and take their medical histories. They order and conduct routine diagnostic tests—for example, breast exams, pelvic exams, and Pap tests—to check for infections or disease, such as sexually transmitted diseases or cancer. They prescribe medications and counsel women on reproductive health, birth control, fertility, menstrual irregularities, and sexual problems. They care for women before, during, and after childbirth, and they perform surgical procedures. Ob-gyns work in hospitals, clinics, and in their own medical offices (**Figure 15.23**).

Training to become an ob-gyn begins with four years of college, followed by four years of medical school. The ob-gyn candidate then completes three or four years of residency training in obstetrics and gynecology. During this time, the medical resident treats patients under the supervision of senior doctors. An

ob-gyn often works long and irregular hours, including nights and weekends. Ob-gyns must be available when their patients are ready to give birth.

Planning for a Health-Related Career

Do some research on the career of an obstetrician-gynecologist or a diagnostic medical sonographer. Otherwise, select a profession from the list of **Related Career Options**. Find answers to the following questions:

1. What are the main tasks and responsibilities of a person employed in this career?
2. What is the outlook for this career? Are workers in demand, or are jobs dwindling?
3. What special skills or talents are required? For example, do you need to be good at science and comfortable with new and ever-changing technologies? Do you need to enjoy interacting with other people?
4. What personality traits do you think are necessary for success in the career that you have chosen to research?
5. Does the work involve a great deal of routine, or are the day-to-day responsibilities varied?
6. Does the career require long hours, or is it a standard, "9-to-5" job?
7. What is the salary range for this job?
8. What do you think you would like about this career? Is there anything about it that you might dislike?

Related Career Options

- Genetic Counselor
- Marriage and Family Therapist
- Medical Laboratory Technician or Technologist
- Neonatal Nurse Practitioner
- Nurse-Midwife
- Reproductive Endocrinologist
- Surgical Technologist
- Urologist

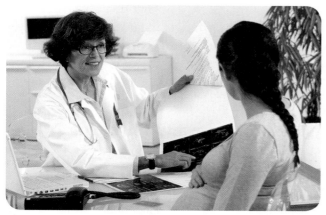

auremar/Shutterstock.com

Figure 15.23 An obstetrician-gynecologist gathers information from a young patient during a routine visit.

Chapter Summaries

Lesson 15.1 **Reproduction and Development of the Human Reproductive Systems**

Build vocabulary with
e-flash cards and games

Key Points

- Of the two types of reproduction—asexual and sexual—sexual reproduction is more complicated.
- Mitosis is the cell division process that occurs in all of the body's tissues throughout life. Meiosis occurs only in the sex organs and produces gametes.
- Unlike other organ systems, the reproductive systems do not become fully functional until later in life, beginning at puberty.
- During puberty, females experience changes such as breast growth, the growth of underarm and pubic hair, and menarche. Males experience growth of the scrotum and testes and growth of underarm, pubic, and facial hair.

Key Terms

centromere
chromatids
chromosomes
crossovers
diploid
fertilization
follicle-stimulating
    hormone (FSH)

gametes
haploid
luteinizing hormone (LH)
meiosis
menarche
zygote

Lesson 15.2 **Male Reproductive System Anatomy and Physiology**

Key Points

- The primary organs of the male reproductive system are the testes.
- Sperm are produced in the testes and then delivered to the external urethral orifice through a series of ducts.
- The penis contains erectile tissue in which blood collects to produce an erection, which makes it possible for the penis to gain entry to the female reproductive tract.
- Semen is ejaculated as a result of nerve impulses that cause peristaltic contractions.

Key Terms

bulbourethral glands
ductus deferens
ejaculation
epididymis
erection
gonads

penis
prostate gland
semen
seminal glands
seminiferous tubules
sperm

Lesson 15.3 **Female Reproductive System Anatomy and Physiology**

Key Points

- The primary organs in the female reproductive system are the ovaries.
- Ovulation occurs when a follicle reaches maturity and the oocyte is released from the ovary.
- The female external genitalia, the vulva, includes the labia, mons pubis, clitoris, and vestibule.

Key Terms

cervix
clitoris
labia majora
labia minora
lactiferous duct

mammary glands
oocyte
oogenesis
ovarian cycle
ovulation

- The female mammary glands produce milk for a newborn baby.
  - During the female's monthly cycle, the ovaries, uterus, and hormones undergo changes.

uterine cycle
uterine tubes

uterus
vagina

Lesson 15.4 Fertilization, Pregnancy, and Birth

Key Points

- Fertilization occurs when the chromosomes of the oocyte and the sperm unite to produce a zygote.
- After fertilization, the zygote travels through the uterine tube and into the uterus, where it implants.
- Fetal vessels carry blood through the umbilical cord to and from the placenta, which grows to meet the nutritional needs of the embryo/fetus.
- The stages of labor are dilation, expulsion, and delivery of the placenta.
- Lactation, the production of milk by the mother, is regulated by hormones.

Key Terms

amniotic fluid
blastocyst
delivery of the placenta
dilation
embryo
expulsion
fetus
human chorionic
  gonadotropin (hCG)

implantation
lactation
let-down reflex
oxytocin
placenta
prolactin
umbilical cord

Lesson 15.5 Disorders and Diseases of the Reproductive System

Key Points

- Infertility is the inability of a couple to conceive after at least one year of unprotected intercourse.
- A sexually transmitted disease is an infection that can be passed from one person to another by sexual intercourse or genital contact.
- Sexually transmitted diseases include acquired immune deficiency syndrome (AIDS), gonorrhea, chlamydia, genital herpes, and HPV.
- Cancers of the reproductive system are some of the most common and deadliest types of cancer.

Key Terms

chlamydia
genital herpes
gonorrhea
human papillomavirus
  (HPV)

infertility
sexually transmitted
  disease

Chapter Assessments

Lesson 15.1

Reproduction and Development of the Human Reproductive Systems

Learning Key Terms and Concepts

1. *True or False?* Homologous chromosomes are the two identical chromosomes that make up one of the 23 pairs in a mother cell.

2. Which of the following helps create genetic diversity?
   A. DNA
   B. mitosis
   C. crossovers
   D. SRY genes

3. Does the presence of a Y chromosome indicate development of a male or a female?

4. Which of the following hormones is *not* involved in stimulating puberty: DNA, FSH, LH, or GnRH?

5. Adolescence officially begins with the appearance of _____ and ends when _____.

6. *True or False?* By the end of puberty, mature sperm are present in semen.

Thinking Critically

7. Imagine that you have been asked to teach a lesson on the differences between mitosis and meiosis to an eighth-grade biology class. How would you explain the differences to the class?

Lesson 15.2

Male Reproductive System Anatomy and Physiology

Learning Key Terms and Concepts

8. Testes are to ovaries as sperm are to _____.

9. At which temperature would you expect sperm production to be most vigorous?
   A. 98.6°F   C. 95°F
   B. 101°F   D. 97°F

10. Identify the functions of the male reproductive system.

11. The _____ glands make the greatest contribution to the production of semen.

12. Does a spermatid have 23 or 46 chromosomes?

13. *True or False?* When a spermatid develops a flagellum and is released into the seminiferous tubule, it is mature.

Thinking Critically

14. Compare sperm cells to other cells in the human body. How are they different? How are they similar?

Lesson 15.3

Female Reproductive System Anatomy and Physiology

Learning Key Terms and Concepts

15. What is an oocyte? Where are oocytes originally located?

16. How many ovarian follicles reach maturity each month?

17. Describe the step-by-step process that occurs during ovulation.

18. Describe where the uterus is located. What is the purpose of the uterus in reproduction?

19. Why is the pH of the vagina acidic in healthy adult women?

20. Identify the functions of the female reproductive system.

21. Which hormone stimulates milk production by the female mammary glands after childbirth?

22. After ovulation, what happens to the levels of estrogen and progesterone in the blood?

Thinking Critically

23. Compare and contrast the anatomy of the ovary and the testis.

24. Compare and contrast the functions of the male and female reproductive systems.

Lesson 15.4

Fertilization, Pregnancy, and Birth

Learning Key Terms and Concepts

25. *True or False?* A gamete has 46 chromosomes.

26. *True or False?* After intercourse, a few thousand sperm may reach the oocyte.

27. What is the function of acrosomal enzymes in sperm?

28. Describe how pregnancy-test kits work.

29. Where is the placenta located and what is its function?

30. Which structure connects the fetus to the placenta?

31. Which stage of labor lasts the longest, and what events occur during this stage?

32. Which hormone stimulates the secretory cells of the mammary glands to produce milk?

Thinking Critically

33. Explain why it is important for pregnant women to avoid drinking alcohol and taking drugs that are illegal or not prescribed. How can these substances reach the developing fetus?

Lesson 15.5

Disorders and Diseases of the Reproductive System

Learning Key Terms and Concepts

34. Why are the male and female reproductive systems vulnerable to infection and disease?

35. Which of the following secretes GnRH?
   A. pituitary   C. hypothalamus
   B. testis   D. ovary

36. What is erectile dysfunction, and what are some common causes?

37. What is in vitro fertilization (IVF)? Briefly describe how it is performed.

38. Which STD is caused by a bacterium?

39. *True or False?* Gonorrhea and chlamydia *cannot* be successfully treated with antibiotics.

40. *True or False?* Genital warts are a symptom of human papillomavirus.

41. What is the most frequently diagnosed cancer of the female reproductive tract?

42. *True or False?* The breast cancer death rate has been declining slowly but steadily.

43. What is the relationship between gene mutation and cancer development?

Thinking Critically

44. Evaluate the cause and effect of the human papillomavirus on the structure and function of the female reproductive system.

45. You are a doctor who treats infertile couples. A new patient complains that she is not pregnant although she and her husband have been trying for six months. What would you tell this patient? Write a "prescription" for lifestyle changes that could help increase their chances of conceiving.

Building Skills and Connecting Concepts

Analyzing and Evaluating Data

Figure 15.24 shows the rate of HPV infection among surveyed females in the United States. Several factors are linked to the rate of infection among certain demographic groups. Use the chart to answer the questions.

46. Which race/ethnicity is most likely to become infected with HPV?

47. What is the difference in HPV infection rate between those at or above the poverty line and those below the poverty line?

48. How much more likely is a woman between 14 and 19 years of age to become infected with HPV than a woman between 50 and 59 years of age?

49. Why do you think that females 20-24 years of age are more likely to become infected with HPV than other age groups?

Fig. 15.24 HPV Infection Rates Among Surveyed U.S. Females

Factor	Demographic Group	Rate of Infection
Age	14-19	40%
	20-24	50%
	25-29	28%
	30-39	37%
	40-49	25%
	50-59	20%
Race/ Ethnicity	African-American	39%
	Caucasian	24%
	Hispanic	24%
Economic Status	Below the poverty line	38%
	At/above the poverty line	24%

Communicating about Anatomy and Physiology

50. **Speaking** Pick a figure in this chapter, such as Figure 15.4, 15.7, or 15.14. Working with a partner, tell and then retell the important information being conveyed by that figure.

51. **Reading and Speaking** Cancer screenings can detect cancer at an early stage, improving the chances of survival. Yet the value of some of these tests for people who have no symptoms and few or no risk factors has recently come into question. As part of a small group, research the debate surrounding either prostate or breast cancer screenings. Choose a position (yes or no) and develop an argument in response to the following question: Do the benefits of cancer screenings outweigh the risks involved?

Lab Investigations

52. Imagine you are studying this photograph of a follicle in an ovary under a microscope.
    A. In which stage of development is the follicle? Explain your answer.
    B. Label the following parts of the follicle.
       oocyte   zona pellucida
       antrum   granulosa cells
    C. Where are chromosomes located in the follicle? How many chromosomes are there?

Expand your learning with additional online resources
- Supplemental Lab Activities
- Interactive Exercises
- Animations

Expand

Companion Website

www.g-wlearning.com/healthsciences

Appendix A Metric Conversion Table

Conversion Table: US Customary to SI Metric*

When You Know	Multiply By:	To Find
Length		
inches	25.4	millimeters
inches	2.54	centimeters
feet	0.3048	meters
feet	30.48	centimeters
yards	0.9	meters
miles	1.6	kilometers
Weight		
ounces	28.0	grams
ounces	.028	kilograms
pounds	0.45	kilograms
short tons	0.9	tonnes
Volume		
teaspoons	5.0	milliliters
tablespoons	15.0	milliliters
fluid ounces	30.0	milliliters
cups	0.24	liters
pints	0.47	liters
quarts	0.95	liters
gallons	3.8	liters
cubic inches	0.02	liters
cubic feet	0.03	cubic meters
cubic yards	0.76	cubic meters
Area		
square inches	6.5	square centimeters
square feet	0.09	square meters
square yards	0.8	square meters
square miles	2.6	square kilometers
acres	0.4	hectares
Temperature		
Fahrenheit	$5/9 \times (F - 32)$	Celsius
Celsius	$(9/5 \times C) + 32$	Fahrenheit

*Note: For all but temperature, when you know the metric measurement, divide by the same numbers given above to determine the US customary measurement.

BMI Calculation	US Customary	SI Metric
	$BMI = \dfrac{wt\ (lb)}{ht\ (in^2)} \times 703$	$BMI = \dfrac{wt\ (kg)}{ht\ (m^2)}$

Appendix B
Anatomy and Physiology Word Elements

Students should learn to recognize word elements that are routinely used in the study of anatomy and physiology. Many of these word parts, which come from Greek and Latin, offer clues to the meanings of words used to describe structures, functions, and processes. For example, the word *physiology* is made up of *physio-* ("function") and *-logy* ("study of"). Thus, *physiology* is the study of how living things function or work. Likewise, the word *anatomy* comes from *ana-* ("apart") and *-tomy* ("cutting"). These word elements are appropriate when you consider that ancient anatomists gained a great deal of knowledge about the structure of tissues and organs through dissection.

The following combining forms, prefixes, and suffixes are used throughout the text. This list is not exhaustive; for the purpose of this introduction to anatomy and physiology, only commonly used forms are presented.

A

ab- away from, off (*abdominal aorta, abduction*)

abdomin(o)- abdomen (*abdominal, abdominopelvic cavity*)

acous/o, acoust/o hearing, sound (*external acoustic meatus*)

acr(o)- extremity, highest or farthest point (*acromegaly, acromioclavicular joint, acromion*)

ad- to, toward, near (*adduction*)

adip(o)- fat or fatty tissue (*adipocyte, adipose tissue*)

af- toward (*afferent nerves, afferent pathway*)

-agon to gather, assemble (*agonist, antagonist, glycagon*)

alb/i-, alb/o-, albin/o- white (*albinism*)

amni- fetal sac (*amnion, amniotic fluid*)

amph-, amphi/- on both sides, around (*amphiarthrosis*)

an- not, without (*anaerobic, anemia*)

ana- apart (*anatomy, anaphase*); up, build up (*anabolism*)

andr/o- male (*androgen*)

angi/o- blood vessel (*angioplasty, angiography, angiotensin*)

antero- forward, from front to back (*anteroposterior*)

anti- against (*antibiotic, antidiuretic hormone, antifungal*)

apo- above, away, off, separated from (*apocrine glands, aponeurosis, apoptosis*)

aque/o- water (*aquaporins, aqueous humor*)

arteri/o- artery (*arterial, arterioles*)

arthr/o- joint (*rheumatoid arthritis, synarthroses, diarthrodial*)

articul/o- joint (*articular fibrocartilage, articulating bones*)

-ase enzyme (*amylase, polymerase*)

ather/o- fat, plaque (*atherosclerosis*)

atri/o- heart, entryway (*atrium, interatrial septum, atrial fibrillation*)

audi/o-, audit/o- hearing (*auditory canal, auditory nerve, audiologist*)

aur/i-, aur/o-, auricul/o- ear, hearing (*auricle*)

aut/o- self (*autoimmune disease, autonomic nervous system*)

axi/o- axis, straight line (*axial skeleton, axon*)

B

bar/o- pressure, weight (*baroreceptors, barometric*)

bi- two, twice, double (*bicarbonate, biceps*)

bi/o- life (*antimicrobial, biopsy, microbial*)

bil/i- bile (*bilirubin*)

blast/o- bud, germ, precursor (*blastocyst, osteoblast*)

brachi/o- arm (*biceps brachii*)

bronch/i, bronch/o- airway (*bronchus, bronchial, bronchodilator*)

C

calc/o-, calci/o- calcium, stone (*hypercalcemia, calcitonin*)

calori- heat (*Calorie, caloric*)

carcin/o- cancer (*carcinogens, carcinogenic*)

cardi/o- heart (*cardiovascular, cardiac*)

carp/o- wrist (*metacarpals, radiocarpal*)

centr/i-, centr/o- middle, center (*centromere, centriole*)

cephal/o- head (*diencephalon, brachiocephalic artery*)

cerebr/o- brain (*cerebrum, cerebral*)

cervic/o- neck, narrow part (*cervical, cervix*)

circ/um- around, about (*circumferential growth, circumduction*)

-clast break (down), destroy (*osteoclasts*)

clavicul/o- hammer, club, key (*clavicle, acromioclavicular joint*)

-cle little (*corpuscle*)

co- with, together (*cotransport*)

col-, col/o-, col/ono- large intestine (*colon, colonoscopy*)

com- with, together (*complement system, compression*)

contus/o- bruise (*contusion*)

coron/o- heart, crown (*coronary, corona radiata*)

corp/o-, corpor/o- body (*corpus luteum, corpus spongiosum, corpora cavernosa*)

corti- covering (*cortex, cortical*)

cost/o- rib (*intercostal nerves, sternocostal joints*)

cox/a-, cox/o- hip (*coxal bone*)

crani/o- skull (*cranium, cranial*)

-crin/o secrete, separate (*endocrine, exocrine*)

cry/o- cold (*cryotherapy, oocyte cryopreservation*)

-cule, -culus small (*molecule, canaliculus*)

cutane/o- skin (*subcutaneous fascia, musculocutaneous*)

cyst/i-, cyst/o- bladder (*cystitis, cholecystectomy, polycystic ovarian syndrome*)

-cyte, cyt/o- cell (*lymphocytes, monocytes, phagocytes, cytoplasm, cytokinesis*)

D

de- down, away from, cessation (*dehydration, defibrillation, deformation*)

dendr/o- tree, branch (*dendrites, oligodendrocytes*)

-derma, dermat/o-, derm/o- skin (*epidermal, dermatologist*)

-desis binding, tying together (*diapedesis*)

desm/o- bond, ligament (*desmosomes, syndesmosis*)

di- two, apart, separate, through (*diuresis, antidiuretic hormone*)

dia- across, separate, through (*diabetes, diaphragm, dialysis*)

dif- apart, separate (*differentiate, diffusion*)

digit- finger (*extensor digitorum, interdigitate*)

dilat/o- widening, expanding, stretching (*dilation, bronchodilator*)

dipl/o- double (*diploid, diplopia*)

dis- apart, separate (*dissect, dislocation*)

dist/o- far, distant (*distal convoluted tubule, distal radioulnar joint*)

dors/i-, dors/o- back, back of body (*dorsal, latissimus dorsi*)

duc-, duct/o- to lead, carry (*ducts, abduction, adduction*)

dynam/o- strength, force, power, energy (*dynamic lung volume, dynamometer*)

dys- bad, abnormal, painful (*muscular dystrophy, dyspnea*)

E

e- out (*ejaculate, eversion*)

-eal pertaining to (*pineal, esophageal, epiphyseal*)

ec-, ect/o- out, outside, away (*ectopic*)

-ectomy incision, surgical removal (*cholecystectomy, mastectomy*)

-edema swelling (*lymphedema, myxedema*)

ef- out, out of (*efferent, effusion*)

-el, -elle small (*organelles, fontanel, micelles*)

electr/o- electricity (*electrocardiogram, electrolytes*)

em- in, within (*embolism*)

-ema condition (*emphysema, myxedema*)

-emia blood condition (*anemia, hyponatremia, leukemia*)

en- in, into (*enzyme*)

encephal/o- brain (*diencephalon*)

end/o- in, inside, within (*endometrium, endoneurium*)

enter/o- intestine (*enteroendocrine cells, gastroenterologist*)

epi- on, upon, above (*epidermis, epididymis, epiphyseal plate*)

epitheli/o- skin (*epithelium, epithelial*)

erythr/o- red (*erythrocytes, erythroblasts*)

-esis action, condition, state of (*erythropoiesis, gluconeogenesis, synthesis*)

estr/o- female (*estrogen*)

ex-, exo- out, out of, away, away from (*exocrine glands, exocytosis, exophthalmos*)

extra- outside (*extracellular*)

F

femor/o- thigh bone (*femur, femoral*)

fer-, -ferent to carry (*afferent, efferent*)

fibr/o fiber (*fibroblast, fibrocartilage*)

fil/i-, fil/o-, filament/o- thread, thread-like (*filament, microfilament, filtration*)

flex/o- bend (*flexion, dorsiflexion*)

fore- before (*forearm*), in front (*forehead*)

-form, -iform having the shape or form of (*fusiform, deformed*)

G

gastr/o- stomach (*gastrointestinal, gastric, gastroesophageal, gastroenteritis*)

-gen, -genic, -genesis producing, bringing about (*gluconeogenesis, spermatogenesis, oogenesis*)

germi- sprout, bud (*germinate, germinal*)

gest/o- to carry (*ingest*); pregnancy (*gestation, progesterone*)

gingiv/o- pertaining to the gums (*gingiva, gingivitis*)

glauc/o- having a blue or blue-gray color (*glaucoma*)

-glia glue (*neuroglia, microglia*)

globu- sphere, ball (*globulin, hemoglobin*)

gloss/o-, glott/o- tongue (*glossopharyngeal*)

gluc/o- sugar, glucose (*glucose, gluconeogenesis, glucocorticoid*)

glyc/o- sugar, glucose (*glycogen, hypoglycemia, glycolysis*)

-gnosis knowledge (*diagnosis, prognosis*)

gon/o-, gonad/o- semen, seed, pertaining to reproduction (*gonad, spermatogonia, gonadotropic*)

gyn/o-, gynec/o- woman, female (*gynecology, gynecologist*)

H

hapl/o- single, simple (*haploid*)

hema-, hemo-, hemat/o- blood (*hematopoiesis, hematocrit, hemoglobin, hemolysis*)

hemi- half (*hemidesmosome, hemisphere*)

-hemia blood condition (*polycythemia*)

hepat/o- liver (*hepatic, hepatocytes, hepatitis*)

hist/o- tissue (*histology*)

hom/o- like, similar (*homologous*)

home/o- unchanging, constant (*homeostasis*)

humer/o- shoulder (*humerus*)

hydr/o- water (*hydrophilic, hydrophobic*)

hyper- above, above normal, excessive (*hypertrophy, hyperextension, hyperopia*)

hypo- under, below normal (*hypothyroidism, hypoxia, hyposecretion*)

I

-ia condition (*anemia, pneumonia*)

-iasis abnormal condition (*psoriasis*)

-iatr/o doctor, medicine (*pediatrician, pediatric*)

-ic, -ical pertaining to (*anatomical, physiological, biological, statistical*)

-icle, -icul small (*ossicle, canaliculus*)

-ics knowledge (*physics, kinetics, genetics*)

-immun/o protection, safety (*immune, autoimmune, immunotherapy*)

in- in, into, not (*inspiration, insertion*)

-in(e) protein, enzyme, chemical compound (*globulin, penicillin, creatinine*)

infra- below, beneath, inferior to (*infraspinous fossa*)

inter- between, among (*interstitial, intermediate, intermembrane, intervertebral*)

intra- within, into (*intracellular, intrapulmonary*)

-ism process (*metabolism, mechanism*); condition or disorder (*gigantism, astigmatism*)

is/o- same, equal (*isometric*)

-ite little (*dendrite*)

-itis inflammation (*gingivitis, arthritis*)

-ium structure, tissue (*cranium, endomysium, epithelium, pericardium*)

J

jaund/o- yellow (*jaundice*)

jug- to join (*jugular*)

juxta- beside, next to (*juxtamedullary nephrons*)

K

kerat/o- hard, horn-shaped tissue (*keratin, keratinized, keratinocytes*)

kin/e-, kin/o, kines/o-, kinesi/o- movement, motion (*kinetic, cytokinesis*)

L

lacrim/o- tear (*lacrimal glands*)

lact/i-, lact/o- milk (*lactic acid, lactation*)

laryng/o- voice box (*larynx, laryngeal*)

later/o- side (*lateral rotation, lateral flexion*)

-lepsy, -leptic seizure (*epilepsy, epileptic*)

-let small (*platelet*)

leuk/o- white (*leukocytes, leukemia*)

lig/o- to tie, bind (*ligament*)

lingu/a-, lingu/o- tongue (*lingual tonsil*)

lip/o- fat (*lipids, lipocytes*)

lith/o- stone (*lithotripsy*)

-logy, -ology study of (*biology, microbiology, physiology*)

-lucent, -lucid clear, light, shining (*zona pellucida, stratum lucidum*)

lumb/o- lower back (*lumbar vertebrae*)

lun- moon, crescent (*semilunar valves*)

lute/o- yellow (*corpus luteum*)

lymph/o- lymph (*endolymph, lymphocytes*)

lys/o-, lyt/o, -lyt/ic separate, break apart, break down, destroy (*lysosome, glycolysis*)

M

macro- large (*macrophage, macronutrients*)

mal/i- bad (*malfunction, malignant*)

mamm(o)- breast (*mammary, mammogram*)

medi/o-, mediastin/o- middle (*medial, intermediate, mediastinum*)

medull/o- middle, deep part, marrow (*medulla, medullary canal, medulla oblongata*)

meg/a-, megal/o-, -megaly large, enlargement (*acromegaly, megakaryocytes*)

melan/o- black color (*melanocytes, melanoma*)

men/o- month, menses, menstruation (*amenorrhea, menarche, menstruation*)

mening/o-, meningi/o- membrane (*meninges, meningitis*)

meta- after, beyond; change (*metaphase, metacarpal, metatarsal, metastasize*)

-meter instrument or device used to measure (*spirometer, sphygmomanometer*)

metri- length, measure (*metric system*)

metri-, metr/o- uterus, womb (*endometrium*)

micro- small; millionth (*microscope, microbiology, micrometer*)

mon/o- one, single (*monomer, monosaccharide, monoglyceride*)

morph/o- form, shape (*polymorphism*)

-mortem, mort/o- death (*mortality, post-mortem*)

muc/o-, mucos/o- mucus (*mucosal*)

multi- many (*multicellular, multipennate*)

muscul/o- muscle (*muscular, musculoskeletal*)

muta- change (*mutation, mutant*)

my/o-, myos/o-, mysi- muscle (*myositis, epimysium*)

myel/o- bone marrow (*myeloid*); spinal cord (*myelin*)

N

nas/o- nose (*nasolacrimal, nasopharynx*)

natr/i-, natr/o- sodium (*hyponatremia, natriuretic*)

neo- new (*gluconeogenesis, neonatal*)

nephr/o- kidney (*nephron*)

neur/o- nerve (*neural, neurons, neuromuscular, neuroscience*)

neutr/o- neutral, neither (*neutrophils, neutralization*)

nucle/o- nucleus (*nuclear membrane, deoxyribonucleic acid*)

nutri/o, nutrit/o- nourish (*nutrients, nutrition*)

O

obstetr/o- pregnancy; birth (*obstetrician*)

ocul/o- eye (*oculomotor, orbicularis oculi*)

odont/o- tooth (*periodontal disease*)

-ole little, small (*arteriole, bronchiole, nucleolus*)

-oma tumor, mass (*carcinoma, hematoma*)

onc/o- tumor (*oncology, oncologist*)

-opia vision condition (*myopia, hyperopia, presbyopia*)

ophthalm/o- eye (*ophthalmologist, exophthalmos*)

-opsy view of (*biopsy*)

optic/o- eye, vision (*optic nerve, optic chiasma*)

or/o- mouth (*oropharynx, oral cavity*)

orbi- circle (*orbicularis, orbital cavities*)

-orexia appetite (*anorexia*)

orth/o- straight (*orthopedic, orthodontist*)

-ose sugar (*glucose, fructose, sucrose*)

-osis process (*mitosis, apoptosis*); disease, abnormal condition (*tuberculosis, cirrhosis*)

osseo- bony (*osseous tissue, interosseous membrane*)

ossi- bone (*ossify, ossification*)

ost/e-, oste/o- bone (*osteoporosis, osteoarthritis*)

ov/o-, ovul/o- egg (*ovum, ovary, ovulation*)

ox/o- oxygen (*hypoxic, oxyhemoglobin*)

P

para- near, next to, beside (*parathyroid, parasites*)

-partum birth; labor (*parturition, postpartum thyroiditis*)

path/o- disease (*pathology, pathogen*); feeling, emotion (*sympathetic*)

pector/o- chest (*pectoral girdle, pectoralis major*)

ped/o- child (*pediatrician*); foot (*tinea pedis*)

pelv/i-, pelv/o- hip (*pelvis, pelvic*)

pend/o- to hang (*appendix, appendicular*)

-penia deficiency (*osteopenia*)

penna- thread (*unipennate, bipennate, multipennate*)

penta- five, fifth (*pentapeptide, pentamer*)

peri- around (*periosteum, peritoneum, periodontal*)

-phage, phag/o- eat, swallow (*esophagus, macrophage, phagocytosis*)

phalang/o- fingers, toes (*phalanges*)

pharyng/o- throat (*pharynx, pharyngeal*)

phil/o- loving, attracted to (*hydrophilic*)

phleb/o- vein (*phlebotomy, phlebotomist*)

-phob/o, -phobia fear (*hydrophobic*)

phon/o-, -phonia voice, sound (*phonetic*)

phot/o- light (*phototherapy*)

physi/o-, physic/o- nature, function (*physiology, physician*)

-physis growth (*diaphysis, epiphysis*)

-plasm shaped, molded (*cytoplasm, endoplasmic, sarcoplasmic*)

-plasty surgical repair (*rhinoplasty*)

-plegia, -plegic   paralysis (*paraplegia, quadriplegia*)

pleur/o-   lung (*pleural sac, pleurisy*)

plex/o-   network of nerves (*brachial plexus, lumbar plexus, sacral plexus*)

-pnea   breath, breathing (*dyspnea*)

pneum/o-, pneumon/o-   lung, air (*pneumonia*)

pod/o-   foot (*podocytes*)

-poiesis   formation (*hematopoiesis, erythropoiesis*)

-poietin   substance that forms (*erythropoietin, thrombopoietin*)

poly-   many, much (*polymer, polysaccharide*)

-porosis   condition of holes, spaces (*osteoporosis*)

post-   after, behind (*postmenopausal, post-mortem*)

poster/o-   back of (the body), behind (*posterior*)

pre-   before, in front of (*precursor, precancerous, preganglionic*)

presby/o-   old age (*presbyopia*)

pro-   before, in front of (*prostate*); promote (*progesterone*)

prot/o-   first (*protoplasm*)

proxim/o-   near (*proximal*)

pseudo-   false (*pseudopod*)

psych/o-   mind (*psychology, psychological*)

pulmon/o-   lung (*pulmonary, cardiopulmonary*)

puls/o-, pulsat/o-   to beat, vibrate, push against (*pulse, propulsion*)

pyr/o-, pyret/o-, pyrex/o-   fire; fever (*pyrogens*)

Q

quadri-   four (*quadriceps*)

quater-   fourth (*quaternary structure*)

R

radiat-   radiating (*corona radiata*)

radi/o-   X-ray; radioactive; (*radiography*)

re-   back, again, backward (*reabsorption, remodeling*)

-receptor, -ceptor   receiver (*sensory receptor*)

ren/o-   kidney (*renal cortex, renal tubule*)

respir/o-   breathe (*respiratory, respiration*)

reti(cul)o-   network (*endoplasmic reticulum, reticular connective tissue*)

retro-   back, backward, behind (*retroperitoneal*)

rhin/o-   nose (*rhinoplasty*)

-rrhage, -rrhagia   bursting forth of blood (*hemorrhagic stroke*)

-rrhea   flow, discharge (*diarrhea, amenorrhea*)

S

sacchar/o-   sugar (*monosaccharide, polysaccharide*)

sacr/o-   posterior section of pelvic bone (*sacrum, sacral curve, sacroiliac joint*)

scapul/o-   shoulder blade (*scapulothoracic joint, subscapular, suprascapular*)

-scope, scop/o-, -scopy   see (*microscope, colonoscope*)

sect/o-   to cut (*dissections, cross section*)

semi-   half (*semicircular canals, semilunar valves*)

semin/i-   semen, seed (*seminal glands, seminiferous tubules*)

-sis   state of, condition (*homeostasis*); process (*mitosis, glycolysis*)

son/o-   sound (*sonogram, sonographer*)

-spasm   sudden contraction of muscles (*muscle spasms, bronchospasms*)

sperm/o-, spermat/o-   sperm cells (*spermatids, spermatic cord, spermatocyte*)

-sphyxia   pulse (*asphyxiation*)

spir/o-   to breathe (*respiration, inspiration, spirometer*)

stas/i-, stat/i-   stop, remain, stay the same (*homeostasis*)

-static   pertaining to stopping or controlling (*homeostatic, hydrostatic*)

sten/o-   narrow, constricted (*valvular stenosis*)

stern/o-   chest, breast (*sternum*)

steth/o-   chest (*stethoscope*)

strept/o-   twisted chains (*streptococcus*)

stri/a-   striped (*striated*)

sub-   under, below (*subcutaneous fascia*)

super-   above, beyond (*superior, superficial*)

sym-   together, with (*symphysis, symmetrical*)

syn-   together, with (*synthesis, synarthroses*)

synaps/o-, synapt/o-   to join, make contact (*synapses, synaptic*)

systol/o-   contraction (*systole, systolic*)

T

tars/i-, tars/o-   ankle, hindfoot (*tarsal, metatarsal*)

tendin/o-, ten/o-   tendon (*tendinitis, tendinosis*)

tens/o-   stretched, strained (*tension, tensile*)

tetra-   four (*tetramers, tetrads*)

therm/o-   heat (*hyperthermia, thermometer*)

thorac/o-, -thorax   chest, pleural cavity (*thoracic cavity, cardiothoracic*)

thromb/o-   blood clot (*thrombosis, thrombocytes*)

tom/o-   to cut (*anatomy, splenectomy, cholecystectomy*)

tox/o-, toxic/o-   poison (*toxins, cytotoxic*)

trans-   across, through (*neurotransmitter, transverse plane, transmembrane*)

tri-   three (*adenosine triphosphate, triglycerides*)

-tropin   to act upon, stimulate (*adrenocorticotropin, gonadotropin, thyrotropin*)

U

-ul, -ule   little, small (*trabecula, microtubules, capitulum, glomerulus*)

ultra-   beyond, excessive (*ultraviolet, ultrasonic*)

-um   structure, tissue, substance (*cerebrum, sodium, stratum granulosum, corpus cavernosum*)

uni-   one (*unipennate, unipolar*)

-uresis   urination (*diuresis*)

ur/i-, ur/o-, -uria, urin/o-   urine, urination (*diuretic, polyuria, urinalysis*)

-us   structure, thing (*fetus, hypothalamus, sartorius, uterus, vastus medialis*)

uter/o-   womb (*uterus, uterine*)

V

valv/o-, valvu/o-   valve (*valvular stenosis*)

vas/o-, vascul/o-   vessel (*vasa recta, vascular, vas deferens*)

ven/i-, ven/o-   vein (*venous, venule, intravenous*)

ventil/o-   to oxygenate (*ventilation, hyperventilation*)

ventr/o-, ventricul/o-   belly side of body, lower part (*ventral, ventricle*)

vers/o, -verse, -version   turning (*eversion, inversion*)

vertebr/o-   spine; backbone (*intervertebral*)

vir/o-   virus (*viral, virology*)

viscer/o-   internal organs (*visceral pleura, visceral pericardium*)

vit/a-, vit/o-   life (*vitamin, vital signs*)

vitr/e-, vitr/o-   glass (*vitreous humor, in vitro*)

Appendix C Common Medical Abbreviations

A

ACTH adrenocorticotropin hormone
AD Alzheimer's disease
ADH antidiuretic hormone
ADP adenosine diphosphate
AED automatic external defibrillator
AIDS acquired immunodeficiency syndrome
ALL acute lymphocytic leukemia
ALS amyotrophic lateral sclerosis
AML acute myeloid leukemia
ANP atrial natriuretic peptide
ANS autonomic nervous system
APC antigen-presenting cell
ATP adenosine triphosphate
AV atrioventricular (node; valves)

B

BMI body mass index
BMR basal metabolic rate
BPM beats per minute

C

CLL chronic lymphocytic leukemia
CML chronic myeloid leukemia
CNS central nervous system
CO$_2$ carbon dioxide
COPD cardiopulmonary disease
CP cerebral palsy
CPR cardiopulmonary resuscitation
CT computed tomography

D

DNA deoxyribonucleic acid
DO doctor of osteopathic medicine
DOMS delayed-onset muscle soreness
DPT doctor of physical therapy

E

ECG electrocardiogram
ED erectile dysfunction
EIB exercise-induced bronchospasms
EKG electrocardiogram (*variant of* ECG)
EMD electromechanical delay
EMT emergency medical technician
EPO erythropoietin
ERV expiratory reserve volume

F

FEV$_1$ forced expiratory volume in one second
FEV$_1$/FVC forced expiratory volume in one second/forced vital capacity
fMRI functional magnetic resonance imaging
FRC functional residual capacity

FSH follicle-stimulating hormone
FT fibers fast-twitch fibers

G

GERD gastroesophageal reflux disease
GFR glomerular filtration rate
GH growth hormone
GI gastrointestinal
GnRH gonadotropin-releasing hormone

H

H$_2$O water
HbA1c glycosylated hemoglobin (test)
hCG human chorionic gonadotropin
HDL high-density lipoprotein
HIV human immunodeficiency virus
HPV human papillomavirus
HR heart rate
HSV-1 herpes simplex virus type 1
HSV-2 herpes simplex virus type 2

I

IRV inspiratory reserve volume
IV intravenous
IVF in vitro fertilization

L

L/min liters per minute
LBP low back pain
LDL low-density lipoprotein
LH luteinizing hormone

M

MAC membrane attack complex
MALT mucosa-associated lymphatic tissue
MAP mean arterial pressure
MD medical doctor; muscular dystrophy
mg/DL milligrams per deciliter
MHC major histocompatibility complex glycoproteins
mL/beat milliliters per beat
mmHG millimeters of mercury
MRA magnetic resonance angiography
MRI magnetic resonance imaging
mRNA messenger RNA (ribonucleic acid)
MS multiple sclerosis

N

NCV nerve conduction velocity
NK cells natural killer cells

O

O$_2$ oxygen
OD optometry degree

P

PA physician assistant
PACs premature atrial contractions
PCOS polycystic ovarian syndrome
PCT proximal convoluted tubule
PD Parkinson's disease
PET positron emission tomography
pH acid-base balance
PID pelvic inflammatory disease
PNS peripheral nervous system
PRO prolactin
PSA test prostate-specific antigen test
PTH parathyroid hormone
PVCs premature ventricular contractions
PVD peripheral vascular disease

Q

Q cardiac output

R

RBC red blood cell
RNA ribonucleic acid
rRNA ribosomal RNA (ribonucleic acid)
RT respiratory therapist
RV pulmonary ventilation residual volume

S

SA sinoatrial (node)
SCID severe combined immune deficiency
SNS sympathetic nervous system
ST fibers slow-twitch fibers
STD sexually transmitted disease
SV stroke volume

T

T$_3$ triiodothyronine
T$_4$ thyroxine
TB tuberculosis
TBI traumatic brain injury
TIA transient ischemic attack
TLC total lung capacity
tRNA transfer RNA (ribonucleic acid)
TSH thyroid-stimulating hormone
TV tidal volume

U

UTI urinary tract infection
UVB ultraviolet B

V

VC vital capacity

W

WBC white blood cell

Photo Credits

All anatomical drawings in this textbook were created by © Body Scientific International.

Figure 2.0 Custom Medical Stock Photo

Figure 2.24 Carolina Biological Supply Company

Figure 2.25 Don W. Fawcett/Science Source

Figure 2.28 Educational Images

Figure 2.29 Science Photo Library

Figure 2.30 Educational Images

Figure 2.31 Custom Medical Stock Photo

Figure 2.32 Custom Medical Stock Photo

Figure 2.33 Manfred Kage/Science Source

Figure 2.34 Science Photo Library

Figure 2.35 Manfred Kage/Science Source

Figure 3.17 Science Photo Library

Figure 4.1 Susumu Nishinaga/Science Photo Library

Figure 4.6 Science Photo Library

Figure 4.33A Science Photo Library

Figure 4.33B Dr. Tony Brain/Science Photo Library

Chapter 4, page 153 NASA/JSC

Figure 5.26A Muscular Dystrophy Association

Figure 5.26B Patrick Landmann/Photo Researchers, Incc

Figure 6.8 Courtesy of Dr. Bill Farquhar

Figure 6.11 Needell MD

Figure 8.0 Phanie / Science Source

Figure 8.12 © RICK WILKING/Reuters/Corbis

Figure 8.13 Biophoto Associates/Photo Researchers, Inc

Figure 8.14 Biophoto Associates/Photo Researchers, Inc

Figure 9.15 SIU BIOMED COMM

Figure 10.19 SPL/Science Source

Figure 11.5 Matt Meadows/Science Source

Figure 11.11 © Brownie Harris/Corbis

Figure 11.29A Biophoto Associates/Photo Researchers, Inc

Figure 11.29B Biophoto Associates/Photo Researchers, Inc

Figure 11.34 Carolyn A. McKeone/Science Source

Figure 12.11 Laurent/Science Source

Figure 12.19 Science Photo Library

Figure 13.22 © Wellcome Image Library/Custom Medical Stock Photo

Figure 13.24 Photo by Scott Bauer

Figure 14.18 Erica Berger for the National Kidney Foundation

Figure 15.18 Gilles Podevins/Science Photo Library/Corbis

Figure 15.20 Russell Kightley Media.

Chapter 15, page 571 Steve Gschmeissner / Science Photo Library / Corbis

Glossary

A

ABCD rule a system for self-determining the presence of melanoma; stands for *Asymmetry, Border irregularity, Color,* and *Diameter*

abdominal aorta term for the left aorta when it reaches the abdomen

abdominal cavity space bounded by the abdominal walls, the diaphragm, and the pelvis

abdominopelvic cavity (ab-DAHM-i-noh-PEHL-vik) continuous internal opening that includes the abdominal and pelvic cavities

abduction movement of a body segment away from the body in the frontal plane

abnormal contractility condition an abnormal heartbeat; *arrhythmia*

absorption the movement of food molecules from the small intestine into the blood

acceleration the change in velocity of the object to which a force is applied

accessory reproductive organs glands and structures other than the ovaries and testes, which are needed for reproduction, such as the prostate gland and vestibular glands

accommodation the process through which contraction of the muscles of the ciliary body makes the lens thicker

acetabulum (as-eh-TAB-yoo-lum) deep socket within each coxal bone that receives the head of the femur to form the hip joint

acetylcholine (a-SEE-til-KOH-leen) a neurotransmitter

acid substance that, when added to water, increases its hydrogen ion concentration

acquired immune deficiency syndrome (AIDS) a disease in which the immune system is greatly weakened due to infection with HIV, making a person more susceptible to rare cancers and opportunistic infections

acromegaly (ak-roh-MEG-a-lee) a rare condition in which the anterior pituitary hypersecretes growth hormone, causing an increase in overall body size; *gigantism*

acromioclavicular joint (a-KROH-mee-oh-kla-VIK-yoo-lar) joint between the acromion process of the scapula and the clavicle

acromion (a-KROH-mee-ahn) bone projection on the top lateral side of each scapula

acrosomal enzymes (AK-roh-sohm-al) enzymes contained in the tip of a sperm's head that allow it to digest the protective glycoproteins surrounding an oocyte

actin a common protein that is the building block for microfilaments and for thin filaments in muscle cells

action potential the electric charge produced in nerve or muscle fiber by stimulation

active immunity immunity in which the blood plasma cells in the body make antibodies as a result of previous exposure to a disease or a vaccine

active process a process that requires the use of muscles

active transport type of membrane transport that requires energy

acute the term used to describe an injury caused by a single force

acute bronchitis a temporary inflammation of the mucous membranes that line the trachea and bronchial passageways; causes a cough that may produce mucus

acute lymphocytic leukemia (ALL) the most common form of leukemia in adults over 70 years of age; characterized by overproduction of lymphocytes

acute myeloid leukemia (AML) the most common form of leukemia in adults; develops when the bone marrow produces too many myeloblasts

adaptive immune system see *immune system*

Addison's disease a condition caused by hyposecretion of adrenal corticoid hormones that causes muscle atrophy, a bronze skin tone, low blood pressure, kidney damage, hypoglycemia, severe loss of fluids and electrolytes, and a general feeling of weakness

adduction movement of a body segment closer to the body in the frontal plane

adenoid see *pharyngeal tonsil*

adenosine triphosphate see *ATP*

adipocyte (AD-i-poh-sight) a fat cell

adipose tissue a type of tissue that is almost entirely fat cells

adrenal cortex outer layer of the adrenal glands, which itself has three layers that secrete steroid hormones

adrenal glands a pair of glands that sits on top of the kidneys; consists of the adrenal cortex and adrenal medulla

adrenaline a hormone that is secreted by the adrenal medulla and is involved in the body's fight-or-flight response; *epinephrine*

adrenal medulla the part of the adrenal glands that functions as a part of the nervous system; it secretes the hormones epinephrine and norepinephrine (catecholamines) during the fight-or-flight response

adrenocorticotropin (ACTH) (a-DREE-noh-KOR-ti-koh-TROH-pin) a tropic hormone secreted by the anterior pituitary that acts on the adrenal cortex to stimulate the release of glucocorticoid hormones like cortisol

adult onset diabetes see *type II diabetes mellitus*

afferent lymphatic vessel vessel that carries lymph into a lymph node

afferent nerves sensory transmitters that send impulses from receptors in the skin, muscles, and joints to the central nervous system

afferent pathway the route on which informational messages travel from a receptor to a control center

agglutination (ah-GLOO-ti-NAY-shun) the process by which red blood cells clump together, usually in response to an antibody; can block small blood vessels and cause hemolysis

agonist (AG-un-ist) role played by a skeletal muscle to cause a movement

agranulocytes (ay-GRAN-yoo-loh-SIGHTS) white blood cells whose cytoplasm lacks granules

albinism (AL-bi-nizm) an inherited condition that prevents the normal production of melanin

aldosterone (al-DAHS-ter-ohn) a steroid hormone produced in the adrenal cortex that regulates salt and water balance in the body by stimulating the kidneys to absorb sodium and water from urine and eliminate potassium

alimentary canal (al-i-MEHN-ter-ee) the passage leading from the mouth to the anus through the pharynx, esophagus, stomach, and intestine; *gastrointestinal tract*

allergen antigen that causes an inappropriately strong immune system response

allergy an inappropriately strong response (hypersensitivity) of the immune system to an environmental antigen that it has previously encountered

all-or-none law the rule stating that the fibers in a given motor unit always develop maximum tension when stimulated

alpha cells cells in the islets of Langerhans that secrete glucagon

alpha interferons (IN-ter-FAIR-ahns) interferons produced by virus-infected leukocytes

alternative pathway one of the two primary ways in which the complement system can be activated; this pathway is triggered when the C3b complement protein binds to foreign material. Compare *classical pathway*

alveolar capillary membrane (al-VEE-oh-lar) gas-exchange structure that contains the alveoli and the capillaries surrounding the alveoli

alveolar ducts (al-VEE-oh-lar) ducts that connect the bronchioles to the alveoli

alveoli (al-VEE-oh-ligh) air sacs in the lungs from which gas is exchanged with the capillaries

Alzheimer's disease condition involving a progressive loss of brain function with major consequences for memory, thinking, and behavior

amblyopia (AM-blee-OH-pee-a) the condition caused when one eye is the extremely dominant eye and the other becomes weak; *lazy eye*

amenorrhea (ay-MEN-oh-REE-a) absence of a menstrual period in women of reproductive age

amino-acid hormones hormones composed of proteins or protein-related substances

amino acids the building blocks of proteins

amnion (AM-nee-ahn) a membrane that forms a closed sac around the embryo and fetus

amniotic fluid (am-nee-AHT-ik) a clear fluid in which the embryo, and then the fetus, is suspended

amphiarthrosis (AM-fee-ar-THROH-sis) joint type that permits only slight motion

amusia a condition characterized by the inability to distinguish differences in pitch

anabolism the process through which complex molecules are constructed from simple ones

anaphylaxis (AN-a-fi-LAK-sis) a severe and potentially life-threatening allergic reaction that may include airway obstruction and very low blood pressure

anatomical position erect standing position with arms at the sides and palms facing forward

anatomy the study of the form or structure of living things, including plants, animals, and humans

androgen the male sex hormone that controls the development and maintenance of masculine characteristics

anemia a condition characterized by a decrease in the number of red blood cells or an insufficient amount of hemoglobin in the red blood cells

aneurysm (AN-yoo-rizm) abnormal ballooning of a blood vessel, usually an artery, due to a weakness in the wall of the vessel

angina pectoris (AN-ji-na) condition characterized by severe, constricting pain or sensation of pressure in the chest, often radiating to the left arm caused by an insufficient supply of blood to the heart

angiotensin (an-jee-oh-TEHN-sin) a polypeptide hormone in the blood that constricts blood vessels and increases blood pressure

angiotensin-converting enzyme an enzyme in the lungs that converts angiotensin I to angiotensin II

anorexia nervosa condition characterized by body weight 15% or more below the minimal normal weight range, extreme fear of gaining weight, an unrealistic body image, and amenorrhea

antagonist (an-TAG-un-ist) role played by a skeletal muscle acting to slow or stop a movement

anterior (ventral) body cavity continuous internal opening that includes the thoracic and abdominopelvic cavities

anterior pituitary one lobe of the pituitary gland that secretes six different hormones: growth hormone, prolactin, adrenocorticotropin hormone, thyroid stimulating hormone, follicle-stimulating hormone, and luteinizing hormone

antibody cells that circulate in plasma and attack red blood cells with foreign antigens, or antigens that are different from those of the host

antibody-mediated immunity see *humoral immunity*

anticodon a set of three bases on tRNA that are complementary to a 3-base codon on mRNA

antidiuretic hormone (ADH) (AN-tee-digh-yoo-REHT-ik) a hormone produced by the hypothalamus and stored in the posterior pituitary that decreases urine output by increasing water reabsorption by the kidneys, which increases body fluid volume; also causes blood vessels to constrict and raises blood pressure; *vasopressin*

antigen (AN-ti-jehn) a molecule on the surface of cells that identifies cells as either "self" or "nonself" (foreign) cells, and which triggers production of antibodies to attack any foreign cells; a protein on the surface of RBCs that is used to identify blood type

antigen-antibody complex antigen combined with a specific antibody

antigenic determinants the distinctive parts of a complex molecule that can be recognized by the immune system

antigen-presenting cells (APCs) cells that process protein antigens and present them on their surface in a form that can be recognized by lymphocytes (white blood cells)

antihistamines (AN-tee-HIS-ta-meenz) medications that work to curb the activity of histamines

anus the lower opening of the gastrointestinal tract

anvil tiny bone within the middle ear that transmits sound from the hammer to the stirrup

aorta a large arterial trunk that arises from the base of the left ventricle and channels blood from the heart into other arteries throughout the body

aortic arch (ay-OR-tik) the curved portion of the aorta between the ascending and descending parts of the aorta

aortic valve (ay-OR-tik) the semilunar valve between the left ventricle and the aorta that prevents blood from flowing back into the left ventricle

apex the pointed end of the heart that lies approximately at the fifth rib and points down toward the left hip

apical (AY-pi-kal) toward the apex; when used to describe an epithelium, it refers to the surface that faces the outside world

aplastic anemia a rare but serious condition in which the bone marrow is incapable of making new red blood cells

apocrine glands (AP-oh-krin) glands that secrete a milky fluid consisting of sweat, fatty acids, and proteins

aponeurosis (AP-oh-noo-ROH-sis) a flat, sheetlike fibrous tissue that connects muscle or bone to other tissues

apophysis (a-PAHF-i-sis) site at which a tendon attaches to bone

apoptosis (AP-ahp-TOH-sis) a programmed process of cellular self-destruction (cell suicide)

appendicular skeleton the bones of the body's appendages; the arms and legs

appendix a small, closed-end extension of the large intestine near the junction of the large and small intestines

aquaporin (ah-kwah-POR-in) a protein in the cell membrane that acts as a channel for water to enter or exit the cell

aqueous and vitreous humors (AY-kwee-us and VIT-ree-us) the watery fluid that fills the anterior and posterior chambers of the eye

arachnoid mater the middle membrane of the brain, which is composed of web-like tissue

areola (a-REE-oh-la) a circular area of pigmented skin that surrounds the protruding nipple

areolar connective tissue a type of tissue that is found throughout the body, typically as a layer under epithelial tissues

arrector pili (ah-REHK-tor PIGH-ligh) tiny muscles that connect either side of a hair follicle to the epidermis

arrhythmia (ay-RITH-mee-a) an irregular heartbeat or rhythm

arteries vessels that carry blood away from the heart

arterioles (ar-TAIR-ee-ohls) microscopic arteries that connect with capillaries

arthritis family of more than 100 common pathologies associated with aging, characterized by joint inflammation accompanied by pain, stiffness, and sometimes swelling

articular cartilage (ar-TIK-yoo-lar) dense, white, connective tissue that covers the articulating surfaces of bones at joints

articular fibrocartilage (ar-TIK-yoo-lar FIGH-broh-KAR-ti-lij) tissue shaped like a disc or partial disc called a meniscus that provides cushioning at a joint

ascending colon the segment of the colon that extends upward from the cecum to the bend on the right side below the liver

ascending limb the final part of the nephron loop through which filtrate flows; is made mostly or entirely of a thick-walled segment

asexual reproduction reproduction that involves only one cell rather than the fusion of two gametes

association cortex the most anterior portion of the frontal lobe, which is believed to be responsible for intellect

asthma (AZ-ma) disease of the lungs characterized by recurring episodes of airway inflammation causing bronchospasms and increased mucus production

astigmatism (a-STIG-ma-tizm) a common eye disorder caused by an irregular curvature of the cornea or lens that results in blurred vision

astrocytes (AS-troh-sights) glial cells that are positioned between neurons and capillaries to transmit nutrients and control the chemical environment

atherosclerosis (ATH-er-oh-skler-OH-sis) hardening of the arteries

atlas the first cervical vertebra; specialized to provide the connection between the occipital bone of the skull and the spinal column

atoms tiny particles of matter

ATP (a-DEHN-oh-seen trigh-FAHS-fayt) a nucleotide composed of an adenine base, a sugar, and three phosphate groups; *adenosine triphosphate*

ATP synthase an enzyme present in large numbers in the inner cell membrane which makes ATP

atrial fibrillation condition in which the atria contract in an uncoordinated, rapid manner (rate above 350 bpm), causing the ventricles to contract irregularly

atrial natriuretic peptide (ANP) (NA-tree-yoo-REHT-ik) a peptide hormone secreted by the atria of the heart that promotes excretion of sodium and water and lowers blood pressure

atrioventricular node (AV node) (AY-tree-oh-vehn-TRIK-yoo-lar) a small mass of tissue that transmits impulses received from the sinoatrial node to the ventricles via the bundle of His

atrioventricular (AV) valves the two valves (tricuspid and mitral) situated between the atria and the ventricles

atrophy decrease in bone mineral density and strength

auditory canal a short, tubelike structure that connects the outer ear to the eardrum

auricle (AW-ri-kuhl) the irregularly shaped outer portion of the ear

auscultation (AWS-kul-TAY-shun) the act of listening to internal sounds of the body using a stethoscope

autoimmune disorder a condition in which the immune system attacks the body's own tissue

autonomic nervous system branch of the nervous system that controls involuntary body functions

autonomic reflexes involuntary stimuli transmitted to cardiac and smooth muscle

axial skeleton central, stable portion of the skeletal system, consisting of the skull, spinal column, and thoracic cage

axis the second cervical vertebra; specialized with an upward projection called the odontoid process, on which the atlas rotates

axon a long, thin fiber connected to the motor neuron cell body

axon terminals offshoots of the axon that branch out to connect with individual muscle fibers

B

B cells see *B lymphocytes*

B lymphocytes lymphocytes that mature in the bone marrow before moving out to the blood and the rest of the body; *B cells*

ball-and-socket joint synovial joint formed between one bone end shaped roughly like a ball and the receiving bone reciprocally shaped like a socket

balloon angioplasty a surgical procedure to open the blocked vessel resulting from a heart attack

baroreceptors (BAIR-oh-ree-SEP-ters) pressure sensitive nerve endings in the atrium, aortic arch, and carotid arteries

basal toward the base; when used to describe an epithelium, it refers to the surface that faces the inside of the body

basal cell carcinoma (KAR-si-NOH-ma) the most common form of skin cancer and the least malignant type

basal metabolic rate the amount of energy required to sustain a person's metabolism for one day if he or she is at complete rest; *BMR*

basal nuclei small regions of gray matter interspersed within the brain's white matter

base (1) the nitrogen-containing part of a nucleotide; (2) the broad end of the heart, which is positioned closer to the neck, at the second rib; (3) the broad end of the lung, which rests on the diaphragm

base pairs pairs of complementary nucleic acid bases; that is, A and T or C and G

bedsores see *decubitus ulcers*

bending a loading pattern created by a combination of off-center forces

benign (bi-NIGHN) term for conditions that involve non-metastasized tumors

beta cells cells in the islets of Langerhans that secrete insulin

beta interferons (IN-ter-FAIR-ahns) interferons produced by virus-infected fibroblasts

bicarbonate an alkaline molecule that neutralizes acidic chyme

bicuspid valve (bigh-KUS-pid) the mitral valve, which has two cusps and is located on the right side of the heart

bile an alkaline fluid made in the liver and secreted into the duodenum; aids especially in the emulsification and absorption of fats

bile canaliculi (kan-a-LIK-yoo-ligh) small ducts in the liver that collect bile

bile salts substances found in bile that aid fat absorption; derived from cholesterol

biochemistry the detailed study of the molecules of life, how they are made, and how they are broken down

bipolar neurons nerve cells that have one axon and one dendrite

birth canal see *vagina*

bitter one of the five basic tastes

bladder a muscular sac in the pelvic cavity where urine from the kidneys is stored before it is excreted

bladder neck location at which the urethra connects to the bladder

blastocyst (BLAS-toh-sist) a fluid-filled cavity

blind spot a tiny area where the optic nerve joins the retina and where there are no rods and cones

blood-brain barrier protective mechanism in the tiny blood vessels supplying the brain that prevents invasion of the brain by many potentially harmful substances

blood glucose test a test for the presence of glucose in the body; a result of 126 mg/dL or higher after an eight-hour fast is considered positive for diabetes

blood pressure cuff device used to measure blood pressure; *sphygmomanometer*

blood vessel capillaries the tiniest blood vessels in the body; they connect the smallest arteries to the smallest veins

bone marrow material with a rich blood supply found within the marrow cavity of long bones; yellow marrow stores fat, and red marrow is active in producing blood cells

bony labyrinth winding tunnels located in the inner ear

brachial artery (BRAY-kee-al) the artery located at the fold of the elbow where the brachial pulse is detected

bradycardia (BRAD-ee-KAHR-dee-a) a normal heart rhythm but with a rate below 60 bpm; a condition common among athletes

breech presentation a position of the fetus in which the buttocks or legs exit the mother's body first, making delivery more difficult

Broca's area a portion of the left frontal lobe that controls the tongue and lip movements required for speech

bronchioles (BRAHNG-kee-ohls) the thin-walled branches of the bronchi; the smallest air-conducting passageways of the bronchi. The terminal bronchioles conduct a small amount of gas exchange in the respiratory zone

bronchospasms (BRAHNG-koh-spazmz) spasmodic contractions of the bronchial muscles that constrict the airways in the lungs during an asthma attack

brush border collective term for the microvilli on the epithelial cells of the small intestine

buffy coat a thin layer of white blood cells and platelets that lies between the red blood cells and plasma in a blood sample that has gone through a centrifuge

bulbourethral glands (BUL-boh-yoo-REE-thral) two small glands at the base of the penis that secrete mucus into the urethra

bulimia nervosa disordered eating that involves a minimum of two eating binges a week for at least three months; an associated feeling of lack of control; use of self-induced vomiting, laxatives, diuretics, strict dieting, or exercise to prevent weight gain; and an obsession with body image

bundle of His a slender bundle of modified cardiac muscle that conducts electrical impulses from the AV node to the left and right bundle branches to Purkinje fibers in the ventricle

burning mouth syndrome a condition that involves a sensation of moderate to severe burning in the mouth that may continue for months or even years

bursae (BER-see) small capsules lined with synovial membranes and filled with synovial fluid; they cushion the structures they separate

bursitis (ber-SIGHT-is) inflammation of one or more bursae

C

calcaneus (kal-KAY-nee-us) the heel bone

calcitonin (kal-si-TOH-nin) hormone secreted by the thyroid gland that works with parathyroid hormone to maintain calcium homeostasis

Calorie the unit that food scientists use to measure the potential energy in foods; the amount of heat required to raise the temperature of 1 kilogram of water by 1°C; *kilocalorie*

canaliculi (kan-a-LIK-yoo-ligh) tiny canals that connect central Haversian canals with cavities called lacunae

cancer the uncontrolled division and growth of abnormal cells

capacitation (ka-pas-i-TAY-shun) the process by which sperm becomes able to fertilize an oocyte

capillaries small, thin-walled vessels where oxygen and carbon dioxide gas exchange occurs between the capillaries and the tissues

capillary beds network of intertwined vessels formed by multiple capillaries

carbaminohemoglobin (kar-BAM-i-noh-HEE-moh-GLOH-bin) molecule that is created when CO_2 attaches to a globin part of the hemoglobin molecule

carbohydrate sugar and starch molecules; *saccharides*

cardiac muscle the major tissue of the heart

cardiac output the amount of blood pumped from the heart per minute

cardiomyopathy (KAHR-dee-oh-migh-AHP-a-thee) heart failure caused by infection and weakening of the myocardium, or heart muscle

cardiopulmonary system the collective name for the respiratory and cardiovascular systems; these systems work together to conduct gas exchange

cardiovascular physiology the study of how the heart functions or works internally

cardioversion (KAHR-dee-oh-VER-zhun) restoration of the heart's rhythm to normal by electrical countershock or by medications

carotid artery the artery located on the side of the neck where the carotid pulse is felt

carpal bones (KAR-pal) bones of the wrist

cartilage a connective tissue that provides support and flexibility to parts of the skeleton

catabolism the process through which complex molecules are broken down into simple ones

cataracts (KAT-uh-rakts) the term used to describe a progressive clouding of the lens of the eye

cavities open chambers inside the human body

cecum (SEE-kum) pouch at the beginning of the large intestine, in between the ileum and the colon

cell body part of an axon that contains a nucleus

cell-mediated immunity see *cellular immunity*

cells the smallest living building blocks of all organisms

cellular immunity immunity that arises from the activation of T lymphocytes (T cells) by antigen-presenting cells; *cell-mediated immunity*

cellulitis (SEHL-yoo-LIGH-tis) a bacterial infection characterized by an inflamed area of skin that is red, swollen, and painful

central chemoreceptors (KEE-moh-ree-SEHP-tor) chemical receptor cells that monitor changes in the pH of the cerebrospinal fluid in an effort to regulate carbon dioxide levels and respiration

central nervous system (CNS) the brain and spinal cord

centrioles (SEHN-tree-ohlz) short cylinders made of nine triplets of parallel microtubules

centromere (SEHN-troh-meer) the point or region on a chromosome that divides the chromosome into two arms and functions as the point of attachment for the sister chromatids; provides movement during cell division

centrosome (SEHN-troh-sohm) an area of the cell near the nucleus

cerebellum (SER-eh-BEHL-um) section of the brain that coordinates body movements, including balance

cerebral cortex (seh-REE-bral) the outer surface of the cerebrum

cerebral hemisphere (seh-REE-bral) term used to describe one-half of the brain; collectively, the two hemispheres make up the cerebrum

cerebral palsy (seh-REE-bral) a group of nervous system disorders resulting from brain damage before or during birth, or in early infancy

cerebrum (seh-REE-brum) the largest part of the brain, consisting of the left and right hemispheres

cerumen (se-ROO-men) the soft, brownish yellow, waxy secretion of the ceruminous glands; *earwax*

ceruminous glands (seh-ROO-mi-nus) secretors of cerumen, or earwax; located in the auditory canal

cervical region (SER-vi-kal) the first 7 vertebrae, comprising the neck

cervix (SER-viks) the narrow, lower end of the uterus that has the opening through which a baby passes during childbirth

channel proteins molecules with a hollow central pore that allows water or small, charged particles of certain substances to pass into or out of the cells

chelation therapy a procedure in which excess metals, such as iron, are removed from the blood

chemical breakdown the breakdown of large food molecules into smaller molecules by enzymes; *digestion*

chest pain angina pectoris

chickenpox a highly contagious, common childhood disease that is characterized by extremely itchy, fluid-filled blisters; *herpes varicella*

chlamydia (kla-MID-ee-a) a sexually transmitted disease that often causes no symptoms, but can damage the female reproductive tract and lead to infertility and increased risk of ectopic pregnancy

cholecystectomy (KOH-leh-sis-TEHK-toh-mee) surgical removal of the gall bladder

chondroblasts (KAHN-droh-blasts) cells that secrete the extracellular matrix of cartilage

chordae tendineae (KOR-dee TEHN-di-nee) thin, fibrous cords, connected to the papillary muscle and the leaflets of the AV valves

chorion the layer of the fetal sac that surrounds the amnion

choroid (KOR-oyd) the middle layer of the eye

chromatids (KROH-ma-tids) paired strands of a duplicated chromosome that become visible during cell division and that are joined by a centromere

chromosomes rod-shaped structures in the nuclei of our body cells that contain individual DNA and genes

chronic bronchitis a long-lasting condition in which the airways of the lungs become obstructed due to inflammation of the bronchi and excessive mucus production

chronic kidney disease a condition defined by evidence of kidney damage or a GFR less than 60 milliliters per minute for at least three months

chronic lymphocytic leukemia (CLL) a form of leukemia characterized by extremely high levels of lymphocytes; most often found in middle-age adults

chronic myeloid leukemia (CML) a form of leukemia characterized by overproduction of granulocytes

chronic obstructive pulmonary disease (COPD) any lung disorder characterized by a long-term airway obstruction, making it difficult to breathe

chyme (kighm) the mixture of food and digestive juice in the stomach and duodenum

cilia (SIL-ee-a) a hair-like projection that actively flexes back and forth to move fluid or mucus across the outside of a cell

ciliary body (SIL-ee-AIR-ee) the structure between the choroid and the iris that anchors the lens in place

ciliary glands (SIL-ee-AIR-ee) modified sweat glands located between the eyelashes

circulatory system the cardiovascular system, which consists of a strong, muscular pump (the heart), an extensive network of pipes (blood vessels), and fluid (blood)

circumduction (SER-kum-DUK-shun) rotational movement of a body segment such that the end of the segment traces a circle

cistern (cisternae) (sis-TER-nee) a flattened, sheet-like chamber in the endoplasmic reticulum

cisterna chyli (sis-TER-na KIGH-ligh) chamber through which lymph flows, situated just in front of the vertebral column in the lumbar (lower back) region

citric acid cycle a reaction that breaks down pyruvate molecules into carbon atoms

class I MHC proteins major histocompatibility complex proteins that are found on the surfaces of all cells that contain nuclei

class II MHC proteins major histocompatibility complex proteins that are found only on the surfaces of certain immune system cells

classical pathway a mode of complement system activation in which a circulating complement protein recognizes an antibody bound to foreign material. Compare *alternative pathway*

clavicle doubly curved long bone that forms part of the shoulder girdle; the *collarbone*

cleft palate a condition that occurs when the parts of the palate do not completely fuse together during a fetus' development in the womb

clitoris (KLIT-or-is) a cylindrical body of erectile tissue that lies at the anterior end of the vulva

clonal selection repeated division of a lymphocyte that produces many exact genetic copies (clones) of itself

clone cell or organism that is a genetic copy of an original cell or organism

coagulation (KOH-ah-yoo-LAY-shun) the process by which the enzyme thrombin and the protein fibrinogen combine to form fibrin, a fiber that weaves around the platelet plug to form a blood clot; takes between 2 and 15 minutes to complete

coccyx (KAHK-siks) 4 fused vertebrae at the base of the spine forming the tailbone

cochlea (KAHK-lee-a) a snail-shaped structure in the inner ear that enables one to hear

cochlear duct (KAHK-lee-ar) the portion of the membranous labyrinth inside the cochlea

codon (KOH-dahn) a set of three bases in DNA or RNA that codes for one amino acid

coenzymes (koh-EHN-zighmz) molecules that are necessary for the action of enzymes

collagen a protein found in skin that provides toughness and binds with water molecules to keep the inner skin moist

collagen fibers fibers of the cytoskeleton that are strong and resistant to stretching

collecting duct a tube that collects urine from several nephrons and carries it to the renal pelvis; urine can become much more concentrated as it flows through the collecting duct

collecting vessels a collection of lymphatic capillaries

colon longest segment of the large intestine

color blindness an inherited condition that affects the cone cells on the retina and impairs the ability to distinguish colors

columnar epithelia tall and skinny epithelia

combined loading the simultaneous action of two or more types of forces

common warts warts that typically appear on the hands or fingers and disappear without treatment

complement proteins proteins in the blood that work with immune system cells and antibodies to defend the body against infection

complement system a system of more than 30 proteins that circulate in the blood plasma through the body and work together to destroy foreign substances; complements, or balances out, the specific and nonspecific defense systems of the body

complex carbohydrate a long chain of simple sugars joined together

compression a squeezing force that creates compression in the structure to which it is applied

compressive strength the ability of a material to withstand compression (inward-pressing force) without buckling

concentric (kun-SEHN-trik) a type of contraction that causes shortening of a muscle

conchae (KAHN-kee) three uneven, scroll-like nasal bones that extend down through the nasal cavity; these bones are divided into the superior, middle, and inferior conchae

conducting zone the zone from the mouth or nose to the terminal bronchioles

conduction the process of conveying or transmitting types of energy, such as electrical impulses

conductivity the ability of a neuron to transmit a nerve impulse

condyloid joint (KAHN-di-loyd) type of diarthrosis in which one articulating bone surface is an oval, convex shape, and the other is a reciprocally shaped concave surface

cones sensory cells in the retina that are sensitive to bright light and provide color vision

conjunctiva (KAHN-junk-TIGH-va) a delicate external membrane that covers the exposed eyeball and lines the eyelid

conjunctivitis (kahn-JUNK-ti-VIGH-tis) a highly contagious inflammation of the conjunctiva; *pink eye*

connective tissue supporting tissue, which consists mainly of an extracellular matrix

connective tissue proper a classification of tissue that includes loose and dense subtypes

constipation condition characterized by difficulty in defecating

contractility the ability to contract or shorten

control center system that receives and analyzes information from sensory receptors, then sends a command stimulus to an effector to maintain homeostasis

contusion the bruises or bleeding within a muscle that result from an impact

convolutions the term used to describe the pattern of gyri and the sulci that appear on the outer surface of the brain

Cooley's anemia a condition that affects the body's ability to produce fully developed hemoglobin and red blood cells; *thalassemia major*

coracoid process (KOR-a-koyd) bony projection on the posterior side of the scapula that serves as a site of muscle attachments

cornea a transparent tissue over the anterior center of the eye

coronary artery disease a narrowing of one or more of the coronary arteries due to a buildup of plaque in the artery; *coronary heart disease*

coronary heart disease see *coronary artery disease*

coronary sinus large venous channel between the left atrium and left ventricle, on the posterior side of the heart that empties into the right atrium at the junction of the four chambers

corpora cavernosa (singular corpus cavernosum) one type of erectile tissue

corpus spongiosum (spun-jee-OH-sum) one type of erectile tissue

cortex outer portion of an organ, for example the outer portion of a lymph node

cortical bone (KOR-ti-kal) dense, solid bone that covers the outer surface of all bones and is the main form of bone tissue in the long bones

cortical nephrons nephrons with short nephron loops that penetrate only slightly into the renal medulla

corticoid hormones hormones of the adrenal cortex

cortisol (KORT-i-sahl) the principal glucocorticoid hormone produced by the adrenal cortex that maintains blood glucose levels by converting fats and amino acids into glucose

cortisone (KOR-ti-sohn) a glucocorticoid hormone produced by the adrenal cortex that is converted into cortisol

coxal bone (KAHK-sal) the hip bone, formed from the fusion of the ilium, ischium, and pubis

cranial cavity opening inside the skull that holds the brain

cranial nerves 12 pairs of nerves that originate in the brain and relay impulses to and from the PNS

craniosacral division (KRAY-nee-oh-SAY-kral) the parasympathetic nervous system, in which nerves originate in the brain stem or sacral region of the spinal cord

cranium fused, flat bones surrounding the back of the head

creatinine (kree-AT-in-een) a normal by-product of muscle metabolism; it is produced by the body at a fairly steady rate and is freely filtered by the glomerulus

Crohn's disease a chronic, inflammatory bowel disease that usually affects the small intestine or colon

cross bridges connections between the heads of myosin filaments and receptor sites on the actin filaments

crossovers connections that form between homologous chromosomes during meiosis, resulting in the swapping of portions of chromosomes

cuboidal epithelia (kyoo-BOYD-al) epithelia whose height is about equal to its width

Cushing's syndrome a disorder of the adrenal cortex caused by hypersecretion of cortisol; symptoms include weight gain, high blood glucose levels, hypertension, and osteoporosis

cutaneous membrane (kyoo-TAY-nee-us) another name for skin

cutaneous sensory receptors specialized receptors that are contained in the skin and are part of the nervous system

cystitis (sis-TIGH-tis) an inflammation of the urinary bladder wall

cytoplasm (SIGH-toh-plazm) the part of a cell that contains everything inside the cell membrane except the nucleus

cytoskeleton a network of proteins that defines the shape of a cell and gives it mechanical strength

cytotoxic T cell T lymphocyte that destroys foreign or virus-infected or cancerous cells; *killer T cell*

D

data systematically collected and recorded observations

deafness the term applied to any loss of hearing, ranging from a slight to a complete inability to hear

debridement the removal of dead tissue using a surgical or chemical procedure

decidua capsularis (di-SIJ-oo-a kap-se-LAR-is) the outermost membrane of the fetal sac

decubitus ulcers (deh-KYOO-bi-tus) skin injuries caused by pressure or shear forces that restrict blood flow to one or more areas of the body; *bedsores*

defecation the discharge of feces from the rectum

defibrillate to stop the heart

defibrillator a device that can deliver a therapeutic dose of electrical current that momentarily stops the heart, allowing its built-in pacemaker—the SA node—to assume control and produce a normal rhythm

deformation the change in shape of the object to which a force is applied

degranulate to release a cell's (especially a mast cell's) intracellular stores of histamine, prostaglandins, and other chemicals

delayed-onset muscle soreness (DOMS) muscle pain that follows participation in a particularly long or strenuous activity, begins 24-73 hours later, and involves multiple, microscopic tears in the muscle tissue that cause inflammation, pain, swelling, and stiffness

delivery of the placenta the last stage of birth in which the placenta detaches from the uterine wall and is expelled

dementia (deh-MEHN-see-a) an organic brain disease involving loss of function in two or more areas of cognition

dendrites (DEHN-drights) branches of a neuron that collect stimuli and transport them to the cell body

dense elastic connective tissue a type of tissue whose extracellular matrix is full of elastic fibers

dentin a material similar to bone that makes up the body of the tooth

depolarize to contract; the atria and ventricles depolarize as the heart beats

depolarized a condition that occurs when the inside of a cell membrane is more positively charged than the outside

dermal papillae (pa-PIL-ee) protrusions from the surface of the dermis into the epidermis

dermis layer of skin between the epidermis and hypodermis; includes nerve endings, glands, and hair follicles

descending colon the segment of the colon that extends from the bend below the spleen to the sigmoid colon

descending limb the first part of the nephron loop through which filtrate flows; usually has a thick-walled segment and a thin-walled segment

detached retina separation of the retina from the underlying support tissue

detrusor (dee-TROO-zer) the smooth muscle that forms most of the bladder wall and aids in expelling urine

deviated septum a large shift in the position of the septum away from the center

diabetes insipidus a disorder resulting from hyposecretion of antidiuretic hormone (ADH) by the posterior pituitary

diabetes mellitus a disease that results from the body's inability to produce sufficient amounts of insulin to regulate blood glucose levels

diabetic nephropathy (neh-FRAHP-a-thee) kidney disease or damage caused by complications from diabetes

diabetic retinopathy (REHT-i-NAHP-a-thee) damage to the retina caused by long-term diabetes

dialyzer (DIGH-a-LIGH-zer) a machine that acts as an artificial kidney

diapedesis (DIGH-a-peh-DEE-sis) the passage of blood, or any of its formed elements, through the blood vessel walls into body tissues

diaphysis (digh-AF-i-sis) the shaft of a long bone

diarrhea the occurrence of frequent, watery bowel movements

diarthrosis (DIGH-ar-THROH-sis) freely movable joints; *synovial joints*

diastole (digh-AS-toh-lee)   the period of relaxation in the heart when the chambers are filling with blood

diencephalon (DIGH-ehn-SEHF-a-lahn)   area of the brain that includes the epithalamus, thalamus, metathalamus, and hypothalamus; the *interbrain*

differentiate   to divide by mitosis to form specialized daughter cells

diffusion   the movement of material from where it is concentrated to where it is less concentrated

dilation   the stage of labor during which the opening of the cervix dilates, or widens

dilator pupillae   a muscle of the iris that causes enlargement of the pupil in the presence of dim light

diploid (DIP-loyd)   a cell having two sets of chromosomes: one set from the mother and one set from the father

diplopia (di-PLOH-pee-a)   the condition that occurs when one eye is misaligned; *double vision*

dislocation   injury involving displacement of a bone from its joint socket

distal convoluted tubule   the last part of a nephron through which urine flows before reaching the collecting duct; some minerals and nutrients are reabsorbed from urine, and some waste products are secreted into urine, through this tubule

distal radioulnar joint (RAY-dee-oh-UHL-nar)   joint between the radius and ulna that is close to the wrist

diuresis (DIGH-yoo-REE-sis)   urine excretion

diuretics   chemicals that stimulate urine production to decrease fluid retention in the body

DNA   a polymer of nucleotides with the bases adenosine, guanine, cytosine, and thymine; *deoxyribonucleic acid*

dorsal ramus (DOR-sal RAY-mus)   the division of posterior spinal nerves that transmit motor impulses to the posterior trunk muscles and relay sensory impulses from the skin of the back

dorsiflexion (DOR-si-FLEHK-shun)   movement of the top of the foot toward the lower leg

downregulated   decreased

dry macular degeneration   a condition caused by progressive thinning of the retina

ductus arteriosus (ar-tair-ee-OH-sus)   a short, broad vessel in the fetus that connects the left pulmonary artery with the descending aorta, allowing most of the blood to bypass the infant's lungs

ductus deferens   the secretory duct of the testis, which extends from the epididymis and joins with the excretory duct of the seminal gland; *vas deferens*

duodenum (DOO-ah-DEH-num)   first segment of the small intestine, which is located between the pyloric valve of the stomach and the jejunum

dura mater (DOO-rah MAY-ter)   the tough, outer membrane of the brain and spinal cord

dwarfism   a condition in which the pituitary gland hypo-secretes growth hormone, resulting in an adult height of less than four feet

dynamic lung volume   lung volume measurements that also measure the rate of flow

E

eardrum   see *tympanic membrane*

earwax   see *cerumen*

eccentric (ehk-SEHN-trik)   a type of contraction that causes lengthening of a muscle

eccrine glands (EK-rin)   the major sweat glands of the body

ectopic pregnancy   the implantation and development of a fertilized egg in the pelvic cavity or uterine tube, rather than in the uterus

effector   unit that receives a command stimulus from the control center and causes an action to help maintain homeostasis

effector cells   short-lived cells that fight an infectious invader

efferent lymphatic vessel   vessel that carries lymph out of a lymph node

efferent nerves   motor transmitters that carry impulses from the central nervous system out to the muscles and glands

efferent pathway   the route on which a command stimulus travels from the control center to an effector

ejaculation   the discharge of sperm from the ejaculatory duct during the male sexual response

ejaculatory duct   the duct through which sperm is carried

elastic   a response that occurs when force is removed and the structure returns to its original size and shape

elastic cartilage   type of cartilage with many elastic fibers

elastic fibers   fibers of the cytoskeleton that can lengthen when stretched and spring back to their original length when released

elasticity   the ability of a material to spring back to its original shape after being stretched

elastic limit   the stretch point beyond which a tissue can no longer return to its original size and shape

electrical synapse   site where communication occurs between cells through direct transfer of electrical charges

electrocardiogram (ee-LEHK-troh-KAHR-dee-oh-gram)   a recording of the electrical activity of the heart; *ECG*

electrochemical event   activity involving conversion of an electrical charge into chemical messengers; an example is the transmission of nerve impulses

embryo   the developing human from the time of implantation to the end of the eighth week after conception

emphysema (EHM-fi-SEE-ma)   chronic inflammation of the lungs characterized by an abnormal increase in the air spaces near the bronchioles; causes an accumulation of carbon dioxide in the lungs

emulsification   the breakdown of large fat particles into much smaller particles, aided by bile

enamel   the substance that forms the coating of each tooth; the hardest material in the body

endocarditis (EHN-doh-kahr-DIGH-tis)   inflammation of the innermost lining of the heart, including the inner surface of the chambers and the valves

endocardium (EHN-doh-KAHR-dee-um)   the innermost layer of the heart, which lines the interior of the heart chambers and covers the valves of the heart

endocrine gland   a gland that secretes its product into the interstitial space

endolymph (EHN-doh-limf)   a thick fluid inside the membranous labyrinth

endometriosis (EHN-doh-MEE-tree-OH-sis)   an abnormal condition in which endometrial cells (cells of the uterine lining) grow outside the uterus, often producing pain and sometimes resulting in infertility

endometrium (ehn-doh-MEE-tree-um)   the mucous membrane that forms the innermost layer of the uterus

endomysium (EHN-doh-MIZ-ee-um)   a fine, protective sheath of connective tissue around a skeletal muscle fiber

endoneurium (EHN-doh-NOO-ree-um)   a delicate, connective tissue that surrounds each nerve fiber

endoplasmic reticulum   a network of membranes in the cytoplasm of a cell

endosteum (ehn-DAHS-tee-um)   tissue lining the medullary cavity

endothelial cells (EHN-doh-THEE-lee-al)   cells that form the walls of lymphatic capillaries; their overlapping structure helps fluid enter the lymphatic capillaries and makes it hard for the fluid to leave

energy   the capacity of a physical system to do work

enzymes   proteins that speed up specific biological reactions

ependymal cells (eh-PEHN-di-mal)   units that form a protective covering around the spinal cord and central cavities within the brain

epicardium (EHP-i-KAHR-dee-um)   the outermost layer of the heart and the innermost layer of the pericardial sac

epidermal dendritic cells   skin cells that initiate an immune system response to the presence of foreign bacteria or viruses

epidermis (EHP-i-DERM-is)   the outer layer of skin

epididymis (EHP-i-DID-i-mis)   a system of small ducts in the testis, in which sperm mature

epiglottis (EHP-i-GLAHT-is)   a flap of cartilaginous tissue that covers the opening to the trachea; diverts food and liquids to the esophagus during swallowing

epilepsy (EHP-i-LEHP-see)   a group of brain disorders characterized by repeated seizures over time

epimysium (EHP-i-MIZ-ee-um)   the outermost sheath of connective tissue that surrounds a skeletal muscle

epinephrine (ehp-i-NEHF-rin)   the chief neurohormone of the adrenal medulla that is used as a heart stimulant, a vasoconstrictor (which narrows the blood vessels), and a bronchodilator (which relaxes the bronchial tubes in the lungs); *adrenaline*

epineurium (EHP-i-NOO-ree-um)   the tough outer covering of a nerve

epiphyseal plate (EHP-i-FIZ-ee-al)   growth plate near the ends of long bones where osteoblast activity increases bone length

epiphysis (eh-PIF-i-seez)   the bulbous end of a long bone

epithalamus (EHP-i-THAL-a-mus)   the uppermost portion of the diencephalon, which includes the pineal gland and regulates sleep-cycle hormones

epithelia (EHP-i-THEE-lee-a)   tissues that cover the body and line cavities within the body

epithelial membranes (EHP-i-THEE-lee-al)   thin sheets of tissue lining the internal and external surfaces of the body

epithelial tissue (EHP-i-THEE-lee-al)   a class of tissue that includes epithelia and glands

erectile dysfunction   the inability to maintain an erection; *impotence*

erectile tissue   tissues that contain spaces in which blood can pool and which, during sexual arousal, become enlarged and rigid from engorgement with blood

erection   the condition of erectile tissue when filled with blood, which permits the penis to gain entry to the female reproductive tract

equilibrium   the condition of being evenly balanced

erythroblastosis fetalis (eh-RITH-roh-blas-TOH-sis fee-TAL-is)   a severe hemolytic disease of a fetus or newborn caused by the production of maternal antibodies against the fetal red blood cell antigens, usually involving Rh incompatibility between the mother and fetus

erythrocytes (e-RITH-roh-sights)   red blood cells

erythropoiesis (eh-RITH-roh-poy-EE-sis)   the process by which red blood cells are produced

erythropoietin (EPO) (eh-RITH-roh-POY-eh-tin)   a hormone secreted by the kidneys that stimulates the production of red blood cells

esophagus (eh-SAHF-a-gus)   the muscular tube that connects the pharynx and stomach

estrogen   the female sex hormone that controls the development and maintenance of female characteristics

ethmoidal sinuses (eth-MOY-dal)   cavities in the lateral masses of the ethmoid bone that are partly completed by adjoining bones and communicate with the nasal cavity

ethmoid bone (EHTH-moyd)   bone of the skull that forms part of the nasal septum

Eustachian tube (yoo-STAY-shuhn)   a channel that connects the middle ear to the nasopharynx (back of the throat) and serves to equalize pressure on either side of the tympanic membrane

eversion   movement in which the sole of the foot is rolled outward

exchange vessels   see *capillaries*

excretory ducts   the channels through which tears are released

exocrine gland   a gland that secretes its product to the outside world

exocytosis (EHK-soh-sigh-TOH-sis)   the process in which cell membranes fuse together and then push debris from the cell vesicles to the outside of the cell

exophthalmos (EK-sahf-THAL-muhs)   a condition in which the eyes bulge outward due to an overactive thyroid gland

expiration   the process by which air is expelled from the lungs; *exhalation*

expiratory reserve volume (ERV)   the additional amount of air that can be exhaled, or forced from the lungs, immediately after a normal exhalation

expulsion   the stage of labor that starts at full dilation and ends when the baby is delivered

extensibility   the ability to be stretched

extension   movement that returns a body segment to anatomical position in the sagittal plane

external acoustic meatus   see *auditory canal*

external genitalia   the reproductive structures on the outside of the body

external otitis (oh-TIGH-tis)   see *swimmer's ear*

external respiration   the process by which gas exchange occurs between the alveoli in the lungs and the pulmonary blood

external urethral orifice   the opening at the end of the urethra

external urethral sphincter   a ring of skeletal muscle that surrounds the intermediate part of the urethra where it passes through the urogenital diaphragm; this muscle is voluntarily controlled during release of urine from the body

extracellular fluid   the fluid—consisting of mostly water—that surrounds a typical cell; *interstitial fluid*

extracellular matrix   the solid or gel-like substance that surrounds a typical cell

extrinsic muscles (ek-STRIN-zik)   muscles attached to the outer surface of the eye that are responsible for changing the direction of viewing

F

facet joints (FAS-eht)   joints that connect the spinous processes of the vertebrae

facial bones bones of the face

facial nerve one of three cranial nerves that is responsible for transmitting taste sensations to the brain

false ribs three ribs that attach only by cartilage to the sternum

fascicle (FAS-i-kuhl) a bundle of muscle fibers

fast-twitch type of muscle that contracts quickly and fatigues quickly

fats substances found in foods that include oils and solid fats; can be classified either as saturated or unsaturated; *lipids*

fatty acid a hydrocarbon chain with a carboxylic acid group at one end

female athlete triad a combination of disordered eating, amenorrhea, and osteoporosis

femur (FEE-mer) thigh bone

fertilization the formation of a single cell that contains the genetic material from two gametes, one from each parent

fetus a developing human from eight weeks after conception to birth

fever the maintenance of body temperature at a higher-than-normal level

fibrin a long, thread-like fiber created by the combination of thrombin and fibrinogen; weaves around the platelet plug to form a blood clot

fibrinogen (figh-BRIN-oh-jehn) a protein that combines with the enzyme thrombin to create fibrin

fibrocartilage (FIGH-broh-KAR-ti-lij) type of cartilage with abundant collagen fibers

fibula (FIB-yoo-la) bone of the lower leg; does not bear weight

filtrate a fluid that has passed through a filter; sometimes used to refer to the fluid in the renal tubule

filtration membrane collective term for the structures through which water passes as it goes from the glomerular capillary into the glomerular capsule; includes capillary endothelial cells, the basement membrane, and the podocytes of the glomerular capsule

fimbriae (FIM-bree-igh) finger-like projections on the end of the uterine tube near the ovary

first-degree burns burns that affect only the epidermal layer of skin

first-degree heart block a heart block in which the impulse from the SA node is delayed

fissures the uniformly positioned, deep grooves in the brain

flagellum (fla-JEHL-um) a tail

flat bones bones that are largely (but not entirely) flat, such as the breast bone, hip bone, skull, and shoulder blades

flexion (FLEHK-shun) forward movement of a body segment away from anatomical position in the sagittal plane

floating ribs the two lowest ribs that do not attach at all to the sternum

flow volume meter a device used for measuring dynamic lung volumes

foam cells white blood cells, which digest LDL particles, become engorged with fat, and create a foamy substance

follicles (FAHL-i-kuhlz) bulb-shaped structures within the dermis that produce hair

follicle-stimulating hormone (FSH) a tropic hormone secreted by the anterior pituitary gland that stimulates the production of eggs in women and sperm in men

follicular phase (fah-LIK-yoo-lar) the phase of the menstrual cycle, lasting from day 1 to day 14, during which the ovarian follicles mature; *proliferative phase*

fontanel (FAHN-ta-NEHL) openings in the infant skull through which the baby's pulse can be felt; these openings enable compression of the skull during birth and brain growth during late pregnancy and early infancy

foramen ovale (foh-RA-men oh-VA-lee) opening in the septal wall between the atria that is normally present only in the fetus

force push or pull acting on a structure

forced expiratory volume in one second (FEV1) the amount of air that a person can expire in one second

forced expiratory volume in one second/forced vital capacity (FEV1/FVC) the overall expiratory power of the lungs

formed elements the solid components of blood; red blood cells, white blood cells, and platelets

fracture any break or disruption of continuity in a bone

frontal bone the bone that forms the forehead

frontal lobes sections of the brain located behind the forehead

frontal plane an invisible, vertical, flat surface that divides the body into front and back halves

frontal plane movements sideways motions of the body or body segments

frontal sinuses two air-filled cavities lined with mucous membrane, each of which lies within the frontal bone above one of the orbits

full-thickness burns see *third-degree burns*

functional layer the layer of the endometrium that is shed during menstruation

functional residual capacity (FRC) the amount of air that remains in the lungs after a normal expiration; ERV + RV

G

gallbladder the digestive organ that stores bile and delivers it to the duodenum when needed

gallstones solid crystals that form from substances in the bile of the gallbladder

gametes (GAM-eets) mature haploid male or female cells that unite with cells of the opposite sex to form a zygote; *eggs* and *sperm*

gamma interferons (IN-ter-FAIR-ahns) interferons produced by natural killer cells and T lymphocytes that have been activated by detection of foreign materials

ganglion (GAYNG-glee-ahn) a mass of nervous tissue composed mostly of nerve-cell bodies

gap junctions synapses where cell communication occurs through direct transfer of electrical charges

gas exchange the process by which oxygen is supplied to the body while carbon dioxide is also eliminated from the body

gastric glands glands in the stomach wall that secrete gastric juice, hormones, and mucus

gastric juice digestive fluid secreted in the stomach

gastric pits tiny openings in the lining of the stomach that each lead to a gastric gland

gastrin (GAS-trin) hormone that regulates digestion; secreted by enteroendocrine cells

gastroenteritis (GAS-troh-ehn-ter-IGH-tis) an inflammation of the stomach or intestine that produces some combination of nausea, vomiting, diarrhea, and abdominal pain

gastroesophageal reflux (GAS-troh-eh-SAHF-a-JEE-al) the movement of chyme from the stomach into the lower esophagus

gastroesophageal reflux disease (GERD) (GAS-troh-eh-SAHF-a-JEE-al) chronic inflammation of the esophagus caused by the upward flow of gastric juice

gastrointestinal tract (GAS-troh-in-TEHS-tin-ahl) the stomach, small intestine, and large intestine; *alimentary canal*

genital herpes a sexually transmitted disease that may cause blisters or sores in the genital or anal area or near the mouth; may cause no symptoms

gestation the period from fertilization to birth; *pregnancy*

gingiva (JIN-ji-vuh) soft tissue that covers the necks of the teeth, the mandible, and the maxilla; *gum*

glands epithelial cells that are organized to produce and secrete substances

glans penis the enlarged end of the penis

glaucoma (glaw-KOH-ma) a condition of increased pressure within the eyeball

glenohumeral joint (GLEH-noh-HYOO-mer-al) joint between the glenoid fossa of the scapula and the humerus; the *shoulder joint*

glenoid fossa (GLEE-noyd) shallow socket on the lateral end of each scapula that forms part of the shoulder joint

glial cells (GLIGH-al) supporting cells that appear in nerve tissue

gliding joint type of diarthrosis that allows only sliding motion of the articulating bones

globin (GLOH-bin) the large protein present in hemoglobin

glomerular capsule (glah-MER-yoo-lar) a thin, membranous, double-walled capsule surrounding the glomerulus of a nephron

glomerular capsule space the hollow space between the inner and outer surfaces of the glomerular capsule

glomerular filtrate the fluid that reaches the glomerular capsular space

glomerular filtration rate (GFR) the total amount of water filtered from the glomerular capillaries into the glomerular capsule per unit of time; usually measured in milliliters per minute

glomerulus (glah-MER-yuh-lus) a cluster of capillaries around the end of a renal corpuscle

glossopharyngeal nerve (GLAHS-oh-feh-RIN-jee-al) one of three cranial nerves that is responsible for transmitting taste sensations to the brain

glottis (GLAHT-is) the opening to the larynx and trachea; includes the vocal cords

glucagon (GLOO-kuh-gahn) hormone secreted by the pancreas that causes the breakdown of glycogen stored in the liver

glucocorticoids (gloo-koh-KORT-i-koids) a group of steroid hormones produced by the adrenal cortex that regulates carbohydrate, fat, and protein metabolism

gluconeogenesis (gloo-koh-nee-oh-JEH-neh-sis) the process by which fats and proteins are converted into glucose by the liver

glucose the main form of sugar that circulates in the blood

glucose tolerance test a test in which glucose is given and blood samples are taken afterwards to determine how quickly blood sugar levels return to normal

glyceride (GLIS-er-ighd) compound composed of a glycerol molecule with one, two, or three fatty acids attached

glycocalyx (GLIGH-koh-KAY-liks) the layer of carbohydrate groups surrounding a cell

glycogen (GLIGH-koh-jehn) a polymer of glucose that is found in animals

glycolysis (gligh-KAHL-i-sis) the breakdown of a glucose molecule into two pyruvate molecules

glycoproteins (GLIGH-koh-PROH-teenz) proteins with carbohydrate groups attached

goiter (GOY-ter) an enlarged thyroid caused by insufficient amounts of iodine or a thyroid disorder

Golgi apparatus (GOHL-jee) a set of membranous discs in the cytoplasm

gonads (GOH-nads) the organs that produce gametes (oocytes and sperm): the ovaries in females and the testes in males

gonorrhea (GAHN-oh-REE-a) a sexually transmitted disease that may cause pain during urination, unusual discharge of fluid from the vagina or penis, or no symptoms at all; can lead to infertility

granulocytes (GRAN-yoo-loh-SIGHTS) white blood cells whose cytoplasm contains granules

granulosa cells (GRAN-yoo-LOH-sa) the supporting cells that surround the oocyte

Graves disease an autoimmune disorder that causes an overactive thyroid gland and outward bulging of the eyes

gray matter tracts of unmyelinated fibers in the central nervous system

greater vestibular glands mucus-secreting glands that lie on either side of the vagina

gross anatomy the study of the body structures that can be seen with the naked eye

growth hormone an anterior pituitary hormone that promotes bone and muscle development

gustatory cells (GUS-ta-TOH-ree) sensory receptors within a taste bud

gustatory hairs (GUS-ta-TOH-ree) threads that emerge from the gustatory cells

gyrus (JIGH-rus) a curved, raised area on the brain

H

hair cells sensory receptors located in the organ of Corti and semicircular canals

hairy tongue a symptom of certain conditions that promote unnatural growth of the gustatory hairs of the tongue

hammer tiny bone in the middle ear that transmits sound from the tympanic membrane (eardrum) to the anvil

haploid (HAP-loyd) having a single set of unpaired chromosomes

hardening of the arteries see *atherosclerosis*

hard palate (PAL-at) the anterior part of the palate that separates the oral and nasal cavities, which is supported by bone

Haversian canals (ha-VER-zhen) major passageways running in the direction of the length of long bones, providing a path for blood vessels

Haversian system includes a single Haversian canal along with its multiple canaliculi, which branch out to join with lacunae, forming a comprehensive transportation matrix for supply of nutrients and removal of waste products; *osteon*

HbA1c test a glucose tolerance test that measures the average blood glucose levels over the course of three months

hearing aids devices that amplify and change sounds so that the wearer can better hear them

heart block   a condition in which the impulses traveling from the SA node to the ventricles are delayed, intermittently blocked, or completely blocked by the AV node

heart murmurs   extra or unusual sounds heard by a stethoscope during a heartbeat that may be harmless or indicative of a problem with one of the heart valves

heat   a sign of inflammation

heat capacity   the quantity of heat required to raise the temperature of 1 gram of material by 1°C

helper T cell   T lymphocyte that helps activate cytotoxic T cells and B cells

hematocrit (hee-MAT-oh-krit)   the percentage of the total blood volume that is composed of red blood cells

hematopoiesis (HEE-ma-toh-poy-EE-sis)   process of blood cell formation

heme (heem)   the iron molecule present in hemoglobin

hemodialysis (HEE-moh-digh-AL-i-sis)   a procedure for removing metabolic waste products from the body; blood is withdrawn from an artery, pumped through a dialyzer, and then returned to the patient through a vein

hemoglobin (HEE-moh-GLOH-bin)   an essential molecule of the red blood cell that serves as a binding site for oxygen and carbon dioxide; composed of two molecules: *globin* and *heme*

hemolysis (hee-MAHL-i-sis)   the rupture of red blood cells as a result of disease or old age

hemophilia (HEE-moh-FIL-ee-a)   a condition in which blood does not clot properly due to the absence of a clotting factor

hemorrhagic stroke (HEM-oh-RAJ-ik)   a stroke that occurs when one of the arteries in the brain ruptures, causing bleeding in the brain

hemostasis (HEE-moh-STAY-sis)   the sequence of events that causes a blood clot to form and bleeding to stop

hepatitis   a disease characterized by inflammation of and damage to the liver

hepatocyte (HEHP-a-toh-sight)   a liver cell

Hering-Breuer reflex (HER-ing BROY-er)   an involuntary impulse triggered by stretch receptors in the bronchioles and alveoli that halts inspiration and initiates exhalation

hernia   a balloon-like section of the lining of the abdominal cavity that protrudes through a hole or weakened section of the muscles in the abdomen

herpes   a viral infection that produces small, painful, blisterlike sores

herpes simplex virus type 1   the form of herpes that generates cold sores or fever blisters around the mouth

herpes simplex virus type 2   the genital form of herpes

herpes varicella (VAIR-i-SEHL-a)   a highly contagious, common childhood disease that is characterized by extremely itchy, fluid-filled blisters; *chickenpox*

herpes zoster (ZAHS-ter)   a disease that involves a painful, blistering rash accompanied by headache, fever, and a general feeling of unwellness; *shingles*

high-risk HPVs   type of HPV infections known to sometimes cause cancer

hilum (HIGH-lum)   the part of an organ, often indented, where vessels enter and exit; found on lymph node, spleen, kidney, lung, and other organs

hinge joint   type of diarthrosis that allows only hinge-like movements in forward and back directions

histamines (HIS-ta-meenz)   molecules that trigger a reaction to irritation of the nasal membranes, which produces nasal congestion and drainage

histology   the study of tissues

histone (HIS-tohn)   a small protein that binds to DNA and helps it coil

homeostasis (HOH-mee-oh-STAY-sis)   a state of regulated physiological balance

homeostatic imbalance   a state in which there is a diminished ability for the organ systems to keep the body's internal environment within normal ranges

homeostatic mechanisms   the processes that maintain homeostasis

homologous chromosomes (hoh-MAHL-uh-gus)   a pair of chromosomes that have the same genes in the same relative positions (and possibly different alleles, alternative forms of the genes that arise through mutation); one member of the pair comes from the mother and one from the father

hormonal control   type of endocrine control in which endocrine organs are stimulated by hormones from other endocrine organs, starting with the hypothalamus

hormones   chemical messengers secreted by the endocrine glands

human anatomy   the study of the form or structure of the human body

human chorionic gonadotropin (hCG) (kor-ee-AHN-ik GOH-nad-oh-TROH-pin)   a hormone secreted by the trophoblast cells of the embryo that prevents deterioration of the corpus luteum and stimulates progesterone production in the placenta

human genome   the DNA sequence of a human

human immunodeficiency virus (HIV)   the virus that causes AIDS

human papillomavirus (HPV)   a sexually transmitted disease that causes warts, especially on the genitals, and that can cause cervical cancer; however, the virus usually is asymptomatic

human physiology   the study of how humans function internally

humerus (HYOO-mer-us)   major bone of the upper arm

humoral control   type of endocrine control in which levels of various substances in body fluids are monitored for homeostatic imbalance

humoral immunity   immunity associated with free antibodies that circulate in the blood; *antibody-mediated immunity*

hyaline cartilage (HIGH-a-lin)   type of cartilage that forms the smooth covering on the ends of long bones

hydrogen bond   electrical interactions between the positive region around the hydrogen atom of a water molecule and the negatively charged region of another molecule

hydrophilic (HIGH-droh-FIL-ik)   term that describes a molecule that can form favorable hydrogen bonds with water

hydrophobic (HIGH-droh-FOH-bik)   term that describes a molecule that cannot form favorable hydrogen bonds with water

hydrostatic pressure   the pressure exerted by a liquid as a result of its potential energy

hypercalcemia (HIGH-per-kal-SEE-mee-a)   a condition caused by the hypersecretion of parathryroid hormone (PTH), leading to increased blood calcium levels and increased calcium absorption by the kidneys

hyperextension   backward movement of a body segment past anatomical position in the sagittal plane

hyperglycemia (HIGH-per-gligh-SEE-mee-a)   a condition in which blood glucose levels become elevated

hyperopia (HIGH-per-OH-pee-a)   the condition that results from a flattened eyeball shape; *farsightedness*

hypertension condition that occurs when the force of blood against the arterial wall remains elevated for an extended period of time; *high blood pressure*

hyperthyroidism a condition characterized by a visibly enlarged thyroid gland in the neck; *overactive thyroid*

hypertrophy (high-PER-troh-fee) increase in bone mineral density and strength

hyperventilation excessive ventilation that leads to an abnormal expulsion of carbon dioxide

hypodermis the layer of skin beneath the dermis, which serves as a storage repository for fat

hypothalamic inhibiting hormones hormones secreted by the hypothalamus that direct the activities of the pituitary gland; *hypothalamic nonreleasing hormones*

hypothalamic nonreleasing hormones hormones produced in the hypothalamus and carried by a vein to the anterior pituitary, where they stop certain hormones from being released; *hypothalamic inhibiting hormones*

hypothalamic releasing hormones hormones produced in the hypothalamus and carried by a vein to the anterior pituitary, where they stimulate the release of anterior pituitary hormones

hypothalamus (HIGH-poh-THAL-a-mus) a portion of the diencephalon and nervous system that is also considered an endocrine gland; includes vital autonomic regulatory centers that control functions such as metabolism, heart rate, and blood pressure

hypothyroidism a condition caused by an underactive thyroid gland

hypoxemia (HIGH-pahk-SEE-mee-a) a condition in which arterial blood oxygen content is lowered

I

IgE antibody a class of antibody that interacts with mast cells and basophils to cause histamine release, inflammation, and, sometimes, allergic reactions

ileocecal valve (IL-ee-oh-SEE-kal) valve located at the end of the ileum that opens in response to gastrin released by the stomach

ileum (IL-ee-um) longest and last portion of the small intestine; between the jejunum and the large intestine

iliac crest (IL-ee-ak) prominent upper edge of the ilium of the hip bone

ilium (IL-ee-um) bone comprising most of each coxal bone, connecting posteriorly to the sacrum at the sacroiliac joint

immune system the cells and chemicals that contribute to the body's specific defenses against disease

immunoglobulins (IM-yoo-noh-GLAHB-yoo-lins) proteins that recognize particular antigens with great specificity; *antibodies*

immunotherapy a long-term, preventive treatment for allergies; *allergy shots*

impetigo (IM-peh-TEE-goh) a bacterial infection common in elementary school children that is characterized by pink, blisterlike bumps, usually on the face

implantation the binding of the blastocyst to the endometrium

incus see *anvil*

inferior term meaning below or under

inferior articular process indentation on the lower side of each vertebra forming a facet joint with the next vertebra

inferior concha (KAHN-ka) bones forming the sides of the nasal cavity

inferior vena cava largest vein in the human body that returns deoxygenated blood to the right atrium of the heart from body regions below the diaphragm

infertility the inability of a couple to get pregnant

inflammatory bowel disease a condition in which the wall of the small and/or large intestine becomes chronically inflamed

inflammatory response physiological response to tissue injury or infection including heat, redness, swelling, and pain; *inflammation*

influenza a viral infection that affects the respiratory system; the *flu*

infundibulum (in-fun-DI-byuh-lum) a short stalk on the underside of the hypothalamus from which the pituitary gland is suspended

ingestion the intake of food and liquids via the mouth

insertion muscle attachment to a bone that tends to move when the muscle contracts

inspiration the process by which air flows into the lungs; *inhalation*

inspiratory reserve volume (IRV) the amount of air that can be inhaled immediately after a normal inhalation

insulin a hormone that promotes glucose uptake in body tissues

insulin resistance a condition common in type II diabetes in which the pancreas secretes insulin, but the body's insulin receptors are downregulated, causing low blood glucose levels

integumentary system (in-TEHG-yoo-MEHN-ta-ree) enveloping organ of the body that includes the epidermis, dermis, sudoriferous and sebaceous glands; also includes nails and hair

interatrial septum (IN-ter-AY-tree-al) the wall that separates the right and left atria in the heart

interferons (IN-ter-FAIR-ahns) proteins released by cells that have been infected with viruses; interfere with virus reproduction

interleukins chemicals that stimulate an immune response

intermediate filament a type of fiber in the cytoskeleton, made of keratin

internal respiration the process of gas exchange between the tissues and arterial blood

internal urethral sphincter a layer of smooth muscle located at the inferior end of the bladder and the proximal end of the urethra; this muscle, which prohibits release of urine, is under involuntary control

interneurons (inter-NOO-rahnz) nerve cells that form bridges to transmit impulses between sensory and motor neurons; *association neurons*

interosseus membrane (IN-ter-AHS-ee-es) tough, fibrous connective tissue that bonds the radius and ulna together and also binds the tibia and fibula together

interphase the phase in the life cycle of a cell when it is not dividing; DNA duplication occurs during this phase

interstitial fluid (IN-ter-STISH-al) fluid in the spaces between cells

interstitial space the space between cells

interventricular septum (IN-ter-ven-TRIK-yoo-lar SEP-tum) thick wall that divides the two ventricles in the heart

intervertebral discs (IN-ter-VER-teh-bral) fibrocartilaginous cushions between vertebral bodies that allow bending of the spine and help to create the normal spinal curves

intestinal trunks lymphatic vessels that carry lymph from abdominal organs toward the cisterna chyli

intrinsic factor   glycoprotein secreted by cells in the stomach that is essential for absorption of vitamin B$_{12}$

inulin   a nontoxic polysaccharide from plants; used to test kidney function

inversion   movement in which the sole of the foot is rolled inward

in vitro fertilization (IVF)   an assisted reproductive technology in which the oocyte is fertilized outside the body

iris   the anterior portion of the choroid, which gives the eye its color

iron-deficient anemia   the most common anemia; caused by an insufficient dietary intake of iron, loss of iron from intestinal bleeding, or iron-level depletion during pregnancy

irregular bones   bones with shapes that do not allow them to be classified as long, short, or flat, including the bones of the pelvic girdle and spinal column

irregular dense connective tissue   type of connective tissue that is composed primarily of collagen fibers that are oriented in random directions

irritability   the ability to respond to a stimulus

ischemia (is-KEE-mee-a)   a lack of blood flow, usually due to the narrowing of a blood vessel

ischemic stroke (is-KEE-mik)   a stroke that occurs when one of the arteries of the brain becomes blocked

ischium (IS-kee-um)   bone forming the inferior (lowest) portion of each coxal bone; supports the weight of the upper body during sitting

islets of Langerhans (IGH-lets of LAHNG-er-hahnz)   cells of the pancreas that secrete insulin and glucagon

isometric (IGH-soh-MEHT-rik)   a type of contraction that causes no change in muscle length

isthmus (IS-mus)   a center band of tissue that connects the two lateral lobes of the thyroid gland

J

jaundice   a blood disorder characterized by yellow-colored skin and whites of the eyes

jejunum (jeh-JOO-num)   middle segment of the small intestine; between the duodenum and the ileum

juvenile onset diabetes   see *type I diabetes mellitus*

juxtamedullary nephrons (JUKS-ta-MEHD-yoo-LAIR-ee)   nephrons located near the boundary between the renal cortex and the renal medulla; have long nephron loops that penetrate deeply into the renal medulla; important regulators of urine concentration

K

keratin (KER-a-tin)   a tough protein found in the skin, hair, and nails

keratinocytes (keh-RAT-i-noh-sights)   cells within the epidermis that produce keratin

ketacidosis (keet-oh-as-i-DOH-sis)   a condition caused by the enhanced production of ketone bodies, which causes the pH of the blood to decrease and become dangerously acidic

kidney stone   solid crystalline mass that can form in the kidney and which may become stuck in the renal pelvis or ureter; usually made of calcium, phosphate, uric acid, and protein

killer T cell   see *cytotoxic T cell*

kinetics   the analysis of the actions of forces

L

labia majora   two skin folds posterior to the mons pubis that lie parallel on either side of the vaginal opening

labia minora   a smaller set of skin folds inside the labia majora

labyrinthitis (LAB-uh-rin-THIGH-tis)   an infection of the inner ear that produces inflammation

lacrimal bones (LAK-ri-mal)   tiny bones connecting to the orbits and surrounding the tear ducts

lacrimal canaliculi (LAK-ri-mal kan-a-LIK-yoo-ligh)   tiny canals where tears are flushed from the eye

lacrimal glands (LAK-ri-mal)   tear secretors; located above the lateral end of each eye

lactation   secretion of milk by the mammary glands

lactiferous duct (lak-TIF-er-us)   a duct through which milk is secreted and which opens at the nipple

lacunae (la-KOO-nee)   tiny cavities laid out in concentric circles around the Haversian canals

lamellae (la-MEHL-ee)   concentric circles of lacunae around the Haversian canals

lamina propria (LAM-in-a PROH-pree-a)   loose, connective tissue under the epithelium of a mucous membrane

large intestine   the portion of the digestive tube between the small intestine and the anus; its major segments are the cecum, colon, rectum, and anal canal

laryngitis (LAIR-in-JIGH-tis)   inflammation of the larynx, or voice box

laryngopharynx (la-RING-goh-FAIR-ingks)   the lower section of the pharynx

larynx (LAIR-ingks)   a triangular-shaped space inferior to the pharynx that is responsible for voice production; the *voice box*

lateral extension   term for the return from a position of lateral flexion to anatomical position

lateral flexion   trunk and neck motions away from anatomical position in the frontal plane

lateral malleolus (mal-LEE-oh-lus)   bony projection on the end of each fibula; the *ankle bone*

lateral rotation   outward (lateral) movement of a body segment in the transverse plane

left bronchomediastinal trunk (BRAHN-koh-MEE-dee-as-tin-al)   duct that drains lymph from the left side of the chest and lower neck

left bundle branches   the left limbs or branches through which electrical impulses are transmitted from the bundle of His through the left ventricle

left jugular trunk   duct that drains lymph from the left side of the head

left lumbar trunk   duct carrying lymph from left lower body toward the cisterna chyli

left subclavian trunk (sub-KLAY-vee-an)   duct that drains lymph from the left arm

lens   a transparent, flexible structure that is curved outward on both sides

let-down reflex   contraction of smooth muscle cells in the mammary glands that allows milk to be squeezed toward and out of the nipple

leukemia   a cancer caused by production of an extremely high number of immature white blood cells in the bone marrow

leukocytes (LOO-koh-sights)   white blood cells

ligaments   bands composed of collagen and elastic fibers that connect bones to other bones

limbic system   a set of structures in the brain that stimulate the sympathetic branch in the cardiac center

lingual tonsils (LING-gwal)   two masses of lymphatic tissue that lie on either side of the base of the tongue

lipids   fatty molecules that dissolve poorly in water but dissolve well in a nonpolar solvent; fats and oils

lipocytes (LIP-oh-sights)   fat-storing cells

lithotripsy (LITH-oh-TRIP-see)   the use of intense, ultrasonic sound waves to break up a kidney stone into pieces small enough to be passed from the body in the urine

lobes   the name for the four regions of the brain—frontal, parietal, occipital, and temporal

long bones   bones that are long in shape, such as the major bones of the arms and legs

longitudinal arch   arch of the foot running lengthwise

loop of Henle (HEN-lee)   see *nephron loop*

loose connective tissue   type of connective tissue that has cells and an extracellular matrix containing fibers running through it

lower extremity   bones of the hips, legs, and feet

low-risk HPVs   type of HPV infection that can cause warts, but are not known to cause cancer

lumbar region (LUM-bar)   low back region of the spine composed of 5 vertebrae

lumen (LOO-mehn)   the hollow inside portion of a body cavity or tube

lunule (LOO-nyool)   the white, crescent-shaped region at the base of the nail

luteal phase   the phase of the menstrual cycle that begins at ovulation and ends with the onset of menstruation

luteinizing hormone (LH) (LOO-tee-in-ighz-ing)   a tropic hormone produced by the anterior pituitary gland that signals the egg's release from the follicle, stimulates the production of progesterone and small amounts of estrogen in women, and stimulates the interstitial cells of the testes to produce testosterone in men

lymph   clear, transparent, sometimes faintly yellow fluid that is collected from tissues throughout the body and flows in the lymphatic vessels

lymph nodes   small, bean-shaped structures found along the lymphatic vessels throughout the body

lymphatic capillaries   the smallest lymphatic vessels that collect lymph in organs and tissues

lymphatic nodules   small, localized clusters of dense tissue formed by lymphocytes and macrophages

lymphatic tissue   loose, connective tissue that contains many lymphocytes and is found in mucous membranes and certain organs throughout the body

lymphatic trunks   large lymphatic vessels that drain lymph from different parts of the body

lymphatic valves   tissue flaps that act as one-way valves inside the lymphatic vessels

lymphatic vessels   vessels that carry lymph

lymphedema (LIMF-eh-DEE-ma)   a buildup of extracellular fluid in the body because of disruption in lymphatic drainage

lymphocytes (LIM-foh-sights)   white blood cells that are abundant in lymphatic tissue

lysosome (LIGH-soh-sohm)   a compartment where reactions involving potentially dangerous enzymes and reactants can be conducted in isolation from the cytoplasm

lysozyme   an enzyme contained in tears that attacks bacteria

M

macronutrients   substances such as carbohydrates, proteins, and fats that the body requires in relatively large quantities

macrophages (MAK-roh-fay-jehz)   cells that phagocytize (surround and destroy) foreign cells, such as bacteria and viruses

macular degeneration (MAK-yoo-lar)   a condition that causes a progressive loss of central vision

major histocompatibility complex glycoproteins (MHCs)   family of proteins found on the surfaces of lymphocytes and other cells; help the immune system recognize foreign antigens and ignore "self" tissues

malignant   term for tumors that are cancerous

malignant melanoma (MEHL-a-NOH-ma)   cancer of the melanocytes; the most serious form of skin cancer

malleus   see *hammer*

mammary glands   the milk-producing glands in the female

mandible (MAN-di-buhl)   jaw bone

manubrium (ma-NOO-bree-um)   upper portion of the sternum (breast bone)

mass   the quantity of matter contained in an object

mast cells   connective tissue cell with granules (particles) that contain histamine, a compound which, when released into surrounding fluid, activates an inflammatory response

matrix   term for a growth zone

maxillary bones (MAK-sil-lair-ee)   two fused bones that form the upper jaw, house the upper teeth, and connect to all other bones of the face, with the exception of the mandible

maxillary sinuses (MAK-sil-lair-ee)   air cavities in the body of the maxilla that communicate with the middle meatus of the nose

mean arterial pressure   the overall pressure within the cardiovascular system, which determines blood flow to various organs

mechanical breakdown   the breakdown of food into smaller pieces, thus increasing its surface area

mechanoreceptors (MEHK-a-noh-ree-SEHP-tors)   chemical receptor cells that detect muscle contraction and force generation during exercise; they quickly increase inspiration rates when exercise begins

medial rotation   inward (medial) movement of a body segment in the transverse plane

mediastinum (MEH-dee-as-TIGH-num)   the area of the thoracic cavity between the lungs; houses the heart, great blood vessels, trachea, esophagus, thoracic duct, thymus gland, and other structures

medulla   deep or middle portion of an organ, for example the deep part of a lymph node

medulla oblongata (meh-DOOL-a AHB-lawn-gah-tah)   the lower portion of the brain stem, which regulates heart rate, blood pressure, and breathing, and controls several reflexes

medullary cavity (MEHD-oo-LAIR-ee)   central hollow in the long bones

meiosis   a type of cell division that produces eggs (in females) or sperm (in males), daughter cells with half the chromosome number of the parent cell

melanin   a pigment that protects the body against the harmful effects of ultraviolet ray damage from the sun

melanin granules   particles of melanin that are pushed into skin cells as more melanin is produced

melanocytes (MEHL-a-noh-sights)   specialized cells in the skin that produce melanin

melatonin   hormone that is released by the pineal gland when the body is exposed to darkness; high levels of melatonin cause the body to feel drowsy or sleepy

membrane attack complex (MAC)   a complex of complement proteins that create a large, lethal hole in the cell membrane

membranes thin sheets or layers of pliable tissue

membranous labyrinth (MEHM-bray-nus) membrane-covered tubes inside the bony labyrinth

memory cells B lymphocytes and T lymphocytes in lymphatic tissues that can respond if a previously encountered antigen invades the body again

memory cytotoxic T cell one of the daughter cells produced by clonal selection of cytotoxic T lymphocytes

memory helper B cell one of the daughter cells produced by clonal selection of helper B lymphocytes

memory helper T cell one of the daughter cells created by clonal selection of helper T lymphocytes

menarche (MEHN-ar-kee) the first menstrual bleeding

Ménière's disease (men-YAIRZ) a condition characterized by chronic inflammation of the semicircular canals of the inner ear

meninges (meh-NIN-jeez) three protective membranes that surround the brain and spinal cord

meningitis (MEHN-in-JIGH-tis) an infection-induced inflammation of the meninges surrounding the brain and spinal cord

menstrual discharge the blood and tissue lost in the menstrual phase

menstrual phase the phase of the uterine cycle during which the endometrium breaks down

Merkel cells touch receptors in the skin

mesentery (MEHS-ehn-TER-ee) a double layer of peritoneum attached to the abdominal wall

messenger RNA single-strand RNA molecule whose base sequence carries the information needed by a ribosome to make a protein

metabolic rate the speed at which the body consumes energy

metabolism (meh-TAB-oh-lizm) the sum of the chemical and physical reactions that occur in an organism to keep it alive

metacarpals (meht-a-KAR-pals) the five interior bones of the hand, connecting the carpals in the wrist to the phalanges in the fingers

metaphase the second stage of cell division, in which chromosomes align along the center of the cell

metastasis (meh-TAS-ta-sis) the spreading of cancerous cells from their original location to other areas of the body

metatarsals (meht-a-TAR-salz) small bones of the ankle

metric system international system of measurement that is used in all fields of science

microfilament a type of fiber in the cytoskeleton; made of actin

microglia (migh-KROHG-lee-a) glial cells that absorb and dispose of dead cells and bacteria

micronutrients vitamins and minerals that are essential to the body in small amounts

microscopic anatomy the study of the tiny parts of the body seen only with a microscope

microtubule (MIGH-kroh-TOO-byool) a type of fiber in the cytoskeleton; made of tubulin

microvilli (MIGH-kroh-VIL-ee) finger-like extensions that increase the surface area of a cell

micturition (mik-choo-RISH-un) urination

midbrain relay station for sensory and motor impulses; located on the superior end of the brain stem

middle ear cavities openings in the skull that serve as chambers for transmitting and amplifying sound

mineralocorticoids (min-eh-ra-loh-KORT-i-koids) a group of steroid hormones produced by the adrenal cortex that regulate the body's sodium and fluid levels

minerals elements that the body needs in relatively small amounts

mitochondria (MIGH-toh-KAHN-dree-a) organelles in the cytoplasm that make ATP

mitosis the division of a cell nucleus and chromosomes into two nuclei, each with its own set of identical chromosomes

mitral valve (migh-tral) the valve that closes the orifice between the left atrium and left ventricle of the heart; *bicuspid valve*

mitral valve prolapse an incomplete closing of the mitral valve, causing blood to flow backward into the left atrium when the left ventricle contracts

modeling process through which new bone is created during growth

molecules chemical combinations of two or more atoms

monocytes (MAHN-oh-sight) leukocytes that develop into phagocytizing macrophages when they migrate out of lymphatic circulation into surrounding tissue

monounsaturated fats one category of unsaturated fatty acids; sources include canola oil and olive oil

mons pubis the region of skin and underlying fat in front of the vaginal opening on which pubic hair grows during puberty

motor neuron a nerve that stimulates skeletal muscle tissue

motor unit a single motor neuron and all of the muscle fibers that it stimulates

mucosa the mucous membrane of the alimentary canal; the innermost layer

mucosa-associated lymphatic tissue (MALT) lymphatic tissue found in mucous membranes that line passageways open to the outside world; these include the respiratory, gastrointestinal, urinary, and reproductive tracts

mucous layer a viscous coating that surrounds the olfactory hairs

mucous membranes thin sheets of tissue lining the body cavities that open to the outside world

multiple myeloma (MIGH-eh-LOH-ma) a cancer of the plasma cells in blood marrow

multiple sclerosis a chronic, slowly progressive disease of the central nervous system that destroys the myelin sheath of nerve cell axons

multipolar neurons nerve cells that have one axon and multiple dendrites

muscle cramps moderate to severe muscle spasms that cause pain

muscle fiber an individual skeletal muscle cell

muscle physiology the study of how muscles function internally

muscle strain an injury that occurs when a muscle is stretched beyond the limits to which it is accustomed

muscle tissue a type of tissue that generates force and allows the body to move

muscular dystrophy (MD) a group of similar, inherited disorders characterized by progressively worsening muscle weakness and loss of muscle tissue

muscularis externa outer layer of smooth muscle in the wall of the esophagus, stomach, small intestine, and large intestine

myelin sheath (MIGH-eh-lin) the fatty bands of insulation surrounding axon fibers

myocardial infarction tissue death that occurs in a segment of heart muscle from blockage of a coronary artery; *heart attack*

myocarditis (MIGH-oh-kahr-DIGH-tis) inflammation of the myocardium, the middle layer of the heart; the *heart muscle*

myocardium (MIGH-oh-KAHR-dee-um) the middle layer of the heart, which makes up about 2/3 of the heart muscle

myometrium (migh-oh-MEE-tree-um) smooth muscle that comprises the bulk of the uterine wall

myopia (migh-OH-pee-a) the condition that results from an elongated eyeball shape; *nearsightedness*

myosin a widely distributed protein that is the major component of thick filaments in skeletal, cardiac, and smooth muscle fibers

myositis ossificans (migh-oh-SIGH-tis ah-SIF-i-kanz) a condition in which a calcium mass forms within a muscle over three to four weeks after a muscle injury

myxedema (MIKS-eh-DEE-ma) a condition in adults with hyperthyroidism that causes weight gain; a swollen, puffy face; low body temperature; dry skin; and decreased mental acuity

N

nail bed a specialized region of the stratum basale under each nail

nail matrix a thickened region of the nail that serves as its growth zone

nares two openings in the nose through which air enters; *nostrils*

nasal bones two bones forming the bridge of the nose

nasal cavity opening within the nose

nasal septum the bony and cartilaginous partition dividing the nasal cavity into two passages

nasolacrimal duct (NAY-zoh-LAK-ri-mal) the channel into which the lacrimal canaliculi drain

nasopharyngitis (NAY-zoh-FAIR-in-JIGH-tis) inflammation of the nasal passages and pharynx; the *common cold*

nasopharynx (NAY-zoh-FAIR-ingks) the upper section of the pharynx

natural killer (NK) cells lymphocytes that play an important role in the nonspecific defense system of the body by killing virus-infected cells and cancer cells

negative feedback mechanism that reverses a condition that has exceeded the normal homeostatic range to restore homeostasis

neonatal hypothyroidism hypothyroidism that occurs in infants and children; may develop congenitally, or following birth

nephron (NEH-frahn) the fundamental excretory unit of each kidney

nephron loop the U-shaped part of the nephron that is between the proximal convoluted tubule and the distal convoluted tubule; has a descending limb and ascending limb; *loop of Henle*

nerve impulse electrical charge that travels along a nerve fiber when stimulated

nerve tissue a type of tissue that conveys information by electrical signaling

net force the single force resulting from the summation of all forces acting on a structure at a given time

neural control type of endocrine control in which nerve fibers stimulate the endocrine organs to release hormones

neurilemma (NOO-ri-LEHM-a) the thin, membranous sheath enveloping a nerve fiber

neuroglia (ner-ROHG-lee-a) non-neural tissue that forms the interstitial or supporting elements of the CNS; *glial cells*

neuromuscular junction the link between an axon terminal and a muscle fiber

neurons the cells that make up nerve tissue

neurotransmitters chemical messengers

neutrophils (NOO-troh-fils) the most common type of white blood cell; can slip out of capillaries and into surrounding tissues, where they destroy bacteria and cellular debris

night blindness a condition that affects the rods in the retina and makes it difficult to see well at night

nitrogenous waste waste substances in urine that contain nitrogen; mainly urea

nocturnal emission the discharge of semen during sleep

nodes of Ranvier (rahn-vee-AY) the uninsulated gaps in the myelin sheath of a nerve fiber where the axon is exposed

non-planar the term used to describe movements that do not occur in the direction of one of the three imaginary planes

noradrenalin a neurotransmitter involved in the body's flight or fight response; *norepinephrine*

norepinephrine (NOR-ehp-i-NEHF-rin) a neurotransmitter released by postganglionic neurons in the sympathetic nervous system; *noradrenalin*

normal contractility condition a normal sinus rhythm of the heart

nuclear envelope a membrane that defines the boundary of the cell's nucleus

nuclear pore an opening in the nucleus through which mRNA can leave

nucleic acids key information-carrying molecules in cells

nucleotides (NOO-klee-oh-tighdz) subunits that make up nucleic acids

nucleus a rounded or oval mass of protoplasm within the cytoplasm of a cell that contains the cell's DNA and is bounded by a membrane

nutrients chemicals that the body needs for energy, growth, and maintenance

O

occipital bone (AHK-sip-i-tal) forms the base and lower back portions of the skull

occipital lobes (AHK-sip-i-tal) sections of the brain located behind the parietal lobes; responsible for vision

odor molecules tiny airborne particles from food that trigger the sense of smell

olfactory bulb (ohl-FAK-toh-ree) the thickened end of the olfactory nerve that sends sensory impulses to the olfactory region of the brain

olfactory filaments (ohl-FAK-toh-ree) fibers in the olfactory nerve that receive impulses from olfactory receptor cells

olfactory hairs (ohl-FAK-toh-ree) threads that extend from the olfactory receptor cells into the nasal cavity

olfactory nerve (ohl-FAK-toh-ree) sensory pathway from the nasal cavity to the olfactory cortex of the brain

olfactory receptor cells (ohl-FAK-toh-ree) the sensors responsible for smell

olfactory receptors (ohl-FAK-toh-ree) sensory cells in the olfactory region that provide the sense of smell

olfactory region (ohl-FAK-toh-ree) a dime-sized area along the mucous membrane on the roof of the nasal cavity where olfactory epithelium and glands are found

oligodendrocytes (AHL-i-goh-DEHN-droh-sights) glial cells that wrap around nerve fibers and produce a fatty insulating material called myelin

oocyte (OH-uh-sight) egg cell

oogenesis (oh-ah-JEHN-eh-sis) the process by which oocytes, or female gametes, are generated

oogonia (oh-uh-GOH-nee-a) diploid stem cells in females that are similar to spermatogonia in males

opportunistic infection an infection that rarely or never occurs in people with a healthy immune system but that may occur in a person with a damaged immune system such as from AIDS

opposition touching any of your four fingers to the thumb; this movement enables grasping of objects

opsonins (AHP-soh-nins) proteins that make cells more attractive to phagocytes

opsonization the process of making cells attractive to phagocytes

optic chiasma (kigh-AZ-ma) the point at which the optic nerves cross

optic disc the junction between the optic nerve and the eye; the location of the blind spot

optic nerve transmitter of visual sensory signals to the occipital lobe of the brain

optic tracts the continuation of the optic nerve fibers beyond the optic chiasma

oral cavity opening within the mouth

orbicularis oris (or-BIK-yoo-LAH-ris) a skeletal muscle located in the lips

orbital cavities openings that hold the eyes

organ body part organized to perform a specific function

organ of Corti a spiral-shaped ridge of epithelium in the cochlear duct lined with hair cells that serve as hearing receptors

organ system two or more organs working together to perform specific functions

origin muscle attachment to a relatively fixed structure

oropharynx (OR-oh-FAIR-ingks) the middle section of the pharynx

osmosis (ahz-MOH-sis) the movement of water molecules from a region of low osmotic pressure to a region of high osmotic pressure

osmotic diuresis (ahs-MAHT-ik) an increase in urine production caused by high osmotic pressure of the glomerular filtrate, which "pulls" more water into the filtrate

osmotic pressure (ahs-MAHT-ik) a pressure created by the presence of dissolved substances in water

osseous tissue (AHS-ee-us) bone tissue

ossicles (AHS-i-kuhls) the body's three smallest bones—the hammer, anvil, and stirrup; found in the middle ear

ossification (AHS-i-fi-KAY-shun) process of bone formation

osteoarthritis degenerative disease of articular cartilage, characterized by pain, swelling, range-of-motion restriction, and stiffness

osteoblasts (AHS-tee-oh-BLASTS) specialized bone cells that build new bone tissue

osteoclasts (AHS-tee-oh-KLASTS) specialized bone cells that resorb bone tissue

osteocytes mature bone cells

osteon a Haversian system

osteopenia (AHS-tee-oh-PEE-nee-a) reduced bone mass without the presence of a fracture

osteoporosis (AHS-tee-oh-poh-ROH-sis) condition in which bone mineralization and strength are so abnormally low that regular, daily activities can result in painful fractures

otitis media (oh-TIGHT-is) an infection of the middle ear caused by bacteria or a virus

oval window a membrane-covered opening that connects the middle ear to the inner ear

ovarian cycle the sequence of events associated with maturation and release of an oocyte

ovaries the female sex glands

ovulation the release of an oocyte, or egg, from the ovarian follicle

oxyhemoglobin (AHK-see-HEE-moh-GLOH-bin) molecule that is created when oxygen combines with the heme part of the hemoglobin molecule

oxytocin (AHK-see-TOH-sin) a hormone that stimulates uterine contractions during labor and milk secretion during breastfeeding

P

pacemaker an important internal control mechanism of the heart; *sinoatrial node*

pain a sign of inflammation

palate (PAL-at) the structure consisting of hard and soft components that separates the oral and nasal cavities; the *roof of the mouth*

palatine bones (PAL-a-tighn) bones that form the posterior part of the hard palate, or roof of the mouth

palatine tonsils two masses of lymphatic tissue that lie in the back of the mouth, on the left and right sides; the largest and most commonly infected tonsils

palpitations sensation of rapid heartbeat

pancreas a long, thin gland located posterior to the stomach. As an endocrine gland, the pancreas secretes insulin and glucagon, which control blood glucose levels; as an exocrine gland, the pancreas secretes digestive enzymes

pancreatic amylase a substance that breaks down starches into chains that are as short as two sugar molecules

pancreatic lipase a substance that breaks down lipids into their constituent fatty acids and monoglycerides

pancreatitis (PAN-kree-a-TIGH-tis) inflammation of the pancreas

papilla the rounded tip of a renal pyramid, through which collecting tubules discharge urine

papillae (pa-PIL-ee) bumps on the surface of the tongue, some of which house taste buds

papillary layer (PAP-i-LAIR-ee) the outer layer of the dermis

papillary muscle (PAP-i-LAIR-ee) one of the small muscular bundles attached at one end to the chordae tendineae and at the other to the innermost or endocardial wall of the ventricles; maintains tension on the chordae tendineae as the ventricle contracts

parallel a type of muscle fiber arrangement in which fibers run largely parallel to each other along the length of the muscle

paraplegia (PAIR-ah-PLEE-jee-a) disorder characterized by loss of function in the lower trunk and legs

parathyroid glands two pairs of glands located on the posterior aspect of the thyroid gland that secrete parathyroid hormone in response to low blood calcium levels

parathyroid hormone (PTH) hormone produced by the parathyroid glands that works with calcitonin to maintain calcium homeostasis

paravertebral ganglia (pair-a-VER-the-bral GAYNG-glee-a) mass of nerve cell bodies close to the spinal cord

parietal bones (pah-RIGH-eh-tal) bones that form the majority of the top and sides of the skull

parietal layer (pah-RIGH-eh-tal) membrane lining the interior of each body cavity

parietal lobes (pah-RIGH-eh-tal) sections of the brain located behind the frontal lobes; integrate sensory information from the skin, internal organs, muscles, and joints

parietal pleura (pah-RIGH-eh-tal) the membrane that lines the thoracic wall and diaphragm

Parkinson's disease a chronic nervous system disease characterized by a slowly spreading tremor, muscular weakness, and rigidity

partial-thickness burns see *first-* and *second-degree burns*

parturition childbirth

passive immunity immunity that comes from antibodies received from an outside source, such as breast milk

passive process a process that does not require the use of muscles

passive transport type of membrane transport that does not require energy

patella (pa-TEHL-a) kneecap

pathogens disease-causing agents

pectoral girdle (PEHK-toh-ral) bones surrounding the shoulder, including the clavicle and scapula; the *shoulder girdle*

pelvic cavity (PEHL-vik) internal opening that holds the reproductive and excretory organs

pelvic girdle (PEHL-vik) bony encasement of the pelvic region, formed by two large, strong coxal bones, (or hip bones), and the sacrum

pelvis bones of the pelvic girdle and the coccyx at the base of the spine

penis the reproductive organ that delivers sperm to the female reproductive tract

pennate a type of muscle fiber arrangement in which each fiber attaches obliquely to a central tendon

peptic ulcer a break in the protective lining of the stomach, duodenum, or lower esophagus that is caused by *Helicobacter pylori*

peptide bond the chemical bond that links two amino acids by connecting the amino group of one amino acid to the acid group of another

perforated septum a condition that causes one or more holes to develop in the septum

perforating (Volkmann's) canals large canals that connect the Haversian canals

perforins (PER-for-ins) proteins made and released by a T lymphocyte that join together to form a lethal pore in a target cell (similar to membrane attack complex)

pericarditis (PER-i-kahr-DIGH-tis) inflammation of the pericardial sac that surrounds the heart

pericardium (PER-i-KAR-dee-um) the membrane that surrounds the heart

perilymph (PER-i-limf) a clear fluid that fills the bony labyrinth

perimetrium (per-i-MEE-tree-um) the thin, membranous outer layer of the uterine wall

perimysium (PER-i-MIZ-ee-um) connective tissue sheath that envelops each primary bundle of muscle fibers

perineurium (PER-i-NOO-ree-um) a protective sheath that surrounds a bundle of nerve fibers

periodontal disease (PER-ee-oh-DAHN-tal) disease that affects the supporting structure of the teeth and the gums

periodontal ligament (PER-ee-oh-DAHN-tal) the fibrous connective tissue that covers the base of a tooth and holds it in place in the jawbone

periosteum (PER-ee-AHS-tee-um) fibrous connective tissue membrane that surrounds and protects the shaft (diaphysis) of long bones

peripheral chemoreceptors sensory receptor cells located in the aortic arch and carotid arteries that are sensitive to changes in blood oxygen level

peripheral nervous system (PNS) all parts of the nervous system external to the brain and spinal cord

peripheral neuropathy (noo-RAHP-a-thee) a disease or degenerative state of the peripheral nerves often associated with diabetes mellitus; marked by muscle weakness and atrophy, pain, and numbness

peripheral vascular disease (PAD) condition caused by a narrowing of the arteries in the legs

peristalsis (PER-i-STAHL-sis) a wave of symmetrical squeezing of the digestive tract walls that occurs during digestion

peritoneal cavity (PER-i-toh-NEE-al) the "empty space" between the parietal and visceral peritoneum

peritoneal dialysis a renal dialysis method that uses the patient's peritoneum to filter fluids and dissolved substances from the blood

peritoneum (PER-i-toh-NEE-um) the membrane that lines the abdominal cavity

peritonitis (PER-i-toh-NIGH-tis) inflammation of the peritoneum, the membrane lining the inner wall of the abdomen and covering the abdominal organs

peritubular capillaries (per-i-TOO-byuh-lar) capillaries that surround the proximal and distal convoluted tubules

pernicious anemia a severe anemia caused by the inability of the intestines to absorb vitamin B_{12}, which is essential for the formation of red blood cells; usually develops in older adults

Peyer's patches clusters of mucosa-associated lymphatic tissue (MALT) in the small intestine

pH a measure of the acidity or alkalinity of a solution

phagocytes (FAG-oh-sights) specialized white blood cells that engulf and consume bacteria, foreign material, and debris; distributed throughout the dermis

phagocytosis the process by which a cell engulfs and destroys foreign matter and cellular debris

phalanges (fa-LAN-jeez) bones of the fingers

pharyngeal tonsil (fa-RIN-jee-al) lymphatic tissue that lies at the back of the nasopharynx, the part of the throat above the palate, and opens into the nasal cavity; the *adenoid*

pharyngitis (FAIR-in-JIGH-tis) inflammation of the pharynx, or *throat*

pharynx (FAIR-ingks) the muscular passageway that extends from the nasal cavity to the mouth and connects to the esophagus; the *throat*

pheochromocytoma (FEE-oh-KROH-moh-sigh-TOH-ma) a tumor on the adrenal medulla, which causes hypersecretion of epinephrine and norepinephrine

phlebotomy (fleh-BAHT-oh-mee) the drawing of blood; a standard treatment for polycythemia

phospholipids a lipid containing phosphate group

phototherapy a medical treatment in which the skin is carefully exposed to ultraviolet light; *light therapy*

physiology (FIZ-ee-AHL-oh-jee) the study of how living things function or work

pia mater (PIGH-ah MAY-ter)   the delicate, innermost membrane of the brain, which attaches directly to the surface of the brain and the spinal cord

pineal gland (PI-nee-al)   a pinecone-shaped gland in the brain that releases the sleep-inducing hormone melatonin

pinna   see *auricle*

pituitary gland (pi-TOO-i-tair-ee)   a pea-sized gland that activates a metabolic response in target tissues or stimulates other endocrine glands to release hormones

pivot joint   type of diarthrosis that permits rotation around only one axis

placenta   the organ that grows in the uterus to meet the nutritional needs of the embryo and fetus

plantar flexion   downward motion of the foot away from the lower leg

plantar warts   warts that develop on the soles of the foot, grow inward, and can become painful

plaque   a sticky mixture of bacteria, food particles, and mucus

plasma   the liquid component of blood

plasma cells   activated B lymphocytes that produce antibodies, which circulate as free proteins in the blood

plasma membrane   the membrane that defines the outer shell of a cell

plastic   a response characterized by some amount of permanent deformation

platelet plug   gathering of platelets that forms a small mass at the site of an injury

platelets   part of the formed elements of the blood; play a vital role in blood clotting

pleura (PLOO-ra)   the membrane that encases the lungs

pleural sac   the thin, double-walled serous membrane that surrounds the lungs

pleurisy (PLOOR-i-see)   inflammation of the pleura, the membrane that encases the lungs

plexuses   complex interconnections of nerves

pneumonia (noo-MOH-nee-ah)   an infection of the lungs that causes inflammation; caused by a virus, bacterium, fungus, or—in rare cases—parasites

podocytes (PAHD-oh-sights)   "foot cells" that wrap around capillaries in the glomerular capsule

polarized   a condition that occurs when the inside of a cell membrane is more negatively charged than the outside

polycythemia (PAHL-ee-sigh-THEE-mee-a)   a condition in which the bone marrow manufactures too many red blood cells; caused by prolonged altitude exposure and a genetic mutation

polydipsia (pahl-i-DIP-see-a)   excessive thirst to replenish water lost through polyuria

polymer   a molecule made of many similar subunits

polypeptide   a long chain of amino acids

polyphagia (pahl-ee-FAY-jee-a)   increased hunger to replace fats and proteins used as fuel sources

polyspermy   fertilization of an oocyte by more than one sperm

polyuria (pahl-ee-YOOR-ee-a)   excessive urination to eliminate glucose from the body

polyunsaturated fats   one category of unsaturated fatty acids; sources include corn oil and soybean oil

pons (pahnz)   the section of the brain that plays a role in regulating breathing

pores of Kohn (kohn)   small openings in the alveolar walls that allow gases and macrophages to travel between the alveoli

positive feedback   mechanism that further increases a condition that has exceeded the normal homeostatic range

posterior (dorsal) body cavity   continuous internal opening located near the back of the body that includes the cranial and spinal cavities

posterior pituitary   one lobe of the pituitary gland that stores two hormones produced by the hypothalamus: antidiuretic hormone and oxytocin

postganglionic neuron (POHST-gayng-glee-AHN-ik)   the second neuron in a series that transmits impulses from the CNS

precapillary sphincter (pree-KAP-i-LAIR-ee SFINGK-ter)   a band of smooth muscle fibers that encircles the capillaries at the arteriole-capillary junctions and controls blood flow to the tissues

precipitation   the formation of an insoluble complex, such as a clump of antigen molecules joined together by antibodies

preganglionic neuron (PREE-gayng-glee-AHN-ik)   the first neuron in a series that transmits impulses from the CNS

premature atrial contractions (PACs)   condition in which an irritable piece of atrial heart tissue fires before the SA node causing the atria to contract too soon

premature ventricular contractions (PVCs)   condition in which Purkinje fibers fire before the SA node, causing the ventricles to contract prematurely

prepuce (PREE-pyoos)   the foreskin of the penis

presbycusis (PREHZ-bee-KYOO-sis)   age-related hearing loss

presbyopia (PREZ-bee-OH-pee-a)   an age-related version of farsightedness

pressure   force distributed over a given area

pressure ulcers   see *decubitus ulcers*

primary bronchi (BRAHNG-kigh)   the two passageways that branch off the trachea and lead to the right and left lungs

primary follicle   an ovarian follicle in which the primary oocyte develops

primary immune response   the initial immune system response to a foreign invader such as a virus or bacterium

primary motor cortex   outer region of the brain in the frontal lobes that sends neural impulses to the skeletal muscles

primary somatic sensory cortex   outer region of the brain in the parietal lobes that interprets sensory impulses received from the skin, internal organs, muscles, and joints

primary spinal curves   those spinal curves present at birth, including the thoracic and sacral curves

primordial follicle   the structure that is formed when the primary oocyte is surrounded by a single layer of follicle cells in the ovarian follicle

progesterone (proh-JES-teh-rohn)   a hormone produced by the ovaries in women to help regulate the menstrual cycle and promote breast development in puberty

prolactin   a trophic hormone that stimulates the growth of mammary glands and milk production in a nursing mother

prolactin-releasing factor   a hormone that triggers the release of prolactin, which stimulates the secretory cells of the mammary glands to produce milk

proliferative phase   the phase of the uterine cycle during which the functional layer of the endometrium grows back after having been shed in the menstrual phase

pronation   medial rotation of the forearm (palm down)

prophase   the first stage of cell division, during which the chromosomes become visible and the nuclear membrane disintegrates

propulsion the movement of food through the gastrointestinal tract that is stimulated by swallowing at the pharynx and peristalsis, muscular contractions that move food through the rest of the GI tract

prostaglandins (PRAHS-ta-GLAN-dins) fatty acids involved in the control of inflammation, smooth-muscle contractions, and body temperature

prostate gland the gland that sits directly under the bladder and surrounds the beginning of the urethra in the male; produces about one-third of the fluid volume of semen

protein a large biological molecule made of chains of dozens to hundreds of amino acids

proteinuria protein in the urine; often a sign of kidney damage

provitamin D3 cholesterol molecules in the skin that are converted into vitamin D when exposed to UVB rays

proximal convoluted tubule the part of the nephron between the glomerular capsule and the nephron loop; minerals, nutrients, and water are reabsorbed from the filtrate here

proximal radioulnar joint joint between the radius and ulna close to the elbow

psoriasis (soh-RIGH-a-sis) a common skin disorder that involves redness, irritation, and scales (flaky, silver-white patches) that itch, burn, crack, and sometimes bleed

pubis (PYOO-bis) anterior portion of each coxal bone

pubis symphysis (PYOO-bis) joint in the center front of the body where the two pubic bones fuse and are joined by a disc of hyaline cartilage

pulmonary circulation (PUL-muh-NAIR-ee) circulation of oxygen-poor blood from the right ventricle, through the lungs, and returning to the left atrium with oxygen-rich blood

pulmonary valve (PUL-muh-NAIR-ee) a valve located at the opening of the pulmonary artery on the right side of the heart

pulmonary ventilation the process of continuously moving air in and out of the lungs

pulp cavity a hollow, central region in the tooth that contains soft tissue, nerves, and blood vessels

pupil the opening through which light rays enter the eye

Purkinje fibers (per-KIN-jee) part of the impulse-conducting network of the heart that rapidly transmits impulses throughout the ventricles causing ventricular contraction

pus a combination of neutrophils, cellular debris, and fluids

pyelonephritis (PIGH-eh-loh-neh-FRIGH-tis) inflammation of the kidney and/or ureter, usually due to the spread of a bacterial infection from the bladder

pylorus (pi-LOR-us) the opening from the stomach into the small intestine

pyrogens (PIGH-roh-jehns) chemicals that tend to cause fever by raising the set-point temperature of the neurons in the hypothalamus

Q

quadriplegia (KWAH-dri-PLEE-jee-a) disorder characterized by the loss of function below the neck

quiescent inactive

R

radial artery the artery located on the thumb side of the wrist where the radial pulse is detected

radial deviation rotation of the hand toward the thumb

radiocarpal joint joint between the radius and the carpal bones of the wrist

radius (RAY-dee-us) smaller of the two bones in the forearm; rotates around the ulna

reabsorption the movement of water and dissolved substances from the filtrate (in a renal tubule) back into the blood

receptor transmitter that senses environmental changes

rectum the short, final segment of the digestive tube; its lower end is the anal canal

red blood cells part of the formed elements of the blood; contain hemoglobin, a protein responsible for oxygen and carbon dioxide exchange; *erythrocytes*

redness a sign of inflammation

reflexes simple, rapid, involuntary, programmed responses to stimuli

refractory period (ree-FRAK-toh-ree) the time between the completion of the action potential and repolarization

regular dense connective tissue a type of connective tissue composed primarily of collagen fibers oriented parallel to one another

remodeling process through which adult bone can change in density, strength, and sometimes shape

renal columns inward extensions of cortex-like tissue that separate the renal pyramids from each other

renal corpuscle (KOR-puh-suhl) the part of a nephron that consists of a glomerular capsule with its included glomerulus

renal cortex the lighter-colored, outer layer of the kidney that contains the glomeruli and convoluted tubules

renal dialysis (digh-AL-i-sis) the removal of wastes from the blood by artificial means

renal hilum (REE-nal HIGH-lum) the indentation on the medial surface of each kidney, where blood vessels and the ureter enter and leave

renal medulla the darker, innermost part of the kidney

renal pelvis a funnel-shaped cavity in the center of the kidney where urine collects before it flows into the ureter

renal pyramids cone-shaped masses that form the medullary substance of the kidney

renal tubule (TOO-byool) the part of a nephron that leads away from a glomerulus and empties into a collecting tubule; consists of a proximal convoluted tubule, nephron loop, and distal convoluted tubule

renin (REE-nin) an enzyme made and secreted by the kidneys; aids in the production of angiotensin

repolarization the reestablishment of a polarized state in a cell after depolarization

repolarize to relax; the atria and ventricles repolarize as the heart beats

research question a question to be answered or a problem to be solved in a research study

residual volume (RV) the volume of air that never leaves the lungs, even after the most forceful expiration

respiration the process by which the lungs provide oxygen to body tissues and dispose of carbon dioxide; *breathing*

respiratory gas transport the process by which oxygen and carbon dioxide are transported to and from the lungs and tissues

respiratory zone the collective name for the respiratory bronchioles, alveolar ducts, and alveoli

reticular connective tissue (reh-TIK-yoo-lar) a type of tissue that contains reticular fibers and is found in lymph nodes, bone marrow, and the spleen

reticular formation (reh-TIK-yoo-lar) a collection of gray matter that extends the length of the brain stem

reticular layer the layer of skin superficial to the papillary layer

retina the innermost layer of the eye, containing light-sensitive nerve endings that send impulses through the optic nerves to the brain

retroperitoneal (REHT-roh-PER-i-toh-NEE-al) located behind the peritoneum, the membrane that lines the abdominopelvic cavity

Rh factor the antigen of the Rh blood group that is found on the surface of red blood cells; people with the Rh factor are Rh⁺ and those lacking it are Rh⁻

rheumatoid arthritis autoimmune disorder in which the body's own immune system attacks healthy joint tissues; the most debilitating and painful form of arthritis

rhinitis (righ-NIGH-tis) inflammation of the mucous membranes that line the nasal passage

rhinoplasty reconstructive or cosmetic surgery of the nose to correct its form or function

RhoGAM an immune serum that prevents a mother's blood from becoming sensitized to foreign antibodies from her fetus

ribosomal RNA the major ingredient in ribosomes (protein is the other ingredient); *rRNA*

ribosomes (RIGH-boh-sohmz) very large enzymes that make polypeptides

right bronchomediastinal trunk (BRAHN-koh-MEE-dee-as-tin-al) duct that drains lymph from the right side of the chest and lower neck

right bundle branches the right leg or branch through which electrical impulses are transmitted from the bundle of His through the right ventricle

right jugular trunk duct that drains lymph from the right side of the head

right lumbar trunk duct carrying lymph from the right lower body toward the cisterna chyli

right subclavian trunk (sub-KLAY-vee-an) duct that drains lymph from the right arm

RNA one of two kinds of information-carrying nucleic acids found in cells; *ribonucleic acid*

RNA polymerase (pahl-IM-er-ays) the enzyme that makes an RNA molecule complementary to a gene on DNA

rods sensory cells in the retina that are activated in dim light

root canal a hollow cavity in the tooth that provides a passageway for nerves and blood vessels to reach the pulp cavity from the jaw bone

rough endoplasmic reticulum membranous network in the cytoplasm that is involved in protein synthesis

round window a membrane-covered opening beneath the oval window of the middle ear

rule of nines a method used in calculating body surface area affected by burns

S

saccharides (SAK-a-righd) sugar and starch molecules; *carbohydrates*

sacroiliac joint (SA-kroh-IL-ee-ak) joint between the sacrum and each ilium

sacrum (SAY-krum) five fused vertebrae that form the posterior of the pelvic girdle

saddle joint type of diarthrosis in which the articulating bone surfaces are both shaped like the seat of a riding saddle

sagittal plane (SAJ-i-tal) an invisible, vertical flat surface that divides the body into right and left halves

sagittal plane movements (SAJ-i-tal) forward and backward motions of the body or body segments

saliva a clear, tasteless, odorless fluid secreted from glands in the oral cavity

salivary glands the saliva-secreting exocrine glands of the oral cavity

saltatory conduction (SAWL-ta-TOH-ree) the rapid skipping of an action potential from node to node on myelinated neurons

salty one of the five basic tastes

sarcolemma (SAR-koh-LEHM-a) the delicate membrane surrounding each striated muscle fiber

sarcomeres (SAR-koh-mairz) units composed of actin and myosin that contract inside the muscle fiber

satellite cells glial cells that provide cushioning and support for a neuron

saturated fatty acids that have all single bonds

scales the flaky, silver-white patches that appear in cases of psoriasis

scapula (SKAP-yoo-la) shoulder blade

scapulothoracic joint (skap-yoo-loh-thoh-RAS-ik) joint between each scapula and the underlying tissues of the thorax; not a true joint

Schwann cells (shwahnn) units that form the fatty myelin sheaths around nerve fibers in the parasympathetic nervous system

science a systematic process that creates new knowledge and organizes it into a form of testable explanations and predictions about an aspect of our universe

scientific method a systematic process that can be used to answer questions or find solutions to problems

scientific research hypothesis an educated guess about what the outcome of a study will be

scientific theory an explanation of some aspect of the natural world that is based on rigorously tested, repeatedly confirmed research

sclera (SKLER-a) the tough, fibrous outer layer of the eye

scrotum a sac that encases the pair of oval testes

sebaceous glands (seh-BAY-shus) glands located all over the body that produce sebum

sebum (SEE-bum) an oily substance that helps to keep the skin and hair soft

secondary bronchi bronchi that arise from the primary bronchi and lead to the tertiary bronchi

secondary follicle a maturing ovarian follicle that contains the oocyte surrounded by layers of granulosa cells

secondary immune response immune system response to an infectious agent that it has encountered before

secondary oocyte a cell produced by division of a primary oocyte in the first stage of meiosis

secondary spinal curves those spinal curves that develop after birth, including the cervical and lumbar curves

second-degree burns burns that involve damage to both the epidermis and the upper portion of the underlying dermis; characterized by blisters

second-degree heart block a heart block in which the impulse from the SA node is intermittently blocked

secretion the active movement of substances from the blood into the filtrate, which will become urine

secretory phase the phase of the uterine cycle after ovulation, during which the uterine glands secrete mucus, under the influence of progesterone secreted by the corpus luteum

self-antigen normal protein antigen on the surface of a body cell; does not normally cause an immune reaction

semen the fluid that contains sperm, which is delivered to the female during intercourse; *penile ejaculate*

semicircular canals (SEHM-ee-SIR-kyoo-lar) inner ear channels containing receptor hair cells that play an important role in balance

semilunar valves (SEHM-ee-LOO-nar) valves situated at the opening between the heart and the aorta and at the opening between the heart and the pulmonary artery; they prevent backflow of blood into the ventricles

seminal glands glands that produce up to 70% of the volume of semen; *seminal vesicles*

seminal vesicles glands that produce up to 70% of the volume of semen; *seminal glands*

seminiferous tubules small tubes in the testes in which sperm form

sensory neurons transmitters that carry impulses from the skin and organs to the spinal cord and brain; *afferent neurons*

separase a protein that splits the sister chromatids by cutting the centromeres in half

septum the structure made of cartilage that divides the left and right air passages in the nose

serosa (seh-ROH-sa) the outermost layer of the alimentary canal

serous fluid a thin, clear liquid that serves as a lubricant between parietal and visceral membranes

serous membranes (ser-us) thin sheets of tissues that line body cavities that are closed to the outside world

sex hormones estrogens (female) and androgens (male)

sexual reproduction a method of reproduction that involves two parents, with each parent contributing half the genetic material for their offspring

sexually transmitted disease an infectious disease transmitted through sexual contact; *sexually transmitted infection*

shear a force that acts along a surface and perpendicular to the length of a structure

shingles a disease that involves a painful, blistering rash accompanied by headache, fever, and a general feeling of unwellness; *herpes zoster*

shin splints the name for pain localized to the anterior lower leg

short bones bones that are nearly cubicle in shape, such as the bones of the wrist and ankle

shoulder complex all joints surrounding the shoulder, including the acromioclavicular, sternoclavicular, and glenohumeral joints

shoulder girdle bones surrounding the shoulder, including the clavicle and scapula; *pectoral girdle*

sickle cell anemia a disease in which the red blood cells are shaped like a sickle, or crescent, rather than a disk; caused by irregularly shaped hemoglobin molecules in the red blood cells

side bending movements within lateral flexion

sigmoid colon (SIG-moyd) final segment of the colon, between the descending colon and the rectum

simple columnar epithelium epithelium with a single layer of columnar cells

simple cuboidal epithelium epithelium with a single layer of cuboidal cells

simple epithelia epithelium with a single layer of cells

simple squamous epithelium (SKWAH-mus) epithelium with a single layer of flattened cells

single nucleotide polymorphism base locations that tend to vary; *SNPs*

sinoatrial node (SA node) (SIGH-noh-AY-tree-al) a small mass of specialized tissue located in the right atrium that normally acts as the pacemaker of the heart, causing it to beat at a rate between 60 and 100 bpm; *pacemaker*

sinuses the air-filled cavities that surround the nose

sinusitis (SIGH-nus-IGH-tis) inflammation of the sinuses

skeletal muscle voluntary muscle that is usually attached to bone and helps us to move

skeletal physiology the study of how the skeleton functions internally

skull the part of the skeleton composed of all of the bones of the head

slow-twitch type of muscle that contracts slowly and is fatigue resistant

small intestine the portion of the digestive tract where most of the chemical breakdown of food, food absorption, and water absorption occurs; the longest segment of the GI tract

smooth ER a site where "replacement" membrane is made for membranous structures in the cell

smooth muscle involuntary muscle found in the walls of hollow organs

soft palate (PAL-at) the posterior part of the palate that is made of muscle

somatic nervous system branch of the nervous system that stimulates the skeletal muscles

somatic reflexes involuntary stimuli transmitted to skeletal muscles from neural arcs in the spinal cord

sour one of the five basic tastes

specific immune system see *immune system*

sperm (singular or plural) the male gamete; a haploid cell that can fertilize an egg to make a zygote

spermatids (SPER-mat-ids) immature sperm cells

spermatogenesis (sper-mat-oh-JEHN-e-sis) sperm formation

spermatogonia (sper-mat-oh-GOH-nee-a) stem cells in the male that undergo mitosis; similar to oogonia in females

sphenoidal sinuses (sfee-NOY-dal) two irregular cavities in the body of the sphenoid bone that communicate with the nasal cavities

sphenoid bone (SFEE-noyd) butterfly shaped bone, centrally located within the skull, that supports part of the base of the brain, forms part of the orbits of the eyes, and is connected to all of the other bones of the skull

sphincter pupillae (pyoo-PIL-ay) a muscle of the iris which causes a contraction of the pupil in bright light

spinal cavity the internal opening that houses the spinal cord

spinal cord a column of nerve tissue that extends from the brain stem to the beginning of the lumbar region of the spine

spinal nerves neural transmitters that branch from the left and right sides of the spinal cord

spinous process bony projections on the posterior of each vertebra

spirometer (spigh-RAHM-eh-ter) a device used for measuring static lung volumes

spleen the largest lymphatic organ in the body, located in the abdomen below the diaphragm; filters blood and activates an immune response if necessary

spongy urethra the longest part of the male urethra

spontaneous abortion the naturally occurring premature termination of pregnancy

sprain injuries caused by abnormal motion of the articulating bones that result in overstretching or tearing of ligaments, tendons, or other connective tissues crossing a joint

squamous cell carcinoma (KAR-si-NOH-ma) a type of rapidly growing cancer that appears as a scaly, reddened patch of skin

squamous epithelia almost–flat epithelia

SRY gene on the Y chromosome that acts as a switch to cause development of male sex organs; *sex-determining region Y*

stapes see *stirrup*

static lung volume lung volume that measures volume only

statistical inference the practice of generalizing the findings of a research study to a large population

statistical significance an interpretation of statistical data indicating that the results of a study can legitimately be generalized to the population represented in the study sample

stent a circular, hollow, wire mesh tube

sternoclavicular joint (STER-noh-kla-VIK-yoo-lar) joint between the sternum (breast bone) and clavicle (collar bone)

sternum (STER-num) breastbone

steroid hormones lipid (fat-based) hormones

steroids a class of lipids with a structure that is different from other lipids; cholesterol, testosterone, and estrogen are three well-known steroids

stirrup tiny bone in the middle ear that attaches to the anvil on one side and the oval window on the other

stomach the reservoir in which food is broken down mechanically and chemically before it enters the small intestine

strabismus (strah-BIZ-mus) a condition that causes one eye to drift in different directions due to the malfunctioning of the extrinsic muscles of the eye

stratified epithelia epithelium with multiple layers of cells

stratified squamous epithelia epithelium with multiple layers of cells, the outermost layer of which are flattened; found where chemical and mechanical protection are most needed

stratum basale the deepest layer of the epidermis

stratum corneum the outer layer of the epidermis

stratum granulosum a layer of somewhat flattened cells lying just superficial to the stratum spinosum and inferior to the stratum lucidum

stratum lucidum the clear layer of thick skin found only on the palms of the hands, fingers, soles of the feet, and toes

stratum spinosum the layer of cells in the epidermis superior to the stratum basale and inferior to the stratum granulosum

stress force distribution inside a structure

stress fracture tiny, painful crack in bone that results from overuse

stretch receptors mechanoreceptors in the bronchioles and alveoli that are sensitive to stretching and prevent over inflation of the alveolar sacs and stimulate expiration

stroke a sudden blockage of blood flow, or rupture of an artery in the brain, that causes brain cells to die from lack of oxygen

stroke volume the volume of blood pumped from the heart per beat

styloid process (STIGH-loyd) bony projection on the distal lateral end of each radius and ulna; easy to see and feel

subcutaneous fascia (sub-kyoo-TAY-nee-us FASH-a) see *hypodermis*

submucosa (SUB-myoo-KOH-sa) a layer of irregular, dense connective tissue containing blood vessels, lymphatic vessels, and nerves

sudoriferous glands (SOO-doh-RIF-er-us) sweat glands that are distributed in the dermis over the entire body

sulcus (SUL-kus) a groove between adjacent gyri on the outer surface of the brain

superior above or over

superior articular processes indentations on the top side of each vertebra that form a facet joint with the above vertebra

superior vena cava second largest vein in the body that returns deoxygenated blood to the right atrium of the heart from the upper half of the body

supination (SOO-pi-NAY-shun) lateral rotation of the forearm (palm up)

suppressor T cell T lymphocyte that prevents the cellular immune response from being too strong or too long-lasting

surfactant a phospholipid that reduces the surface tension in the alveoli and prevents them from collapsing

suspensory ligaments tiny structures that attach the lens of the eye to the ciliary body

sutures joints in which irregularly grooved, articulating bone sheets join closely and are tightly connected by fibrous tissues

sweet one of the five basic tastes

swelling a sign of inflammation

swimmer's ear a bacterial or fungal infection of the auditory canal caused by immersion in contaminated water

symphysis (SIM-fi-sis) type of amphiarthrosis joint in which a thin plate of hyaline cartilage separates a disc of fibrocartilage from the bones

synapse (SIN-aps) the intersection between a neuron and another neuron, a muscle, a gland, or a sensory receptor

synaptic cleft (si-NAP-tik) a microscopic gap that separates axon terminals from other neurons or muscle fiber

synarthrosis (SIN-ar-THROH-sis) fibrous joint that can absorb shock, but permits little or no movement of the articulating bones

synchondrosis (SIN-kahn-DROH-sis) type of amphiarthrosis joint in which the articulating bones are held together by a thin layer of hyaline cartilage

syndesmosis (SIN-dehz-MOH-sis) joint at which dense fibrous tissue binds the bones together, permitting extremely limited movement

synovial fluid (si-NOH-vee-al) a clear liquid secreted by synovial membranes that provides cushioning for and reduces friction in synovial joints

synovial joint (si-NOH-vee-al) a diarthrodial joint

synovial membrane (si-NOH-vee-al) the lining of the synoival joint cavity that produces synovial fluid

systemic circulation circulation of oxygenated blood through the arteries, capillaries, and veins of the circulatory system, from the left ventricle to the right atrium

systole (SIS-toh-lee) a period of contraction when the chambers are pumping blood out of the heart

T

T cells see *T lymphocytes*

T lymphocytes group of white blood cells that are part of the immune system; complete their maturation in the thymus before moving into the blood and the rest of the body; *T cells*

tachycardia (TAK-i-KAHR-dee-a) a normal rhythm, but with a rate above 100 bpm

talus (TAY-lus) second largest of the tarsal bones of the ankle (next to the calcaneus)

tanning the result of exposure to sunlight and the production of melanin

tarsal glands (TAR-sal) secretors of an oily substance; located in the eyelids

tarsals (TAR-salz) bones of the ankle

tartar hardened plaque

tastants (TAYS-tehnts) compounds that stimulate the gustatory hairs to send nerve impulses to the brain

taste buds sensory receptors for taste

taste pores very small openings in the top of the taste buds through which gustatory hairs project

tectorial membrane (tek-TOR-ee-al) a gelatinous covering over the surface of the organ of Corti

temporal bone (TEHM-poh-ral) bone that surrounds the ear

temporal lobes (TEHM-poh-ral) the most inferior portions of the brain; responsible for speech, hearing, vision, memory, and emotion

tendinitis inflammation of a tendon, usually accompanied by pain and swelling

tendinosis degeneration of a tendon believed to be caused by microtears in the tendon connective tissue

tendon tissue band composed of collagen and elastic fibers that connects a muscle to a bone

tendon sheaths double-layered synovial structures surrounding tendons subject to friction given their position close to bones; secrete synovial fluid to promote free motion of the tendons during joint movement

tensile strength the ability to withstand tension (outward pulling force) without tearing or breaking

tension a pulling force that creates tension in the structure to which it is applied

tertiary bronchi bronchi that arise from the secondary bronchi and lead to the bronchioles

testes (TEHS-teez) the male sex glands

testosterone male sex hormone that is primarily secreted by the testes in men and ovaries in women and is responsible for the development of male sex characteristics

tetanus a sustained, maximal level of muscle tension that occurs with high-frequency stimulation

tetany (TET-a-nee) a condition of sustained muscular contraction

thalamus (THAL-a-mus) the largest portion of the diencephalon, which communicates sensory and motor information between the body and the cerebral cortex

third-degree burns burns that destroy the entire thickness of the skin

third-degree heart block a heart block in which the impulse from the SA node is completely blocked

thoracic cage (thoh-RAS-ik) bony structure surrounding the heart and lungs in the thoracic cavity; composed of the ribs, sternum, and thoracic vertebrae

thoracic cavity (thoh-RAS-ik) the internal opening that houses the heart and lungs

thoracic region (thoh-RAS-ik) the twelve vertebrae in the middle of the back

thoracolumbar division (THOH-rah-koh-LUM-bar) the sympathetic system of nerves that lies near the thoracic and lumbar regions of the spine

thrombin (THRAHM-bin) an enzyme that combines with the protein fibrinogen to create fibrin

thrombocytes platelets

thrombopoietin (THRAHM-boh-POY-eh-tin) a hormone that regulates platelet production

thymosin (THIGH-muh-sin) a hormone secreted by the thymus that is essential for the development of white blood cells (T cells)

thymus gland a gland that secretes thymosin, a hormone vital to the body's immune system; functions as both an endocrine gland and a lymphatic organ

thyroid cartilage the largest cartilaginous plate in the larynx; *Adam's apple*

thyroid gland gland located below the larynx, or *Adam's apple,* that secretes thyroid hormones (T_3 and T_4) and calcitonin

thyroid hormone hormone secreted by the thyroid gland that is responsible for the regulation of metabolism

thyroiditis (thigh-royd-IGHT-is) inflammation of the thyroid gland

thyroid-stimulating hormone (TSH) a tropic hormone secreted by the anterior pituitary that acts on the thyroid gland to release two thyroid hormones, thyroxine and triiodothyronine

thyroxine (T_4) (thigh-RAHK-seen) hormone found in thyroid hormone that is responsible for controlling the rate of energy metabolism and heat production

tibia (TIB-ee-a) major weight-bearing bone of the lower leg

tidal volume (TV) the amount of air inhaled in a normal breath

tinea (TIN-ee-a) a fungal infection that tends to occur in areas of the body that are moist

tinea corporis a fungal infection that is characterized by a red, ring-shaped rash with a pale center; *ringworm*

tinea cruris a fungal infection that primarily affects males around the groin and scrotum; *jock itch*

tinea pedis the most common fungal infection, characterized by cracked, flaky skin between the toes or on the side of the foot; *athlete's foot*

tinea unguium a fungal infection under the nails of the fingers or toes; *fungal nail infection*

tinnitus (TIN-i-tus) a condition that causes a sound like ringing to be heard in the ear

tissues organized groups of similar cells

tolerance reduction or elimination of the allergic response, which may occur after immunotherapy

tonsils clusters of lymphatic tissue in the pharynx that function as the first line of defense against infection

tonsillitis (TAHN-si-LIGH-tis) inflammation of the tonsils

torque (TORK) the rotary effect of a force

torsion (TOR-shun) a loading pattern that can cause a structure to twist about its length

total lung capacity (TLC) a combination of the vital capacity plus the residual volume; IRV + FRV + RV

trabecular bone (tra-BEHK-yoo-lar) interior, spongy bone with a porous, honeycomb structure

trachea (TRAY-kee-a) the air tube that extends from the larynx into the thorax, where it splits into the right and left bronchi; *windpipe*

transcription factor a protein that controls when genes are switched on or off

transfer RNA a molecule that binds to the mRNA- ribosome complex and helps assemble amino acids into polypeptides

transient ischemic attack (TIA) (is-KEE-mik) a temporary lack of blood flow to the brain

transitional epithelium stratified epithelium found in the lining of hollow organs that can stretch

trans-unsaturated fats one category of unsaturated fatty acids that are artificially produced; *trans fats*

transverse arch arch running sideways across the bottom of the foot

transverse colon the mostly horizontal segment of the colon between the ascending and descending colon

transverse plane an invisible, horizontal flat surface that divides the body into top and bottom halves

transverse plane movements rotational motions of the body or body segments

transverse processes bony projections on the lateral sides of the vertebral arches

traumatic brain injury mild or severe trauma that can result from a violent impact to the head

tricuspid valve (trigh-KUS-pid) the valve that closes the orifice between the right atrium and right ventricle of the heart; composed of three cusps

triglycerides (trigh-GLIS-er-ighdz) compounds composed of a glycerol molecule with three fatty acids attached

trigone (TRIGH-gohn) the triangular region of the bladder formed by the two ureteric orifices and the urethra

triiodothyronine (T$_3$) (trigh-ah-doh-THAIR-oh-neen) hormone found in thyroid hormone that is responsible for controlling the rate of energy metabolism and heat production; a more potent hormone than *thyroxine*

trophoblast cells (TROH-foh-blast) cells on the outer layer of the blastocyst that nourish the embryo and aid in implantation

tropic hormones (TROH-pik) pituitary hormones that act on other endocrine glands; *tropins*

true ribs ribs having a bony articulation with the sternum

tuberculosis a highly contagious bacterial infection caused by *Myobacterium tuberculosis*

tunica externa (TOO-ni-ka) the outermost layer of a blood vessel composed mostly of fibrous connective tissue that supports and protects the vessel

tunica intima (TOO-ni-ka) the innermost layer of a blood vessel composed of a single layer of squamous epithelial cells over a sheet of connective tissue; its smooth, frictionless surface allows blood to flow smoothly through the vessel

tunica media the thicker middle layer of a blood vessel that contains smooth muscle cells, elastic fibers, and collagen; its muscle cells are directed by the sympathetic nervous system to increase or decrease blood flow to tissues as needed

tympanic cavity (tim-PAN-ik) see *middle ear cavities*

tympanic membrane (tim-PAN-ik) a sheet of tissue at the end of the auditory canal; the *eardrum*

type I diabetes mellitus a form of insulin-dependent diabetes in which the body produces an insufficient amount of insulin or no insulin at all; *juvenile-onset diabetes*

type II diabetes mellitus a form of diabetes (typically non-insulin-dependent) that develops most often in obese individuals and results from the body's inability to efficiently move glucose from the bloodstream; *adult-onset diabetes*

U

ulcer a break in the lining of the stomach, duodenum, or lower esophagus

ulcerative colitis (koh-LIGH-tis) an inflammatory bowel disease that usually affects the colon and the mucosal layer of the intestinal wall

ulna (UHL-nuh) larger bone of the lower arm

ulnar deviation rotation of the hand toward the little finger

umami one of the five basic tastes

umbilical cord the cord that connects the fetus to the placenta

unicellular exocrine gland isolated secretory cells in an epithelium

unipolar neurons nerve cells that have a single axon with dendrites on the peripheral end and axon terminals on the central end

universal donor a person with type O blood; type O blood has no antigens that can be attacked by the host's blood, so it can be donated to anyone

universal recipient a person with type AB blood; type AB blood has neither A nor B antibodies, so a universal recipient can safely receive a transfusion of any blood type

unsaturated term that describes fatty acids that have one or more double bonds

upper extremity bones of the shoulders, arms, and hands

upregulated increased

ureter (YOOR-eht-er) a duct through which urine travels from the kidney to the bladder

ureteric orifices the two openings of the ureters into the bladder; one opening lies at each corner of the trigone

urethra (yoo-REE-thra) a thin tube that connects the urinary bladder to the outside environment

urinalysis laboratory analysis of urine to test for the presence of disease

urinary bladder a hollow, muscular organ that stores urine; *bladder*

urinary system the organs involved in the formation, storage, and excretion of urine; includes the kidneys, ureters, bladder, and urethra

urinary tract infection (UTI) an infection of the urethra, bladder, ureters, and/or kidney, usually caused by bacteria that enter the urethra at its outside opening

urine specific gravity the density (mass per unit volume) of urine, divided by the density of pure water

urogenital diaphragm (yoor-oh-JEHN-i-tal) a double layer of pelvic muscle that encircles the urethral sphincters

uterine cycle the monthly cycle of changes that the uterus undergoes; includes the menstrual, proliferative, and secretory phases

uterine fibroids benign tumors of the muscular layer of the uterus

uterine tubes (YOOT-er-in) tubes in which the oocyte is fertilized; begin at the lateral end of the ovary and curve up and around the ovary to terminate at the top lateral portion of the uterus

uterus (YOOT-er-us) a hollow, muscular organ located in front of the rectum and behind the bladder; the *womb*

uvula (YOO-vyoo-la) a fleshy mass at the end of the oral cavity that helps prevent food from entering the nasal cavity

V

vaccination the introduction of a foreign substance to the body for the purpose of inducing immunity

vacuum-assisted closure treatment for a bedsore that involves a vacuum drawing moisture from the ulcer

vagina a thin-walled, tubular structure below the uterus; *birth canal*

vagus nerve (VAY-gus) one of three cranial nerves that is responsible for transmitting taste sensations to the brain

valvular stenosis a narrowing of the heart valve due to stiff or fused valve cusps

vas deferens (vas DEHF-eh-rehnz) see *ductus deferens*

vasa recta thin-walled blood vessels that begin and end near the boundary between the renal cortex and the renal medulla, and which extend deep into the renal medulla, running parallel to the nephron loops; play a role in the formation of concentrated urine

vasoconstrict (VA-soh-KUN-strikt) to decrease the opening of the lumen

vasoconstriction (VA-soh-kun-STRIK-shun) narrowing of the lumen of the blood vessels, which decreases blood flow

vasodilate (VA-soh-DIGH-layt) to increase the opening of the lumen

vasodilation (VA-soh-digh-LAY-shun) widening of the lumen of blood vessels, which increases blood flow

vasopressin see *antidiuretic hormone (ADH)*

veins vessels that carry blood to the heart

ventral ramus (VEHN-tral RAY-mus) the anterior division of spinal nerves that communicate with the muscle and skin of the anterior and lateral trunk

ventricular fibrillation a life-threatening condition in which the heart ventricles quiver at a rate greater than 350 bpm

ventricular tachycardia (ven-TRIK-yoo-lar tak-i-KARD-ee-a) a life-threatening arrhythmia in which the ventricles, rather than the SA node, initiate the heartbeat; the heart rate is between 150 and 250 bpm, requiring swift medical attention

venules (VEN-yools) the smallest veins that connect the capillaries with the larger systemic veins

vertebra (VER-teh-bra) one of the bones making up the spinal column

vertebral arch (VER-teh-bral) round projection of bone on the posterior aspect of the vertebra which surrounds a hole known as the *vertebral foramen*, through which the spinal cord passes

vertebral body (VER-teh-bral) solid, disc-shaped portion on the anterior side of a vertebra, which bears most of the weight positioned above it

vertebral foramen (VER-teh-bral foh-RAY-mehn) hole in the center of the vertebral arch, through which the spinal cord passes

vertex presentation normal position of the fetus in which the head exits the mother's body first

vertigo severe dizziness

vesicular follicle a mature ovarian follicle that contains a fluid-filled cavity and that ruptures during ovulation to release an egg

vestibular region the area at the front of the nasal cavity, just inside the naris

vestibule (VEHS-ti-byool) (1) a chamber in the inner ear that contains the three semicircular canals; (2) the recessed area in which the vaginal and urethral openings lie

vestibulocochlear nerve (vehs-TIB-yoo-loh-KAHK-lee-ar) a cranial nerve comprised of the cochlear nerve and the vestibular nerve

visceral layer membrane covering each organ within a body cavity

visceral pleura (PLOO-ra) the membrane that lines the lungs and dips into the fissures

vital capacity (VC) the total amount of air that can be forcibly expired from the lungs after a maximum inspiration

vital signs measurements of pulse and blood pressure

vitamin deficiency the long-term lack of a particular vitamin in one's diet; may result in certain health problems

vitamins organic chemicals needed by the body for normal functioning and good health

vitreous floaters small, irregularly shaped specks that appear to drift within the field of vision

vocal cords a pair of folds in the mucous membrane of the larynx

vomer (VOH-mer) plow–shaped bone, comprising most of the bony nasal septum

vulva the external female genitalia; includes the labia, mons pubis, clitoris, and vestibule

W

weight force equal to the gravitational acceleration exerted on the mass of an object

wet macular degeneration a condition that involves leakage of small blood vessels within the eye

white blood cells formed elements present in blood; fight infection and protect the body through various mechanisms; *leukocytes*

white matter the term that describes tracts of myelinated fibers within the central nervous system

womb see *uterus*

Z

zona pellucida (peh-LOO-si-da) a clear, extracellular glycoprotein coat that develops on the oocyte

zygomatic bones (ZIGH-goh-MAT-ik) cheek bones, which also form much of the sides of the orbits, or eye sockets

zygote (ZIGH-goht) a diploid cell produced by the fusion of a sperm with an egg; a fertilized egg

Index

A